PHYSIOLOGY AND PATHOBIOLOGY OF AXONS

This handsome volume is a thorough compendium of the principles of structure and function of normal and pathological axons, together with a lucid account of the clinical correlates of laboratory findings. The material has been drawn from the fields of ultrastructure and freeze-fracture, physiology, biochemistry, immunology, neuropathology, and clinical neurology. The illustrations include 112 highly detailed electron micrograph plates, plus hundreds of diagrams. There is also a carefully selected bibliography with over 2,000 references. The clear explanation of the physiology, pathology, and pathophysiology of axons will be especially useful to students, and should be an essential tool in the working library of neuroscientists, neurologists, neurosurgeons, and neuropathologists concerned with such clinical disorders as multiple sclerosis, peripheral neuropathies, and traumatic nerve lesions.

Title entry

Physiology
and
Pathobiology
of Axons

Editor

Stephen G. Waxman, M.D., Ph.D.

Associate Professor of Neurology
Harvard Medical School
Boston, Massachusetts
and
Visiting Associate Professor
Neural Ultrastructure Laboratory
Harvard–MIT Division of Health Sciences and Technology
Research Laboratory of Electronics
Massachusetts Institute of Technology
Cambridge, Massachusetts

Raven Press ▪ New York

Raven Press, 1140 Avenue of the Americas, New York, New York 10036

Made in the United States of America

Library of Congress Cataloging in Publication Data

Main entry under title:

Physiology and pathobiology of axons.

    Includes bibliographical references and index.
    1. Axons—Diseases. 2. Axons. I. Waxman,
Stephen G. [DNLM: 1. Axons—Physiology.
2. Axons—Pathology. WL102.5 P578]
RC347.P53   616.8   77–17751
ISBN 0–89004–215–2

Foreword

Erasistratus of Chios (circa 300 B.C.) may be considered the father of axonology since it was he who first pointed out the role of nerve fibers in the transport of animal spirits (pneuma) from the cerebral ventricles to the rest of the body. Although Pneumatist theories are now medical mythology the concept that axons convey vital substances to and from the brain and spinal cord survives today as a well established principle of neurobiology. The 'animal spirits' of the Pneumatists are the electrical and chemical signals of current concern. The mechanisms by which these signals are generated, the identity and functions of the various chemical species transported in axons, and the mode of interaction between electrical and chemical signals in axons and related cellular elements are problems of central importance for understanding the normal and abnormal functions of the nervous system.

The present volume arrives at a critical time in the development of new ideas about axons that will undoubtedly alter traditional views of axonal structure, function, and pathobiology. If there is one unifying theme in the following chapters it is surely that axons ought to be accorded greater respect than is usually implied by analogizing their functions with transmission cables and conveyer belts. Axons have not of late enjoyed the prestige of dendrites and particularly synapses as key components of neurons involved in information processing. Perhaps one reason for this is that neurobiologists have generally assumed that basic mechanisms subserving learning, memory, and other higher nervous activities are likely to reflect transactions involving modifiable components of neurons. The variable geometrical and functional properties of dendrites and the plastic responsiveness of synaptic operations have tended to attract more attention in this regard than axons with their seemingly monotonous, all-or-none impulses. One of the more provocative aspects of the present volume is its advocacy of axons as candidate elements in complex signal processing. Structural and functional heterogeneity are demonstrable in axonal systems and single axonal trajectories and these diverse properties can be expected to exert effects on output signals perhaps to a degree not encountered with variations in dendritic morphology at input ends of the neuron. This heterogeneity is detectable at overt structural and molecular levels and is reflected in part in variations in ionic channel density, axon–Schwann cell or glial relations and effects of neurotoxins, metabolic, genetic, and other environmental perturbations that affect axonal properties at spatially different sites.

In the past 25 years since Hodgkin and Huxley elucidated the role of membrane voltage in controlling ionic permeability in the genesis of the nerve impulse, knowledge concerning voltage sensitive ionic conductances, as well as related aspects of the structural and functional basis of electrogenesis has accumulated at an extraordinary rate. Advances in the analysis of pathobiological processes in axons have further contributed to the burgeoning field of axonology. The present volume exemplifies what can be done to make the essential advances in this field available to student and expert alike by judicious selection of topic areas and more importantly, choice of contributors. The data reviewed are something more than cogent examinations of the state-of-the-art in axonology. They are stepping stones to the next major advances in neurobiology. After all, it is hardly a coincidence that most of the principles of neuronal operations have been gleaned from studies of axons.

Dominick P. Purpura
New York, New York
January, 1978

Preface

The last decade has seen a re-awakening of interest in, and a remarkable expansion of our understanding of, the conductile process of the nerve cell—the axon. This development reflects a number of factors. One has been the development of new techniques, such as freeze-fracture and optical methods for studying nerve activity. A second factor has been the refinement of existing methods for studying nervous tissue, exemplified by recent improvements in the fixation of nerve cells for electron microscopy, and the application of voltage clamp methods to single nodes of Ranvier. Still another factor has been the appreciation that diseased axons are amenable to study by this armamentarium of sophisticated techniques. Thus, for the first time we are approaching an understanding of some neurological disorders at a cellular, or even molecular, level.

This book was written to meet the need for a volume that would treat, in close juxtaposition, the biology of both normal and diseased axons. Because of the breadth of the field, it was decided that a multi-authored approach would be best. In choosing this approach, we have, at least in part, sacrificed the comfort of a "unitary" treatment of the subject. But such a treatment, by any single author, would necessarily have implied some conceptual biases and a second-hand discussion of certain methodologies and research strategies. We have tried, in this collaborative effort, to provide a comprehensive and first-hand treatment that surveys our contemporary understanding of the physiology and pathobiology of the axon.

Stephen G. Waxman

Acknowledgments

Each of the contributors to this volume, I am sure, owes a great debt to his teachers. Some of my own teachers are among the authors of the chapters of this book. The others have included George Park Sellmer, who taught me to respect living systems, and Howard Hermann, J. David Robertson, J. Z. Young, George Pappas, Dominick Purpura, and Michael Bennett, who, each in a distinctive way, taught me about the nervous system. I wish to thank Portia Tholl and Arbella Chase for their typing and re-typing of many of the chapters, and my assistant, Erika Hartwieg, for hours of her meticulous labor. I am indebted to Dr. Diana Schneider of Raven Press for her encouragement and counsel during the planning for, and preparation of, this volume.

Last, but certainly not least, I express my appreciation to my wife Merle and my sons Matthew and David, for their patience during the editing of this volume.

Contents

Contributors

Jerald J. Bernstein
Departments of Neuroscience and Ophthalmology
University of Florida College of Medicine
Gainesville, Florida 32610

Mary E. Bernstein
Departments of Neuroscience and Ophthalmology
University of Florida College of Medicine
Gainesville, Florida 32610

Claes-H. Berthold
Department of Anatomy
Karolinska Institute
S 104–01 Stockholm 60, Sweden

Murray B. Bornstein
Department of Neurology and
Rose F. Kennedy Center for Research in Mental Retardation and Human Development
Albert Einstein College of Medicine
Bronx, New York 10461

Michael Cahalan
Department of Physiology
University of California at Irvine
Irvine, California 92664

Herbert M. Dembitzer
Division of Neuropathology
Department of Pathology
Montefiore Hospital and Medical Center and
Albert Einstein College of Medicine
Bronx, New York 10461

Marshall Devor
Neurobiology Unit
Institute of Life Sciences
The Hebrew University of Jerusalem
Jerusalem, Israel

Norman Geschwind
Department of Neurology
Harvard Medical School
Beth Israel Hospital
Boston, Massachusetts 02215

Steven S. Goldstein
Zimmerman Medical Clinic and
Department of Neurology
University of Texas
Medical School at Houston
Houston, Texas 77054

Asao Hirano
Division of Neuropathology, Department of Pathology
Montefiore Hospital and Medical Center and
Albert Einstein College of Medicine
Bronx, New York 10467

J. Y. Lettvin
Departments of Biology and Electrical Engineering
Research Laboratory of Electronics
Room 36–889
Massachusetts Institute of Technology
Cambridge, Massachusetts 02139

Gen Matsumoto
Electrotechnical Laboratory
Optoelectronics Section
Tanashi, Tokyo 188, Japan

John W. Moore
Department of Physiology and Pharmacology
Duke University Medical Center
Durham, North Carolina 27710

Enrico Mugnaini
Laboratory of Neuromorphology
Department of Biobehavioral Sciences
University of Connecticut
Storrs, Connecticut 06268

Norman S. Namerow
Department of Neurology
Reed Neurological Center
University of California at Los Angeles Center for the Health Sciences
Los Angeles, California 90024

S. Ochs
Department of Physiology
Indiana University School of Medicine
Indianapolis, Indiana 46202

A. S. Paintal
Department of Physiology
Vallabhbhai Patel Chest Institute
Delhi University
Delhi–110007, India

Donald C. Quick
Department of Neurology
Harvard Medical School
Beth Israel Hospital
Boston, Massachusetts 02215

Cedric S. Raine
Departments of Pathology (Neuropathology)
and Neuroscience
Rose F. Kennedy Center for Research in Mental Retardation and Human Development
Albert Einstein College of Medicine
Bronx, New York 10461

Michael Rasminsky
Division of Neurology
Montreal General Hospital and Department of Neurology and Neurosurgery
McGill University
Montreal, Quebec, H3G 1A4 Canada

S. A. Raymond
Research Laboratory of Electronics
Room 36–889
Massachusetts Institute of Technology
Cambridge, Massachusetts 02139

Thomas D. Sabin
Neurological Unit
Boston City Hospital
Boston, Massachusetts 02118

Herbert H. Schaumburg
Departments of Neurology, Pathology (Neuropathology) and Neuroscience
Rose F. Kennedy Center for Research in Mental Retardation and Human Development
Albert Einstein College of Medicine
Bronx, New York 10461

Bruce Schnapp
Laboratory of Neuromorphology
Department of Biobehavioral Sciences
University of Connecticut
Storrs, Connecticut 06268

Peter S. Spencer
Departments of Neuroscience and Pathology (Neuropathology)
Rose F. Kennedy Center for Research in Mental Retardation and Human Development
Albert Einstein College of Medicine
Bronx, New York 10461

Austin Sumner
Department of Neurology
University of Pennsylvania School of Medicine
Philadelphia, Pennsylvania 19174

Kunihiko Suzuki
Department of Neurology, Department of Neuroscience, and
Rose F. Kennedy Center for Research in Mental Retardation and Human Development
Albert Einstein College of Medicine
Bronx, New York 10461

Harvey A. Swadlow
Department of Neurology
Harvard Medical School
Beth Israel Hospital
Boston, Massachusetts 02215

Ichiji Tasaki
Laboratory of Neurobiology
National Institute of Mental Health
Bethesda, Maryland 20014

P. D. Wall
Cerebral Functions Research Group
Department of Anatomy
University College London
London W.C. 1E 6BT England
and
Neurobiology Unit
Institute of Life Sciences
The Hebrew University of Jerusalem
Jerusalem, Israel

Stephen G. Waxman
Department of Neurology
Harvard Medical School
Beth Israel Hospital
Boston, Massachusetts 02215
and
Harvard–MIT Program in Health Sciences and Technology
Massachusetts Institute of Technology
Cambridge, Massachusetts 02139

Harold J. Weinberg
Departments of Neuroscience and Pathology
Albert Einstein College of Medicine
Bronx, New York 10461

Michael R. Wells
Department of Neuroscience and Ophthalmology
University of Florida College of Medicine
Gainesville, Florida 32610

R. M. Worth
Department of Neurosurgery
Indiana University School of Medicine
Indianapolis, Indiana 46202

Physiology and Pathobiology of Axons, edited by
S. G. Waxman. Raven Press, New York © 1978.

Introduction and Perspectives

Stephen G. Waxman

*Department of Neurology, Harvard Medical School,
Beth Israel Hospital, Boston, Massachusetts 02215*

The axon of the nerve cell, interposed between perikaryon and presynaptic ending, occupies a crucial site in the path traversed by neural information. Yet despite this fact and the fact that axons and their supporting cells may represent a major site of pathology in a large number of clinical entities, knowledge concerning the structure and function of axons remained relatively rudimentary until this century. Our current understanding of the functional architecture of the axon rests in large part on progress made during the past 10 years, using morphological techniques such as electron microscopy and freeze-fracture, as well as modern electrophysiological methodology. Our knowledge of the mechanisms underlying axonal impulse conduction rests on more basic concepts of biological membrane biophysics, which have also been recently refined. The pathobiology of axonal disease has only recently been explored with this armamentarium of techniques and concepts, and is currently being pursued to the cellular and subcellular levels.

This book represents an attempt to provide a survey of experimental and theoretical approaches in contemporary research on axons. It includes chapters on both normal and pathological axons. Emphasis is placed on those areas in which recent progress has been made, reflecting either the development of new techniques or analytical methods, or the application of existing techniques to previously unexplored areas. A complete survey of axonology could easily fill several volumes. In the present instance, we have chosen not to present an encyclopedic compendium, but rather to present the *principles* of structure and function

of normal and diseased axons. The inclusion of chapters on normal and pathological axons in the same volume was deliberate and reflects the belief that pathobiology is not a separate endeavor but requires a firm basis in, shares areas of mutual interest with, and motivates questions for the study of normal cellular function.

The first part of this volume concentrates on the biology of nonpathological axons. The initial chapter serves not only to delineate the morphology of normal peripheral axons but also as a guide to the cell biology of axonal organelles. The next two chapters treat the ultrastructure of normal central axons and the structure of axons as revealed by recently developed freeze-fracture techniques. Subsequent sections focus on the physiology of nonpathological axons from phenomenological (what are the conduction properties of axons?) and mechanistic (what basic membrane characteristics determine these properties?) points of view. It has become clear in recent years that, from an informational standpoint, axons do not necessarily function as simple conduits. Attention is therefore turned to the aftereffects of impulse transmission, to mechanisms of differential transmission of neural messages in axonal branches, and to the mechanisms and strategies underlying axonal coding. The next topic covered is optical probes of axonal activity; these methods, which have been developed and refined primarily over the past 10 years, promise to be of great importance because they provide a technology for the *noninvasive* monitoring of axonal activity. Finally, attention is focused on the metabolic maintenance of the axon and the biochemical interplay between axon, cell body, and synaptic terminals as mediated by the various modes of axonal transport.

The second part of this volume concentrates on the pathobiology of axons. Here we are not concerned so much with nosology as with the pathogenetic and pathophysiological basis of disorders of axons, and of the relation of cellular pathology to clinical presentation, diagnosis, and treatment. The pathology of two illustrative classes of axonal disorder—the dying-back neuropathies and the demyelinating diseases—is first discussed. Next, we turn to the immunobiology and biochemistry of demyelination and the mechanisms which control remyelination. Attention is then turned to the physiology of axons in various disease states and to the clinical implications of altered electrical function. Finally, there are discussions of regeneration and of clinical aspects of axonal pathobiology, as studied in the evoked potential laboratory and at the bedside.

It should soon become apparent to the reader that the "basic" chapters, nominally devoted to normal axons, hold many lessons for the pathobiologist and that, in turn, the chapters on pathobiology hold many lessons for the "basic" axonologist.

Lest the casual reader be lulled into a false sense of security, it should be stated at the outset that many questions remain unanswered. The molecular structure of the axon membrane and the mechanisms controlling ionic permeability and excitability remain exciting areas for investigation. The conduction properties of central axons, in contrast to those of their peripheral counterparts, remain relatively elusive. The mechanisms which determine specificity in neuroglial relations and in myelinogenesis are being carefully studied, but the detailed nature of the chemical messages mediating this specificity has not yet been determined. With respect to diseased axons, one need only to recall that there are, at any given time, in excess of 100,000 identifiable cases of multiple sclerosis, mostly in young adults, in the United States alone. Clearly, many questions remain unanswered, and many challenges remain.

Despite the fact that a multiplicity of techniques—morphological, physiological, pharmacological, biophysical, biochemical—has yielded important information about the properties of normal and diseased axons, it would be imprudent to predict that the remaining problems will be solved easily or quickly. Nevertheless, if the last decade of research can be used as a guide, these advances will continue in the near future, and we may fully expect that as our understanding of the nervous system continues to grow there will develop not only a fuller understanding of the structure and function of axons but also an increasingly wide range of therapies for diseases of axons in the peripheral and central nervous system.

Physiology and Pathobiology of Axons, edited by
S. G. Waxman. Raven Press, New York © 1978.

Morphology of Normal Peripheral Axons

Claes-H. Berthold

Department of Anatomy, Karolinska Institute, Stockholm, Sweden

The axon is a more or less cylindrical nerve cell elongation that effects point-to-point transmission of electrically and chemically coded information. Propagation of electrically coded messages is in practice unidirectional and nondecremental. It involves the plasma membrane of the axon and proceeds somatofugally at a velocity that depends on axon diameter and varies from approximately 10^{-1} meters/sec in thin axons to more than 10^2 meters/sec in thick axons. Transmission of chemical signals (Ochs and Worth, *this volume*) is bidirectional and takes place inside the axon simultaneously at several different velocities, independent of axon size, varying from approximately 1 mm/day to more than 400 mm/day (212,325).

Most axons reside in the central nervous system (CNS). In mammals, fewer than 1 per 1,000 appear in the peripheral nervous system (PNS). Of these, most cross the PNS–CNS border and should, strictly speaking, be regarded as PNS–CNS compound axons. Genuine peripheral axons (i.e., axons that wholly remain outside the CNS) are the thin, usually unmyelinated axons of autonomic postganglionic neurons. This chapter deals with the morphology of PNS axons, referring to the broader meaning of the term.

Since the first comprehensive presentation of the morphology of PNS nerve fibers by Ranvier (230), the subject has been treated in a number of reviews (46,55,58,104,137,170, 183,203,220,279,281,332). In view of the many modern treatises and in particular the recent and thorough presentations of myelinated nerve fibers by Landon and Hall (172) and of unmyelinated fibers by Ochoa (207, 208), the present work is largely restricted to mammalian nerves and especially to feline myelinated axons. Aspects of comparative axonal morphology may be found in the articles by Bunge (55) and Gray (137). Rosenberg (239) gives a summary of the biology of squid giant axon, and Tasaki and Sisco recently reviewed methods for studying excitability of the axon membrane (287). The maturation of peripheral mammalian axons is briefly commented on in the final part of this chapter.

GENERAL ORGANIZATION AND CLASSIFICATION OF PNS AXONS

Peripheral axons are always accompanied by Schwann cells, which separate them from the endoneural space with their basement membranes. According to the organization of the attending Schwann cells, peripheral axons are classified as unmyelinated or myelinated. In the former case several axons are more or less submerged in longitudinal troughs on the outside of Schwann cells. A string of longitudinally arranged and closely apposed Schwann cells and the axons lodging therein constitute an unmyelinated fiber (207). In myelinated fibers one single axon is associated with a string of longitudinally arranged Schwann cells. Each Schwann cell supports the integrity of a well-defined segment of the myelin sheath, a highly ordered lipid–protein–water layer coating the axon. In addition, Schwann cells serve the axons in several trophic, but so far little-clarified ways (e.g., refs. 47,172). Axon diameter is commonly referred to as *"d,"* the myelin sheath thickness as *"m,"* and the myelinated fiber diameter as *"D"* ($D = d + 2m$). The caliber spectrum of peripheral mammalian axons is between 0.1 and ~16 μm, unmyelinated axons being less than 1–2 μm and myelinated ones being more. Length of PNS axons varies from less than 1 cm to several meters, maximum length depending on animal size. In most neurons with axons in the PNS, more than 90% of cell volume is axonal.

Branching of PNS axons is more or less restricted to effector and receptor fields (183, 234). The degree of branching is nil or very small in spinal roots, increases gradually along the proximodistal course of the axon, and becomes high close to or inside the effector and receptor fields (93,133). According to Thiel's (291) observations, average axon diameter remains fairly constant between branch points. On the other hand, Thiel found considerable individual and unsystematic variation around the average diameter. Since axon branches in most cases are thinner than their parent fiber, the shift to the left of the caliber spectrum, noted when tracing a peripheral nerve trunk in the distal direction, should depend on branching rather than tapering (228,234,283).

The main axon types in mammalian PNS are shown in Fig. 1, which also gives the commonly used classification systems. The part of an axon which extends between CNS or autonomic ganglia and the field of termination is referred to as the *stereotype axon segment*. The stereotype segment discloses a monotonously repeated segmental pattern in-

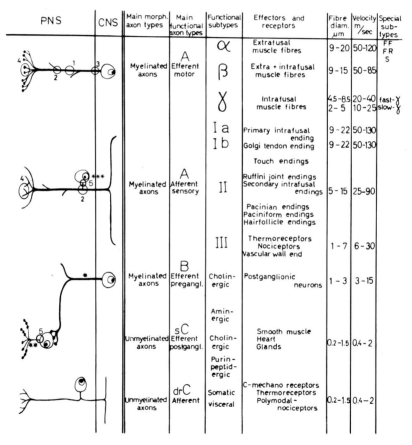

FIG. 1. Classification of mammalian PNS axons. The classification is mainly based on that of J. A. Boyd and M. R. Davey (50a). 1: Stereotype part of axon. 2: Branching point. 3: PNS–CNS transition. 4: Terminal receptor or effector field. 5: Initial segment. 5***: Crus commune of spinal ganglion neuron. The crus commune divides in one central branch, the original axon, and one peripheral branch (245). Ontogenetically the latter is a dendrite which grows into the receptor field and adopts the morphological characteristics and the conduction mode of an axon. However, like a dendrite it conveys nerve impulses in the cellulipetal direction. In this way an afferent axonal transmission line is established which bypasses the parent cell body (48,172,184,245). *Some preganglionic axons are unmyelinated (121). **Some postganglionic axons are myelinated (121).

terrupted only by a few branch points. As indicated by the numbered circles in Fig. 1, morphological interest centers at five sites: (a) the repeating unit of the stereotype axon, i.e., the part related to one Schwann cell; (b) branch points; (c) the PNS–CNS transition; (d) terminal branches of the effector and receptor fields, including motor end-plates (127, 290), terminals of pre- and postganglionic autonomic axons (102,103,121,290), and receptor terminals (20); and (e) axon hillock–initial segment regions of sensory and autonomic neurons. Morphology of effector and receptor fields are only briefly mentioned, and the works just referred to should be consulted for reviews and further references. Neither is morphology of the axon hillock and initial segment dealt with in any detail. Both regions are difficult to identify in autonomic ganglia (102,103,121).

COMPONENTS OF A PNS AXON

Axolemma

According to current concepts the axolemma corresponds to the excitable membrane of nerve fibers. It is ~8 nm thick and appears as an asymmetrical triple-layered unit membrane after fixation with OsO_4, $KMnO_4$, or glutaraldehyde; the inner leaflet of the membrane is thicker and most osmiophilic, features not shown by the Schwann cell plasma membrane, which is symmetrical (99,101). Differences in the outside–inside osmiophilia of cell membranes have been discussed on the background of different affinities to K^+ and Na^+ (163). One aspect of the difference between Schwann cell plasma membrane and axolemma is well illustrated in feline unmyelinated fibers after incubation in a hypotonic solution: The axons shrink and Schwann cells swell (100; see also 236).

Neither the patchy septate organization of the axolemma of squid giant axons (298) nor the inside Ca^{2+} accumulations of this axolemma have so far been observed in mammals (151, 289). There are in the axolemma of crayfish giant axons local patches of globular units (221). The axolemma carries on its inside small, irregular accumulations of electron-dense material, and shows various degrees of corrugation and irregularities most obvious at the nodes of Ranvier in myelinated fibers. Endocytotic vesicles are comparatively common (302). Under the influence of its Schwann cells, the axon becomes involved in peristaltic activities (135,143,313,319,320).

A thick, long axon has a plasma membrane many times the mantle area of its cell body. In a large spinal motoneuron (soma = 50 μm; axon: $d = 15$ μm, length = 1 meter) the axon membrane area is 6,000 times that of the soma, the latter area being reproduced by each 170-μm long axon segment. It is not surprising that many axonal activities take part in the maintenance of such a comparatively enormous plasma membrane.

Isolation of axon plasma membranes pure enough to allow biochemical analysis is difficult because of contamination by myelin and satellite cell membranes. Roughly 30% of total axonal protein is part of the axolemma (166). The "axolemma" fraction of bovine white matter is enriched in Na^+-K^+-activated ATPase, 5-nucleotidase, acetylcholinesterase, and tetrodotoxin-binding elements (80,166). Only minor differences have so far been noted in the phospholipid and fatty acid composition of axonal and periaxonal membrane fractions (64).

Axoplasm

The axoplasm constitutes the fluid compartment in which formed elements are suspended. Whether the wispy material of moderate electron density, as found directly inside the axolemma and outside most of the formed elements, represents artifactually condensed axoplasmic material (172) or depicts true matrix substance coats (329) remains obscure (Plates 1 and 2). Axoplasm of squid giant axons has the consistency of a strong gel (78). The viscosity of mammalian axoplasm, as estimated by electron spin resonance analysis (142), is five times that of water.

The purification of mammalian axoplasm requires several hours (81), and little is known about its composition. The presence in *Myxicola* axons—whose axoplasm can be extruded and put to analysis within approximately 10 sec (14,130,131)—of a Ca^{2+}-activated thiol proteinase prompts cautious interpretation of molecular weight estimations of axoplasmic proteins and of *in vitro* axoplasmic gel–sol transformations (14,132).

Axoplasm constitutes the medium within which bidirectional axoplasmic flow takes place at several velocities (Ochs and Worth, *this volume*). Proteins rapidly transported in the somatofugal direction have been separated in several classes ranging from 18,000 to 130,000 daltons (23). Among those considered to be propagated in the axoplasm at a rate of 1–2 mm/day, Droz (83) lists: unspecified soluble proteins, tubulin, neurofilament subunits, and several enzymes (see also refs. 84,109,154).

Formed Axoplasmic Elements

Mitochondria

Axonal mitochondria are 0.1–0.3 μm in diameter, 0.5–8 μm in length, and oriented longitudinally. They contain conspicuous matrix substance and round or flat cristae which extend longitudinally inside the organelle (Plates 15 and 33). Dense intramitochondrial granules are not seen (289). Concentration of mitochondria decreases with increasing axon size, from an average of 2–5/μm² in small axons to 0.1/μm² in large ones (32,82,338) (Tables 1 and 2).

Axonal mitochondria have been observed in association with neurotubules. This arrangement, which is less common in dorsal root axons, has been taken to mean a transport of mitochondria along neurotubules and/or an energy coupling between neurotubules and mitochondria (73,121,211,229,273). Mito-

chondria are considered to be continuously generated in the perikaryon (246) and then to enter the axon, being slowly propagated distally as a consequence of axoplasmic bulk movement. The cross section of an average axon is passed by some 1,000 mitochondria/day (315). The situation becomes more complex when the obviously viable status of mitochondria in the axon terminals and the fact that mitochondrial proteins are rapidly transported distally inside the axon (83,84) are considered.

Vital microscopy of vertebrate axons has revealed two types of circumscribed axoplasmic bodies: round bodies 0.2–0.5 μm in diameter and rod-shaped bodies 0.2–0.3 × 1.8 μm (29,73,164). In *Xenopus laevis* (73) members of the former group, in a ratio of 1:10, move both somatofugally and somatopetally. The movements are jerky and saltatory, and net velocities of transport are 85 and 114 mm/day, respectively. Rod-shaped bodies, on the other hand, remain more or less stationary; some move in either direction by saltatory jerks, and a very small number drift distally approximately 1.5 mm/day (29,164). Presumably the rod-shaped bodies are mitochondria. The round, shorter bodies form a heterogeneous group (see below) that should include small mitochondria and other axonal bodies.

Smooth Endoplasmic Reticulum

The smooth endoplasmic reticulum (SER) of axons lacks ribosomes. In electron micrographs the SER forms a discrete system of

TABLE 1. *Concentration of formed axoplasmic elements in feline unmyelinated lumbar dorsal root axons*

Element	Axon: 0.21–0.40 μm		Axon: 0.41–0.60 μm		Axon: 0.61–0.80 μm		Axon: 0.81–1.00 μm	
	Animal		Animal		Animal		Animal	
	I	II	I	II	I	II	I	II
Number of fibers	20	36	78	92	45	19	4	0
Mitochondria/μm²	1.4	1.4	2.0	2.0	1.8	1.3	0.8	—
SER profiles/μm²	17	24	11	13	8	11	7	—
Neurofilaments/μm²	162	346	189	313	163	283	178	—
Neurotubules/μm²	84	105	50	53	40	43	33	—

Perfusion fixation with phosphate-buffered 5% glutaraldehyde. Vestopal embedding (31,32).
The concentration values are calculated from the total number of the various axoplasmic elements observed in a fiber group divided by the total cross sectional area of the fibers in that group.

TABLE 2. *Axon size, no of myelin lamellae and occurrence of axoplasmic elements in myelinated feline ventral root axons of different sizes*

	Axon I	Axon II	Axon III	Axon IV	Axon V	Axon VI
Mean d_{circ} μm[a]						
1	1.6 ± 0.3 (1)[b]	3.1 ± 0.4 (1.7)	4.2 ± 0.6 (2.2)	8.6 ± 0.8 (3)	14.4 ± 0.9 (3.2)	12.5 ± 0.8 (2.7)
2	2.3 ± 1.1 (3.2)	3.1 ± 0.4 (1.7)	4.2 ± 0.6 (2.2)	8.7 ± 0.9 (3.9)	14.4 ± 0.9 (3.2)	12.7 ± 0.8 (2.7)
3	3.5 ± 1.0 (2.9)	3.3 ± 0.7 (1.3)	4.9	10.5	14.1	13.5
4	0.7 ± 0.00 (0)	1.2 ± 0.06 (0.1)	1.8 ± 0.1 (0.1)	3.5 ± 0.08 (0.1)	5.4 ± 0.07 (0.1)	5.5 ± 0.07 (0.1)
Mean d_{area} μm[c]						
1	1.3 ± 0.1 (0.5)	2.6 ± 0.4 (1.2)	3.6 ± 0.5 (1.8)	7.8 ± 1.1 (4.3)	13.4 ± 0.8 (3)	11.6 ± 0.8 (2.5)
2	1.4 ± 0.2 (0.7)	2.6 ± 0.3 (1.2)	3.6 ± 0.5 (1.8)	7.9 ± 1.2 (5.1)	13.4 ± 0.8 (3)	11.6 ± 0.8 (2.5)
3	1.5 ± 0.2 (0.6)	2.4 ± 2 (0.3)	4.4	9.7	13.8	12.8
4	0.7 ± 0.00 (0)	1.2 ± 0.00 (0)	1.7 ± 0.1 (0.1)	3.4 ± 0.00 (0)	5.3 ± 0.00 (0)	5.4 ± 0.07 (0.1)
Mean no. myelin lamellae[e]	25 ± 2.3 (7)	66 ± 5 (13)	94 ± 3.5 (10)	131 ± 6.5 (15)	142 ± 1.5 (7)	150 ± 4.4 (10)
Mitochondria (STIN)/μm[2d]	0.6	0.7	0.3	0.16	0.13	0.13
(Node)	2.6	2.9	1.8	0.7	0.3	0.6
Neurotubules (STIN)/μm[2d]	30	47.2	31	13	11	16.5
(Node)	120	216	130	85	72	62
Neurofilaments (STIN)/μm[2d]	150	125	125	125	126	153
(Node)	100	73	90	116	130	130
SER profiles/μm[2d]	7.8	6.4	4.7	1.9	2.2	2.5
SER profiles associated to the axolemma No/μm of circumference[d]	1.2	1.1	1.3	0.9	1.5	1.4

Glutaraldehyde-OsO$_4$ fixation and embedding in Vestopal W. (cf. 31,32): The data derive from an analysis of 23,000 consecutive ultrathin cross sections covering a length of about 2 mm. The analyzed fibers are presented in Fig. 4.

1: Estimations exclude Schwann cell nuclear levels; $n = 20$, 2: Estimations include Schwann cell nuclear levels, 3: Only Schwann cell nuclear levels; $n = 4$: Nodal levels; n: see Fig. 4.

[a] d_{circ} axon diameter calculated from axon circumference.

[b] Values in parenthesis represent ranges.

[c] d_{area} axon diameter calculated from axon cross section area.

[d] The figures represents the mean value of two estimations performed in the first and the last section of the series.

[e] The figures were obtained from the mean values of the total occurrence in several cross sections (n: see Fig. 4) by division with the average axon cross section area.

more-or-less flattened tubes 60 × 100 nm in size (Plates 1, 2, 4, and 8). In some profiles part of the SER membrane appears septated, consisting of globular units (Plate 1).

The SER occupies less than 2.5% of the axon cross section (338), and its full visualization requires serial reconstructions. It is more developed in peripheral nerves and ventral roots than in dorsal roots (338). In amphibian PNS axons the SER appears quite distinct after incubation in ruthenium red, forming longitudinal varicose tubes 20–60 nm thick. It has been speculated that endocytotic vesicles generated at nodes of Ranvier might be the vehicle interconnecting the endoneural space and SER (262).

Droz et al. (85), using high-voltage electron microscopy (EM) on rat spinal and chick ciliary ganglia, depicted the SER as an extensive and continuous reticular meshwork of 20- to 120-nm thick tubules extending uninterrupted from the axon hillock out into the axon terminals. At sites during its course along the axon, the SER forms dilated "subaxolemmal" plates (Plate 8). In preterminal branches the SER separates into a primary system of thicker tubes and a secondary system of thinner ones. The primary SER system runs just inside the plasma membrane and extends into the terminals toward the presynaptic grids. The secondary SER system occupies the core of the axon and breaks up into spherical units the size of synaptic vesicles (83).

For obvious reasons the SER has attracted interest as a possible route in axoplasmic transport. Droz (83) suggests that bidirectional fast transport is connected to the SER. Among the somatofugally transported substances have been mentioned axolemmal proteins, glycoproteins, mitochondrial and lysosomal proteins, acetylcholinesterase, mucopolysaccharides, gangliosides, and phospholipids (83,136). Among somatopetally transported substances might be mentioned exogenously administered horseradish peroxidase (169,182,274) and nerve growth factor (256).

Neurotubules

Neurotubules belong to a group of organelles referred to as cytoplasmic microtubules (25, 278). They appear as thin, hollow cylinders 24–25 nm in diameter. The wall consists of 12–15 (usually 13) protofilaments. The protofilaments are arranged in a three-start helix and consist of tubulin subunits 4 nm in size. Tubulin (a dimeric GTP-binding protein 110,000–120,000 daltons in weight) in the appropriate milieu self-assembles into microtubules (11,107,278). Microtubules are particularly well visualized electron microscopically after glutaraldehyde–tannic acid fixation (56).

Neurotubules are unbranched, and some are considered to extend uninterrupted from cell body to axon terminals. At branch points new neurotubules add to those derived from the parent fiber (335). At some sites there are 5-nm granules in the neurotubular lumen (Plate 4) (218,229). Axoplasmic neurotubules often appear in groups, together with mitochondria and SER profiles, in clearings of the neurofibrillar latticework (Plate 2) (272,329). Outside the neurotubules there are radiations of wispy material (Plates 1 and 2) (329) which occasionally join similar material coating a mitochondrion, a SER profile, or a neurofilament. A few neurotubules show distinct arms 8 nm thick and 20 nm long by which separate tubules are interconnected or attach to mitochondria (Plate 2). Negatively stained neurotubules show coarse irregular side projections 100 nm or less in length (329). Whether these are related to the dynein arms of ciliary microtubules, there playing a role in ciliary movements, has not been clarified (329).

On the average, there are 50–100 neurotubules/μm^2 in unmyelinated axons (Table 1) and 10–20/μm^2 in large myelinated ones (82, 119) (Table 2). Zenker et al. (338,339) reported that in the rat there are significant differences in neurotubular densities when comparing: (a) sensory and motor axons of peripheral nerve; (b) peripheral and central (i.e., dorsal root) axons of a spinal ganglion; and (c) small and large ventral root axons with small and large dorsal root axons. A similar situation is seen in *Xenopus laevis*: In ventral root small ($D = 5$ μm) and large ($D = 20$ μm) fibers contain 30 and 10 neurotubules/μm^2, respectively, whereas in dorsal root axons the corresponding figures are 5 and 1 (273). However, neurotubules and dissolved tubulin units exist in labile equilibrium in the axoplasm (54). Several factors may disturb this balance and bring about disassembling of tubules (19,257,278): colchicine, Ca^{2+}, increased hydrostatic pressure, and cold. This, together with the observation that the yield of microtubules and their association to other organelles after glutaraldehyde fixation is influenced also by composition of the fixative buffer (168,188), indicates that the number of neurotubules must be cautiously evaluated (54). Functionally, microtubules have been suggested to maintain shape in anisotropic cells, to bring about intracellular movements like chromosome transportation and axoplasmic flow (278), to be associated with synaptic vesicles (18,138), and to participate in subaxolemmal arrangements at the initial axon segment (317); and they are suspected of involvement in transmembranous ionic shifts (214) and in cell-surface site distribution (108,301).

Axonal Filaments

Axons contain two types of filament, actin-like microfilaments ~5 nm in diameter and conventional neurofilaments ~10 nm in diameter. The former filaments are found inside the pseudopods of axonal growth cones (288). It is noteworthy that 10–15% of total neuronal protein appears to be actin (52), compared to 25% in striated muscle. A description of the interplay between actin filaments and membrane proteins is given in refs. 198 and 293.

Conventional neurofilaments (196,197,329) are longitudinally arranged structures of undetermined length. At fairly regular intervals of 50 nm, 1–8 spokes radiate from the shafts of the neurofilaments. The spokes (~10 nm thick and 30–60 nm long) interconnect groups of neighboring filaments into a complex three-dimensional latticework showing a mixture of triangular, rhombic, and quadratic patterns in cross section. In the longitudinal view this gives a characteristic ladder-like pattern (195) (Plates 1 and 2).

Longitudinally viewed neurofilaments appear beaded (Plate 1) at a 50-nm interval. Presumably this is a superposition effect. Isolated negatively stained neurofilaments appear smooth without spokes (329). Neurofilaments tend to

form clusters of units that interconnect to latticeworks as described above and that probably take a spiral course down the axon (314, 331). The neurofilaments are reported to consist of globular subunits 3–3.5 nm in diameter, which in cross section reveal a rhombic arrangement, and in longitudinal view a helical assembly (328,330) (Plate 1). The need for cautious evaluation of data on neurofilament monomeres was recently stressed, in view of axoplasmic proteinases (14,132). Recent data also indicate that neurofilaments might actually be lipoprotein structures relatively rich in galactolipid (254).

In mammals and amphibia there are, irrespective of axon size, 100–300 neurofilaments/μm^2 cross-cut axoplasm. There is a tendency toward slightly higher values in dorsal root axons compared to ventral root axons (273,338).

The functional significance of neurofilaments is obscure. They may cooperate with neurotubules in promoting axonal flow (110, 171). In this connection it should be mentioned that there are invertebrate axons that appear to lack neurotubules but contain neurofilaments, and other species that appear to lack the filaments but contain tubules (329). Neurofilaments, microfilaments, and neurotubules are now recognized as separate proteins (226). Colchicine, vinblastine, cytochalasin B, and related compounds have during recent years found common use for investigating the involvement of microtubules, neurofilaments, and microfilaments in growth, maintenance of shape, and axoplasmic transport (e.g., refs. 28, 120,199).

Miscellaneous Membrane-Bound Bodies

There are miscellaneous membrane-bound bodies that constitute a heterogeneous group of obscure functional significance: multivesicular bodies 0.5–2 μm in diameter containing 50–100 nm vesicles (215,237); oblong dense lamellated or compact bodies 0.2–0.3 × 0.3–1 μm; empty-looking vesicular entities 0.05–0.5 μm; and large and small dense-core vesicles 0.1–0.2 μm and 0.05–0.08 μm in diameter, respectively. Small dense-core vesicles, when observed in unmyelinated postganglionic axons, presumably represent catecholamine-containing synaptic granules (159). The lamellated and compact bodies might correspond to lysosomes (155).

Ribosomes

Ribosome units that are parts of typical Nissl bodies are common in the initial segment of primary rat sensory neurons and cat spinal motoneurons (71,333,334). More distally, in the myelinated part of the crus commune and its peripheral branch, granules interpreted as ribosomes are free in the axoplasm or connected to mitochondria and SER. In particular, such observations have been made close to nodes of Ranvier. When searched for, solitary ribosome-like particles occur in the constricted nodal parts of some axons (32; also see below). The observation of axonal ribosome-like particles far from the cell body is interesting in view of speculations of a local axonal protein synthesis (49,50,94).

Axonal Inclusions

Glycogen granules have been found in, among other sites, cultured spinal ganglion axons (191) and afferent axons of autumn frogs (30). Glycogen is noted in various receptor–axon and effector–axon terminals. There are randomly scattered glycogen granules in motor end-plates (22). In axon receptor terminals and preterminals there might be observed the gamut, from scattered glycogen granules to granular clusters and glycogen bodies where the granules are associated with whorls of SER (75,295). Lipid droplets do not seem to occur in the normal mammalian axoplasm but are at hand in the axons of invertebrates, e.g., the horseshoe crab (86).

UNMYELINATED PNS AXONS

In mammals there are approximately 75% unmyelinated axons in cutaneous nerves and dorsal spinal roots (174,209), 50% in muscle nerves (174), and 30% in ventral roots (17, 67,68,297). Visceral nerve trunks (e.g., inferior cardiac nerve, gray rami communicantes) contain but few myelinated fibers (69, 106). White rami communicantes contain approximately two-thirds unmyelinated axons (69).

Stereotype Part of the Axon

Axonal Components

The axolemma of unmyelinated axons lacks particular morphological characteristics. Axons dwelling in the same Schwann cell trough are often separated by a space less than 20 nm. At many of these sites one or both of the facing axolemmas reveal an irregular 5- to 20-nm thick inside coating of diffuse electron-dense material (Plate 3).

No major differences have been reported between unmyelinated and myelinated axons concerning their formed elements. However, neurofilament latticeworks are less conspicuous in unmyelinated fibers, and their SER is sometimes very discretely represented by a solitary profile 20 nm in size (Plate 4). The occurrence of formed axoplasmic elements in feline dorsal root unmyelinated axons is given in Table 1. There are, on the average, 2 and 0.8 mitochondria, 20 and 9 SER profiles, and 100 and 35 neurotubules/μm^2 cross-cut small ($d = <0.5$ μm) and large (0.7–1.0 μm) axons, respectively. Concentration of these elements decreases as the d-value increases. The occurrence of neurofilaments is 100–300/μm^2, small and large fibers alike. Postganglionic axons contain vesicles of various kinds: small, dense-cored vesicles considered to represent catecholamine storage units (159); large dense-cored vesicles discussed in connection with "purinergic" and "peptidergic" neurons (72); and empty-looking vesicles suggested to be cholinergic (105,127). A presentation of axonal heterogeneity in visceral innervation based on different transmitter substances is given by Olsson et al. (213).

Axon Shape and Caliber

The *in vivo* cross-sectional shape of unmyelinated axons is not known. Immersion fixations employing KMnO$_4$ or OsO$_4$ give more-or-less circular contours (96,209,316), a shape enhanced by use of methylmethacrylate as an embedding medium (cf. Fig. 2 in ref. 96 with Fig. 2 in ref. 97). After perfusion fixation with glutaraldehyde and embedding in Araldite, Epon, or Vestopal W, the axons appear irregular but basically rounded with smooth corners. Angulated and densely packed profiles probably develop as an effect of an osmotically unbalanced fixative vehicle (100,208). It has been suggested that unmyelinated axons are thicker at the levels of the Schwann cell nuclei than at points where consecutive Schwann cells join (79).

The caliber spectrum of unmyelinated fibers has an unimodal distribution, with the peak at 0.4–1.0 (1.6) μm and a range of 0.15–2 (3) μm (53,90,91,124,126,165). Values given in parentheses refer to human cutaneous nerves, which have a maximum diameter of approximately 3 μm (26,209,316). Dyck's observations in human sural nerves do not confirm the higher values (89). With few exceptions, fewer than 15% of unmyelinated axons measure more than 1 μm. As found in serial section analysis (7) the diameters of individual axons, measured at 5-μm intervals, varied from the mean value by an average range of 16%; a variation of 20–30% was common, and in approximately 1% of fibers it was 50%. It is likely that mean values of several estimates along individual fibers should be used for accurate caliber spectrum analysis, and that the use of mean values would decrease the span of the spectrum and shift its upper limit toward 1 μm, the controversial borderline value between unmyelinated and myelinated PNS axons (115,311,312).

Periaxonal Space

Most axons in an unmyelinated fiber lodge superficially in the Schwann cell. The axons are separated from the endoneural space by the Schwann cell basement membrane and Schwann cell cytoplasm, interrupted by the 20- to 30-nm wide mesaxon (Plate 3). Some axons reside deep in the Schwann cell, their mesaxons being long and winding. Other axons run superficially in shallow furrows, covered by just the basement membrane. Although most axons when changing from one fiber track to another are invested by the Schwann cell, some undertake the transposition surrounded only by basement membrane (Plate 3).

The narrow space between the axolemma and the plasma membrane of the Schwann cell (the periaxonal space) is 20–30 nm in width; it either contains a diffuse, finely granular

material of low electron density or is more-or-less empty (208). However, restricted parts of the axolemma joining the Schwann cell membrane may form five- or seven-layered membrane complexes (99,189). These relations become more frequent after freeze drying (101) and freeze substitution (189). The use of freeze drying sometimes renders a completely obliterated periaxonal space (101).

The periaxonal space, which communicates with the outside of the Schwann cell via the mesaxon, has attracted great interest: It constitutes the immediate exterior of the excitable membrane in unmyelinated axons. Although the periaxonal space appears to be freely accessible to penetration by horseradish peroxidase (57), it cannot be concluded that the space is open to free diffusion. This is illustrated by the accumulation of K^+ outside the excitable membrane in mammalian unmyelinated axons during sustained impulse propagation as well as by the comparatively slow clearing of this K^+ surplus (139). The diffusion properties and functional significance of the periaxonal space were discussed in detail by Adelman and Palti (4) and Landon and Hall (172).

Accumulations of electron-dense material—claimed to represent enzymatic reaction products—appear in the periaxonal space outside afferent and efferent axons after histochemical incubation for various esterases and phosphatases (206,271), particularly acetylcholinesterases (21,160,247).

Axons Per Schwann Cell

The number of axons per Schwann cell in an unmyelinated fiber is variable and difficult to estimate. The difficulties depend on the frequent interchange of axons between adjacent fibers (7). Defined as the number of axons per Schwann cell in cross sections at the level of the Schwann cell nucleus, there are 1 to ~100 (mean 23) axons in cat dorsal root unmyelinated nerve fibers (38; Berthold and Carlstedt, *unpublished*). Schwann cells that attend one or just a few axons are common in human cutaneous nerves (26,209).

It is possible to estimate the number of "Schwann cell units" per cross-sectional area and the number and size of axons related to such units (e.g., refs. 5,26). "Schwann cell unit" refers to a cell profile representing a cross section through any part of a Schwann cell. A feline dorsal root Schwann cell unit containing 82 axons of different sizes is shown in Plate 3. In rabbit mesenteric nerves (5), 35.4% of all Schwann cell units contain only 1 axon and 1.6% contain 10 or more axons. In mouse sural nerve 16.5% and 13.4% of the units contain 1 and 10 or more axons, respectively (5). Based on analyses of Schwann cell units, it has been suggested that human unmyelinated axons degenerate spontaneously with increasing age and that regenerative events are initiated (89,210). Whether this in fact is the result of minor trauma—normal axons remaining intact if they are left undisturbed (26)—is an open question.

In view of the small size and close packing of unmyelinated axons, it is obvious that morphometric analysis must depend on electron microscopy. The presence of collagen pockets (122) necessitates a comparatively high magnification. Frequent changes in position within the individual Schwann cell and between adjacent ones, as well as variation of diameter along individual axons, demand analyses of serial sections at close intervals. In a study of unmyelinated fibers in prenatal kittens, an interval between serial sections not exceeding 1 μm had to be used if serious mistakes were to be avoided in tracing individual axons (Berthold and Nilsson, *in preparation*).

Schwann Cells

The length of Schwann cells in unmyelinated fibers is difficult to assess by direct observation. The extent of the joints between consecutive Schwann cells is imperceptible unless high-magnification serial section analysis is performed, since Schwann cell processes accompany axons that change fiber track. Instead, Schwann cell internuclear distance (224) along a fiber is used as a measure of Schwann cell length. In adult rat cervical sympathetic trunks and sural nerves, the average Schwann internuclear distance is 90 μm (range 20–250) and 108 μm (range 20–310), respectively, as estimated light microscopically in teased specimens (223). In contrast to this is the statistical

calculation of a Schwann cell length of 200–500 μm based on observations in electron micrographs of human sural nerve (60). The diversity in the estimates is probably explained partly by species differences and partly by the better resolution of individual fibers in electron micrographs.

There are no particular axonal arrangements at the Schwann cell joints in unmyelinated fibers (92). Consecutive Schwann cells simply interdigitate or telescope into one another. The intervening gaps are empty-looking and measure 10–30 μm in width. Some interdigitating processes show desmosome-like structures, and at some places the cytoplasm of one of the meeting Schwann cells reveals an increased electron density (92).

One much-discussed question is whether there is a fundamental difference between "unmyelinated" and "myelinated" Schwann cells. Cross-innervation experiments show that the regenerating axons of myelinated fibers grow into the distal stump of an unmyelinated nerve trunk where they subsequently become myelinated and vice versa (148,259). The question arises: Do surviving "unmyelinated" Schwann cells manufacture myelin, or do "myelinated" Schwann cells of the proximal stump accompany the regenerating axons and manufacture the myelin? It was recently demonstrated that Schwann cells indeed are multipotent as regards their being myelin-producing or non-myelin-producing units (6,8,311,312), and that they seem to operate accurately when transplanted to homologous organisms, provided immunodepression is used (9). This topic is discussed more fully by Spencer and Weinberg (*this volume*).

Branching Points

On the basis of light microscopy and neurophysiological evidence, it is clear that extensive terminal branching is common in unmyelinated axons (63,208,294,310). As shown by means of light microscopy by Ha (141), the branching in the spinal ganglion of the crus communis of unmyelinated neurons gives rise to one thin dorsal root branch and one considerably thicker peripheral branch. At the branch point the axon shows a triangular dilatation. Lieberman (184) recently discussed the issue of the number of spinal ganglion nerve cell bodies versus the number of peripheral and central branches.

PNS–CNS Transition

In cat S_1 dorsal roots the axons become segregated by size as they reach within a few hundred micrometers from the spinal cord junction (38). Unmyelinated axons are directed to a superficial position in the ventro-lateral part of the rootlets. In order to reach this position, the axons criss-cross extensively in the rootlets (62).

PNS axons 0.7–0.8 μm or more in diameter acquire myelin as they enter the CNS (62). These myelin sheaths consist of 10–15 lamellae and show internodes 10–40 μm in length (Plate 41). There is a gap 1–3 μm in length between termination of the Schwann cell and the beginning of the CNS myelin, partly occupied by astrocytic processes that reach close to the axolemma and partly by the continuation of the Schwann cell basement membrane. There are distinct accumulations of electron-dense material on the axoplasmic side of the axolemma at sites where it faces the astrocytic processes. The CNS organization of some axons 0.6–0.8 μm in diameter is best described as "segmental myelination;" there are irregularly spaced CNS myelin segments 3–20 μm in length interrupted by unmyelinated stretches 3–20 μm in length.

Axons less than 0.6–0.7 μm in diameter aggregate into densely packed bundles on the CNS side of the borderline (62). Before they enter the bundles, these axons show astrocytic contacts of the type given above. Only the smallest unmyelinated axons (0.1–0.3 μm) enter the CNS without some specialized astrocytic contact. Many small axons run for several micrometers in the endoneural space just covered by a basement membrane. Branching of unmyelinated axons at the CNS entrance has not been observed. However, it is well known that branching takes place deeper inside the CNS (284). Branching probably means a decreased diameter and (in this part of the spectrum) an increased probability of an unmyelinated condition of the axons.

Three points are noteworthy regarding the borderline passage of unmyelinated fibers: (a) extensive redistribution of the axons; (b) special axolemma–astrocytic contacts; and (c) myelination of large axons. Whether the redistribution takes place according to the sensory quality of the axons is unknown. The significance of axolemma–astrocytic relations noted at the borderline is obscure. The arrangements are reminiscent of those of CNS nodes of Ranvier. Myelination of some axons means that certain members of the slowly propagating population of C-fibers suddenly, at the CNS entrance, become comparatively fast conducting lines. In view of axon size the sensory quality thus promoted should emanate from low-threshold mechanoreceptors (43). Regardless of its functional implications, the arrangements at the transition are noteworthy in view of the utterly monotonous picture offered by the stereotype part of unmyelinated axons.

MYELINATED PNS AXON

In view of the well-documented functional heterogeneity of myelinated fibers (briefly indicated to the right in Fig. 1), one expects that information should have accumulated that would enable correlation between axon morphology, neurophysiology, and molecular biology (140,149,150,153,156,161,235,286). However, most textbooks and reviews refer to very small fibers (1–4 μm in diameter) of unknown functional quality. Statements regarding the organization of larger fibers are based on extrapolations from the small fibers. As was indicated by Gasser (125) and by Hess and Lansing (145) in the pioneer works on nerve fiber ultrastructure, and later demonstrated by Williams and Landon (175,322; see also refs. 32,225), there does indeed exist an involved morphological organization at nodal regions of large axons, an organization that very well might accommodate a number of functionally significant differences. This precludes the use of data based on extrapolations. Preparatory difficulties and technical shortcomings of the early EM era are obvious parts of the explanation for the careless use of extrapolations. Less obvious are the roles played by physiological doctrines dealing with propagation of the nerve impulse.

These doctrines use concepts such as "nerve

membrane" and "excitable membrane," terms easily taken to mean the axolemma. A consideration of methods of the neurophysiologists reveals that what they referred to as a "membrane" actually meant the tissue layer between their "inside" and "outside" electrodes. In squid giant axon this layer includes, beside the axolemma, a comparatively thick multicellular Schwann cell layer and an external basement membrane. The significance of these outer components of the "excitable membrane" have been much discussed and just recently put to experimental tests (3,248,290,292,299).

In myelinated fibers the "membrane" separating the "inside" of a nerve fiber from its "outside" during physiological experiments is more complex. Besides the axon plasma membrane, it includes the myelin sheath sandwiched between strata of Schwann cell cytoplasm. At a few sites of restricted length, the axon plasma membrane is free of myelin but still covered by the basement membrane and the constituents of the node gap (see below). Some properties of the "excitable membrane" may therefore, in fact, depend on elements outside the axolemma (202).

All classic neurophysiological doctrines dealing with axonal dimensions assume a cylindrical axon shape. This facilitates calculations of a number of fiber parameters. A still more simplified situation seems to emerge when adopting the ideas suggested by others, including Rushton (241), who calculated that all electrically important axonal dimensions of differently sized myelinated fibers varied in accordance with the axon diameter.

Osmic acid and potassium permanganate were the favorite fixatives in early EM studies of nerve. Both rendered comparatively well-preserved small fibers, which in most cases showed circular cross sections. It so appeared that theoretical demands on axon shape were easily satisfied. In view of the physiological concepts, it then appeared safe to extrapolate nerve fiber morphology from small to large units. However, permanganate is poor for the preservation of large myelinated fibers, and osmic acid as a first fixative brings about disarrangements at nodes and Schmidt–Lanterman incisures (31). It is noteworthy that Rushton excluded fibers less than 5 μm in diameter from his concept of axonal dimensional similarity, i.e., precisely the fiber sizes on which morphological extrapolations have been based. The introduction of glutaraldehyde as a fixative (242) meant an improved preservation of peripheral fibers (31,307); myelin splitting decreased, and microtubules appeared intact and well preserved. The use of embedding media like epon and Vestopal W (70) added to improved preservation. These and other methodological progress encouraged morphometric studies, and quantitative axon morphology began for the first time to reach beyond the frontiers set at the beginning of the century (7,32,38,39,89,111–114,118,305, 309,336,338). During the last decade ultrastructural morphometric data have accumulated that emphatically invalidate the idea of morphological similarity in axons (see below; Waxman, *this volume*).

The principal features of morphology of a

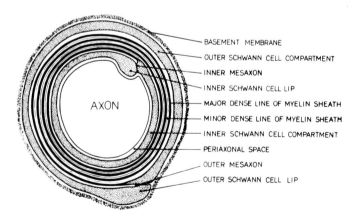

FIG. 2. A small cross-cut myelinated axon illustrating some terms used in the text.

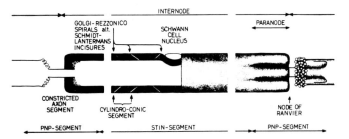

FIG. 3. A large myelinated axon as viewed longitudinally, illustrating some terms used in the text. The myelin sheath is "removed" from the internodes to the extreme right and left of the figure.

myelinated fiber emerge out of one axon and its row of attending Schwann cells, each separate Schwann cell by a process of continuous spiral wrapping and infolding of its cell membrane generating the myelin sheath outside the axon. Short unmyelinated segments are left between consecutive Schwann cells: the *nodes of Ranvier*. Figures 2 and 3 schematically present the myelinated axon and define the terminology to be used.

Stereotype Part of the Axon

The major repeating unit of the myelinated nerve fibers is the internode, the length of which depends primarily on axon diameter. During saltatory conduction the internodes act as passive myelin-insulated core conductors that interconnect the regularly spaced and comparatively narrow stripes of excitable axon membrane situated at the nodes of Ranvier (Waxman, *this volume;* Cahalan, *this volume*).

As indicated in Fig. 3, the organization of the Schwann cell and its myelin sheath—which is not a major subject of this chapter—indicates that internodes might be subdivided into a number of smaller segments. We can separate the axon into stereotype internodal (STIN) segments and paranode–node–paranode (PNP) segments (Fig. 3).

STIN Segment

The axolemma forms a fairly smooth contour. Coated vesicles and invaginations are common in large fibers and sparse in small ones (302; Berthold, *unpublished observations*). The inner Schwann cell lip indents the

axolemma, sometimes to a considerable depth. Similar indentations are also formed by local invaginations of the inner Schwann cell compartment.

Average packing density of formed axoplasmic elements is low. It can be calculated (Table 2) for a large fiber that approximately 95% of the axon cross section is "empty." The elements lie scattered at random or form clusters where a mitochondrion, several neurotubules, and a few SER profiles associate in a clearing of a surrounding neurofilament latticework. The mitochondrion occurrence is 0.7 and $0.1/\mu m^2$ in small and large axons, respectively. The corresponding figures for neurotubules are ~ 50 and $\sim 10 \mu m^2$. There are 100–200 neurofilaments/μm^2 in large and small axons alike.

Longitudinally cut SER tubes are rarely seen regardless of the direction of sectioning, which is consistent with a reticular distribution. The SER organization as described by Droz et al. (85) in preterminal axons seems to be present in feline spinal root fibers: a primary tubular system closely adapted to the inside of the axolemma and a secondary tubular system branching in the axon core (Plate 8). The SER profiles average 1–2/μm of axon circumference. Occurrence of the secondary system seems less constant (Table 2; Fig. 4).

The primary SER system is particularly noteworthy in relation to studies of incorporation of metabolites into various nerve fiber compartments. Thus if it is assumed that the SER communicates with the endoneural space via the node gaps (262) and that SER connected transport takes place in either direction at 200–400 mm/day, the primary SER system offers a route that during a delay of less than

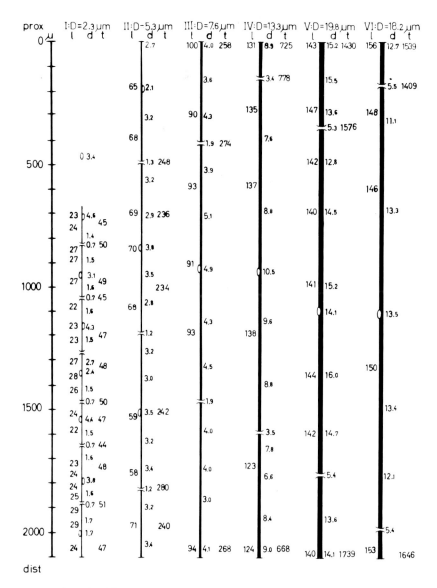

FIG. 4. Reconstruction of 6 feline myelinated ventral root axons obtained from 23,000 consecutive ultrathin sections. The fibers are drawn to scale with the exception of the size of the Schwann cell nuclei and the width of the node gaps. The D values are calculated from the mean axon cross-sectional area and the mean number of myelin lamellae, assuming an average shrinkage of 10% and a lamellar periodicity in the myelin of 18 nm. The d values at different axon levels were calculated directly from axon circumferences as estimated by a map reader. (t) Number of neurotubules found in the cross-cut axon. (l) Number of myelin lamellae. For further data see Table 2.

10 min joins the immediate vicinity of the total axolemma of any fiber and the endoneural space (260).

Miscellaneous bodies and granular material occur rarely and randomly in the STIN segment.

Shape

The shape of the STIN axon is greatly influenced by the preparative procedure. The generally accepted view of a circular axon contour is probably based on an artifact. In cross sections through frozen fresh or glutaraldehyde-fixed specimens, the nerve fibers lay closely packed, their cross-cut contours basically round but mutually adapted as an effect of crowding (31). Fresh fibers often appear notched or "cog wheel"-like, reflecting depressions caused by distribution of the outer Schwann cytoplasm like longitudinal stripes (31,32). Preparatory procedures no doubt enhance the dimensions of originally shallow furrows as the myelin sheath must adapt its shape to a complex situation where it shrinks approximately 10% in the longitudinal and circumferential directions but more than 30% in the radial direction (31,61). On the other hand, corrugated, notched, and noncircular axons show nearly perfect circular contours when sectioned at the level where a Golgi–Rezzonico spiral enters the myelin sheath (Plate 5). In view of the many Golgi–Rezzonico spirals present along an internode and a 5- to 10-μm thickness of paraffin sections, a circular shape hidden at some level of most fibers in such a section may give the illusion of circularity (32). Most STIN segments are deformed at their midpoints by the impression

of the Schwann cell perikaryon. This deformation is most obvious in small fibers (Plates 6 and 7; Fig. 4).

Caliber

The diameter of myelinated axons varies considerably when measured at several sites along the same fibers (157). Table 2 (see also Fig. 4) gives a range of 50% of the mean value in small and 25% in large fibers, provided paranodal and nuclear regions are excluded. If these are included, the variation increases considerably. The fact that the mean axon diameter calculated from an axon cross-sectional area shows smaller *SD*-values and narrower ranges than mean *d*-values calculated from axon circumference seems to indicate that the former method for approximating axon diameter is to be preferred. Variation in size and shape along individual fibers makes measurements uncertain, particularly of teased specimens. Here size and shape are judged from a mere silhouette. There is also risk of uncontrollable flattening (231) and artifacts as a result of a differential resistance to longitudi-

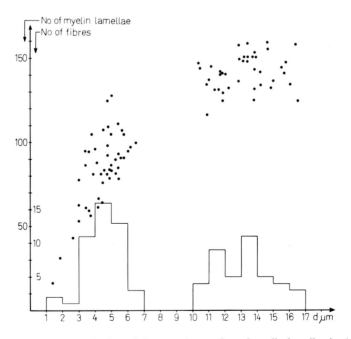

FIG. 5. Axon caliber spectrum and plotting of *d* versus the number of myelin lamellae in the L$_6$ ventral root of an adult cat. Glutaraldehyde–OsO$_4$ fixation; Vestopal embedding.

nal stretch, the node–paranode regions being more resistant than the main part of the internodes (249).

The caliber spectrum of myelinated axons is typically bimodal, with one peak in the lower range ($d = 4$–5 μm) and one peak in the upper range ($d = 13$–15 μm). As shown in Fig. 5, feline axons 7–10 μm are virtually absent in the ventral root L_6.

Caliber Versus Myelin Sheath Thickness

Based on light microscopic analysis of fresh, frozen (318) and cross-sectioned peripheral nerves and spinal roots of the rabbit (324) and on ultrastructural observations in the rat, mouse, and dog (116,117,255), it has been claimed that axon diameter throughout the spectrum correlates rectilinearly with myelin thickness, i.e., with the number of myelin lamellae. Calculations of axon diameter from a cross-sectional area and circumference as obtained by electron microscopy of feline ventral roots (39) give a logarithmic plot between d and the number of lamellae (Fig. 5). A tentatively drawn graph would rise rapidly and "rectilinearly" between $d = 1$ μm and $d = 7$ μm, corresponding to approximately 20 and 120 lamellae, respectively. In larger axons the graph flattens at the level of 130–140 lamellae. Consequently it appears as if g (d/D) should increase in the upper part of the spectrum and, not as commonly suggested, reach a steady state of 0.6–0.7 at $D > 10$ μm.

A comparison between the data of Williams and Wendell-Smith (324) and the present data (Fig. 5) reveals a good correspondence for axons more than 6 μm in diameter. In smaller axons the discrepancies are great, and they increase with decreasing size: Williams and Wendell-Smith observed a myelin sheath thickness of 2.25 μm outside axons 1–2 μm in diameter (Figs. 1 and 5 in ref. 324). Using a lamellar periodicity of 18 nm in fresh PNS myelin, one obtains a lamellar number of 125, a figure never observed in electron microscopically studied 1- to 2-μm normal PNS axons. These are commonly surrounded by 20–30 lamellae. Assuming that myelin thickness in small fibers has been considerably overestimated, the data of Williams and Wendell-Smith that concern large ventral root fibers

seem to support the idea of a nonlinear plot between axon diameter and myelin thickness (see also refs. 252,253).

The linear plottings between d and the number of myelin lamellae for rat and mouse (116,117) sciatic and vague nerves are simply explained by the fact that there are too few axons large enough in these species to reveal whether there is linearity or nonlinearity beyond a d-value of 6 μm or more. In rat spinal roots there is no clear-cut linearity (258); Boyd and Kalu (51) obtained an exponential plotting similar to the one of Fig. 5 when examining cat hind limb nerves.

Caliber Versus Internodal Length

The internodal length ("il") of mammalian A-fibers measure 200–300 μm in small axons and approximately 2,000 μm in large axons (172,324). The considerable species and local variations noted in the correlation between fiber size and "il" are usually explained by variations in longitudinal growth after myelination has started (324). Internodes as short as 90 μm have been noted on small axons in feline ventral roots L_{6-7} (Berthold and Rydmark, *in preparation*), and myelinated fibers in the paravertebral sympathetic chain show "il" values which are consistently approximately a third of that of somatic nerves (15,300).

There is general agreement that little variation exists in internodal length when measured along an individual axon (172,183,281; see, however, ref. 186 and fiber 1 in Fig. 4 herein). The differences commonly noted in the "il" values *between* axons of similar dimensions are illustrated by fibers IV, V, and VI in Table 2. The observation that the relation between conduction velocity and internodal length is linear on a semilogarithmic plot (74) suggests linearity also in the semilogarithmic plot between D and internodal length, a relation similar to that between D and the number of lamellae. This may indicate a linearity between number of myelin lamellae and internodal length (161) (Fig. 4).

Periaxonal Space

During microinjection of saline between an axon and its myelin sheath in large frog fibers, de Renyi (232) noted "contacts" that offered remarkable resistance before they yielded to the advancing fluid. Greatest resistance was offered by contacts at nodes of Ranvier. In view of the ultrastructure of the periaxonal space, it is not unlikely that de Renyi's micropipettes had entered this region. The axolemma and plasma membrane of the inner Schwann cell compartment form either five-layered membrane complexes reminiscent of dense junctions (134) or seven-layered complexes, the intermembranous space being 2–4 nm (i.e., the dimensions of a gap junction) or there is a substantial gap of 15–20 nm. All types of arrangements are seen outside the individual axon after glutaraldehyde–OsO_4 fixation, substantial gaps being more common in small fibers and five- and seven-layered complexes the rule outside large axons (99,101). The seven-layered complexes are similar to those found close to the node (see below) and are often seen at sites where SER profiles lie close to the axolemma (Plates 8 and 9).

According to freeze-fracture studies (Schnapp and Mugnaini, *this volume*), the periaxonal space is sealed off from the intermediate myelin sheath space by a zona occludens at the inner mesaxon (200,251). In small fibers surrounded by a few myelin lamellae, lanthanum (La^{3+}) enters the outer mesaxon, penetrates along the intermediate line of the myelin, and may appear in the periaxonal space (233). In fibers with more than some 10 lamellae, La^{3+} penetrates the first turns of the myelin sheath but does not reach the periaxonal space (233). Ferritin and ruthenium red do not seem to enter the periaxonal space of STIN segments (144,262). These tracers penetrate along the axon from the nodes for just a few micrometers. Horseradish peroxidase, on the other hand, has been demonstrated in the periaxonal space of adult myelinated newt nerve fibers (340).

The observations that there is a substantial periaxonal space outside all myelinated CNS axons (216), that this space may be penetrated by horseradish peroxidase (152), and that CNS axons during teasing are often accidentally pulled out from their myelin tubes (Berthold, *unpublished observations*)—a phenomenon never observed in PNS fibers—emphasize the danger in extrapolating PNS fiber morphol-

ogy from observations in the CNS and vice versa. Moreover, they suggest that there might be differences in the mode of impulse propagation along the PNS and CNS parts of an axon (Paintal, *this volume;* Swadlow and Waxman, *this volume*).

In some fibers the inner Schwann cell compartment and a few (one to five) of the innermost myelin lamellae attach at long intervals to the STIN segment, hundreds of micrometers from the node (112). This probably explains the variation in number of lamellae along individual internodes (Fig. 4). The arrangement also implies that the periaxonal space might be divided into a series of bulkheads.

The inner Schwann cell compartment is 10–25 nm thick. It contains a diffuse granular material, receives the cytoplasm of the Golgi–Rezzonico spirals, and may contain dense accumulations of fibrillar material (162).

PNP Segment

The regularly distributed PNP segments, which exhibit a spectacular morphology, are of obvious neurophysiological interest (Cahalan, *this volume;* Rasminsky, *this volume*).

Paranode

"Paranode" denotes either of the two ends of an internode. The length of the paranodal segment varies from 10 μm in small to 40–50 μm in large fibers. This segment is characterized by a system of myelin furrows that, with increasing depth, extend up to the node (Plates 10 and 11). The furrows, filled with mitochondrion-rich Schwann cytoplasm, and the intervening myelin ridges often disclose a spiral course. Fibers less than 3–4 μm in diameter seem to lack both ridges and mitochondrion aggregations (39). The number of myelin furrows varies from three in small to seven in large fibers.

The two bulbous ends of consecutive paranodes may come very close together (Plate 12). Each is equipped with a central opening at the node of Ranvier, where the myelin sheath turns sharply toward the axon. Particularly in large fibers, the axon is constricted to between one-half and one-third of its internodal diameter along that part which receives the in-turning myelin and passes the gap between consecutive internodes.

That constricted part of a paranodal axon segment along which the myelin sheath attaches is referred to as the *myelin sheath attachment* (MySA) *segment*. The proximal and distal MySA segments, together with the intervening nodal segment, constitute the constricted axon segment (Fig. 3; Plate 12). The two paranodal fiber segments that meet at a node constitute a paranodal pair. (The MySA segment, particularly among workers interested in freeze-fractured nerve fibers, is referred to as the paranodal segment. This classification is not used here.)

Paranodes are commonly portrayed as bulbiform dilated parts demarcated from the rest of the internode by a slightly constricted fiber segment (187,321,322). Paranodal dilations have been reported in living rat fibers (119). In cats and rabbits all teased fibers seem to show paranodal dilatations. In the rabbit the

paranodal pairs in peripheral nerve trunks are polarized with a larger cranial and small caudal member, an arrangement valid also in the descending and ascending limbs of the recurrent branch of the vagal nerve (321). In the spinal root the pairs are polarized in either direction, a few being nonpolarized but still dilated. The *in vivo* presence of paranodal dilatations has been doubted (59), and de Rényi (231) observed that dilatations developed as teased fibers adhered to a glass surface and flattened out, an observation possibly explained by the increased cross-sectional length of the paranodal myelin sheath (Fig. 6). Clear-cut paranodal bulbs were not noted in glutaraldehyde perfusion-fixed and teased fibers (40), and neither the total fiber cross-sectional area nor its circumference changed when passing from internode into paranode of large feline ventral root fibers (Fig. 6). Moreover, fixed and teased human PNS nerve fibers, as depicted comprehensively by Dyck (89), either

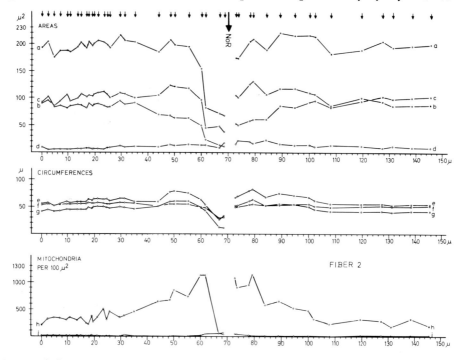

FIG. 6. Numerical values of parameters estimated in series of consecutive cross sections through the node–paranode region of a large feline ventral lumbar spinal root fiber ($D = \sim 15 \ \mu m$). **a**: Cross-sectional area of the whole fiber. **b**: Cross-sectional area of the myelin sheath. **c**: Cross-sectional area of the axon. **d**: Cross-sectional area of the outer cytoplasmic Schwann cell compartment. **e**: Circumference of the myelin sheath. **f**: Circumference of the whole fiber. **g**: Circumference of the axon. **h**: Calculated number of mitochondria per 100 μm^2 cross-cut Schwann cell cytoplasm. **i**: Calculated number of mitochondria per 100 μm^2 cross-cut axoplasm. (From ref. 32.)

lacked or showed only very moderate para-nodal dilatations.

The paranodal axon segment is a cast of the myelin sheath. Its cross-sectional area decreases gradually in the nodal direction as a consequence of the indenting myelin furrows. Thus the axon discloses an increasingly deeper fluting with a shrinking central core decorated by radiating high and delicate crests often less than 0.5 μm in width (Fig. 6; Plates 10 and 11). The axon has lost half its cross-sectional area at a level less than 10 μm from the node. As the myelin turns to the MySA segment, the axon crests disappear rather suddenly, whereby only 15–20% of the original axon cross-sectional area is left in some fibers.

The most developed paranodal axon crests are seen in axons 4–6 μm in diameter. In many large fibers the myelin ridges extend beyond the level of the node and turn more than 90° to reach the MySA segment (32,88). Inside such ridges there are blind pockets filled by the axon Schwann cell network (Plates 11, 14, and 15) (see below).

At some paranodes the ridges decrease in height before reaching the level of the node, and cross sections close to the node show a small axon (actually the MySA segment) surrounded by a comparatively thick myelin sheath (actually the in-turning part of it). Up to the level where the constricted axon segment begins, the axolemma of the paranodes shows the same five- and seven-layered membrane contacts with the inner Schwann cell compartment as seen elsewhere along the internode. A similar arrangement is noted in several commonly used experimental mammals (36). However, in rat and mouse the paranodal crenation is more irregular, the myelin exhibiting pits and short grooves rather than longitudinal furrows.

Axon–Schwann Cell Network

The axon–Schwann cell network (275) is normally seen close to the nodes of Ranvier. It develops inside the in-turning myelin ridges as subjacent axon crests "fragment" into a number of winding processes embedded in parts of the inner Schwann cell compartment (Plates 11, 12, 14, and 15). This gives a pattern of axonal profiles surrounded by granular Schwann cell cytoplasm rich in multivesicular, lamellar, and dense bodies, as well as profiles reminiscent of damaged mitochondria (Plates 15 and 16). Axoplasm in the crests close to the networks contains mitochondria as well as some miscellaneous bodies and neurofilaments; and it is practically devoid of neurotubules. Five- and seven-layered membrane complexes separate the axoplasm and Schwann cell (32). Spencer and Thomas (275) demonstrated this network in normal individuals and also identified it in a much more developed state in all parts of an internode in animals suffering from neuropathological conditions, e.g., dying-back toxic diseases. They suggest that the axon–Schwann cell network, normally restricted to paranodal regions, reflects phagocytotic and sequestering activity of the Schwann cell whereby wornout parts of the axon can be eliminated, an activity greatly enhanced when abnormal constituents appear in the axoplasm (see also ref. 261).

Constricted Axon Segment

See Fig. 3 and Plate 12.

Axolemma of the MySA Segment

The myelin sheath attaches to the MySA segments and uncoils along them in a helical manner (237). The end of each myelin lamella, as seen in longitudinal section, splits into two leaflets that enclose a drop-shaped Schwann cell terminal cytoplasmic pocket (Plates 9 and 13). The pockets represent the same helical cord of Schwann cell cytoplasm, which at each internodal end interconnects the outer and inner Schwann cell compartments. The pocket of the innermost lamella attaches furthest from the node, and subsequent lamellae terminate in subsequent order up to the node. The pockets depress the axolemma to bring about a serrated contour of the MySA segments. Each pocket requires a 100- to 200-nm axolemma segment for its attachment. Small myelinated fibers contain approximately 25 lamellae, and large fibers 150–160 lamellae. Measurements in fibers of all sizes show that the MySA segments measure some 2–4 μm irrespective of fiber size and myelin thickness (32,33). This again illustrates the danger in extrapolating the organization of small fibers to that of large ones. Many textbooks state that all lamellae contact the axon, and even that part of longitudinal internodal growth depends on the increased length required by the increasing number of myelin lamellae. In fibers approximately 3 μm in size, far from all pockets reach the axolemma; and in large fibers less than 20% do.

As revealed by a longitudinal section (Plates 12 and 13) the terminal pockets, instead of arranging in a longitudinal row, pile up on top of and then beneath each other. This gives—in successful preparations—the characteristic picture of ear-like elements; the pockets correspond to the kernels which symmetrically, on the two sides of a MySA segment, evaginate deep into the surrounding myelin. This pattern indicates that the arrangement of the terminal pockets as seen ultrastructurally explains the much-discussed spinous bracelets of Nageotte (9,32,146,172,203).

In feline fibers fixed in glutaraldehyde and OsO₄, the axolemma of the MySA segment and the Schwann cell membrane of the pockets form seven-layered membrane complexes approximately 17 nm in thickness (Plates 9, 13, and 17). The intervening space measures 2–3 nm and contains granular material of high electron density. In fibers treated *en bloc* with uranyl acetate before dehydration, the interlamellar substance closest to the node gap appears most electron-dense (33). The regular arrangement of 15-nm long, evenly spaced bands merging with the outer leaflets of the facing cell membranes and found all along the MySA segments in rat and in CNS fibers (216) have not been observed in feline fibers. However, as shown in Plate 9, there seems to be some periodicity within the seven-layered complexes of feline axons.

The MySA segments of CNS axons have been studied extensively using freeze-fracture techniques (185,243,250). The observations indicate the presence of specialized membranous arrangements, evoking speculations regarding an ionic coupling between the axon and the Schwann cells. It has also been suggested that the close-to-node arrangements mean that the myelin is locked onto the axon in a joint of high mechanical stability. As suggested by Rosenbluth (240), the membrane relations might constitute a "bottleneck" whereby the

specialized components of the nodal axon membrane are prevented from drifting away into the MySA STIN segments (see also Schnapp and Mugnaini, *this volume*).

Axolemma of the Node of Ranvier

The nodal axolemma delineates the nodal axon segment and extends between the last closely attached myelin pocket of one internode and the first closely attached pocket of the next internode (Plates 12 and 17). Its length is approximately 1 μm in small fibers and 1.5 μm in large fibers (32). The nodal axolemma exhibits a corrugated contour and an electron-dense layer coating its axoplasmic side. The extent of this coat coincides with that part of the axolemma that shows ATPase positivity immunohistochemically (327) and is related on its inside to an ion-binding layer (227). The amplitude of the corrugations is 10–100 nm. The nodal axon segment is usually slightly bulging and barrel-shaped (Plates 12 and 17).

At many nodes the axolemma evaginates and forms 0.1- to 0.5-μm high spines or crests (32). The crests run across the long axis of the fiber. They are sometimes approximately 10 μm long, and their surface may add considerable area to that of the nodal axolemma. A nodal axon segment may carry many crests and spines, which explains its often irregular shape as seen in cross sections. Coated invaginations are particularly common along the nodal axolemma (Plate 20).

Nodal Undercoating

The axolemma receives its nodal undercoating at the very spot where the seven-layered membrane complex between the MySA segment and the myelin pockets cease (Plate 17). The thickness of the undercoating is commonly reported to be 20–30 nm (e.g., refs. 98,172, 237). A detailed study in feline fibers shows that the coat is of uneven thickness (Plates 18 and 19). It measures up to 80 nm at one site, is absent at another, and shows an average thickness of approximately 30 nm. In the thicker parts of the coat, the dense material has an irregular distribution (Plate 18). Thin condensations of diffuse material interconnect the coat with adjacent axoplasmic elements, particularly neurofilaments and SER profiles. Mature feline fibers of 15–20 lamellae ($d = 1$ μm) (very rare in adult cats) lack the nodal coating but show a few solitary patches of dense subaxolemmal substance (Plate 34).

Conclusive electron micrographs showing the organization of the nodal coating are difficult to obtain, perhaps as a consequence of axolemmal corrugation. At high magnification the coat resolves into high-, medium-, and low-contrast regions (Plates 18–21). The latter often appear like round spots 7–10 nm in size surrounded by medium-contrast rims 2–4 nm in width and dispersed in a high-contrast matrix. Whether this should be interpreted as globular osmiophobic units distributed irregularly in an osmiophilic matrix just inside the nodal axolemma, or whether it represents a lattice of amorphous high-contrast material enclosing small empty spaces cannot be decided. In my opinion the former interpretation seems to correspond fairly well with the pattern noted in tangentially cut parts of the nodal axolemma (Plate 21).

At some places in most feline nodes, there is a low-contrast space 8–10 nm wide between the inner leaflet of the axolemma and the coating. At some sites these clearings are distinctly separated; when found in combination with pyramidiform accretions of the coating material, this gives a picture similar to that described by Chan-Palay (65) in the initial segment of Purkinje cell axons (Plates 18 and 19).

Detailed freeze-fracture studies of the organization of the nodal axolemma of small CNS fibers have now appeared (185,240,250; see also ref. 238). Rosenbluth (240) demonstrated aggregations of irregularly distributed globular particles approaching 20 nm in diameter attached to the outer leaflet of the axolemma. He emphasized that the globules were too large to be accommodated within the axolemma; and since particles assumed to represent ATPase should attach to the inner membrane leaflet, he suggested that the nodal outer-leaflet particles might correspond to ionophores containing a sodium channel.

Axoplasm and Axoplasmic Elements

Axoplasm of the constricted nodal segments stains intensely with heavy metal salts (146,

230). AgNO$_3$ treatment gives rise to the crosses of Ranvier, where the horizontal bar corresponds to the deeply black-stained constricted axon segment. The axoplasm of this part of the axon is of a peculiar consistency. It forms a hindrance for the progression of injected fluid (232) and, as observed by Ranvier (230; see also refs. 146,172), can, like a plug, be removed and transferred into adjacent paranodal parts of the axon. The qualities of the nodal axoplasm suggested that there was a transverse septum in the nodal axon (201), an opinion now conclusively refuted by electron microscopy.

As one passes along the paranode toward the node, there is a concentration of formed elements to the axoplasmic core region and a successive depletion of outer axoplasmic regions. Packing density of axoplasmic elements is high all along the constricted axon segment (Table 2). Neurotubules reach a concentration similar to that of the average unmyelinated fiber and disclose a higher concentration in the peripheral zone as compared to the core of the constricted segment (Plates 22, 24, and 25). Neurotubules are arranged in bundles of 2–10 members (Plate 2), an arrangement reminiscent of that in the initial axon segment (71, 322). The concentration of mitochondria is approximately five times that of the STIN segment (Table 2), a value that agrees fairly well with a situation where any level of an axon is passed by an equivalent number of mitochondria per unit time. The concentration of neurofilaments is roughly the same as internodally. All along the constricted axon segment there are conspicuous neurofilamentous latticeworks.

The occurrence of SER profiles is high in the constricted nodal segment, and longitudinal profiles are dominant. This indicates a reorganization from a reticular pattern to a longitudinal one as the SER enters the constricted segment. SER profiles often reach close to the nodal coating and project into nodal crests and spines (Plates 17 and 24).

In the constricted axon segments there is added a formed axoplasmic element not seen elsewhere, i.e., a beaded tube 0.5–3 μm long and 0.05–0.5 μm thick. The beaded tubes seem to bud off vesicles at their distal ends. Longitudinal SER tubes often appear in close connection to the beaded tubes (Plate 24). However, a direct transformation of SER membrane into membrane of a beaded tube has not been observed. It is suggested as a working hypothesis that parts of the SER take part in building up the nodal system of beaded tubes.

In large fibers, bundles of neurotubules, mitochondria, SER profiles, and beaded tubules form clusters that extend in a peripheral zone throughout the proximal MySA segment and partly into the nodal segment. Such clusters are rare in the distal part of the node and in the distal MySA segment (Plates 25 and 26).

Granular Material

The appearance of granular material (Plates 27–30) in some constricted nodal axon segments is rather enigmatic. Most nodal segments contain a few scattered electron-dense granules 15–30 nm in size. Whether they represent glycogen granules, ribosomes, or some other material is unknown. Typical glycogen-like granules—round, stippled, and ~30 nm in size—are noted at the entrance of the proximal MySA segments in some fibers (Plate 28).

The most spectacular observation concerning granular material in the constricted axon segment is that of diffusely granulated proximal MySA segments. The granular material may be organized in either of two main patterns:

1. Round stippled granules of low-to-medium contrast, 10–20 nm in size, fill out the proximal MySA segment. There is a sharp demarcation between granulated and nongranulated axoplasm in the proximal nodal segment (32). At the demarcation between the MySA segment and the fluted paranodal axon, the transition between granular and nongranular axoplasm is diffuse. The granularity obscures microtubules and neurofilaments (Plate 27).

2. The second pattern is characterized by condensation of granular material to a central core, leaving a 0.2- to 0.5-μm zone of ordinary looking axoplasm. There are granules of medium and high contrast. In contrast to a homogeneous granulation obscuring neurotubules and neurofilaments, these elements are easily identified in the second type of granular organization, where tubules and filaments are surrounded by a clear zone 10–40 nm in width (Plates 31 and 32). It might be suspected that the clear zones develop as a consequence of

some low-contrast material coating the tubules and filaments. There are also intermediate patterns, e.g., where high-contrast granules lay scattered on a background of medium-contrast granularity. Diffusely granulated axoplasm is rich in SER profiles. Characteristic as well are 2- to 10-nm thick, homogeneous, high-density layers that coat mitochondria, SER profiles, and miscellaneous bodies (Plate 30). Neither axon tubules and filaments nor the axolemma reveal such an electron-dense coating. High-contrast coats are noted in some nongranulated axons and even in the STIN segments, usually outside SER profiles.

The occurrence of granules in the PNP segments is noteworthy, especially in view of their inconsistency: In one animal it is absent, in a second most axons reveal granulated PNP segments, and in others all variations are encountered. One possible working hypothesis is that the different granular patterns reflect various functional stages or phases of some physiological process.

The occurrence of high-contrast layers outside membrane-demarcated axoplasmic organelles should also be emphasized. A similar material was noted in unmyelinated crayfish axons fixed in glutaraldehyde during impulse propagation (222). Biochemical experiments (222) indicate that the osmiophilia might reflect SH groups unmasked during activity. Similar osmiophilia appeared after asphyxiation (222). In view of this, the high-contrast layering and granularity might signify variation in oxygenation of tissue during preparation for fixation.

At the paranodal outlet of distal MySA segments, all kinds of membrane-demarcated miscellaneous bodies, particularly lamellar and dense ones, are numerous.

Node of Ranvier

Axonal Dimensions

The cross-sectional area of the node of Ranvier axon is approximately one-third and one-fifth to one-sixth times the internodal area in small and large fibers, respectively (Table 2). Recalculating the observed values to presumably "fresh" values shows, for instance, that a 20-μm feline ventral root fiber has an

TABLE 3. *Some nodal parameters in feline ventral spinal roots*

No. of nodal regions analyzed	Approx. fiber size (μm)	Diameter of nodal axon segment (μm)	Mean length of nodal axon segment (range) (μm)	Area of nodal axon segment (μm²)	Height of node gap (μm)	Total area of microvilli-like processes (μm²)	Area of lateral node gap walls (μm²)	Total membranous Schwann cell area facing node gap (% of nodal axon segment area)	Mean length of MYSA segment (μm)
1	15	4.7	1.5 (1.7–1.3)	22.3	0.9	147.3	31.6	800	3.4 (3.2–3.7)[a]
1	14	3.7	1.4 (1.6–1.1)	15.8	1.1	105.5	32.9	880	3.2 (3.1–3.3)[a]
1	6	1.3	1.0 (1.1–0.8)	4.1	0.9	33.2	13.9	1150	—
1	6	1.5	0.9 (1.0–0.6)	4.0	0.9	33.3	12.3	1130	—
1	14	4.8	1.5 (1.7–1.1)	22.5	1.1	210.6	40.4	1120	3.0 (2.8–3.2)[a]
1	13	3.9	1.2 (1.5–0.9)	14.4	0.8	112.7	24.0	950	3.3 (2.9–3.4)[a]
1	5	1.8	0.9 (1.1–0.8)	5.1	0.7	33.7	10.0	850	—
1	5	1.4	0.83 (1.0–0.76)	3.6	0.6	19.4	7.9	750	—
10[a]	13–16	—	1.3 (1.7–1.1)	—	—	—	—	—	3.4 (2.8–4.0)
1	15	4.8	1.7 (1.9–1.4)	25.3	1.3	278.6	47.6	1290	3.2 (3.1–3.5)[a]
1	14	4.5	1.3 (1.5–1.2)	18.8	1.1	179.0	38.6	1160	3.2 (2.8–3.4)[a]
1	5	1.4	0.9 (1.0–0.7)	3.7	0.7	30.3	8.5	1050	—
10[a]	13–16	—	1.3 (1.5–1.1)	—	—	—	—	—	3.0 (2.3–3.4)

[a] Measurements performed only in median section through node.
From ref. 32.

axon with a mean diameter of 14.7 μm and a nodal axon diameter of 5.3 μm. Table 2, moreover, shows that there is practically no variation in the nodal axon diameter when examining consecutive nodes on individual fibers. The present data suggest that morphometric analysis of myelinated fibers should use nodal axon diameter instead of *d,* an idea that seems reasonable, not least with respect to the role of the nodes in saltatory conduction.

The dimensions of cross-cut axons should also be considered in connection with bulk axoplasmic flow. The velocity of a fluid in a tube depends on the fourth power of the radius. Thus bulk flow of axoplasm through nodal segments of large feline fibers should be approximately 40 times the internodal velocity. A factor of 40 and observations which state that axoplasmic granules pass along constricted axon segments at a velocity not different from the internodal one (73) appear rather compromising for the current concepts regarding axoplasmic bulk flow; it may not even exist, all transportation following preformed tracks at different velocities, tracks that focus at the nodes of Ranvier.

Estimations of the area of the nodal axolemma based on electron microscopy of serial sections of feline ventral (32) and dorsal (39) roots give 4–5 μm² in small fibers (*D* = 5–6 μm) and 20–25 μm² in large ones (*D* = 15–20 μm). These values fit Rushton's (241; see also ref. 146) calculations regarding dimensional similarity, and agree with neurophysiological considerations (280). The recent studies of Moore et al. (197a) suggest that conduction velocity, while strongly dependent on fiber diameter, may be relatively insensitive to small changes in nodal area. Calculations of nodal axon area based on light microscopy should be avoided, as discussed below. Hess and Young (146), in view of the small size of the nodal axon area in large fibers (calculated from the light microscopic image), speculated that the whole constricted axon segment might be actively involved in impulse transmission. This idea was recently revived by Dun (87) in a theoretical study, and by Livingston et al. (185) in a freeze-etch study of the "node–paranode" region (i.e., of the constricted axon segment). Dun's calculations are based on the erroneous assumption that the

nodal segment measures 20 μm in length and 9 μm in diameter in large vertebrate axons, and are hence somewhat uninteresting. Livingston et al. (185) refer to work (1,147) in which the heat generated by the nervous impulse was calculated to require an active membrane area more than 10 times that of a nodal axon segment; and they suggest, in view of their own observations regarding the specialization of the MySA segment, that this might enlarge the active region of the node. However, Livingston et al. (185) do not mention the area offered by the Schwann cell microvilli, which is 10 times the axon nodal area (32) (Table 3).

Node Gap

The node gap is a ring-shaped space surrounding the nodal axolemma bordered proximally and distally by the myelin sheaths of two meeting internodes (Plate 17). Its external demarcation toward the endoneural space is formed by the Schwann cell collars (Plates 33 and 34); and where the collars leave openings between them, the Schwann cell basement membrane forms the node gap cover. The endoneural space outside the node gap and between the internodal ends is called the perinodal space. The perinodal space in large fibers is a narrow gap, sometimes less than 0.2 μm in width and 5–7 μm in depth. Its Schwann cell walls show several specializations (32). The height of the gap is 0.5–1.5 μm and its base length 0.3–0.7 μm. The remaining part of the nodal axolemma (1–1.5 μm in length) faces narrow lateral node gap recesses, 50 nm in height and covered by overhanging terminal myelin pockets (Plate 17). This organization means that node gap lengths cannot be measured correctly in large fibers using light microscopy. In small fibers where the myelin sheath often turns to the axon with an internodal tilt (32,146), the node gaps appear more open, and the length of the nodal axon can be approximated with light microscopy.

The node gap is occupied by Schwann cell microvilli projecting from the nodal collars. In very small fibers (*D* <3–4 μm) the microvilli are few and randomly arranged (Plate 34). In larger fibers they form a corona of densely packed units outside the nodal axon (Plates 33 and 35). A high degree of morphological order exists in the node gaps of cat, rabbit, and dog, and a somewhat lower degree in rat and mouse (36). At many sites the tips of the nodal microvilli come close to the axolemma, the separation being 3–5 nm. In frog (13) and mouse (Plate 23) nodes there are seven-layered membrane complexes, the intervening space being 2–4 nm.

Node Gap Matrix Substance

Even in conventionally treated specimens the ultrastructure of the gap matrix is variable (Plates 36 and 37). It is suggested, as a working hypothesis, that the variation in the electron-dense material indicates various functional stages. Langley and Landon (173, 176–180) suggested that the node gap substance is a complex mucopolysaccharide containing two types of polyions, one carboxylated and one also containing sulfate esters. The gap substance was portrayed as polyanionic with the properties of a cation exchanger, properties that make it metallophilic and disturb histochemical reactions that employ heavy metal ions. Thus the use of Cu and Pb in the demonstration of acetylcholinesterase, ATPase, and various phosphatases requires meticulous control experiments (2,167,181). Prolonged staining in solutions of heavy metal ions gives rise to the crosses of Ranvier: a horizontal bar representing local metallophilia of the constricted axon segment and a vertical bar representing the node gap. The capriciousness of the staining properties of the gap substance is illustrated by distinct variations in density even

at the same node gap (167) as well as by the observation that a brief cacodylate-buffered aldehyde fixation before osmication and staining with ferric ion and ferrocyanide renders the node gap substance inactive but the nodal axolemma and subjacent axoplasm highly reactive (227).

Paranodal Apparatus

The term "paranodal apparatus" was introduced by Williams and Landon (175,322), who emphasized the possible functional interconnection between the nodal axolemma and the mitochondrion-rich paranodal Schwann cell cytoplasm (32,323). In the PNP segments of PNS myelinated fibers there are, close to the axolemma, large numbers of mitochondria (77). The mitochondrion-rich compartments are connected to the immediate outside of the nodal axolemma partly via microvilli, instruments known to engage in absorption and receptor-transducing phenomena (244), and partly via node gap substance. Certainly this is a picture (Fig. 7) that invites speculation regarding functional significance. Unfortunately, it suffers the lack of quantitative data and data from physiological and biochemical experiments. However, recent studies in squid giant axons indicate a Schwann cell–axon coupling during impulse transmission (190). Tasaki and Carbone (286) pointed out that the functional properties of the excitable membrane require a polyanionic exterior, and Müller-Mohnssen et al. (202) suggest, on the basis of experiments testing the action potential

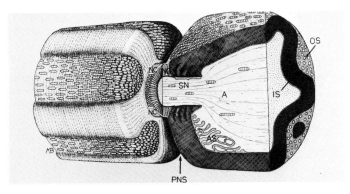

FIG. 7. Node–paranode region, illustrating the arrangement of the elements of the paranodal apparatus. (OS) Outer Schwann cell compartment. (IS) Inner Schwann cell compartment. (AS) Axon–Schwann cell network. (SN) MySA segment. (NC) Nodal collar. (A) Axon. Arrow and PNS indicate the perinodal space.

of myelinated axons locally damaged by a microlaser beam, that the electrophysiological properties of a node of Ranvier might be partly "controlled by a paranodal organ" localized outside the axolemma. The morphological similarity between the paranodal apparatus and elements of the ion-secreting salt glands of certain birds was pointed out by Landon and Hall (172).

Polarization of the PNP Segment

Regardless of the phenomena underlying the appearance of the granule-containing constricted axon segments, their polarization is quite obvious. So far it appears that the proximal MySA segments (the ones closest to the cell bodies) are granulated. The large number of beaded tubes in proximal MySA segments and the aggregation of miscellaneous membrane-bound bodies at the outlet of distal MySA segments add to the polarized state of the constricted axon segments of large fibers.

An additional illustration of this polarization is found in PNS axons transporting horseradish peroxidase (HRP) in a retrograde direction. Thirty-six hours after administration of HRP in cat soleus muscle, nodes 4–6 cm proximal to the muscle appear after histochemical treatment as shown in Plate 38. The outlet from the distal MySA segment is crowded by HRP-positive bodies. A few of these have penetrated half way along the nodal segment. Proximal to this level, HRP-positive bodies are rare and the proximal MySA segment is crowded by a longitudinally arranged tubular membranous system with a sharp proximal demarcation. These observations (Berthold and Mellstrom, *to be published*) infer that the PNP segments are polarized in a way that might have implications for nodal and axonal functions, and reveal a considerable *de novo* synthesis of membranous tube-shaped elements (Plate 39).

Branching Points

Branching of the stereotype axon segment takes place at nodes of Ranvier (93,282). Both di- and polychotomous branching is noted in the terminal fields (336). In rat sternomastoideus nerve the ratio between the cross-sectional area of a main A-α-axon and that of all its terminal branches is 1:11 (336). As a rule, each of the branches is thinner than the stem fiber. An exception seems to be the bifurcation of the crus commune of spinal ganglion neurons, where the peripheral and central branches are of approximately equal size (141,234; see, however, ref. 193).

Ultrastructural descriptions of branch points in terms of the paranodal apparatus or in morphometric terms are not available. Ha (141), who goes into some detail on the ultrastructure of the bifurcation of crus commune in the cat, remarks that the myelin sheath arrangements are similar to those of other parts of a myelinated fiber. Of significance is the observation that neurotubules and neurofilaments never pass from the peripheral branch into the central one (141). All tubules and filaments originate in the perikaryon, pass along the crus commune, and are delivered partly into the central and partly into the peripheral axon branches. There is a clear-cut difference between peripheral and central spinal ganglion processes, the former showing the higher concentration of neurotubules. The arrangement suggests one way in which a soma, its axonal branches, and peripheral domains might be differentiated. Andersson and McClure (12) showed that different protein species are transported along peripheral and central spinal ganglion axon branches. The detailed design of branch points becomes particularly interesting when discussing nervous function in terms of the "multiplex neuron" (303; Waxman, *this volume*). The impulse filtering noted at axon branching points was recently discussed by Chung (66).

Crus Commune "Axon"

It is questionable, ontogenetically and morphologically, whether the crus commune of primary sensory neurons should be classified as an axon (245,276,337). A brief description is included here because recent observations suggest that the perikaryon–crus commune unit in certain situations might influence the propagation of impulses along the bypassing axon (285).

Ontogenetically the crus commune is a part of the perikaryon that attenuates during development of an originally bipolar neuron into a pseudounipolar one. The crus commune contains Nissl substance (334,337), microtubules, SER profiles, and clusters of mitochondria-containing granules (276,337). Proximally the crus commune is unmyelinated. It shows the principal features of an initial axon segment adjacent to the level at which it gets a myelin sheath. The distal, myelinated part of the crus commune shows internodes of increasing length and of increasing myelin thickness (276). Since the size of the myelinated part of the crus roughly corresponds to that of its branches (141), its g (d/D) value is exceptionally high, a phenomenon used as an argument against the idea that the axon, by its size, determines the degree of myelination (276).

PNS–CNS Transition in Myelinated PNS Axons

The only detailed ultrastructural data derive from a study in feline S_1 dorsal spinal roots (38,39). The transition between the PNS and CNS parts of an axon takes place at a node of Ranvier (Plate 40): the transitional node (38, 39,123,192,277). In less than 1% of all myelinated axons the transitional node is missing (39). Instead, the CNS myelin sheath projects for a few hundred micrometers into the PNS, where it is covered by a PNS myelin sheath.

There is no significant difference between the PNS and CNS D values of individual axons as seen 100μm on either side of the transitional node (39). Figure 8 shows PNS D values plotted against CNS D values of individual fibers. On the whole, the plotted values distribute according to $x = y$. However, in very small axons the higher number of PNS myelin lamellae (39) becomes crucial, and PNS D values are constantly higher than CNS D values in this group. This seems to explain the current idea (123,192) that fiber size decreases at the CNS entrance. Again, the organization of large fibers has been erroneously extrapolated from that of small ones. At a deeper level in the CNS the axons branch and the individual branches should be smaller than the stem axon (284).

The most proximal PNS internodes are 25% shorter than their more distal companions (39). Exceptionally large numbers of Schwann

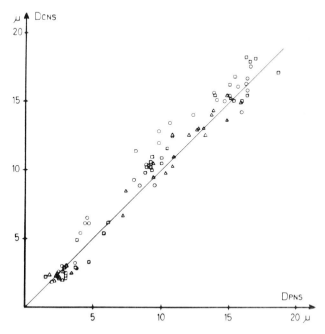

FIG. 8. Fiber size of feline S_1 dorsal root myelinated axons as seen on the PNS side of the PNS–CNS borderline (D_{PNS}) plotted against the fiber size of the same axons as found on the CNS side of the borderline (D_{CNS}). The symbols ($\square$, $\triangle$, $\bigcirc$) refer to three adult cats. The solid line indicates $D_{PNS} = D_{CNS}$. (From ref. 39.)

cell mitochondria occur close to the transitional node gap, which is occupied by both microvilli and astrocytic processes (Plate 40). As at ordinary PNS nodes, Schwann cell mitochondria are scarce in fibers less than 4 μm in size, and the nodal axon membrane varies from 4 to 25 μm² in small and large fibers, respectively. The number of astrocytic perikarya related to the transitional nodes and the CNS paranodes are surprisingly high: more than 50 times the number expected from the content in the membrane glia limitans externa in general (39).

Morphological Differences Between Myelinated Axons

There are now several observations which support the idea that myelinated axons can be separated according to morphological criteria other than fiber size. Thus the design of the paranodal apparatus distinguishes between axons 1–3 μm in diameter and those that are larger (32,39,225). Small and large fibers may also be differentiated with regard to the cyclic AMP content after activity (16). Afferent and efferent axons can be distinguished with respect to acetylcholinesterase content (336) and the capacity to transport HRP (45). Ventral root axons contain more mitochondria, more SER, and more neurotubules than dorsal root fibers (273,338,339). It may be added that afferent and efferent axons differ in their K⁺ sensitivity (27) and their accommodation properties (264,296).

MATURATION OF PNS AXONS

The axon differentiates from a neuronal process that grows away from the soma guided by the mobile and probing growth cone. During early phases of development, axons are thin (~0.1 μm in diameter) and lie closely packed without intervening cytoplasmic septa. Axon bundles are surrounded by primitive sheath cells. Separation and isolation of the axons then begin: The original axon bundles become separated into families of axons by invading Schwann cells (76,217,306,308,309). By intense mitotic activity among the Schwann cells, the original families are further sepa-

rated into smaller axon–Schwann cell units. This finally gives Schwann cell units containing only one isolated axon and units where most axons are grouped into separate compartments in the Schwann cell. The latter are considered to represent future unmyelinated axons, and their increase in diameter finally ceases somewhere between 0.2 and 1.5 μm.

In Schwann cell units that contain one axon and reach a size of more than 1 μm, the Schwann cells generally fold themselves around the axon in a continuous helical wrapping to manufacture the myelin sheath (128). Nodes of Ranvier develop at sites where consecutive Schwann cells join along the axon (129). Myelination has been thoroughly reviewed (see, e.g., refs. 172,219,263) and is not further commented on here. Instead, the maturation process that gives rise to the paranodal apparatus and a final number of nodes in large feline fibers is briefly summarized.

Nodalization

As already mentioned, morphology of large nerve fibers has often been extrapolated from that of small fibers. In the same way, because the appearance of very small ($D < 4$ μm) mature fibers is similar to that of future large fibers early during postnatal development, myelination was taken to be a final fundamental step in fiber maturation, the appearance of nodes of Ranvier then being a mere consequence of the segmental node of myelination. Thus the just-myelinated fiber was considered to be a miniature of its fully developed counterpart, development following the concept of dimensional similarity.

In contrast, in kittens there is a remarkable functional development that could not be explained just by increasing fiber size. This maturation takes place during the first postnatal weeks, and the future large fibers show nearly mature properties as they reach a size of approximately 4–5 μm (95,158,194,204,205,265–269,326). The maturation is reflected in an increase in conduction velocity unaccompanied by a similar increase in fiber size (in fact, future large fibers increase very little in diameter during the first 2 postnatal weeks) (270), a marked decrease in leg length conduction time, a decrease in relative refractory period, and an increased ability to mediate sustained activity at a high frequency (158).

The major morphological development concerning the future large fibers during the first postnatal weeks is a profound reorganization of the node–paranode regions, denoted "nodalization." The term includes the development of paranodal myelin sheath crenation (9,41,42), Schwann cell paranodal mitochondrion clusters (40), a densely packed corona of node gap microvilli (10,33), a terminal myelin cuff consisting of compact myelin (33), and a fixed number of nodes and Schwann cells along a given axon length (35–37).

During nodalization the Schwann cells are involved in local segmental myelin sheath degeneration, giving rise to numerous Marchi-positive bodies aggregated in the paranodes. There are three types of internodes in the newborn kitten: long internodes 150–400 μm in length with a "complex" dilated and strongly Marchi-positive paranode at one end (Plate 42), short internodes 50–150 μm in length carrying complex paranodes at both ends, and very short internodes 10–50 μm in length revealing a general occurrence of Marchi-positive bodies (34). Electron microscopy has shown that in addition to two types of very short internode—myelinated and unmyelinated —there also are numerous node–paranode regions that carry solitary juxtaposed Schwann cells rich in myelin debris (Plate 43). The occurrence of juxtaposed Schwann cells and short and very short internodes declines rapidly during the first 2 postnatal weeks. They are not seen in kittens more than a month of age (35,41,42). Axon segments connected to Schwann cells engaged in myelin disintegration often contain dense lamellar bodies (42), an arrangement which when observed in a random cross section might suggest neuronal degeneration. Examination of adjacent, normal-looking segments of the same axon, however, disproves this suggestion.

Since the Schwann cells of future large spinal root axons are approximately 100 μm long at the beginning of myelination (Berthold and Nilsson, *in preparation*) and approximately 1,200 μm in the fullgrown cat (35), it is obvious that Schwann cell length (or internodal length) has increased approximately 12 times. On the other hand, during the same period the root L_6 increases from 5 to 30 mm

in length, a sixfold increase. Consequently, the large axons of the L_6 root can accommodate only 50% of the Schwann cells that originally tried to myelinate them, and the surplus Schwann cells must leave the axons. The occurrence of paranodal Marchi positivity of internodes of highly variable size and juxtaposed Schwann cells may then be a result of internodal crowding that develops consequent to a discrepancy in longitudinal growth of axons and their internodes. Schwann cell elimination is less obvious in feline hind limb nerve trunks where the postnatal longitudinal growth is approximately twice that of the L_6 root (35). The idea of internodal crowding as the cause behind myelin destruction and Schwann cell elimination along developing axons becomes still more attractive when it is found that Marchi positivity is weak and signs of Schwann cell elimination very rare in rat spinal root fibers. In this animal in L_6 spinal root length from the start of myelination to adulthood increases approximately 10 times, a factor consistent with an original internodal length of 100 μm and a final one of $\sim$1,000 μm (37).

Neurophysiological tests of developing feline fibers that take the events of the nodalization process into consideration have not yet been performed. In view of the decreased conduction velocity and increased conduction time noted during segmental demyelination, we suggest that the improvements in these parameters as noted in the kitten depend on the elimination of certain Schwann cells occupying unmyelinated axon segments and on the appearance of compact myelin cuffs. It remains to be investigated whether the development of the elements of the paranodal apparatus are significant for the length of the relative refractory period and the ability to maintain activity at high frequencies. Finally, the nodalization process may be noteworthy when discussing the integrative properties of the axon (66,304; Waxman, *this volume*).

The references for this chapter are on pages 52–53, following the plates.

ACKNOWLEDGMENT

This work was supported by the Swedish Medical Research Council (project No. 12x-03157) and by funds from the Karolinska Institute.

Abbreviations used in plates and legends to plates.

AsN	= astrocyte nucleus	NR	= node of Ranvier
Ax	= axon	PAx	= paranodal axon
Bt	= beaded tube	PM	= paranodal Schwann cell mitochondria
CoAx	= constricted axon segment	prox.	= proximal
dist.	= distal	Sc	= Schwann cell
ES	= endoneural space	ScCo	= Schwann cell collar
F	= neurofilament	ScJ	= juxtaposed Schwann cell
IScC	= inner Schwann cell compartment	ScN	= Schwann cell nucleus
LDV	= large dense-core vesicle	SER	= smooth-surfaced endoplasmic reticulum
M	= mitochondrion	STIN	= stereotype internodal segment
myl	= myelinated	T	= neurotubule
MySA	= myelin sheath attachment	Tp	= terminal pocket
NG	= node gap	V	= microvilli

The plates show glutaraldehyde–OsO$_4$-fixed specimens embedded in Vestopal, the sections having been stained with uranyl acetate and lead citrate. Plates with a magnification of more than ×100,000 represent sections that showed a dark-gray interference "color" and which were mounted on 400-mesh grids without supporting film.

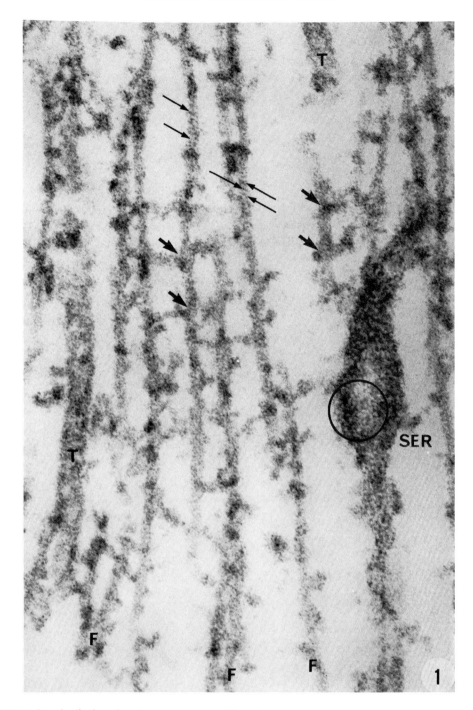

PLATE 1. Longitudinal section through a group of formed axoplasmic elements in a large myelinated feline ventral root axon. The neurofilaments form a typical ladder-like pattern and disclose a helically arranged filamentous substructure (*small arrows*). The tangentially cut SER membrane discloses a globular substructure (*encircled*). Large arrows point at sites where spokes radiate from the shafts of the neurofilaments. ×300,000.

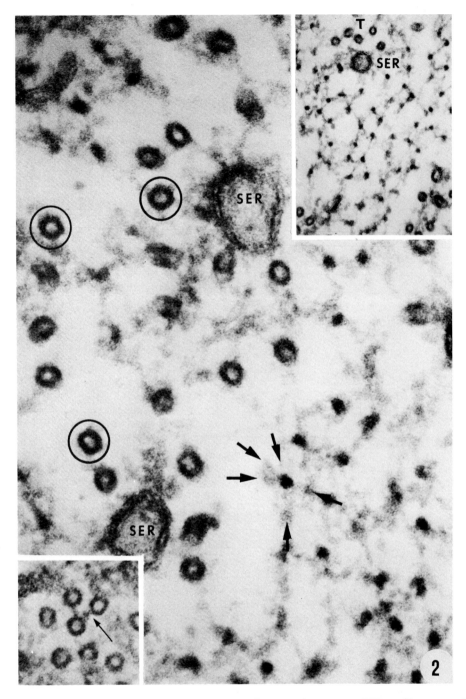

PLATE 2. Cross-cut MySA segment of large myelinated feline ventral root axon. SER profiles, neurotubules, and neurofilaments interconnect with thin bridges of a diffuse, moderately dense material. Protofilament units are discernible in the walls of the encircled neurotubules. Spokes radiate from the neurofilaments (*arrows*). ×300,000. **Lower inset:** A neurotubular fascicle where the three members interconnect via distinct short rods. ×194,000. **Upper inset:** A typical neurofilament latticework and a group of formed elements consisting of one SER profile and five neurotubules. ×94,000.

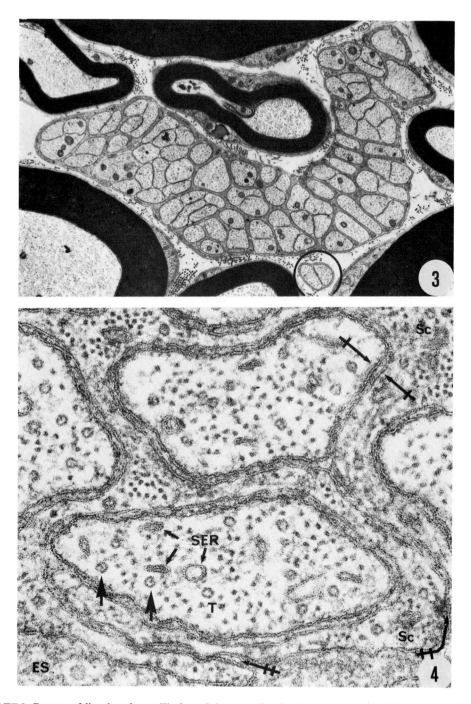

PLATE 3. Cross-cut feline dorsal root. The large Schwann cell unit at the center contains 82 unmyelinated axons. The two encircled axons in the lower part of the figure lack surrounding Schwann cell cytoplasm and are demarcated by just a basement membrane. ×10,000.

PLATE 4. Cross-cut unmyelinated feline dorsal root axons. Single-barred arrows indicate periaxonal space. Double-barred arrows point into mesaxons. Arrowheads mark neurotubules containing a dense granulum. ×119,000.

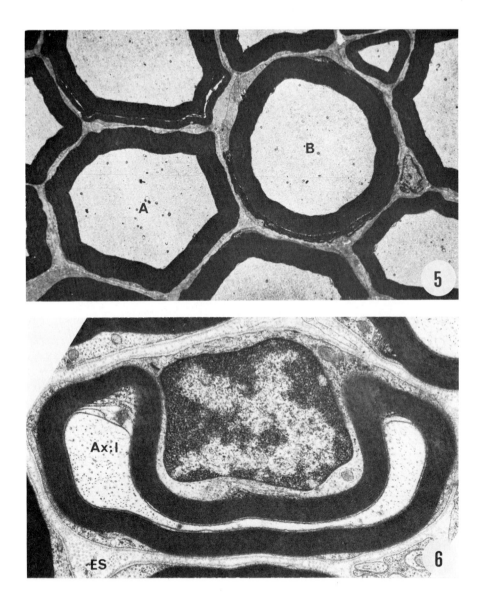

PLATE 5. Cross-cut feline ventral root. The two myelinated fibers (A and B) are cut through their STIN segments. Fiber A appears polygonal whereas fiber B, which has been cut at a level where a Golgi–Rezzonico spinal leaves the outer Schwann cell compartment, displays a more-or-less circular contour. ×5,500.

PLATE 6. Small myelinated feline ventral root axon (fiber I of Fig. 4 and Table 2) cross cut at the level of a Schwann cell nucleus. Note the extended and deeply indented myelin sheath contour. ×19,500.

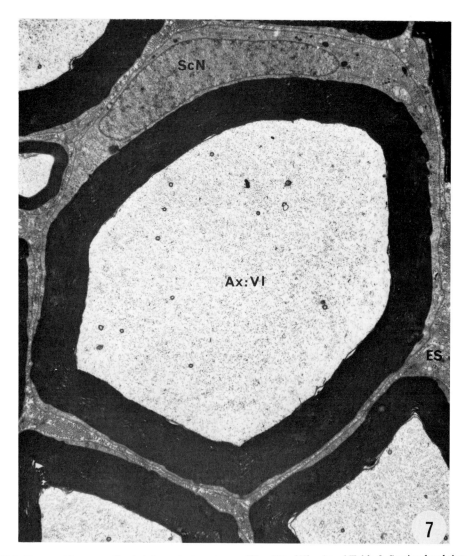

PLATE 7. Cross-cut large myelinated A. ventral root axon (fiber VI of Fig. 4 and Table 2. Section level through Schwann cell nucleus. ×6,500.

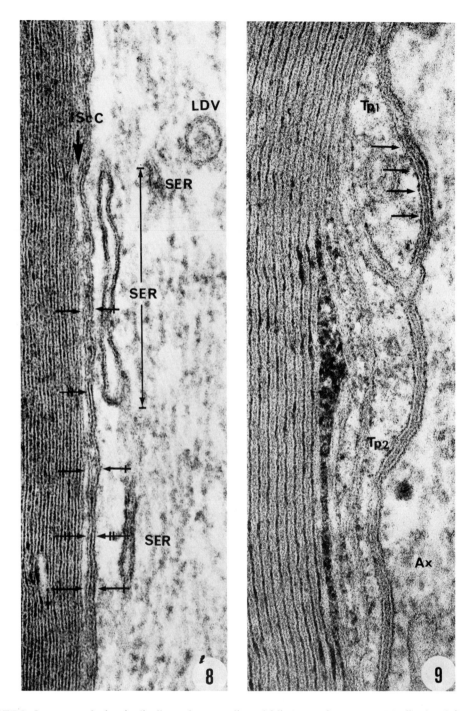

PLATE 8. Outer part of a longitudinally cut large myelinated feline ventral root axon. Myelin sheath is to the left. The plasma membrane of the inner Schwann cell compartment forms five-layered (*double-barred arrows*) and seven-layered (*single-barred arrows*) membrane complexes together with the axolemma. The extended SER profile reaches within less than 10 nm from the axolemma. There is a large dense-core vesicle in the axoplasm. ×176,000.

PLATE 9. Longitudinally cut MySA segment of a small myelinated feline dorsal root axon. The major dense line of the myelin sheath (*at left*) splits into terminal cytoplasmic pockets, which attach to the axolemma, so forming a seven-layered membrane complex. A certain degree of periodicity in this membrane complex is indicated by the arrows. ×194,000.

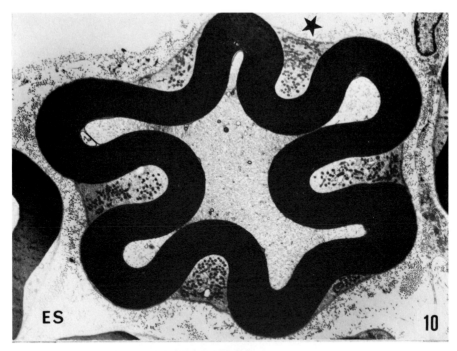

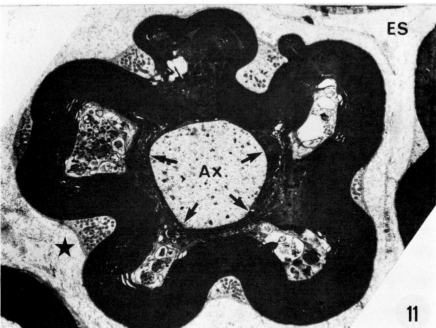

PLATE 10. Cross-cut large myelinated ventral root axon. The paranodal level is approximately 10 μm from the node. The myelin sheath is deeply crenated. Mitochondrion-rich cords of Schwann cell cytoplasm occupy the myelin furrows (*star*). ×4,000 (From ref. 32.)

PLATE 11. Cross-cut large myelinated ventral root axon. The paranodal level is approximately 2 μm from the node. The axon crests occupying the inside of the myelin ridges of Plate 10 have disappeared. Arrows point at the blind pockets of the myelin ridges in which there are well-developed axon–Schwann cell networks. ×3,600 (From ref. 32.)

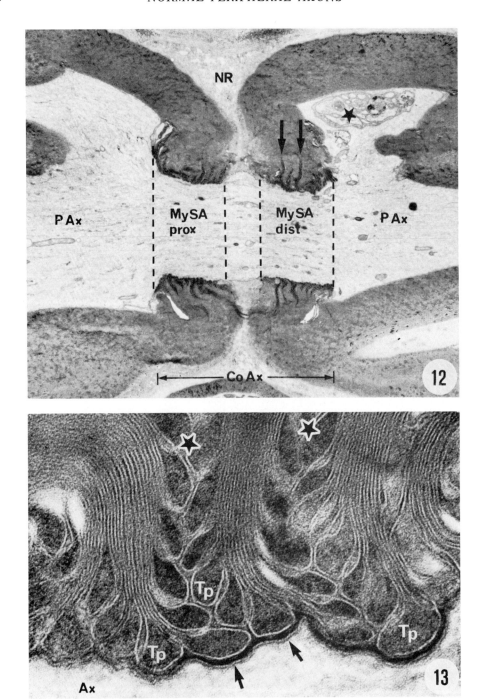

PLATE 12. Longitudinal section through the node–paranode region of a large myelinated feline ventral root axon. The constricted axon segment transforms proximally and distally into the more dilated parts of the paranodal axon. The nodal axon segment is bordered bilaterally by the MySA segments. Arrows indicate ears of terminal cytoplasmic pockets. The axon–Schwann cell network is at the star. ×6,000.

PLATE 13. Detail of myelin sheath attachment in a large longitudinally cut ventral root fiber. Stars mark the points of two ears of terminal pockets. There is a highly electron-dense material between the pockets and the axolemma (*arrows*). The light intermediate stratum of the cell membrane of the pockets appears particularly distinct. ×200,000.

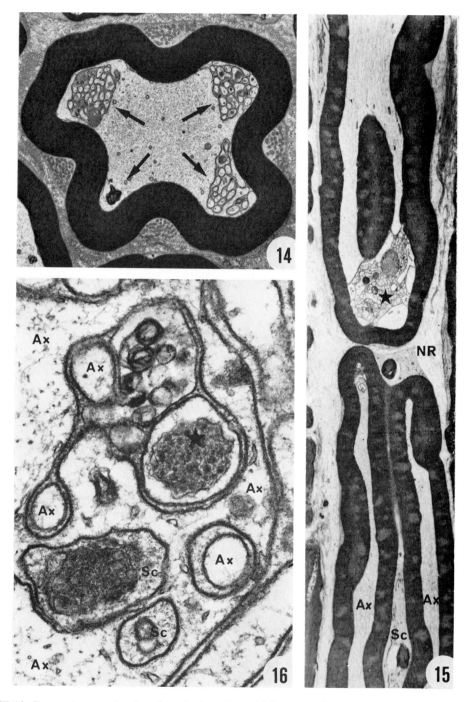

PLATE 14. Cross-cut paranode of medium-sized myelinated feline ventral root axon. Arrows indicate axon–Schwann cell networks. ×5,800.

PLATE 15. Longitudinal section through the node–paranode region of a large myelinated feline ventral root fiber. The nodal axon segment is outside the sectioning plane. The upper paranode contains a well-developed axon-Schwann cell network. ×2,200 (From ref. 32.)

PLATE 16. Detail of axon–Schwann cell network. Both axon and Schwann cell profiles contain dense multivesicular bodies (*star*). ×44,000.

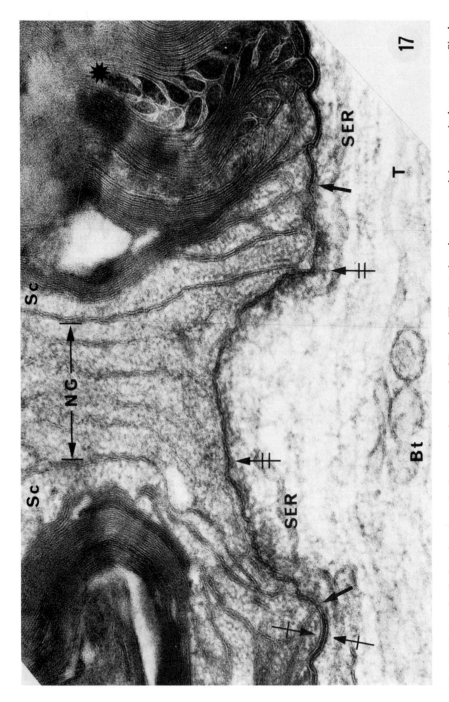

PLATE 17. Longitudinal section through a large ventral root node of Ranvier. The coated axolemma extends between the large arrows. Single-barred arrows indicate a seven-layered membrane complex between axolemma and Schwann cell membrane of a terminal pocket. The ax-olemma of the nodal recesses extends between the large and the double-barred arrows. The star is at the ear of the terminal pockets. ×124,000.

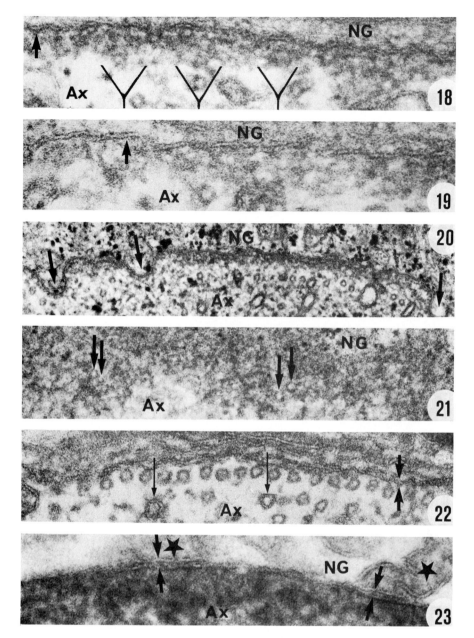

PLATE 18. Cross-sectioned nodal axon of a large myelinated feline ventral root fiber. Arrow indicates the axolemma. The subcoating is of a variable thickness forming pyramid-like clumps (Y). Note the round low-contrast regions of the coat. ×185,000.

PLATE 19. Cross-sectioned nodal axon of a myelinated feline dorsal root fiber. Arrow points at the axolemma. There are numerous round empty-looking spaces in the axolemmal subcoating. ×240,000.

PLATE 20. Cross-sectioned nodal axon of large feline ventral root fiber. The axolemma shows three coated invaginations (*arrows*). There are clumps of an electron-dense material in the node gap. ×80,000.

PLATE 21. Tangentially sectioned nodal axon of large feline ventral root fiber. In the subcoating there are numerous circular low-contrast regions 7–11 nm in diameter (*arrows*). ×132,000.

PLATE 22. Large myelinated feline dorsal root axon. Cross-sectioned MySA segment. Short arrows indicate the axolemma. On the axoplasmic side of the axolemma there is a "layer" of neurotubules. Long arrows point at SER profiles. ×144,000.

PLATE 23. Rat ventral root. Cross-sectioned nodal axon. The nodal axolemma and the cell membrane of node gap Schwann cell microvilli (*stars*) form seven-layered membrane complexes 17 nm thick (*arrows*). ×180,000.

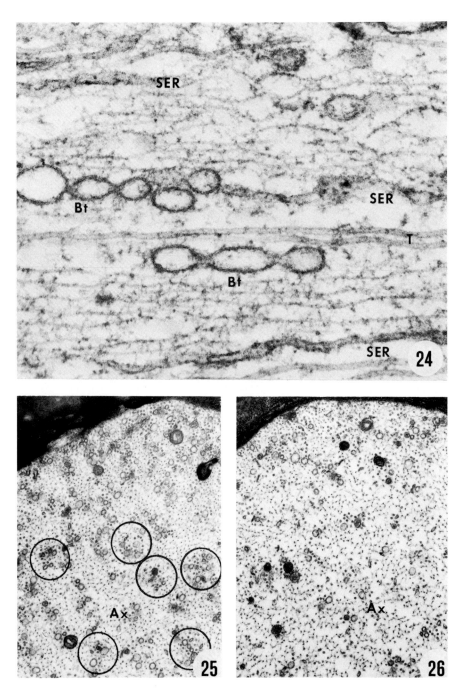

PLATE 24. Large feline ventral root axon. Longitudinal section through the proximal MySA segment of a constricted axon segment. There are two beaded tubes, several longitudinally cut SER profiles, a neurotubular fascicle of two members, and numerous interconnecting neurofilaments. ×81,000.

PLATE 25. Large feline ventral root axon. Cross section of proximal MySA segment. The axoplasm is crowded with neurotubules, beaded tubes, neurofilaments, and SER profiles. At some sites these elements lie clustered (*encircled*). ×24,000.

PLATE 26. Same constricted axon segment as in Plate 25. The cross section passes through the distal MySA segment approximately 5 μm from the level shown in Plate 25. Note the comparatively low concentration of beaded tubes. ×24,000.

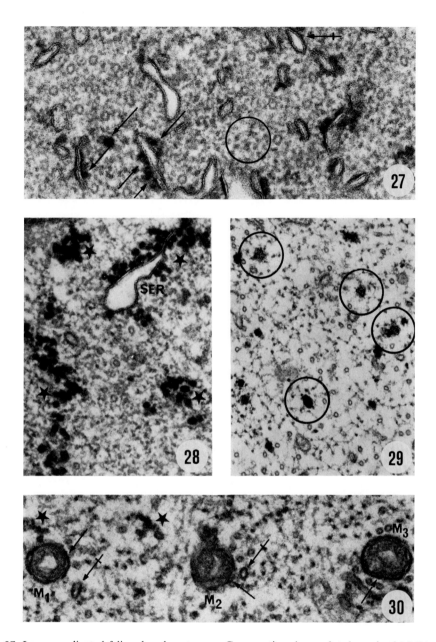

PLATE 27. Large myelinated feline dorsal root axon. Cross-sectioned granulated proximal MySA segment. Plain arrows indicate 30-nm glycogen-like granules, some of which attach to SER profiles. The barred arrow points at a SER profile coated with a thin layer of electron-dense material. The axoplasm is crowded with granules 10–20 nm in size and of moderate contrast (see *encircled area*). Neurotubules and neurofilaments are difficult to identify. ×108,200.

PLATE 28. Large myelinated feline dorsal root axon. Cross-sectioned proximal MySA segment. There are four clusters of 30-nm granules in the axoplasm (*stars*). The upper right cluster is associated with a comparatively large SER profile. ×69,100.

PLATE 29. Large myelinated feline ventral root axon. Cross section through nodal axon segment. Besides the familiar axoplasmic elements, there are scattered, irregularly shaped clumps of dense material (*encircled areas*). Some clumps are 100 nm in size and have a "moth-eaten" appearance. ×48,200.

PLATE 30. Large myelinated feline ventral root axon. Cross-cut nodal segment. The three mitochondria (M₁, M₂, and M₃) are partly covered by a thin layer of a substance of high electron density (*plain arrows*). Barred arrows point at SER profiles. Stars appear at small clusters of 20- to 30-nm granules. ×75,500.

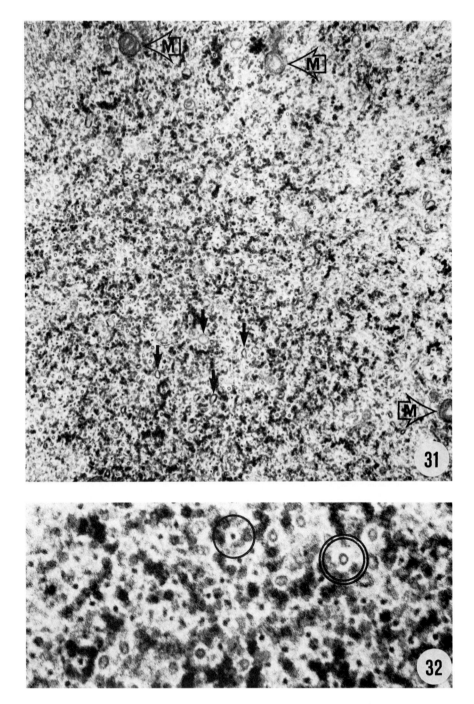

PLATE 31. Large myelinated feline dorsal root axon. Cross section through a proximal granulated MySA segment. Distinct neurotubules, neurofilaments, SER profiles (*arrows*), and 20- to 30-nm granules are suspended in the axoplasm. ×38,000.

PLATE 32. Detail from section shown in Plate 30. Neurofilaments (*single circle*) and neurotubules (*double circle*) are surrounded by an empty-looking zone. ×119,000.

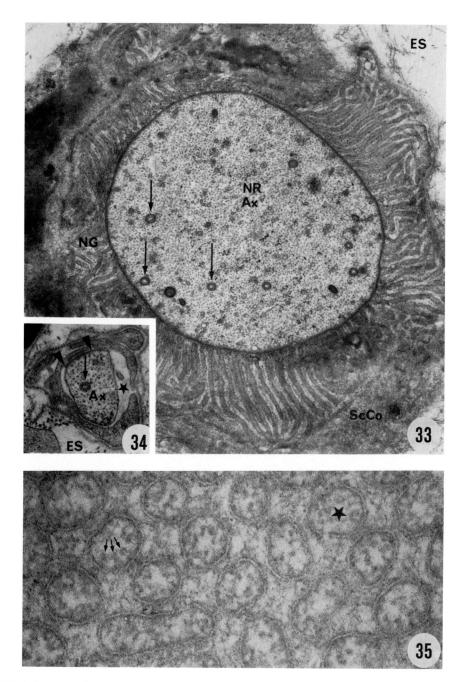

PLATE 33. Large myelinated feline dorsal root axon internodally equipped with 150 myelin lamellae ($D = 16$ μm). Cross section through the node of Ranvier. The nodal axolemma is distinctly coated on its axoplasmic side and faces a node gap containing matrix substance and radially arranged microvilli that derive from the Schwann cell collars of the two meeting internodes. Arrows point at mitochondria in the nodal axoplasm. $\times$16,000.

PLATE 34. Very small myelinated feline dorsal root axon internodally equipped with 15 myelin lamellae (D = 1.5μm). The node gap (star) contains only one microvillus (on top of the star). Arrow points at a mitochondrion in the nodal axoplasm. The axolemma has a subcoating only between the two arrowheads. $\times$ 22,000.

PLATE 35. Longitudinal section through the node gap of a large myelinated feline ventral root axon. The nodal axon segment is outside the plane of the section. The node gap is occupied by radially arranged Schwann cell microvilli (*star*), which here are shown cross sectioned. Arrows point at microfilaments inside a microvillus. $\times$170,000.

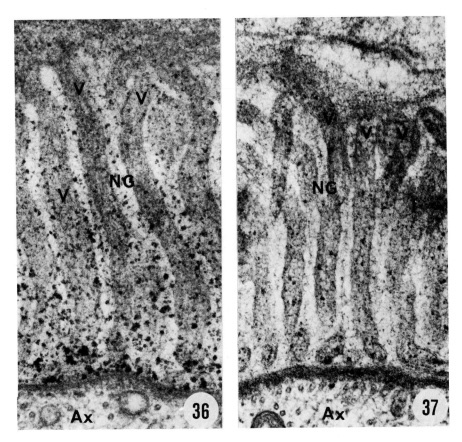

PLATE 36. Large myelinated feline ventral root axon. Part of cross section through a node gap. The node gap matrix substance contains numerous electron-dense clumps. The dense clumps seem to aggregate along the node gap microvilli and outside the nodal axolemma. ×65,000.

PLATE 37. Large myelinated feline ventral root axon of the same specimen as shown in Plate 35. Part of cross-sectioned node gap where the node gap matrix contains few clumps of electron-dense material, of which the main parts are associated with the microvilli. ×65,000.

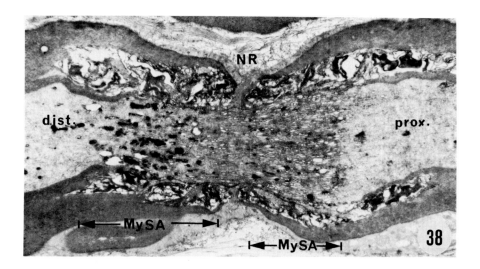

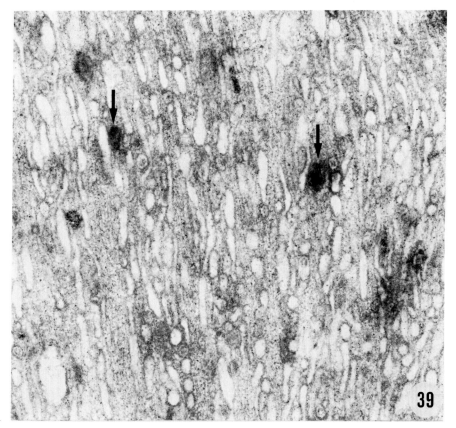

PLATE 38. Longitudinal section through a nodal region of a large myelinated feline axon of the nerve to the soleus muscle. The muscle had been injected with horseradish peroxidase (HRP) 36 hr before immersion fixation in 5% glutaraldehyde, teasing, incubation in Graham–Karnowsky medium, and OsO₄ postfixation. The constricted axon segment reveals a clear polarization in a distal MySA segment containing many HRP-positive bodies and a proximal MySA segment containing a densely packed tubular system. Note the sharp demarcation between the proximal MySA segment and the subsequent part of the paranodal axon. ×6,500. (From Berthold and Mellström, *in preparation*.)

PLATE 39. Detail of the proximal MySA segment of the axon in Plate 37. Arrows indicate HRP-positive membrane-bound bodies. ×44,000. (From Berthold and Mellström, *in preparation*.)

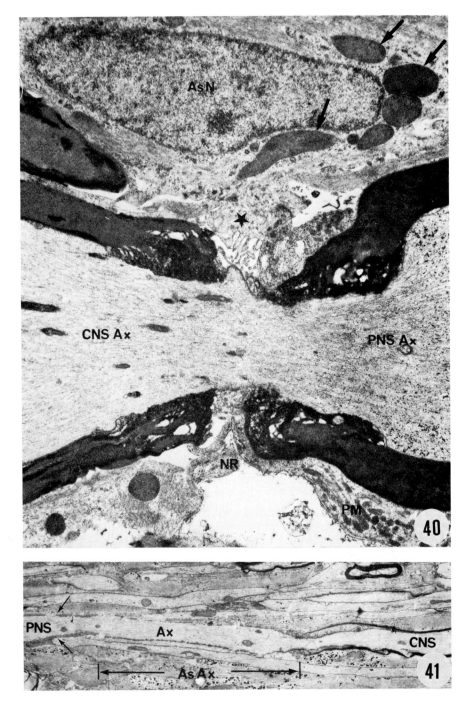

PLATE 40. Transitional node of Ranvier of a large myelinated feline S₁ dorsal root axon. An astrocyte is connected to the node. The astrocyte contains a nucleus and several large gliosomes (*arrows*); it projects (*star*) a tuft of thin processes into the node gap. Notice the electron-dense granules in the PNS part of the axon. ×6,800. (From ref. 39.)

PLATE 41. PNS–CNS transition of a large unmyelinated feline S₁ dorsal root axon. Arrows to the left indicate genuine PNS part of axon invested by Schwann cell cytoplasm. The subsequent part of the axon (AsAx) is related to astrocytic folia for a length of several micrometers and then becomes myelinated (CNS). ×13,000. (From ref. 62.)

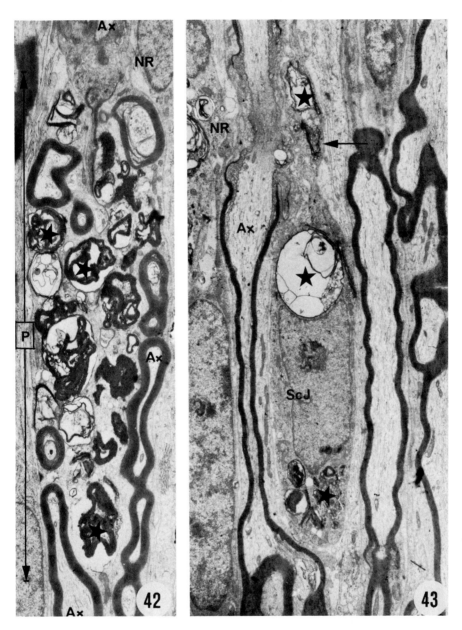

PLATE 42. Zero-day-old kitten. Ventral root. Longitudinal section through a complex paranode of a future large fiber. The node of Ranvier is at the top of the picture. The paranodal Schwann cell cytoplasm contains many irregularly shaped lamellar bodies (*star*) similar in appearance to clumps of degenerating myelin. ×5,600. (From ref. 33.)

PLATE 43. Seven-day-old kitten. Ventral root. Longitudinal section through a nodal region carrying a juxtaposed Schwann cell. The Schwann cell cytoplasm contains numerous lamellar bodies (*stars*). Arrow indicates the node of Ranvier. ×4,200. (From ref. 33.)

REFERENCES

1. Abbot, B. C., Hill, A. V., and Howarth, J. V. (1958): The positive and negative heat associated with a nerve impulse. *Proc. R. Soc. B.,* 148:149–187.
2. Adams, C. W. M., Bayliss, O. B., and Grant, R. T. (1969): Copper-binding and cholinesterase activity around the node of Ranvier. *J. Histochem. Cytochem.,* 17:125–127.
3. Adelman, W. J., and Palti, Y. (1969): The influence of external potassium on the inactivation of sodium currents in giant axons of the squid, Loligo paelei. *J. Gen. Physiol.,* 53:685–703.
4. Adelman, W. J., Jr., and Palti, Y. (1972): The role of periaxonal and perineuronal spaces in modifying ionic flow across neural membranes. In: *Current Topics in Membrane and Transport,* Vol. III, edited by F. Bronner and A. Kleinzeller, pp. 199–235. Academic Press, New York.
5. Aguayo, A. J., and Bray, G. M. (1975): Pathology and pathophysiology of unmyelinated nerve fibers. In: *Peripheral Neuropathy,* Vol. I, edited by P. J. Dyck, P. K. Thomas, and H. L. Lambert, pp. 363–390. Saunders, Philadelphia.
6. Aguayo, A. J., Charron, L., and Bray, G. M. (1976): Potential of Schwann cells from unmyelinated nerves to produce myelin: A quantitative ultrastructural and radiographic study. *J. Neurocytol.,* 5:565–573.
7. Aguayo, A. J., Bray, G. M., Terry, L. C., and Sweezey, E. (1976): Three dimensional analysis of unmyelinated fibres in normal and pathologic autonomic nerve. *J. Neuropathol. Exp. Neurol.,* 35:136–151.
8. Aguayo, A. J., Epps, J., Charron, L., and Bray, G. M. (1976): Multipotentiality of Schwann cells in cross-anastomosed and grafted myelinated and unmyelinated nerves: Quantitative microscopy and radioautography. *Brain Res.,* 104:1–20.
9. Aguayo, A. J., Attiwell, M., Trecarten, J., Perkins, S., and Bray, G. M. (1977): Abnormal myelination in transplanted trembler mouse Schwann cells. *Nature (Lond),* 265:73–75.
10. Allt, G. (1969): Ultrastructural features of the immature peripheral nerve. *J. Anat.,* 105:283–293.
11. Amos, L. A. and Klug, A. (1974): Arrangements of subunits in flagellar microtubules. *J. Cell Sci.,* 14:523–549.
12. Andersson, L. E., and McClure, W. O. (1973): Differential transport of proteins in axons: Comparisons of sciatic nerves and dorsal columns in cats. *Proc. Natl. Acad. Sci. USA,* 70:1521–1525.
13. Andersson-Cedergren, E., and Karlsson, U. (1966): Demyelination regions of nerve fibres in frogs muscle spindles as studied by serial sections for electron microscopy. *J. Ultrastruct. Res.,* 14:212–239.
14. Anderton, B. H., Bell, C. W., Newby, B. J., and Gilbert, D. S. (1976): Neurofilaments. *Biochem. Soc. Transact.,* 4:544–547.
15. Appenzeller, O., and Ogin, G. (1973): Myelinated fibres in the human paravertebral sympathetic chain: Quantitative studies on white rami communicantes. *J. Neurol. Neurosurg. Psychiatry,* 36:777–785.
16. Appenzeller, O., Ogin, G., and Palmer, G. (1976): Fibre size spectra and cyclic AMP content of sciatic nerves: Effect of muscle hypoactivity and hyperactivity. *Exp. Neurol.,* 50:595–604.
17. Applebaum, M. L., Clifton, G. L., Coggeshall, R. E., Coulter, J. D., Vance, W. H., and Willis, W. D. (1976): Unmyelinated fibres in the sacral 3 and caudal 1 ventral roots of the cat. *J. Physiol. (Lond),* 256:557–572.
18. Banks, P. (1976): Microtubules and vesicle migration in neurons. *Biochem. Soc. Transact.,* 4:548–551.
19. Banks, P., Mayor, D., and Owen, T. (1975): Effects of low temperatures on microtubules in the non-myelinated axons of post ganglionic sympathetic nerves. *Brain Res.,* 83:277–292.
20. Bannister, L. H. (1976): Sensory terminals of peripheral nerves. In: *The Peripheral Nerve,* edited by D. N. Landon. Chapman and Hall, London.
21. Barajas, L., Wang, P., and De Santis, S. (1976): Light and electron microscopic localization of acetylcholinesterase activity in the rat renal nerves. *Am. J. Anat.,* 147:219–234.
22. Barker, D., Stacey, M. J., and Adal, M. N. (1970): Fusimotor innervation in the cat. *Philos. Trans. R. Soc. Lond. [Biol.],* 258:315–346.
23. Barker, J. L., Neale, J. H., and Gainer, H. (1976): Rapidly transported proteins in sensory, motor and sympathetic nerves of the isolated frog nervous system. *Brain Res.,* 105:497–515.
24. Baumgarten, H. G., Holstein, A. F., and Stelzner, F. (1973): Nervous elements in the human colon of Hirschsprungs disease. *Virchows Arch. [Pathol. Anat.],* 358:113–136.
25. Behnke, O., and Zelander, T. (1967): Filamentous substructures in microtubules of the marginal bundle of mammalian blood platelets. *J. Ultrastruct. Res.,* 19:147–165.
26. Behse, F., Buchthal, F., Carlsen, F., and Knappeis, G. G. (1975): Unmyelinated fibres and Schwann cells of sural nerve in neuropathy. *Brain,* 98:493–510.
27. Bergman, C., and Stämpfli, R. (1966): Difference de perméabilité des fibres nerveuses myélinisées sensorielles et motrices á l'ion potassoin. *Helv. Physiol. Acta,* 24:247–258.

28. Berl, S. (1976): The actomyosin-like system in nervous tissue. In: *The Nervous System,* Vol. I, edited by D. B. Tower. Raven Press, New York.

29. Berlinrood, M., McGee-Russell, S. M., and Allen, R. D. (1972): Patterns of particle movement in nerve fibres in vitro—an analysis by photokymography and microscopy. *J. Cell Sci.,* 2:875–886.

30. Berthold, C-H. (1966): Ultrastructural appearance of glycogen in the B-neurons of the frog. *J. Ultrastruct. Res.,* 14:254–267.

31. Berthold, C-H. (1968): A study on the fixation of large mature feline myelinated ventral lumbar spinal root fibres. *Acta Soc. Med. Uppsala (Suppl. 9),* 78:1–36.

32. Berthold, C-H. (1968): Ultrastructure of the node-paranode region of mature feline ventral lumbar spinal root fibres. *Acta Soc. Med. Uppsala (Suppl. 9),* 73:37–70.

33. Berthold, C-H. (1968): Ultrastructure of postnatally developing peripheral nodes of Ranvier. *Acta Soc. Med. Uppsala,* 73:145–168.

34. Berthold, C-H. (1973): Histochemistry of postnatally developing feline spinal roots. I. A study with the OTAN-method. *Neurobiology,* 3:271–290.

35. Berthold, C-H. (1973): Local "demyelination" in developing feline nerve fibres. *Neurobiology,* 3:339–352.

36. Berthold, C-H. (1974): A comparative morphological study of the developing node-paranode region in lumbar spinal roots. I. Electron microscopy. *Neurobiology,* 4:82–104.

37. Berthold, C-H. (1974): A comparative morphological study of the developing node-paranode region in lumbar spinal roots. II. Light-microscopy after OTAN-staining. *Neurobiology,* 4:117–131.

38. Berthold, C-H., and Carlstedt, T. (1977): Observations of the morphology at the transition between the peripheral and the central nervous system in the cat. II. General organisation of the transitional region in S₁ dorsal rootlets. *Acta Physiol. Scand.* [*Suppl.*] 446:23–42.

39. Berthold, C-H., and Carlstedt, T. (1977): Observations on the morphology at the transition between the peripheral and the central nervous system in the cat. III. Myelinated fibers in S₁ dorsal rootlets. *Acta Physiol. Scand.* [*Suppl.*], 446:43–60.

40. Berthold, C-H., and Skoglund, S. (1967): Histochemical and ultrastructural demonstration of mitochondria in the paranodal region of developing feline spinal roots and nerves. *Acta Soc. Med. Uppsala,* 72:37–70.

41. Berthold, C-H., and Skoglund, S. (1968): Postnatal development of feline paranodal myelin sheath segments. I. Light microscopy. *Acta Soc. Med. Uppsala,* 73:113–126.

42. Berthold, C-H., and Skoglund, S. (1968): Postnatal development of feline paranodal myelin sheath segments. II. Electron microscopy. *Acta Soc. Med. Uppsala,* 73:127–144.

43. Bessou, P., and Perl, E. R. (1969): Response from sensory cutaneous units with unmyelinated fibres to noxious stimuli. *J. Neurophysiol.,* 32:1025–1043.

44. Biondi, R. J., Levy, M. J., and Weiss, P. A. (1972): An engineering study of the peristaltic drive of axonal flow. *Proc. Natl. Acad. Sci. USA,* 69:1732–1736.

45. Bisby, M. A. (1977): Retrograde axonal transport of endogenous protein: Differences between motor and sensory axons. *J. Neurochem.,* 28:249–251.

46. Bischoff, A., and Thomas, P. K. (1975): Microscopic anatomy of myelinated nerve fibres. In: *Peripheral Neuropathy,* Vol. 1, edited by P. J. Dyck, P. K. Thomas, and E. H. Lambert, pp. 104–130. Saunders, Philadelphia.

47. Bittner, G. D., and Mann, D. W. (1976): Differential survival of isolated portions of crayfish axons. *Cell Tissue Res.,* 169:301–311.

48. Bodian, D. (1962): The generalized vertebrate neuron. *Science,* 137:323–326.

49. Bondy, S. C., and Purdy, J. L. (1975): Migration of ribosomes along the axons of the chick visual pathway. *Biochim. Biophys. Acta,* 390:332–341.

50. Bonnet, K. A., and Bondy, S. C. (1976): Transport of RNA along the optic pathway of the chick: An autoradiographic study. *Exp. Brain Res.,* 26:185–191.

50a. Boyd, J. A., and Davey (1968): *Composition of Peripheral Nerves.* Livingstone, Edinburgh.

51. Boyd, J. A., and Kalu, K. U. (1973): The relation between axon size and number of lamellae in the myelin sheath for afferent fibres in groups I, II and III in the cat. *J. Physiol. (Lond),* 232:P31–33.

52. Bray, D. (1976): Actin and myosin: Their role in the growth of nerve cells. *Biochem. Soc. Transact.,* 4:543–544.

53. Bray, G. M., and Aguayo, A. J. (1974): Regeneration of peripheral unmyelinated nerves: Fate of the axonal sprouts which develop after injury. *J. Anat.,* 117:517–529.

54. Bryan, I. (1976): A quantitative analysis of microtubule elongation. *J. Cell Biol.,* 71:749–767.

55. Bunge, R. P. (1968): Glial cells and the central myelin sheath. *Physiol. Rev.,* 48:197–251.

56. Burton, P. R., Hinkley, R. E., and Pierson, G. B. (1975): Tannic acid-stained microtubules with 12, 13 and 15 protofilaments. *J. Cell Biol.,* 65:227–233.

57. Böck, P., Hanak, H., and Stockinger, L. (1970): The penetration of exogenous protein into mesaxonal and periaxonal space:

An electron microscopic study on unmyelinated nerves using horseradish peroxidase as a tracer. *J. Submicr. Cytol.,* 2:189–192.

58. Cajal, S. R. (1928): *Degeneration and Regeneration of the Nervous System,* Vol. I. Oxford University Press, New York.

59. Causey, G. (1960): *The Cell of Schwann.* Livingstone, Edinburgh.

60. Carlsen, F., Knappeis, G. G., and Behse, F. (1974): Schwann cell length in unmyelinated fibres of human sural nerve. *J. Anat.,* 117:463–467.

61. Carlstedt, T. (1977): Observations on the morphology at the transition between the peripheral and the central nervous system in the cat. I. A preparative procedure useful for electron microscopy. *Acta Physiol. Scand. [Suppl.],* 446:5–22.

62. Carlstedt, T. (1977): Observations on the morphology at the transition between the peripheral and the central nervous system in the cat. IV. Unmyelinated fibres in S_1 dorsal rootlets. *Acta Physiol. Scand. [Suppl.],* 446:61–72.

63. Cauna, N. (1973): The free penicillate nerve endings of the human hairy skin. *J. Anat.,* 115:277–288.

64. Chacko, G. K., Barnola, F. V., and Villegas, R. (1976): Phospholipid and fatty acid compositions of axon and periaxonal cell plasma membranes of lobster leg nerve. *J. Neurochem.,* 28:445–447.

65. Chan-Palay, V. (1972): The tripartite structure of the undercoat in initial segments of Purkinje cell axons. *Z. Anat. Entwicklungsgesch.,* 139:1–10.

66. Chung, S-H. (1976): Intermittent nerve conduction. *Nature (Lond),* 264:313–314.

67. Coggeshall, R. F., Coulter, J. D., and Willis, W.D., Jr. (1973): Unmyelinated fibers in the ventral root. *Brain Res.,* 57:229–233.

68. Coggeshall, R. E., Coulter, J. D., and Willis, W. D., Jr. (1974): Unmyelinated axons in the ventral roots of the cat lumbosacral enlargement. *J. Comp. Neurol.,* 153:39–58.

69. Coggeshall, R. E., Hancock, M. B., and Applebaum, M. L. (1976): Categories of axons in mammalian rami communicantes. *J. Comp. Neurol.,* 167:105–124.

70. Condie, R. M., Howell, A. E., and Good, R. A. (1961): Studies on the problem of preservation of the myelin sheath ultrastructure: Evaluation of fixation, dehydration and embedding techniques. *J. Biophys. Biochem. Cytol.,* 9:429–443.

71. Conradi, S. (1969): On motoneuron synaptology in cats and kittens. III. Observations on the ultrastructure of the axon hillock and initial axon segment of lumbosacral motoneurons in the cat. *Acta Physiol. Scand. [Suppl.],* 332:65–84.

72. Cook, R. D., and Burnstock, G. (1976): The ultrastructure of Auerbacks plexus in

the guinea pig. I. Neuronal elements. *J. Neurocytol.,* 5:171–194.

73. Cooper, P. D., and Smith, R. S. (1974): The movement of optically detectable organelles in myelinated axons of Xenopus laevis. *J. Physiol. (Lond),* 242:77–97.

74. Coppin, C. M. L., and Jack, J. B. B. (1972): Internodal length and conduction velocity of cat muscle afferent nerve fibres. *J. Physiol. (Lond),* 222:91–93.

75. Corvaja, N., Magherini, P. C., and Pompeiano, O. (1971): Ultrastructure of glycogen-membrane complexes in sensory nerve fibres of cat muscle spindles. *Z. Zellforsch.,* 121:199–217.

76. Cravioto, H. (1965): The role of Schwann cells in the development of human peripheral nerves. *J. Ultrastruct. Res.,* 12:634–651.

77. Crompton, M., Capano, M., and Carafoli, E. (1976): The sodium-induced efflux of calcium from heart mitochondria: A possible mechanism for the regulation of mitochondrial calcium. *Eur. J. Biochem.,* 69:453–462.

78. Davison, P. F. (1970): Microtubules and neurofilaments: Possible implications of axoplasmic transport in biochemistry of simple neuronal models. *Adv. Biochem. Psychopharmacol.,* 2:289–302.

79. De la Motte, D. (1973): Cited as a personal communication in ref. 208.

80. De Vries, G. H. (1976): Isolation of axolemma-enriched fractions from bovine central nervous system. *Neurosci. Lett.,* 3:117–122.

81. De Vries, G. H., Eng, L. F., Lewis, D. L., and Hadfield, M. G. (1976): The protein composition of bovine myelin-free axons. *Biochim. Biophys. Acta,* 439:133–145.

82. Donoso, J. A., Illanes, J-P., and Samson, F. (1977): Dimethylsulfoxide action on fast axoplasmic transport and ultrastructure of vagal axons. *Brain Res.,* 120:287–301.

83. Droz, B. (1976): Synthetic machinery and axoplasmic transport: maintenance of neuronal connectivity. In: *The Nervous System,* Vol. I, edited by B. D. Tower. Raven Press, New York.

84. Droz, B., Koenig, H. L., and Giamberardino, L. (1973): Axonal migration of protein and glycoprotein to nerve endings. I. Radioautographic analysis of the renewal of protein in nerve endings of chicken ciliary ganglion after intra cerebral injection of (^{3}H)lysine. *Brain Res.,* 60:93–127.

85. Droz, B., Rambourg, A., and Koenig, H. L. (1975): The smooth endoplasmic reticulum: Structure and role in the renewal of axonal membrane and synaptic vesicles by fast axonal transport. *Brain Res.,* 93:1–13.

86. Dumont, J. N., Anderson, E., and Chomyn, E. (1965): The anatomy of the peripheral nerve and its ensheathing artery

in the horseshoe crab, Xiphosura (Limulus) polyphemus. *J. Ultrastruct. Res.,* 13:38–64.

87. Dun, F. T. (1970): The length and diameter of the node of Ranvier. *IEEE Trans. Biomed. Engin.,* BME-17 No. 1:21–24.

88. Düllmann, J., and Wulfhekel, U. (1970): Über Schmidt-Lantermannsche einkerbungen und paranodale bulbi des n. ischiadicus. *Z. Anat. Entwicklungstgesch.,* 132:350–358.

89. Dyck, P. J. (1975): Pathologic alterations of the peripheral nervous system of man. In: *Peripheral Neuropathy,* Vol. I, edited by P. J. Dyck, P. K. Thomas, and E. H. Lambert, pp. 296–336. Saunders, Philadelphia.

90. Dyck, P. J., and Lambert, E. H. (1969): Dissociated sensation in amyloidosis. *Arch. Neurol.,* 20:490–507.

91. Dyck, P. J., Lambert, E. H., and Nichols, P. C. (1971): Quantitative measurements of sensation related to compound action potential and number and sizes of myelinated and unmyelinated fibres of sural nerve in health, Friedreich's ataxia, hereditary neuropathy and tabes dorsalis. *Electroencephalogr. Clin. Neurophysiol.,* 9:83–118.

92. Eames, R. A., and Gamble, H. J. (1970): Schwann cell relationship in normal human cutaneous nerves. *J. Anat.,* 106:417–435.

93. Eccles, J. C., and Sherrington, C. S. (1930): Numbers and contraction values of individual motor-units examined in some muscles of the limb. *Proc. R. Soc. B.,* 106:326–357.

94. Edström, A. (1969): RNA protein synthesis in Mauthner nerve fibre components of fish. In: *Cellular Dynamics of the Neuron.* Symp. Internat. Soc. Cell Biol., 8:51–72.

95. Ekholm, J. (1967): Postnatal changes in cutaneous reflexes and in the discharge pattern of cutaneous and articular sense organs. *Acta Physiol. Scand [Suppl.],* 297.

96. Elfvin, L. G. (1958): The ultrastructure of unmyelinated fibres in the splenic nerve of the cat. *J. Ultrastruct. Res.,* 1:428–454.

97. Elfvin, L. G. (1961): Electron microscopic investigation of filament structures in unmyelinated fibers of cat splenic nerve. *J. Ultrastruct. Res.,* 5:51–64.

98. Elfvin, L-G. (1961): The ultrastructure of the nodes of Ranvier in cat sympathetic nerve fibres. *J. Ultrastruct. Res.,* 5:374–387.

99. Elfvin, L-G. (1961): Electron microscopic investigation of the plasma membrane and myelin sheath of autonomic nerve fibres in the cat. *J. Ultrastruct. Res.,* 5:388–407.

100. Elfvin, L. G. (1962): Electron microscopic studies on the effect of anisotonic solutions on the structure of unmyelinated splenic nerve fibers of the cat. *J. Ultrastruct. Res.,* 7:1–38.

101. Elfvin, L-G. (1963): The ultrastructure of the plasma membrane and myelin sheath of peripheral nerve fibres after fixation by freeze-drying. *J. Ultrastruct. Res.,* 8:283–304.

102. Elfvin, L-G. (1963): The ultrastructure of the superior cervical sympathetic ganglion of the cat. I. *J. Ultrastruct. Res.,* 8:403–440.

103. Elfvin, L-G. (1963): The ultrastructure of the superior cervical sympathetic ganglion of the cat. II. A study of the praeganglionic endfibres as studied by serial sections. *J. Ultrastruct. Res.,* 8:441–476.

104. Elfvin, L-G. (1968): The structure and composition of motor sensory and autonomic nerves and nerve fibres. In: *The Structure and Function of Nervous Tissue,* Vol. I, edited by G. H. Bourne, pp. 325–377. Academic Press, New York.

105. Elfvin, L-G. (1976): The ultrastructure of neuronal contacts. *Prog. Neurobiol.,* 8:45–79.

106. Emery, D. G., Foreman, R. D., and Coggeshall, R. E. (1976): Fiber analysis of the feline inferior cardiac sympathetic nerve. *J. Comp. Neurol.,* 166:457–468.

107. Erickson, H. P. (1974): Assembly of microtubules from preformed, ring-shaped proto filaments and 6-s tubulin. *J. Supramol. Struct.,* 2:393–411.

108. Feit, H., and Barondes, S. H. (1970): Colchicine-binding activity in particulate fractions of mouse brain. *J. Neurochem.,* 17:1355–1364.

109. Feit, H., Dutton, G. R., Barondes, S. H. and Shelanski, M. L. (1971): Microtubule protein: Identification in and transport to nerve endings. *J. Cell Biol.,* 51:138–147.

110. Forbes, M. S., and Dent, J. N. (1974): Filaments and microtubules in the gonadotrophic cell of the lizard Anolis carolinensis. *J. Morphol.,* 143:409–434.

111. Fraher, J. P. (1972): A quantitative study of anterior root fibres during early myelination. *J. Anat.,* 112:99–124.

112. Fraher, J. P. (1973): A quantitative study of anterior root fibres during early myelination. II. Longitudinal variation in sheath thickness and axon circumference. *J. Anat.,* 115:421–444.

113. Fraher, J. P. (1974): A numerical study of cervical and thoracic ventral nerve roots. *J. Anat.,* 118:127–142.

114. Fraher, J. P. (1976): The growth and myelination of central and peripheral segments of ventral motoneurone axons: A quantitative ultrastructural study. *Brain Res.,* 105:193–211.

115. Friede, R. L. (1972): Control of myelin formation by axon calibre (with a model of the control mechanism). *J. Comp. Neurol.,* 144:233–252.

116. Friede, R. L., and Martinez, A. J. (1970): Analysis of the process of sheath expansion

in swollen nerve fibres. *Brain Res.,* 19:165–182.

117. Friede, R. L., and Somorajski, T. (1967): Relation between the number of myelin lamellae and axon circumference in fibres of vagus and sciatic nerves of mice. *J. Comp. Neurol.,* 130:223–232.

118. Friede, R. L., and Samorajski, T. (1968): Myelin formation in the sciatic nerve of the rat. *J. Neuropathol. Exp. Neurol.,* 27:546–570.

119. Friede, R. L., and Samorajski, T. (1970): Axon caliber related to neurofilaments and microtubules in sciatic nerve fibres of rats and mice. *Anat. Rec.,* 167:379–387.

120. Furcht, L. T., and Scott, R. E. (1975): Effect of vinblastine sulfate, colchicine and lumicolchine on membrane organization of normal and transformed cells. *Exp. Cell Res.,* 96:271–282.

121. Gabella, G. (1976): Ganglia of the autonomic nervous system. In: *The Peripheral Nerve,* edited by D. N. Landon, pp. 355–395. Chapman and Hall, London.

122. Gamble, H. J. (1964): Comparative electronmicroscopic observations on the connective tissues of a peripheral nerve and a spinal root in the rat. *J. Anat.,* 98:17–25.

123. Gamble, H. J. (1976): Spinal and cranial nerve roots. In: *The Peripheral Nerve.* Chapman and Hall, London, pp. 330–354.

124. Gasser, H. S. (1950): Unmedullated fibres originating in dorsal root ganglia. *J. Gen. Physiol.,* 33:651–690.

125. Gasser, H. S. (1952): The hypothesis of saltatory conduction. *Cold Spring Harbor Symp. Quant. Biol.,* 17:32–36.

126. Gasser, H. S. (1955): Properties of dorsal root unmedullated fibres on the two sides of the ganglion. *J. Gen. Physiol.,* 38:709–728.

127. Gauthier, G. F. (1976): The motor endplate structure. In: *The Peripheral Nerve,* edited by D. N. Landon, pp. 464–494. Chapman and Hall, London.

128. Geren, B. B. (1954): The formation from the Schwann cell surface of myelin in the peripheral nerves of chick embryos. *Exp. Cell Res.,* 7:558–562.

129. Geren Uzman, B., and Nogueira-Graf, G. (1957): Electronmicroscope studies of the formation of nodes of Ranvier in mouse sciatic nerves. *J. Biophys. Biochem. Cytol.,* 3:589–597.

130. Gilbert, D. S. (1975): Axoplasm architecture and physical properties as seen in the Myxicola giant axon. *J. Physiol. (Lond),* 253:257–301.

131. Gilbert, D. S. (1975): Axoplasm chemical composition in Myxicola and solubility properties of its structural proteins. *J. Physiol. (Lond),* 253:303–319.

132. Gilbert, D. S., and Newby, B. (1975): Neurofilament disguise, destruction and discipline. *Nature (Lond),* 256:586–589.

133. Gilliatt, R. W. (1966): Axon branching in motor nerves. In: *Control and Innervation of Skeletal Muscle,* edited by B. L. Andrew, pp. 53–60. Livingstone, Edinburgh.

134. Gilula, N. B. (1976): Junctional membrane structure. In: *The Nervous System,* Vol. 1, edited by D. B. Tower, Raven Press, New York.

135. Gitlin, G., and Singer, M. (1974): Myelin movements in mature mammalian peripheral nerve fibers. *Morphology,* 143:167–176.

136. Grafstein, B. (1975): Axonal transport: The intracellular traffic of the neuron. In: *Handbook of the Nervous System, Vol. 1: Cellular Biology of Neurons,* edited by E. R. Kandel. American Physiological Society, Washington, D.C.

137. Gray, E. G. (1970): The fine structure of nerve. *Comp. Biochem. Physiol.,* 36:419–448.

138. Gray, E. G. (1975): Presynaptic microtubules and their association with synaptic vesicles. *Proc. R. Soc. B,* 190:369–372.

139. Greengard, P., and Straub, R. W. (1958): Afterpotentials in mammalian non-myelinated nerve fibres. *J. Physiol. (Lond),* 144:442–462.

140. Grundfest, H. (1971): The varieties of excitable membranes. In: *Biophysics and Physiology of Excitable Membranes,* edited by Adelman, Van Nostrand Reinhold, New York, pp. 22, 477–505.

141. Ha, H. (1970): Axonal bifurcation in the dorsal root ganglion of the cat: A light- and electron-microscopic study. *J. Comp. Neurol.,* 140:227–240.

142. Haak, R. A., Kleinhaus, F. W., and Ochs, S. (1976): The viscosity of mammalian nerve axoplasm measured by electron spin resonance. *J. Physiol. (Lond),* 263:115–137.

143. Hall, S. M., and Williams, P. L. (1970): Studies on the incisures of Schmidt and Lanterman. *J. Cell Sci.,* 6:767–791.

144. Hall, S. M., and Williams, P. L. (1971): The distribution of electron-dense tracers in peripheral nerve fibres. *J. Cell Sci.,* 8:541–555.

145. Hess, A., and Lansing, A. J. (1953): The fine structure of peripheral nerve fibres. *Anat. Rec.,* 117:175–200.

146. Hess, A., and Young, J. Z. (1952): The nodes of Ranvier. *Proc. R. Soc. B,* 140:301–320.

147. Hill, A. V., and Howarth, F. V. (1958): The initial heat production of stimulated nerve. *Proc. R. Soc. B,* 149:167–175.

148. Hillarp, N., and Olivecrona, H. (1946): The role played by the axon and the Schwann cells in the degree of myelination

of the peripheral nerve fibre. *Acta Anat.,* 2:17–32.

149. Hille, B. (1975): Ionic selectivity of nerve membranes. In: *Membranes—A Series of Advances,* Vol. 3, edited by C. Eisenman, pp. 232–255, Marcel Dekker, New York.

150. Hille, B. (1976): Gating in sodium channels of nerve. *Annu. Rev. Physiol.,* 38:139–152.

151. Hillman, D. E., and Llinas, R. (1974): Calcium-containing electron-dense structures in the axons of the squid giant synapse. *J. Cell Biol.,* 61:146–155.

152. Hirano, A., Becker, N. H., and Zimmerman, H. M. (1969): Isolation of the periaxonal space of the central myelinated nerve fibre with regard to the diffusion of peroxidase. *J. Histochem. Cytochem.,* 17:512–516.

153. Hodgkin, A. L. (1967): *The Conduction of the Nervous Impulse.* Liverpool University Press, Liverpool.

154. Hoffman, P. N., and Lasek, R. J. (1975): The slow component of axonal transport: Identification of major structural polypeptides of the axon and their generality among mammalian neurons. *J. Cell Biol.,* 66:351–366.

155. Holtzman, E., and Novikoff, A. B. (1965): Lysosomes in the rat sciatic nerve following crush. *J. Cell. Biol.,* 27:651–669.

156. Hope, A. B. (1971): *Ion Transport and Membranes: A Biophysical Outline.* Butterworths, London.

157. Hursh, J. B. (1939): Conduction velocity and diameter of nerve fibres. *Am. J. Physiol.,* 127:131–139.

158. Hursh, J. B. (1939): The properties of growing nerve fibres. *Am. J. Physiol.,* 127:140–153.

159. Hökfelt, T. (1969): Distribution of noradrenaline storing particles in peripheral adrenergic neurons as revealed by electronmicroscopy. *Acta Physiol. Scand.,* 76:427–440.

160. Iurato, S., Luciano, L., Franke, K., Pannese, E., and Reale, E. (1974): Histochemical localization of acetylcholinesterase activity in the cochlear and vestibular ganglion cells. *Acta Otolaryngol.,* 78:28–35.

161. Jack, J. J. B. (1976): Electrophysiological properties of peripheral nerve. In: *The Peripheral Nerve,* edited by D. N. Landon, Chapman and Hall, London.

162. Jacobs, J. M., and Cavanagh, J. B. (1972): Aggregations of filaments in Schwann cells of spinal roots of the normal rat. *J. Neurocytol.,* 1:161–167.

163. Karlsson, U. L., Schultz, R. L., and Hooker, W. M. (1975): Cation-dependent structures associated with membranes in the rat central nervous system. *J. Neurocytol.,* 4:537–542.

164. Kirkpatrik, J. B., Bray, J. J., and Palmer, S. M. (1972): Visualization of axoplasmic flow in vitro by nomarski microscopy: Comparison to rapid flow of radioactive proteins. *Brain Res.,* 43:1–10.

165. Knowles, J. F. (1976): An electron microscope study of the unmyelinated nerve fibres in normal baboon median nerves: Negative effect of vitamin-B_{12} depletion. *J. Anat.,* 121:461–474.

166. Koenig, E. (1970): Membrane protein synthesizing machinery of the axon: Biochemistry of simple neuronal models. *Adv. Biochem. Psychopharmacol.,* 2:303–315.

167. Krammer, E. B., and Lischka, M. F. (1973): Schwermetallaffine Strukturen des peripheren Nerven. *Histochemie,* 36:269–282.

168. Krammer, E. B., and Zenker, W. (1975): Effekt von Zinkionen auf Struktur und Verteilung der Neurotubuli. *Acta Neuropathol. (Berl),* 31:59–69.

169. Kristensson, K., and Olsson, Y. (1976): Retrograde transport of horseradish peroxidase in transected axons. 3. Entry into injured axons and subsequent localization in perikaryon. *Brain Res.,* 115:201–213.

170. Krücke, W. (1974): Patologie der peripheren Nerven. In: *Handbuch der Neurochirurgie,* Vol. 7, edited by H. Olivekrona, W. Tönnis, and W. Krenkel, pp. 1–242, Springer Verlag, Berlin.

171. Lacy, P. E., Howell, S. L., Young, D. A., and Fink, C. S. (1968): New hypothesis of insulin secretion. *Nature (Lond),* 219:1177–1179.

172. Landon, D. N., and Hall, S. (1976): The myelinated nerve fibre. In: *The Peripheral Nerve,* edited by D. N. Landon, pp. 1–105. Chapman and Hall, London.

173. Landon, D. N., and Langley, O. K. (1971): The local chemical environment of nodes of Ranvier: A study of cation binding. *J. Anat.,* 108:419–432.

174. Landon, D. N., and Preston, G. M. (1963): Cited as unpublished observations in ref. 208.

175. Landon, D. N., and Williams, P. L. (1963): Ultrastructure of the node of Ranvier. *Nature (Lond),* 199:575–577.

176. Langley, O. K. (1969): Ion-exchange at the node of Ranvier. *Histochem. J.,* 1:295–309.

177. Langley, O. K. (1970): The interaction between peripheral nerve polyanions and alcian blue. *J. Neurochem.,* 17:1535–1541.

178. Langley, O. K. (1971): A comparison of the binding of alcian blue and inorganic cations to polyanions in peripheral nerve. *Histochem. J.,* 3:251–260.

179. Langley, O. K. (1973): Local anaesthetics and nodal polyanions in peripheral nerve. *Histochem. J.,* 5:79–86.

180. Langley, O. K., and Landon, D. N. (1967): A light and electronmicroscopical approach to the node of Ranvier and myelin of pe-

ripheral nerve fibres. *J. Histochem. Cytochem.*, 15:722–731.

181. Langley, O. K., and Landon, D. N. (1969): Copper binding at nodes of Ranvier: A new electronhistochemical technique for the demonstration of polyanions. *J. Histochem. Cytochem.*, 17:66–69.

182. LaVail, M., and LaVail, J. (1975): Retrograde intraaxonal transport of horseradish peroxidase in retinal ganglion cells of the chick. *Brain Res.*, 85:273–280.

183. Lehman, H. J. (1959): Die Nervenfaser in V. von Möllendorffs. In: *Handbuch der mikroskopischen Anatomie des Menschen*, Vol. 4. Springer Verlag, Berlin.

184. Lieberman, A. R. (1976): Sensory ganglia. In: *The Peripheral Nerve*, edited by D. N. Landon. Chapman and Hall, London.

185. Livingston, R. B., Pfenninger, K., Moor, H., and Akert, K. (1973): Specialized paranodal and interparanodal glial-axonal junctions in the peripheral and the central nervous system: A freeze etching study. *Brain Res.*, 58:1–24.

186. Lubinska, L. (1958): Short internodes "intercalated" in nerve fibres. *Acta Biol. Exp.*, 18:117–136.

187. Lubinska, L., and Lukaszewska, I. (1956): Shape of myelinated nerve fibres and proximo-distal flow of axoplasm. *Acta Biol. Exp.*, 17:115–133.

188. Luftig, R. B., McMillan, P. N., Weatherbee, J. A., and Weihing, R. R. (1976): Increased visualization of microtubules by an improved procedure. *J. Cell Biol.*, 70:228a.

189. Malhotra, S. K., and van Harreveld, A. (1965): Dorsal roots of the rabbit investigated by freeze-substitution. *Anat. Rec.*, 152:282–292.

190. Martin, R., and Rosenberg, P. (1968): Fine structural alterations associated with venom action on squid giant nerve fibres. *J. Cell Biol.*, 36:341–353.

191. Masurowsky, E. B., Bunge, M. B., and Bunge, R. P. (1967): Cytological studies of organotypic cultures of rat dorsal root ganglia following x-irradiation in vitro. II. *J. Cell Biol.*, 32:497–518.

192. Maxwell, D. S., Kruger, L., and Pineda, A. (1969): The trigeminal nerve root with special reference to the central peripheral transition zone: An EM-study in the macaque. *Anat. Rec.*, 164:113–126.

193. Mei, N., Boyer, A., and Condamin, M. (1971): Etude comparée des deux prolongements de la cellule sensitive vagale. *C. R. Soc. Biol.*, 165:2371–2374.

194. Mellström, A. (1971): Postnatal excitability changes of the ankle monosynaptic reflexes in the cat. *Acta. Physiol. Scand.*, 82:477–489.

195. Metuzals, J. (1966): Electron microscopy of neurofilaments. In: *Sixth International Congress on E. M., Kyoto*. Maruzen, Tokyo.

196. Metuzals, J. (1969): Configuration of a filamentous network in the axoplasm of the squid (Loligo Pealli L.) giant nerve fibre. *J. Cell Biol.*, 43:480–505.

197. Metuzals, J., and Izzards, C. S. (1969): Spatial patterns of threadlike elements in the axoplasm of the giant nerve fibre of the squid (Loligo Pealli L.) as disclosed by differential interference microscopy and electronmicroscopy. *J. Cell Biol.*, 43:456–479.

197a. Moore, J. W., Joiner, R. W., Brill, M., Waxman, S. G., and Najaar-Joa M. (1977): Simulations of conduction in uniform myelinated fibers: kelatine sensitivity to changes in nodal and internodal parameters. *Biophys. J.* (*in press*).

198. Mooseker, M. S., and Tilney, L. G. (1975): Organization of an actin filament-membrane complex: Filament polarity and membrane attachment in the microvilli of intestinal epithelial cells. *J. Cell Biol.*, 67:725–743.

199. Mraz, P., and Kapeller, K. (1976): Die Wirkung des Kolchicins und Lumi-Kolchicins auf die Feinstruktur markloser Axone in autonomen Nerven der Katzen in vitro. *Z. Mikrosk. Anat. Forsch.*, 90:352–359.

200. Mugnaini, E., and Schnapp, B. (1974): Possible role of zonula occludens of the myelin sheath in demyelinating conditions. *Nature (Lond)*, 251:725–727.

201. Muralt, A. V. (1946): *Die Signalübermittlung in Nerven*. Verlag Birkhäuser, Basel.

202. Müller-Mohnssen, H., Tippe, A., Hillenkamp, F., and Unsöld, E. (1974): Is the rise of the action potential of the Ranvier node controlled by a paranodal organ? *Naturwissenschaften*, 61:1.

203. Nageotte, J. (1911): Betrachtung über den Tatsachlichen Bau und die künstlisch hervorgerufenen Deformationen der markhaltigen Nervenfaser. *Arch. Mikrosk. Anat.*, 77:245–279.

204. Naka, K. (1964): Electrophysiology of the fetal spinal cord. I. Action potentials of the motoneuron. *J. Gen. Physiol.*, 47:1003–1022.

205. Naka, K. (1964): Electrophysiology of the fetal spinal cord. II. Interaction among peripheral inputs and recurrent inhibition. *J. Gen. Physiol.*, 47:1023–1038.

206. Novikoff, A. B., Wuintana, N., Villaverde, H., and Forschirm, R. (1966): Nucleoside phosphatase and cholinesterase activities in dorsal root ganglia and peripheral nerve. *J. Cell Biol.*, 29:525–545.

207. Ochoa, J. (1975): Microscopic anatomy of unmyelinated nerve fibres. In: *Peripheral Neuropathy*, Vol. I, edited by P. J. Dyck, P. K. Thomas, and E. H. Lambert, pp. 131–150. Saunders, Philadelphia.

208. Ochoa, J. (1976): The unmyelinated nerve fibre. In: *The Peripheral Nerve,* edited by D. N. Landon, pp. 106–158. Chapman and Hall, London.

209. Ochoa, J., and Mair, W. G. P. (1969): The normal sural nerve in man. I. Ultrastructure and numbers of fibers and cells. *Acta Neuropathol.,* 13:197–216.

210. Ochoa, J., and Mair, W. G. P. (1969): The normal sural nerve in man. II. Changes in the axons and Schwann cells due to ageing. *Acta Neuropathol.,* 13:217–239.

211. Ochs, S. (1972): Fast transport of materials in mammalian nerve fibres. *Science,* 1976: 252–260.

212. Ochs, S. (1975): Axoplasmic transport— a basis for neural pathology. In: *Peripheral Neuropathy,* Vol. I, edited by P. J. Dyck, P. K. Thomas, and E. H. Lambert, pp. 213– 230. Saunders, Philadelphia.

213. Olsson, L., Ålund, M., and Norberg, K-A. (1976): Fluorescence-microscopical demonstration of a population of gastro-intestinal nerve fibres with a selective affinity for quinacrine. *Cell Tissue Res.,* 171:407–423.

214. Palay, S. L., Sotelo, C., Peters, A., and Orkland, P. M. (1968): The axon hillock and the initial segment. *J. Cell Biol.,* 38: 193–201.

215. Pappas, G. D., and Purpura, D. P. (1961): Fine structure of dendrites in the superficial neocortical neuropil. *Exp. Neurol.,* 4:507– 530.

216. Peters, A. (1968): The morphology of axons of the central nervous system. In: *The Structure and Function of Nervous Tissue,* Vol. I, edited by G. H. Bourne, pp. 141–186. Academic Press, New York.

217. Peters, A., and Muir, A. R. (1959): The relationship between axons and Schwann cells during development in peripheral nerves in the rat. *Q. J. Exp. Physiol.,* 44: 117–130.

218. Peters, A., and Vaughn, J. E. (1967): Microtubules and filaments in the axons and astrocytes of early postnatal rat optic nerve. *J. Cell Biol.,* 32:113–119.

219. Peters, A., and Vaughn, J. E. (1970): Morphology and development of the myelin sheath. In: *Myelination,* edited by A. N. Davison, and A. Peters, pp. 3–79. Charles C Thomas, Springfield, Ill.

220. Peters, A., Palay, S. L., and Webster, H. de F. (1976): *The Fine Structure of the Nervous System.* Saunders, Philadelphia.

221. Peracchia, C. (1974): Excitable membrane ultrastructure. I. Freeze fracture of crayfish axons. *J. Cell Biol.,* 61:107–122.

222. Peracchia, C., and Robertson, J. D. (1971): Increase in osmiophilia of axonal membranes of crayfish as a result of electrical stimulation, asphyxia, or treatment with reducing agents. *J. Cell Biol.,* 51:223–239.

223. Peyronnard, J-M., Aguayo, A. J., and Bray, G. M. (1973): Schwann cell internuclear distances in normal and regenerating unmyelinated nerve fibres. *Arch. Neurol.,* 29: 56–59.

224. Peyronnard, J. M., Terry, L. C., and Aguayo, A. J. (1975): Schwann cell internuclear distances in developing unmyelinated nerve fibres. *Arch. Neurol.,* 32:36– 38.

225. Phillips, D. D., Hibbs, R. G., Ellison, J. P., and Shapiro, H. (1972): An electron microscopic study of central and peripheral nodes of Ranvier. *J. Anat.,* 111:229–238.

226. Pleasure, D. E. (1975): The structural proteins of peripheral nerve. In: *Peripheral Neuropathy,* Vol. I, edited by P. J. Dyck, P. K. Thomas, and E. H. Lambert. Saunders, Philadelphia.

227. Quick, D. C., and Waxman, S. G. (1977): Specific staining of the axon membrane at nodes of Ranvier with ferric ion and ferrocyanide. *J. Neurol. Sci.,* 31:1–11.

228. Quilliam, T. A. (1956): Some characteristics of myelinated fibre populations. *J. Anat.,* 90:172–187.

229. Raine, C. S., Ghetti, B., and Shelanski, M. L. (1971): On the association between microtubules and mitochondria within axons. *Brain Res.,* 34:389–393.

230. Ranvier, L. (1888): *Technisches Lehrbuch der Histologie,* translated by W. Nicati and H. von Wyss. Verlag von F. C. W. Vogel, Leipzig.

231. Rényi, G. de (1928): The structure of tissues as revealed by microdissection. II. The physical properties of the axis cylinder in the myelinated nerve fibre of the frog. *J. Comp. Neurol.,* 47:405–425.

232. Rényi, G. de (1929): The structure of cells in tissues as revealed by microdissection. III. Observations on the sheaths of myelinated nerve fibres of the frog. *J. Comp. Neurol.,* 48:293–310.

233. Revel, J. P., and Hamilton, D. W. (1969): The double nature of the intermediate dense line in peripheral nerve myelin. *Anat. Rec.,* 163:7–16.

234. Rexed, B., and Sourander, P. (1949): The caliber of central and peripheral neurites of spinal ganglion cells and variations in fiber size at different levels of dorsal spinal roots. *J. Comp. Neurol.,* 91:297–306.

235. Ritchie, J. M. (1971): Electrogenic ion pumping in nervous tissue. *Curr. Top. Bioenergetics,* 4:327–356.

236. Robertson, J. D. (1958): Structural alterations in nerve fibres produced by hypotonic and hypertonic solutions. *J. Biophys. Biochem. Cytol.,* 4:349–364.

237. Robertson, J. D. (1959): Preliminary observations on the ultrastructure of nodes of Ranvier. *Z. Zellforsch.,* 50:553–560.

238. Robertson, J. D. (1976): Membrane models: theoretical and real. In: *The Nerv-*

ous System, Vol. I, edited by D. B. Tower. Raven Press, New York.

239. Rosenberg, P. (1973): The giant axon of the squid: A useful preparation for neurochemical and pharmacological studies. *Methods Neurochem.,* 4:97–160.

240. Rosenbluth, J. (1976): Intramembranous particle distribution at the node of Ranvier and adjacent axolemma in myelinated axons of the frog brain. *J. Neurocytol.,* 5:731–745.

241. Rushton, W. A. H. (1951): A theory of the effect of fibre size in medullated nerve. *J. Physiol. (Lond),* 115:101–122.

242. Sabatini, D. D., Bensch, K., and Barnett, R. J. (1963): The preservation of cellular ultrastructure and enzymatic activity by aldehyde fixation. *J. Cell Biol.,* 17:19–58.

243. Sandri, C., Van Buren, J. M., and Akert, K. (1977): Membrane morphology of the vertebrate nervous system: A study with freeze-etch technique. *Prog. Brain. Res.,* Vol. 43, Elsevier, Amsterdam.

244. Satir, P. (1977): Microvilli and cilia: surface specializations of mammalian cells. In: *Mammalian cell membranes, Vol. 2: The Diversity of Membranes,* edited by G. A. Jamieson and D. M. Robinson. Butterworths, London.

245. Scharf, J-H. (1958): Sensible Ganglien. In: *von Möllendorffs Handbuch der Mikroskopischen Anatomie des Menschen,* Vol. IV/3. Springer Verlag, Berlin.

246. Scharf, J. H., and Blume, R. (1964): Über die abhängigkeit den axonalen Mitochondrienzahl vom Kaliber der segmentierten Nervenfaser auf grund einer Regressions analyse. *J. Hirnforsch.,* 6:361–376.

247. Schlaepher, W. W. (1968): Acetylcholinesterase activity of motor and sensory nerve fibres in the spinal nerve roots of the rat. *Z. Zellforsch.,* 88:441–456.

248. Schmitt, F. O., and Geschwind, N. (1957): The axon surface. *Prog. Biophys. Lond.,* 8:217–240.

249. Schneider, D. (1952): Die Dehnbarkeit der markhaltigen Nervenfasern des Frosches in Abhängigkeit von Funktion und Struktur. *Z. Naturforsch. [C],* 7:38–48.

250. Schnapp, B., and Mugnaini, E. (1975): The myelin sheath: electron microscopic studies with thin sections and freeze-fracture. In: *Golgi Centennial Symposium: Proceedings,* pp. 209–233.

251. Schnapp, B., Peracchia, C., and Mugnaini, E. (1976): The paranodal axo-glial junction in the central nervous system studied with thin sections and freeze-fracture. *Neuroscience,* 1:181–190.

252. Schnepp, P., and Schnepp, G. (1971): Faseranalytische Untersuchungen an peripheren Nerven bei Tieren verschiedener Grösse. II. Verhältnis Axondurchmesser/Gesamtdurchmesser und Internodallänge. *Z. Zellforsch.,* 119:99–114.

253. Schnepp, G., Schnepp, P., and Spaan, G. (1971): Faseranalytische Untersuchungen an peripheren Nerven bei Tieren verschiedener Grösse. I. Fasergesamtzahl, Faserkaliber und Nervenleitungsgeschwindig keit. *Z. Zellforsch.,* 119:77–98.

254. Schook, W. J., and Norton, W. T. (1976): Neurofilaments account for the lipid in myelin-free axons. *Brain Res.,* 118:517–522.

255. Schröder, J. M. (1972): Altered ratio between axon diameter and myelin sheath thickness in regenerated nerve fibres. *Brain Res.,* 45:49–65.

256. Schwab, M. E., and Troenen, H. (1976): Electron microscopic autoradiographic and cytochemical localization of retrogradely transported nerve growth factor (NGF) in the rat sympathetic ganglion. *J. Cell Biol.,* 70:289.

257. Shelanski, M. L. (1973): Microtubules: In: *Protein of the Nervous System,* edited by D. J. Schneider, pp. 227–241. Raven Press, New York.

258. Sima, A. (1974): Relation between the number of myelin lamellae and axon circumference in fibres of ventral and dorsal roots and optic nerve in normal undernourished and rehabilitated rats. *Acta Physiol. Scand. [Suppl.],* 410.

259. Simpson, S. A., and Young, J. Z. (1945): Regeneration of fibre diameter after cross-unions of visceral and somatic nerves. *J. Anat.,* 79:48–65.

260. Singer, M. (1968): Penetration of labelled amino acids into the peripheral nerve fibre from surrounding body fluids. In: *Growth of the Nervous System,* edited by G. E. W. Wolstenholme and M. O'Connor, pp. 200–215. Churchill, London.

261. Singer, S., and Steinberg, M. C. (1972): Wallerian degeneration: A reevaluation based on transected and colchicine poisoned nerves in the amphibian Triturus. *Am. J. Anat.,* 133:51–84.

262. Singer, M., Krishnan, N., and Fyfe, D. A. (1972): Penetration of ruthenium red into peripheral nerve fibers. *Anat. Rec.,* 173:375–390.

263. Sjöstrand, F. S. (1964): The structure and formation of the myelin sheath. In: *Mechanisms of Demyelination,* pp. 1–43. McGraw-Hill, New York.

264. Skoglund, C. R. (1942): The response to linearly increasing currents in mammalian motor and sensory fibres. *Acta Physiol. Scand. [Suppl. 12],* 4.

265. Skoglund, S. (1960): On the postnatal development of postural reflexes as revealed by electronmyography and myography in decerebrate kittens. *Acta Physiol. Scand.,* 49:299–317.

266. Skoglund, S. (1960): The spinal transmission of proprioceptive reflexes and the

postnatal development of conduction velocity in different hindlimb nerves in the kitten. *Acta Physiol. Scand.*, 49:318–329.

267. Skoglund, S. (1960): Central connections and functions of muscle nerves in the kitten. *Acta Physiol. Scand.*, 50:222–237.

268. Skoglund, S. (1960): The reactions to tetanic stimulation of the two-neuron arc in the kitten. *Acta Physiol. Scand.*, 50:238–253.

269. Skoglund, S. (1966): Muscle afferents and motor control in the kitten. In: *Nobel Symposium I*, edited by R. Granit, pp. 45–59. Almqvist & Wiksell, Stockholm.

270. Skoglund, S., and Romero, C. (1965): Postnatal growth of spinal roots and nerves. *Acta. Physiol. Scand.* [*Suppl.* 260], 66.

271. Sluga, E., and Tomanaga, M. (1970): Darstellung und lokalisation der Mg-ATPase im peripheren Nerven. *Histochemie*, 22:187–197.

272. Smith, D. S., Järlfors, U., and Cameron, B. F. (1975): Morphological evidence for the participation of microtubules in axonal transport. *Ann. NY Acad. Sci.*, 253:472–506.

273. Smith, R. S. (1973): Microtubule and neurofilament densities in amphibian spinal root nerve fibres: Relationship to axoplasmic transport. *Can. J. Physiol. Pharmacol.*, 51:798–806.

274. Sotelo, C., and Riche, D. (1974): The smooth endoplasmic reticulum and the retrograde and fast orthograde transport of horseradish peroxidase in the nigro-striato-nigral loop. *Anat. Embryol.*, 146:209–218.

275. Spencer, P. S., and Thomas, P. K. (1974): Ultrastructural studies of the dying-back process. II. The sequestration and removal by Schwann cells and oligodendrocytes of organelles from normal and diseased axons. *J. Neurocytol.*, 3:763–783.

276. Spencer, P. S., Raine, C. S., and Wisniewski, H. (1973): Axon diameter and myelin thickness—unusual relationships in dorsal root ganglia. *Anat. Res.*, 176:225–244.

277. Steer, J. M. (1971): Some observations on the fine structure of rat dorsal spinal nerve roots. *J. Anat.*, 109:467–485.

278. Stephens, R. E., and Edds, K. T. (1976): Microtubules: Structure chemistry and function. *Physiol. Rev.*, 56:709–777.

279. Stoeckenius, W., and Zeiger, K. (1956): Morphologie der segmentierten Nervenfaser. *Ergeb. Anat.*, 35:420–534.

280. Stämpfli, R. (1952): Bau und Funktion isolierter markhaltiger Nervenfasern, *Ergeb. Physiol.*, 47:70–165.

281. Sunderland, S. (1968): *Nerves and Nerve Injuries*. Livingstone, Edinburgh.

282. Sunderland, S., and Lavarack (1953): Branching of nerve fibres. *Acta Anat.*, 17:46–59.

283. Sunderland, S., and Roche, A. F. (1958):

Axon-myelin relationships in peripheral nerve fibres. *Acta Anat.*, 33:1–37.

284. Szentagothai, J. (1964): Neuronal and synaptic arrangements in the substantia geletinosa Rolandi. *J. Comp. Neurol.*, 122:219–239.

285. Tagini, G., and Camino, E. (1973): T-Shaped cells of dorsal ganglia can influence the pattern of afferent discharge. *Pfluegers Arch.*, 344:339–347.

286. Tasaki, I., and Carbone, E. (1974): A macromolecular approach to nerve excitation. In: *Current Topics in Membranes and Transport*, Vol. 5, edited by F. Bronner and A. Kleinzeller. Academic Press, New York.

287. Tasaki, I., and Sisco, K. (1975): Electrophysiological and optical methods for studying the excitability of the nerve membrane. In: *Methods in Membrane Biology, Vol. 5: Transport*, edited by E. D. Korn. Plenum Press, New York.

288. Tennyson, V. M. (1970): The fine structure of the axon and growth cone of the dorsal root neuroblast of the rabbit embryo. *J. Cell Biol.*, 44:62–79.

289. Theron, J. J., Meyer, B. J., Boekkooi, S., and Ldots, J. M. (1975): Ultrastructural localisation of calcium in peripheral nerves of the rat. *S. Afr. Med. J.*, 49:1795–1798.

290. The synapse (1976): *Cold Spring Harbor Symp. Quant. Biol.*, 40.

291. Thiel, W. (1957): Morphologische Ergebnisse an einzelnen markhaltigen Nervenfasern und ihre funktionelle Bedeutung. *Acta Anat.*, 31:156–192.

292. Thomas, R. C. (1972): Electrogenic sodium pump in nerve and muscle cells. *Physiol. Rev.*, 52:563–594.

293. Tilney, L. G., and Mooseker, M. S. (1976): Actin filament-membrane attachment: Are membrane particles involved? *J. Cell Biol.*, 71:402–416.

294. Torebjörk, H. E., and Hallin, R. G. (1970): C-Fibre units recorded from human sensory nerve fascicles in situ. *Acta Soc. Med. Uppsala*, 75:81–84.

295. Tranum-Jensen, J. (1975): The ultrastructure of the sensory endorgans (baroreceptors) in the atrial endocardium of young mini-pigs. *J. Anat.*, 119:255–275.

296. Vallbo, Å. (1964): Accommodation related to inactivation of sodium permeability in single myelinated nerve fibres of Xenopus laevis. *Acta Physiol. Scand.*, 61:429–444.

297. Vance, W. H., Clifton, G. L., Applebaum, M. L., Willis, W. D., Jr., and Coggeshall, R. E. (1975): Unmyelinated preganglionic fibres in frog ventral roots. *J. Comp. Neurol.*, 164:117–126.

298. Villegas, G. M., and Villegas, R. C. (1968): Ultrastructural studies of the squid nerve fibres. *J. Gen. Physiol.*, 51:44–60.

299. Villegas, J., Sevicik, C., Barnola, F. V., and Villegas, R. (1976): Grayanotoxin veratrine

and tetrodoxin-sensitive sodium pathways in the Schwann cell membrane of squid nerve fibres. *J. Gen. Physiol.,* 67:369–380.

300. Voegtli, J. (1954): Über Markgehalt und Segmentierung der Nervenfasern. *Acta Anat.,* 21:366–385.

301. Walters, B. B., and Matus, A. I. (1975): Tubulin in postsynaptic junctional lattices. *Nature (Lond),* 257:496–498.

302. Waxman, S. G. (1968): Micropinocytotic invaginations in the axolemma of peripheral nerves. *Z. Zellforsch.,* 86:571–573.

303. Waxman, S. G. (1972): Regional differentiation of the axon: A review with special reference to the concept of the multiplex neuron. *Brain Res.,* 47:269–288.

304. Waxman, S. G. (1975): Integrative properties and design principles of axons. *Int. Rev. Neurobiol.,* 18:1–39.

305. Webster, H. de F. (1971): The geometry of peripheral myelin sheaths during their formation and growth in rat sciatic nerves. *J. Cell Biol.,* 48:348–367.

306. Webster, H. de F. (1975): Development of peripheral myelinated and unmyelinated nerve fibres. In: *Peripheral Neuropathy,* Vol. I., edited by P. J. Dryck, P. K. Thomas, and E. H. Lambert. Saunders, Philadelphia.

307. Webster, H. de F., and Collins, G. H. (1964): Comparison of osmium tetroxide and glutaraldehyde perfusion fixation for the electronmicroscopic study of the normal rat peripheral nervous system. *J. Neuropathol. Exp. Neurol.,* 23:109–126.

308. Webster, H. de F., and Martin, J. R. (1973): Mitotic Schwann cells in developing nerve: Their changes in shape fine structure and axon relationship. *Dev. Biol.,* 32:417–431.

309. Webster, H. de F., Martin, J. R., and O'Connell, M. F. (1973): The relationships between interphase Schwann cells and axons before myelination: A quantitative electronmicroscopic study. *Dev. Biol.,* 32:401–416.

310. Weddell, G. (1941): The pattern of cutaneous innervation in relation to cutaneous sensibility. *J. Anat.,* 75:346–367.

311. Weinberg, H. J., and Spencer, P. S. (1975): Studies on the control of myelinogenesis. I. Myelination of regenerating axons into a foreign unmyelinated nerve. *J. Neurocytol.,* 4:395–418.

312. Weinberg, H. J., and Spencer, P. S. (1976): Studies on the control of myelinogenesis. II. Evidence for neuronal regulation of myelin production. *Brain Res.,* 113:363–378.

313. Weiss, P. (1967): Neuronal dynamics—an essay. *Neurosci. Res. Prog. Bull.,* 514:371–345.

314. Weiss, P. A., and Mayr, R. (1971): Organelles in neuroplasmic "axonal" flow: Neurofilaments. *Proc. Natl. Acad. Sci. USA,* 68:846–850.

315. Weiss, P., and Pillai, A. (1965): Convection and fate of mitochondria in nerve fibres: Axonal flow as vehicle. *Proc. Natl. Acad. Sci. USA,* 54:48–56.

316. Weller, R. O. (1967): An electron microscopic study of hypertrophic neuropathy of Dejerine-Sottas. *J. Neurol. Neurosurg. Psychiatry,* 30:111–125.

317. Westrum, L. E., and Gray, E. G. (1976): Microtubules and membrane specializations. *Brain Res.,* 105:547–550.

318. Williams, P. L. (1959): Sections of fresh mammalian nerve trunks for quantitative studies: A rapid freezing technique. *Q. J. Micr. Sci.,* 100:425–431.

319. Williams, P. L., and Hall, S. M. (1970): In vivo observations on mature myelinated nerve fibres of the mouse. *J. Anat.,* 107:31–38.

320. Williams, P. L., and Hall, S. M. (1971): Prolonged in vivo observations of normal peripheral nerve fibres and their acute reactions to crush and deliberate trauma. *J. Anat.,* 108:397–408.

321. Williams, P. L., and Kashef, R. (1968): Asymmetry of the node of Ranvier. *J. Cell Sci.,* 3:341–356.

322. Williams, P. L., and Landon, D. N. (1963): Paranodal apparatus of peripheral nerve fibres of mammals. *Nature (Lond),* 198:670–673.

323. Williams, P. L., and Landon, D. N. (1964): The energy source of the nerve fibre. *New Scientist,* 374:166–169.

324. Williams, P. L., and Wendell-Smith, C. P. (1971): Some additional parametric variations between peripheral nerve fibre populations. *J. Anat.,* 109:505–526.

325. Williard, M., Cowan, W. M., and Vagelos, P. R. (1974): The polypeptide composition of intra-axonally transported proteins: Evidence for four transport velocities. *Proc. Natl. Acad. Sci. USA,* 71:2183–2187.

326. Wilson, V. J. (1962): Reflex transmission in the kitten. *J. Neurophysiol.,* 25:263–275.

327. Wood, J. G., Jean, D. H., McLaughlin, B. J., and Wayne Albers, R. (1976): Immunocytochemical localization of the Na^+-K^+-ATPase in electronmicroscopic preparations of fish brain. *J. Cell Biol.,* 70:257a.

328. Wuerker, R. B. (1970): Neurofilaments and glial filaments. *Tissue Cell,* 2:1–9.

329. Wuerker, R. B., and Kirkpatrick, J. B. (1972): Neuronal microtubules, neurofilaments and microfilaments. *Int. Rev. Cytol.,* 33:45–75.

330. Wuerker, R. B., and Palay, S. L. (1969): Neurofilaments and microtubules in anterior horn cells of the rat. *Tissue Cell,* 1:387–402.

331. Yamada, M. K., Spooner, B. S., and Wessells, N. K. (1971): Ultrastructure and function of growth cones and axons of

cultured nerve cells. *J. Cell Biol.,* 49:614–635.

332. Young, J. Z. (1945): The history of the shape of a nerve fibre. In: *Essays on Growth and Form,* edited by W. E. le Gros Clark and P. B. Medawar, pp. 41–93. Clarendon Press, Oxford.

333. Zelená, J. (1970): Ribosome-like particles in myelinated axons of the rat. *Brain Res.,* 24:359–363.

334. Zelená, J. (1972): Ribosomes in myelinated axons of dorsal root ganglia. *Z. Zellforsch.,* 124:217–229.

335. Zenker, W., and Hohberg, E. (1973): A-α-nerve-fibre: Number of neurotubules in the stem fibre and in the terminal branches. *J. Neurocytol.,* 2:143–148.

336. Zenker, W., and Hohberg, E. (1973): α-Motorische nervenfaser: Axonquerschnittsfläche von stammfaser und endnästen. *Z. Anat. Entwicklungesch.,* 139:163–172.

337. Zenker, W., and Högl, E. (1976): The prebifurcation section of the axon of the rat spinal ganglion cell. *Cell Tissue Res.,* 165:345–363.

338. Zenker, W., Mayr, R., and Gruber, H. (1972): Axoplasmic organelles: Quantitative differences between ventral and dorsal root fibres of the rat. *Experientia,* 29:77–78.

339. Zenker, W., Mayr, R., and Gruber, H. (1974): Neurotubules: Different densities in peripheral motor and sensory nerve fibres. *Experientia,* 31:318–320.

340. Krishnan, N., and Singer, M. (1973): Penetration of peroxidase into peripheral nerve fibers. *Am. J. Anat.,* 136:1–14.

Physiology and Pathobiology of Axons, edited by
S. G. Waxman. Raven Press, New York © 1978.

Morphology of Normal Central Myelinated Axons

Asao Hirano and Herbert M. Dembitzer

Division of Neuropathology, Department of Pathology, Montefiore Hospital and Medical Center, and Albert Einstein College of Medicine, Bronx, New York 10461

Several excellent, comprehensive reviews of the anatomy of the central myelinated axon appeared in the recent past (15,16,51,94,109, 110,113). The purpose of this relatively short review is to add some recent observations and to summarize what we feel are the more important general fine structural features which may serve as a morphological framework for the present volume. Most of our considerations are based on observations derived from thin sections. The new and exciting data from freeze-fracture material (25,26,86,96,118,121, 123,124,134) is reviewed by Schnapp and Mugnaini elsewhere in this volume.

GENERAL CONSIDERATIONS OF THE RELATIONSHIP BETWEEN THE CENTRAL AXON AND MYELIN

The central myelinated axon usually originates from a neuronal perikaryon within the central nervous system and may extend for considerable distances. Unlike the dendrites, the axons characteristically maintain their diameter throughout their length (109; but see ref. 35) and, except for certain neurons, do not branch or show synaptic contact until they terminate. Some axons do branch and give rise to collaterals at the nodes (73,82,85,100,144). Occasionally the nodes of Ranvier also become the sites of synapses where presynaptic vesicles accumulate at a junction with a postsynaptic element (14,73,78,102,131,140,141). Axo-axonal synapses have been occasionally reported where a postsynaptic element is present at the initial segment or in a terminal branch (110). Even spine formation, normally regarded as being limited to dendrites and soma,

has been described in the initial segments of axons in the prepyriform cortex in the rat (151). Postsynaptic specializations have not generally been observed at the nodes of Ranvier (110). Septate junctions between axons have also been reported in the cerebellar cortex of the cat (40).

Within the central nervous system almost all axons above a certain diameter are myelinated (18,64,87,88,122,142,143,145,148). As described by light microscopists, the myelin is arranged in segments separated by the nodes of Ranvier along the length of the axon, reminiscent of beads on a string. In general, the length of the internode is roughly proportional to the diameter of the axon (13,92), although some exceptions are reported even under normal conditions (138,139,146). The thickness of the sheath, too, corresponds to the caliber of the axon (143,145). In general, the thickness of the myelinated fiber increases as it passes from the central into the peripheral nervous system (90,98).

Unlike the dendritic processes of the neuron, the axons are generally found in bundles of parallel cell processes, forming the well-known tracts of the white matter of the central nervous system. Within these tracts lie the interfascicular oligodendroglia oriented roughly in chains of closely arranged cells. Astrocytes are often intercalated within the chain.

The myelin internodes within the central nervous system are the product of glia, the equivalent of the Schwann cells of the peripheral nervous system. Most workers today believe that the myelin-forming cell in the central nervous system is the oligodendroglial cell, although some investigators are of the opinion that in some instances, at least, astrocytes assume this function (12,150).

Although it was suspected from a rather early date, it has been difficult to demonstrate a clear-cut connection between the oligodendroglial cell and the myelin sheath in the adult animal (Figs. 1 and 2). Such a relationship has, however, been demonstrated in the developing animal (17,97,107) and even rarely in the adult (48). The explanation generally offered for this difficulty is that the process connecting a myelin sheath with the cell body of an oligodendroglial cell is a long and tortuous one, virtually impossible to include within

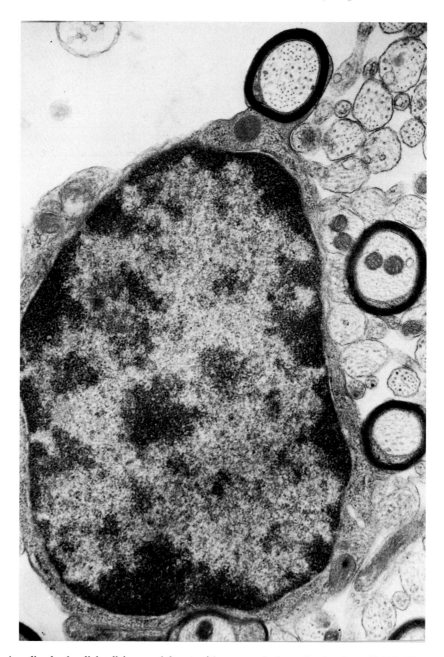

FIG. 1. An oligodendroglial cell in an adult rat with an attached myelin sheath. ×22,500. (From ref. 48.)

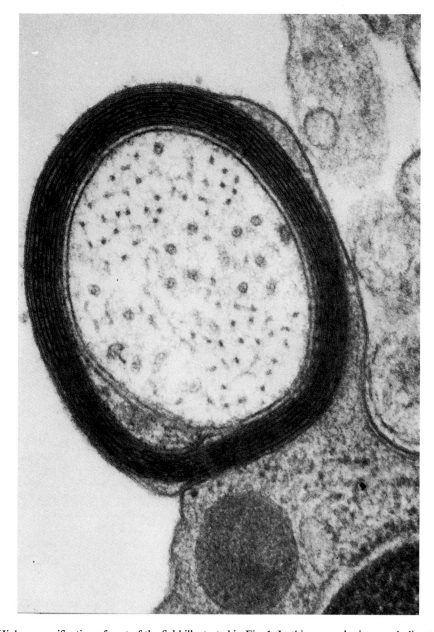

FIG. 2. Higher magnification of part of the field illustrated in Fig. 1. In this unusual micrograph direct continuity between the oligodendroglial cytoplasm and the myelin sheath is clearly visible. ×96,000. (From ref. 48.)

a single thin section. This kind of connection is better understood when one realizes that, unlike the neuron which gives rise to only a single axon, the oligodendroglial cells apparently form numerous internodes, presumably on many axons within the bundle (Fig. 3). It has been estimated that in the optic nerve (111) and spinal cord (88) of the rat a single oligodendroglial cell can form a few dozen internodes. In other areas only two or three internodes are formed by a single glial cell (93). This is in sharp distinction to the peripheral nervous system wherein a single Schwann cell forms a single internode.

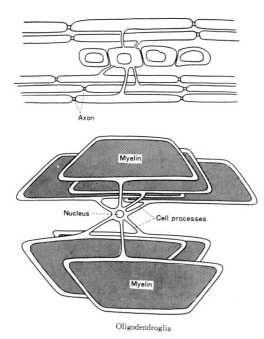

Axon

Myelin

Nucleus

Cell processes

Myelin

Oligodendroglia

FIG. 3. **Top:** Relationship between the oligodendroglia and the myelinated axon in the central nervous system. **Bottom:** A single oligodendroglial cell and its several hypothetically unrolled myelin sheaths attached to it. (Modified from refs. 16,52.)

The developmental processes giving rise to myelin formation are not well understood and are discussed later. In general, however, it can be said that in the vast majority of cases myelin formation is confined to axons. Thus the presence of a surrounding myelin sheath is almost a certain indication that the enclosed cell process is an axon. On the other hand, in pathological conditions and even occasionally in apparently normal tissue, myelin sheaths have been observed around other cell processes or even perikarya (5,11,22,23,60,72,74,83, 120). It is not clear whether the latter occurrence is a permanent or transient phenomenon in normal central nervous tissue. Conceivably also, these unusual observations may have been made on animals with an occult injury or disease. It is known, however, that the perikarya of certain peripheral ganglia are myelinated in the normal, mature animal (110), and certain dendrites in the olfactory bulb are reported to be myelinated in the central nervous system of normal adults (115,153).

AXONAL FINE STRUCTURE

Clearly the most striking aspect of the axon is the enormous length it sometimes achieves. A single axon arising in an anterior horn cell, for example, may reach a length of a few feet. The axon is cylindrical so that accurate cross sections are invariably circular (Fig. 4), and they seem to maintain a fairly constant diameter over relatively long distances. Over almost all of its length, the myelinated axon is closely invested by other cells or processes.

As in other cells and cell processes, the axon is surrounded by a triple-layered plasma membrane, the axolemma, approximately 80 Å thick. This thickness has been reported to increase to approximately 120–150 Å in crayfish abdominal nerve cord during excitation as well as during asphyxia, and in other experimental conditions which affect other membranes within the axon in a similar fashion (104). Compared to many other cell processes, the axonal cytoplasm is relatively lucent and simple. The most prominent features are the neurofilaments and microtubules. These structures are roughly parallel to the long axis of the axon. They are usually not gathered in bundles but instead are more or less evenly scattered in the axonal cytoplasm. The smaller the axon, the greater is the ratio of microtubules to filaments (37,110). The filaments are 100 Å in diameter and show an electron-lucent core in cross section (50,156,157). Their length is indeterminate. Occasionally short, indistinct side arms radiating into the adjacent cytoplasm can be detected (49,135). The microtubules, referred to in the earlier literature as neurotubules, are essentially identical to those seen in many other cell types, and their characteristic reaction to the application of mitotic spindle inhibitors is also similar (63,155). They are approximately 240 Å in diameter and, when viewed in cross section, display a prominent lucent core. Their length has not been determined, and they do not seem to branch. As in the neurofilaments, microtubules too are decorated with short side arms. The wall of the tubule is apparently composed of discrete globular particles arranged in a helical fashion. High-resolution studies reveal approximately 13 globular units

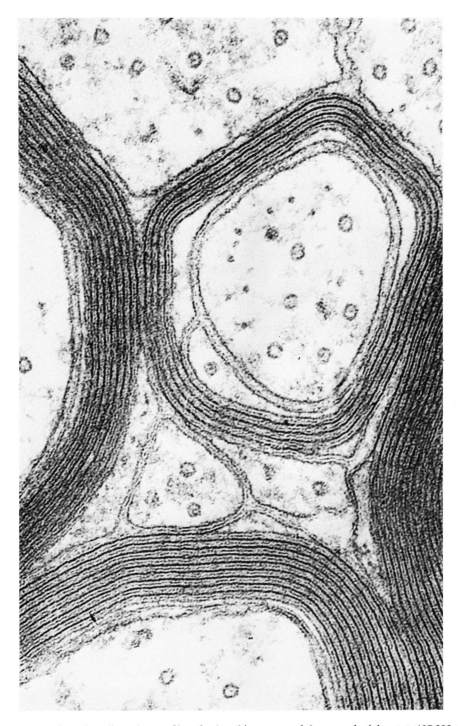

FIG. 4. Cross section of myelinated nerve fibers in the white matter of the normal adult rat. ×187,000. (From ref. 52.)

per turn of the helix (38,136). Often one can detect a 50 Å density within the lucent core. The number of microtubules per unit of cross-sectional area in the accessory nerve of the rat remains constant throughout its length. Since the total area increases at the terminal branches, one must assume that new microtubules are added in this region (161).

The function of these organelles is not completely understood. Most workers suspect that they play a role in maintaining the shape of the elongated axon or are related to axonal transport, or both. Occasionally one may detect mitochondria or other organelles surrounded by a ring of microtubules, suggesting a transport function (64,99,117,129,130).

Other organelles are less prominent in the relatively simple axonal cytoplasm. Small elements of the smooth endoplasmic reticulum are frequently seen. Their function is also questionable, but some evidence exists indicating that it may be related to axonal transport (28,29,110). They differ from microtubules by their irregular, sometimes branching shape and their limiting membrane, which is of typical unit membrane construction. Often their overall configuration is cisternal rather than tubular. In some animals the axonal smooth endoplasmic reticulum forms an elaborate apparatus consisting of flat, fenestrated horizontal cisternae almost occluding the axonal interior (30,34,46,69,84,103). When this occurs other organelles are restricted to the pores penetrating the flattened cisternae. Occasionally, even under normal conditions, such well-developed smooth endoplasmic reticulum can form either whorl-like configurations or complicated honeycomb-like arrangements (2,24,31,49,51, 58,61,62,100,132,137). These are particularly well known in Purkinje cell axons as they pass through the granule cell layer of the cerebellum.

Ribosomes are usually not found in the axons outside the initial segment. Certainly one does not find ribosomes attached to membranes as in rough endoplasmic reticulum. Although the presence of a small amount of RNA has been detected by chemical means, aggregates of ribosomes within the axons have been reported only in very exceptional instances (159,160).

Occasional mitochondria are found in the axon. They are generally cylindrical and ori-ented parallel to the long axis of the axon. Their morphology is unremarkable, but their cristae, embedded in a relatively dense matrix, are generally elongated in the same direction as the mitochondria.

Even less common are the multivesicular bodies, which are sometimes seen within the axoplasm. Similarly, one occasionally detects a coated pinocytotic vesicle at the axonal surface (64,110).

The fine structure of the initial segment of the axon (i.e., that portion of the axon between the axon hillock and the first myelin internode) differs in three respects from that of most of the remainder of the axon (47,70, 101,110,112,151). At 60–100 Å beneath the plasma membrane of the initial segment there is a finely granular undercoating material approximately 200 Å thick showing moderate electron density. When stained with phosphotungstic acid, the undercoating has a dentate appearance (127), which may be explained by assuming a tripartite configuration of its elements (21). According to Westrum and Gray (152) there is a distinct association between the undercoating material and microtubules. The undercoating is interrupted at the sites of synapses in the initial segment (110,142). The microtubules of the initial segment, instead of being scattered as in other parts of the axon, are apparently joined by means of their side arms into fascicles of parallel elements. Finally, free ribosomes are present in the cytoplasm, often forming small, polysome-like clusters.

MYELIN FINE STRUCTURE

Whether viewed in longitudinal or in cross section, the most striking aspect of the myelin sheath is its regular lamellar structure (33). The myelin lamellae consist of alternating dense and less-dense bands with a periodicity of approximately 110 Å, although a certain variability, depending on sheath thickness, has been reported (45). When seen in cross section (Fig. 4), the outside of the sheath displays a tongue of cytoplasm, the outer loop. The compact myelin begins as the inner leaflets of the plasma membrane of the outer loop fuse, excluding all the cytoplasm and forming the major dense line. This prominent, dense line winds a spiral path (19,89,105) around the axon, finally splitting once more to form the inner leaflets of another cytoplasmic tongue situated between the myelin sheath and the axon, the inner loop. For some unknown reason, in approximately 75% of the central myelinated fibers, the inner and outer loops occupy the same quadrant of the circle described by a cross section of the fibers (106). The interiors of the inner and outer loops are essentially identical. They are generally devoid of formed organelles except for microtubules and occasional, small membranous vesicles. Significant numbers of filaments are sometimes seen in the inner loop (65). The inner and outer loops are joined to their respective adjacent myelin lamellae by means of a tight junction (25,95, 117,122).

The outer leaflets of the cytoplasmic loops accompany the major dense line, and when the leaflets of adjacent lamellae approach one another they virtually obliterate the extracellular space and form the so-called intraperiod line, or minor dense line. In well-preserved tissue sectioned in an ideal plane, one can sometimes detect the double nature of the intraperiod line (66).

In the quadrant of the sheath which includes the inner and outer loops, the intraperiod line appears to form a number of dense thickenings described as the "radial component of the central sheath" (110). Freeze-fracture studies have been reported which describe zonulae occludentes at these regions (110).

One of the more striking features of the central nervous system in general is the extremely close arrangement of the cells and processes in the parenchyma. Extracellular space is minimal even around small vessels. The white matter is no exception to this rule and in it, myelin sheaths are found in close juxtaposition. In some areas adjacent sheaths seem to come into actual contact, forming a structure indistinguishable from the intraperiod line seen within a single sheath.

The myelin of the central nervous system is fundamentally the same as that of the peripheral system. It does differ in several respects, however. The periodicity of peripheral myelin is approximately 10% greater (6,68,71), and the intraperiod line is always resolvable into two outer leaflets except in regions of tight junction formation (25,96,118,123). In addition, peripheral myelin sheaths are covered by a collar of Schwann cell cytoplasm, which in turn is surrounded by a basal lamina. Unlike the central nervous system, substantial extracellular space surrounds each myelin sheath. Other differences between central and peripheral myelin are reviewed elsewhere (61,68, 110).

When the central myelin sheath is viewed in longitudinal sections, one can distinguish three regions along the axon. First, there is the myelin internode, which consists of a series of parallel major and minor dense lines. In the longitudinal view the dense lines are arranged in stacks of parallel densities, on both sides of the axon. On either side of the internode lie the paranodal regions. These consist of that part of the sheath in which each major dense line opens to form the two inner leaflets of another cytoplasmic tongue, the lateral loop, which is almost identical to the inner and outer loops seen in the cross-sectional view. Unlike the outer and inner loops, however, the lateral loops are arranged in a slightly overlapping chain closely applied to the axolemma on either side of the axon (Fig. 5). At the region of overlap the lateral loops are joined to one another by tight junctions (96). Sometimes in pathological conditions some lateral loops are not in contact with the axonal surface (110, 114).

As mentioned above, the outer and inner loops are connected to their adjacent myelin lamellae by means of tight junctions (25,96, 118,123) so that there exists a tight junctional seal separating the potential interlamellar spaces from the extracellular parenchymatous and the periaxonal spaces. In certain pathological conditions—e.g., experimental allergic encephalomyelitis (49,81) or certain peripheral neuropathies (27,54,77)—this seal is apparently broken, leading to edema fluid accumulation between the lamellae and eventually to demyelination.

The third region of the axon visible in longitudinal sections is the node of Ranvier itself, which separates adjacent paranodal regions. At this point the axon is directly exposed to the meager extracellular space of the central nervous system. The length of the node is apparently variable (110). In this respect, too,

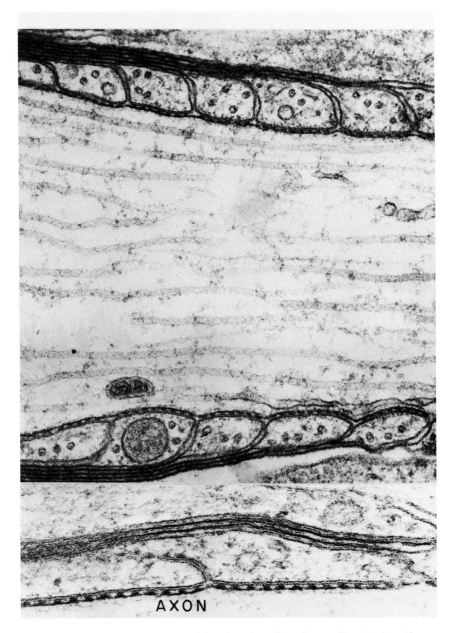

FIG. 5. Longitudinal section through the paranodal region of myelinated nerve fibers in the white matter of the adult rat. The transverse bands are visible at the interface of the lateral loops and the axon. **Top:** ×85,000. **Bottom:** ×136,000. (From ref. 55.)

the central nervous system differs from the peripheral nervous system where the Schwann cell cytoplasm loosely covers the axonal surface between paranodal regions. In these areas the adjacent Schwann cells interdigitate, and they are covered by a continuous basal lamina.

The fundamental architecture of the myelin sheath can best be understood by hypothetically unrolling the sheath from around the axon (43,55,125,126,128,149). When this is done, it becomes clear that the cytoplasmic portions of the sheath form a continuous rim

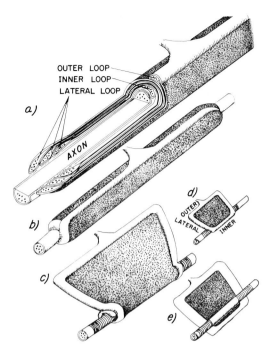

a)

OUTER LOOP
INNER LOOP
LATERAL LOOP

AXON

b)

c)

d)

(OUTER)
LATERAL
INNER

e)

FIG. 6. Relationship between the myelin sheath and the axon in the central nervous system. (From ref. 55.)

around a shovel-shaped membrane of myelin (Fig. 6).

FINE STRUCTURAL AXON—MYELIN RELATIONSHIPS

As mentioned earlier in the chapter, myelin forms almost exclusively around axons. Thus it is not unreasonable to expect that a very special relationship exists between the oligodendroglial cells and the axons. This is indeed the case, and the morphological expressions of this relationship in the mature myelinated fiber are among the most intriguing revealed to us by the electron microscope.

There are two important morphological expressions of axon–myelin interaction. Each involves opposite aspects of the axolemma.

The first is the undercoating material (108) similar to the structure already described at the cytoplasmic surface of the axolemma covering the initial segment. This material is not present under the internodal or paranodal regions of the myelin sheath. It is invariably found, however, under the node of Ranvier, where no overlying myelin or oligodendroglial

processes are present. The only exceptions to this rule are those occasions where a synapse occurs at the node of Ranvier or where collaterals arise (110,142). In such rare instances the undercoating is absent and the thickened postsynaptic membrane is present instead. On the basis of its distribution, the undercoating material has been implicated in the generation and propagation of action potentials since it is present in all areas which, according to the physiologists, are regions important for this process (101). Interestingly, some nodes of peripheral myelinated fibers of the electric organ in the knife fish are devoid of undercoating material, and no spike potentials are generated at those sites (147). How the morphology of the undercoating material is related to action potential generation is not understood.

The second feature which expresses the unique relationship between the axon and myelin sheath in the mature fiber is the "transverse bands" (2,4,15,55,79,108,109). These are differentiations at the surface of the axolemma directly opposite the lateral loops. In these areas, and nowhere else, the axolemma is not the simple, trilaminar density seen in other parts of the axon. Instead, in conventional preparations, there is a series of small, 150 Å long densities separated by approximately 100–150 Å which almost fill the space between the lateral loop and the inner leaflet of the axolemma (Fig. 5). Frequently, however, one can detect an electron-lucent area approximately 20 Å wide between a transverse band and the outer leaflet of the lateral loop. The bands also approach the inner leaflet of the axolemma much closer than the usual distance (20–25 Å) found between inner and outer leaflets (see Fig. 6 in ref. 51). According to Schnapp and Mugnaini (123), however, the outer leaflet of the axolemma always remains continuous and can be stained with special methods. It is their view that the transverse bands are extracellular structures between undulations of the apposing membranes rather than differentiations of the axolemmal outer leaflet. In this regard they consider the junction between the glial and axonal membranes as a variant of the septate junction. It is important to note two additional facts concerning these bands. First, the transverse bands are not seen in regions of the axolemma

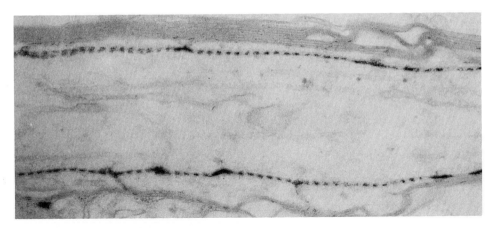

FIG. 7. An unstained longitudinal section of a myelinated fiber in the white matter of a rat brain in which lanthanum nitrate had been implanted. The dense lanthanum fills the space between the lateral loops and between transverse bands. ×76,000. (From ref. 56.)

which appose those areas between lateral loops (Fig. 5) or at the surface of lateral loops not in contact with the axon. Second, the transverse bands are seen in almost all well-oriented sections through the paranodal region of mature myelin sheaths. On these bases it was concluded that the transverse bands consist of

continuous, helically arranged structures which circle the axon parallel to the lateral loops. Tracer studies using lanthanum nitrate (Figs. 7 and 8) and microperoxidase indicate that the spaces between transverse bands are permeable (32,53,56). Grazing sections through lanthanum-treated fibers also suggest that these

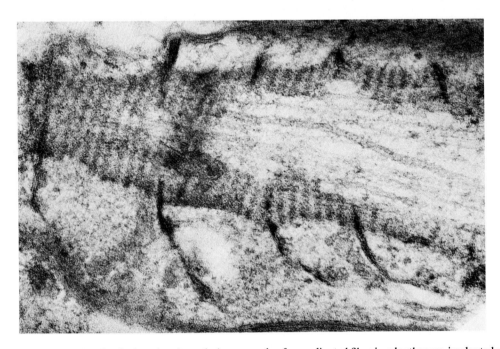

FIG. 8. A grazing longitudinal section through the paranode of a myelinated fiber in a lanthanum-implanted rat brain. Dense deposits of lanthanum between the transverse bands are oriented parallel to the direction described by the lateral loops around the axon. ×104,000. (From ref. 56.)

spaces, and therefore the transverse bands themselves, are parallel to the lateral loops (56). On the other hand, we must point out that recent data from freeze-fracture preparations suggest that the transverse bands are not parallel to the lateral loops but, instead, are short, parallel, linear protrusions arranged at an angle to the helical path traced by the lateral loops (124).

It should also be noted that Schnapp and Mugnaini reported that the transverse bands are not seen after certain preparative techniques, e.g., *en bloc* uranyl acetate staining. Instead, after these procedures the axolemma in the paranodal region displays a typical unit membrane construction. Nevertheless, of course, one cannot ignore its highly atypical appearance when prepared by conventional methods.

MYELIN FORMATION IN THE CENTRAL NERVOUS SYSTEM

During normal development myelination begins and proceeds at differing rates in different parts of the central nervous system. Recent evidence (3,8,9,19,39,42,60,80,91,110,116,119, 133,154) indicates that regeneration of myelin also can occur within the central nervous system, although it may be slow and incomplete.

Myelin formation requires the simultaneous presence of both an axon and a myelin-forming cell. The axon must be of certain minimum diameter, although not necessarily its adult caliber. The myelin-forming cell, presumably an oligodendroglial cell in most cases, must have also achieved a certain level of development.

Once these conditions are met, the oligodendroglial cell sends forth a finger-like process which contacts the axon and then spreads over it in sheet-like fashion, finally wrapping around the axon. The sheet of glial cytoplasm proceeds to wind around the axon and forms areas of compact myelin. Thus in cross sections of myelinating fibers, one may observe lamellae composed of either myelin or glial cytoplasm where the inner leaflets have not yet come together to exclude the cytoplasmic contents.

Early in the wrapping process the direction of the winding may differ at different levels of the same internode (75,76). During this period

it is possible that processes from several myelin-forming cells may compete with one another for the same axonal segment (110). Eventually, however, only one oligodendroglial cell succeeds in forming a single internode, and within it the lamellae all spiral in the same direction. Apparently during this process some abortive internodes, as well as some oligodendroglia, degenerate (44).

Presumably the myelin sheath grows by the elaboration of myelin at one of the cytoplasmic areas abutting the growing myelin membrane, finally leading to the mature sheath. It is not clear, however, precisely where this process occurs. Since, as already pointed out, the oligodendroglial perikaryon is attached via its processes to a number of sheaths, we can rule out the possibility of the myelin-forming cell itself spiraling around the axon. On the other hand, if we assume that the inner loop winds its way around the axon, trailing newly formed myelin behind it, one would expect that very soon the periaxonal space would fill with myelin, thereby preventing the further progress of the inner loop. This difficulty may be overcome by assuming that the myelin lamellae can slip over one another much as the mainspring of a clock unwinds, thereby maintaining the size of the periaxonal space (55). A similar mechanism has been proposed to explain the formation of the large intramyelinic splits seen as the result of certain intoxications, e.g., triethyltin (49,57,67). The same explanation may also serve to permit us to understand the method by which the axon can increase in diameter even after myelination, either during normal growth (36) or as the result of pathological alterations (59).

The outer loop, too, may be responsible for myelin formation. In this case, however, one must then assume that the entire thickening myelin sheath rotates around the axon as the myelin is formed at the outer loop.

Presumably the lateral loops also can form myelin, thus elongating the internode. In this connection we must point out that occasionally during remyelination in the central nervous system one can observe structures very similar to the Schmidt–Lanterman clefts which are normally considered limited to the peripheral nervous system (7,43,68). Their orientation would make them good candidates for sites of myelin formation, which would result in elongation of the internodes (20,41).

Thus it is possible that any of the cytoplasmic areas abutting the myelin itself may be responsible for myelin formation. This is perhaps more easily understood if one reconsiders the model of the unrolled sheath presented above (Fig. 6). Since the cytoplasmic loops are actually all sections through a continuous rim of cytoplasm, which is connected to the oligodendroglial perikaryon, it is not unreasonable to believe that myelin formation can occur in any of the loops.

The special relationship between the axon and the myelin-forming cells is very clear during myelination since in almost all instances only axons become myelinated. On the other hand, at least one of the morphological expressions of that relationship, the transverse bands, does not seem to appear until after myelin sheath formation is well under way (64). In longitudinal sections through the paranodal region of developing white matter, the axolemma apposed to the lateral loops displays typical unit membrane construction, even after conventional preparative procedures.

The apparent function of the transverse bands is to provide at least a partial seal between the extracellular and periaxonal space. Generally, in looking for significant pathological changes the pathologist considers only those situations in which there has been gross demyelination or dysmyelination, or clear changes in the axoplasm itself. It may be that relatively subtle changes in the transverse bands result in a separation between the lateral loops and the axolemmal surface such as is seen in some experimental or pathological conditions (1,10,54,158). This may ultimately produce confluency between the periaxonal and the extracellular spaces at the node, which may render an otherwise intact sheath useless.

ACKNOWLEDGMENT

The authors are grateful to Dr. Leopold G. Koss, Professor and Chairman, Department of Pathology, Albert Einstein College of Medicine at Montefiore Hospital and Medical Center, for his invaluable help in the preparation of this manuscript.

REFERENCES

1. Allt, G., and Cavanagh, J. B. (1969): Ultrastructural changes in the region of the node of Ranvier in the rat caused by diphtheria toxin. *Brain,* 92:459–468.
2. Andres, K. H. (1965): Über die Feinstruktur besonderer Einrichtungen in markhaltigen nervenfasern des Kleinhirns der Ratte. *Z. Zellforsch.,* 65:701–712.
3. Andrews, J. M. (1972): The ultrastructural neuropathology of multiple sclerosis. In: *Multiple Sclerosis. Immunology, Virology and Ultrastructure,* edited by F. Wolfgram, G. W. Ellison, J. G. Stevens, and J. M. Andrews, pp. 23–52. Academic Press, New York.
4. Bargmann, W., and Lindner, E. (1964): Über den Feinbau des Nebennierenmarkes des Igels (Erinaceus europeus L). *Z. Zellforsch.,* 64:868–912.
5. Bignami, A., and Ralston, H. J., III (1968): Myelination of fibrillary astroglial processes in long term wallerian degeneration: The possible relationship to 'status marmoratus.' *Brain Res.,* 11:710–713.
6. Bischoff, A., and Moor, H. (1967): Ultrastructural differences between the myelin sheaths of peripheral nerve fibers and CNS white matter. *Z. Zellforsch.,* 81:303–310.
7. Blakemore, W. F. (1969): Schmidt-Lantermann incisures in the central nervous system. *J. Ultrastruct. Res.,* 29:496–498.
8. Blakemore, W. F. (1973): Remyelination of the superior cerebellar peduncle in the mouse following demyelination induced by feeding cuprizone. *J. Neurol. Sci.,* 20:73–83.
9. Blakemore, W. F., and Patterson, R. C. (1975): Observations on the interactions of Schwann cells and astrocytes following x-irradiation of neonatal rat spinal cord. *J. Neurocytol.,* 4:573–585.
10. Blank, W. F., Bunge, M. B., and Bunge, R. F. (1974): The sensitivity of the myelin sheath, particularly the Schwann cell-axolemmal junction, to lowered calcium levels in cultured sensory ganglia. *Brain Res.,* 67:503–518.
11. Blinzinger, K., Anzil, A. P., and Muller, W. (1972): Myelinated nerve cell perikaryon in mouse spinal cord. *Z. Zellforsch.,* 128:135–138.
12. Blunt, M. J., Baldwin, F., and Wendell-Smith, C. P. (1972): Gliogenesis and myelination in kitten optic nerve. *Z. Zellforsch.,* 124:293–310.
13. Bodian, D. (1951): A note on nodes of Ranvier in the central nervous system. *J. Comp. Neurol.,* 94:475–484.
14. Bodian, D., and Taylor, H. (1963): Synapse arising at central node of Ranvier, and note

on fixation of the central nervous system. *Science,* 139:330–332.

15. Bunge, R. P. (1968): Glial cells and the central myelin sheath. *Physiol. Rev.,* 48: 197–251.

16. Bunge, R. P. (1970): Structure and function of neuroglia: some recent observations. In: *The Neurosciences. Second Study Program,* edited by F. O. Schmitt, pp. 782–797. Rockefeller University Press, New York.

17. Bunge, M. B., Bunge, R. P., and Pappas, G. D. (1962): Electron microscopic demonstration of connections between glia and myelin sheaths in the developing mammalian central nervous system. *J. Cell Biol.,* 12: 448–453.

18. Bunge, M. B., Bunge, R. P., Peterson, E. R., and Murray, M. R. (1967): A light and electron microscopic study of long-term organized culture of rat dorsal root ganglia. *J. Cell Biol.,* 32:439–466.

19. Bunge, M. B., Bunge, R. P., and Ris, H. (1961): Ultrastructural study of remyelination in an experimental lesion in adult cat spinal cord. *J. Biophys. Biochem. Cytol.,* 10:67–94.

20. Celio, M. R. (1976): Die Schmidt-Lantermannschen Einkerbungen der Myelinscheide des Mauthner-axons: Orte longitudinalen Myelinwachstums? *Brain Res.,* 108:221–235.

21. Chan-Palay, V. (1972): The tripartite structure of the undercoat in initial segments of Purkinje cell axons. *Z. Anat. Entwicklungsgesch.,* 141:125–150.

22. Cook, R. D. (1974): Observations on glial cells within myelin sheaths in degenerating optic nerves. *J. Neurocytol.,* 3:737–751.

23. Cooper, M., and Beal, J. A. (1977): Myelinated granule cell bodies in the cerebellum of the monkey (Saimiri sciureus). *Anat. Rec.,* 187:249–256.

24. Del Cerro, M. P., and Snider, R. S. (1969): Cerebellar alteration resulting from dilantin intoxication: an ultrastructural study. In: *The Cerebellum in Health and Disease, Dallas Neurological Symposium,* edited by W. S. Fields and W. D. Willis, Jr., pp. 380–411. Warren H. Green, St. Louis.

25. Dermietzel, R. (1974): Junctions in the central nervous system of the cat. I. Membrane fusion in central myelin. *Cell Tissue Res.,* 148:565–576.

26. Dermietzel, R. (1974): Junctions in the central nervous system of the cat. II. A contribution to the tertiary structure of the axonal-glial junctions in the paranodal region of the node of Ranvier. *Cell Tissue Res.,* 148:577–586.

27. Dropp, R. P., Means, E., Deibel, R., Sherer, G. T., and Barron, K. (1975): Waldenstrom's macroglobulinemia and neuropathy: Deposition of M-component on myelin sheaths. *Neurology (Minneap),* 25:980–988.

28. Droz, B. (1975): Synthetic machinery and axoplasmic transport: maintenance of neuronal connectivity. In: *The Nervous System, Vol. 1: The Basic Neurosciences,* edited by R. O. Brady, pp. 111–127. Raven Press, New York.

29. Droz, B., Bennett, G., DiGiamberardino, L., Koenig, H. L., and Rambourg, A. (1975): Contribution of electron microscopy to the study of the axonal flow. In: *VIIth International Congress of Neuropathology, Proceedings,* Vol. II, edited by St. Kornyey, St. Tariska, and G. Gosztonyi, pp. 299–304. Excerpta Medica, Amsterdam.

30. Ducros, C. (1974): Ultrastructural study of the organization of axonal agranular reticulum in octopus nerve. *J. Neurocytol.,* 3:513–523.

31. Duncan, D., and Williams, V. (1962): On the occurrence of a precise order in axoplasm. *Texas Rep. Biol. Med.,* 20:503–505.

32. Feder, N. (1971): Microperoxidase: An ultrastructural tracer of low molecular weight. *J. Cell Biol.,* 51:339–343.

33. Fernandez-Morán, H., and Finean, J. B. (1957): Electron microscope and low-angle x-ray diffraction studies of the nerve myelin sheath. *J. Biophys. Biochem. Cytol.,* 3:725–748.

34. Follenius, E. (1970): Organisation scalari forme du reticulum endoplasmique dans certains processus nerveus de l'hypothalamus de Gasteroteus aculeatus L. *Z. Zellforsch.,* 106: 61–68.

35. Friede, R. L. (1970): Determination of neurofilament and microtubule density in nerve fibres (what factors control axon calibre?). In: *Alzheimer's Disease and Related Conditions. A Ciba Foundation Symposium,* edited by G. E. W. Wolstenholme and M. O'Connor, pp. 209–222. Churchill, London.

36. Friede, R. L., and Miyagishi, T. (1972): Adjustment of the myelin sheath to change in axon caliber. *Anat. Rec.,* 172:1–14.

37. Friede, R. L., and Samorajski, T. (1970): Axon caliber related to neurofilaments and microtubules in sciatic nerve fibers of rats and mice. *Anat. Rec.,* 167:379–388.

38. Frisch, D. (1969): A photographic reinforcement analysis of neurotubules and cytoplasmic membranes. *J. Ultrastruct. Res.,* 29: 357–372.

39. Gledhill, R. T., Harrison, B. M., and McDonald, W. I. (1973): Pattern of remyelination in the CNS. *Nature (Lond),* 244: 443–444.

40. Gobel, S. (1971): Axo-axonic septate junctions in the basket formations of the cat cerebellar cortex. *J. Cell Biol.,* 51:328–333.

41. Hall, S. M., and Williams, P. L. (1970): Studies on the 'incisures' of Schmidt and Lanterman. *J. Cell Sci.,* 6:767–791.

42. Harrison, B. M., McDonald, W. I., and

Ochoa, J. (1972): Remyelination in the central diphtheria toxin lesion. *J. Neurol. Sci.*, 17:293–302.

43. Hildebrand, C. (1971): Ultrastructural and light microscopic studies of the nodal region on large myelinated fibers of the adult feline spinal cord white matter. *Acta Physiol. Scand. [Suppl.]*, 364:43–80.

44. Hildebrand, C. (1971): Ultrastructural and light microscopic studies of the developing feline spinal cord white matter. II. Cell death and myelin sheath disintegration in the early postnatal period. *Acta Physiol. Scand. [Suppl.]*, 364:109–144.

45. Hildebrand, C. (1972): Evidence for a correlation between myelin period and number of myelin lamellae in fibers of the feline spinal cord white matter. *J. Neurocytol.*, 1:223–232.

46. Hinds, J. W. (1972): Early neuron differentiation in the mouse olfactory bulb. II. Electron microscopy. *J. Comp. Neurol.*, 146:253–276.

47. Hinds, J. W., and Ruffett, T. L. (1973): Mitral cell development in the mouse olfactory bulb: Reorientation of the perikaryon and maturation of the axon initial segment. *J. Comp. Neurol.*, 151:281–305.

48. Hirano, A. (1968): A confirmation of the oligodendroglial origin of myelin in the adult rat. *J. Cell Biol.*, 38:637–640.

49. Hirano, A. (1969): The fine structure of brain in edema. In: *The Structure and Function of Nervous Tissue*, Vol. 2, edited by G. H. Bourne, pp. 69–135. Academic Press, New York.

50. Hirano, A. (1970): Neurofibrillary changes in conditions related to Alzheimer's disease. In: *A Ciba Foundation Symposium: Alzheimer's Disease and Related Conditions*, edited by G. E. W. Wolstenholme and M. O'Connor, pp. 185–207. Churchill, London.

51. Hirano, A. (1972): The pathology of the central myelinated axon. In: *The Structure and Function of Nervous Tissue*, Vol. V, edited by G. H. Bourne, pp. 73–162. Academic Press, New York.

52. Hirano, A. (1976): *An Outline of Neuropathology.* Igaku Shoin Ltd., Tokyo.

53. Hirano, A., Becker, N. H., and Zimmerman, H. M. (1969): Isolation of the periaxonal space of the central myelinated nerve fiber with regard to the diffusion of peroxidase. *J. Histochem. Cytochem.*, 17:512–516.

54. Hirano, A., Cook, S. D., Whitaker, J. N., Dowling, P. C., and Murray, M. R. (1971): Fine structural aspects of demyelination in vitro: The effects of Guillain-Barré serum. *J. Neuropathol. Exp. Neurol.*, 30:249–265.

55. Hirano, A., and Dembitzer, H. M. (1967): A structural analysis of the myelin sheath in the central nervous system. *J. Cell Biol.*, 34:555–567.

56. Hirano, A., and Dembitzer, H. M. (1969): The transverse bands as a means of access to the periaxonal space of the central myelinated nerve fiber. *J. Ultrastruct. Res.*, 28:141–149.

57. Hirano, A., Dembitzer, H. M., Becker, N. H., and Zimmerman, H. M. (1969): The distribution of peroxidase in the triethyltin-intoxicated rat brain. *J. Neuropathol. Exp. Neurol.*, 28:507–511.

58. Hirano, A., and Kochen, J. A. (1976): Experimental lead encephalopathy: Morphological studies. In: *Progress in Neuropathology*, Vol. 3, edited by H. M. Zimmerman, pp. 319–342. Grune & Stratton, New York.

59. Hirano, A., Levine, S., and Zimmerman, H. M. (1967): Experimental cyanide encephalopathy: Electron microscopic observations of early lesions in white matter. *J. Neuropathol. Exp. Neurol.*, 26:200–213.

60. Hirano, A., Levine, S., and Zimmerman, H. M. (1968): Remyelination in the central nervous system after cyanide intoxication. *J. Neuropathol. Exp. Neurol.*, 27:234–245.

61. Hirano, A., Sax, D. S., and Zimmerman, H. M. (1969): The fine structure of the cerebella of Jimpy mice and their "normal" litter mates. *J. Neuropathol. Exp. Neurol.*, 28:388–400.

62. Hirano, A., Rubin, R., Sutton, C. H., and Zimmerman, H. M. (1968): Honeycomb-like tubular structure in axoplasm. *Acta Neuropathol. (Berl)*, 10:17–23.

63. Hirano, A., and Zimmerman, H. M. (1970): Some effects of vinblastine implantation in the cerebral white matter. *Lab. Invest.*, 23:358–367.

64. Hirano, A., and Zimmerman, H. M. (1971): Some new pathological findings in the central myelinated axon. *J. Neuropathol. Exp. Neurol.*, 30:325–336.

65. Hirano, A., and Zimmerman, H. M. (1971): Glial filaments in the myelin sheath after vinblastine implantation. *J. Neuropathol. Exp. Neurol.*, 30:63–67.

66. Hirano, A., Zimmerman, H. M., and Levine, S. (1966): Myelin in the central nervous system as observed in experimentally induced edema in the rat. *J. Cell Biol.*, 31:397–411.

67. Hirano, A., Zimmerman, H. M., and Levine, S. (1968): Intramyelinic and extracellular spaces in triethyltin intoxication. *J. Neuropathol. Exp. Neurol.*, 27:571–580.

68. Hirano, A., Zimmerman, H. M., and Levine, S. (1969): Electron microscopic observations of peripheral myelin in a central nervous system lesion. *Acta Neuropathol. (Berl)*, 12:348–365.

69. Holz, A., and Weber, W. (1970): Periodische auftrettende Querstrukturen in Nevenfasern des Bulbus Olfactorius des Eltrize Phoxinus laevis. *Experientia*, 26:1349–1350.

70. Jones, E. G., and Powell, T. P. S. (1969): Synapses on the axon hillocks and initial segments of pyramidal cell axons in the cerebral cortex. *J. Cell Sci.*, 5:495–507.

71. Karlsson, U. (1966): Comparison of the myelin period of peripheral and central origin by electron microscopy. *J. Ultrastruct. Res.*, 15:451–468.

72. Kemali, M. (1974): An ultrastructural analysis of myelin in the central nervous system of an amphibian. *Cell Tissue Res.*, 152:51–67.

73. Khattab, F. I. (1966): Synaptic contacts at nodes of Ranvier in central nervous tissue. *Anat. Rec.*, 156:91–97.

74. Kim, S. U. (1970): Observations on cerebellar granule cells in tissue culture: A silver and electron microscopic study. *Z. Zellforsch.*, 107:454–465.

75. Knobler, R. L., and Stempak, J. G. (1973): Serial section analysis of myelin development in the central nervous system of the albino rat: An electron microscopical study of early axonal ensheathment. *Prog. Brain Res,.* 40:407–423.

76. Knobler, R. L., Stempak, J. G., and Laurencin, M. (1974): Oligodendroglial ensheathment of axons during myelination in the developing rat central nervous system: A serial section electron microscopical study. *J. Ultrastruct. Res.*, 49:34–49.

77. Koeppen, A. H., Messmore, H., and Stehbens, W. E. (1971): Interstitial hypertrophic neuropathy: Biochemical study of the peripheral nervous system. *Arch. Neurol.*, 24:340–352.

78. Kohno, K., Nakai, Y., and Yamada, H. (1972): Synaptic contacts from nodes of Ranvier in the granular layer of the frog cerebellum. *J. Neurocytol.*, 1:255–262.

79. Laatsch, R. H., and Cowan, W. M. (1966): A structural specialization at nodes of Ranvier in the central nervous system. *Nature (Lond)*, 210:757–758.

80. Lampert, P. W. (1965): Demyelination and remyelination in experimental allergic encephalomyelitis. *J. Neuropathol. Exp. Neurol.*, 24:371–385.

81. Lampert, P. W. (1968): Fine structural changes of myelin sheaths in the central nervous system. In: *The Structure and Function of Nervous Tissue*, Vol. V, edited by G. H. Bourne, pp. 187–204. Academic Press, New York.

82. Lange, W. (1976): The myelinated parallel fibers of the cerebellar cortex and their regional distribution. *Cell Tissue Res.*, 166:489–496.

83. Leonhardt, H. (1970): Myelinisierte Oligodendrozyten in der Wand der Eminentia mediana des Kaninchens. *Z. Zellforsch.*, 103:420–428.

84. Lieberman, A. R. (1971): Microtubule-associated smooth endoplasmic reticulum in the frog's brain. *Z. Zellforsch.*, 116:564–577.

85. Lieberman, A. R., Webster, K. E., and Spacek, J. (1972): Multiple myelinated branches from nodes of Ranvier in the central nervous system. *Brain Res.*, 44:652–655.

86. Livingston, R. B., Pfenninger, K., Moor, H., and Akert, K. (1973): Specialized paranodal and interparanodal glial-axonal junctions in the peripheral and central nervous system: A freeze-etching study. *Brain Res.*, 58:1–24.

87. Matthews, M. A. (1968): An electron microscopic study of the relationship between axon diameter and the initiation of myelin production in the peripheral nervous system. *Anat. Rec.*, 161:337–351.

88. Matthews, M. A., and Duncan, D. (1971): A quantitative study of the morphological changes accompanying the initiation and progress of myelin production in the dorsal funiculus of the rat spinal cord. *J. Comp. Neurol.*, 142:1–22.

89. Maturana, H. R. (1960): The fine anatomy of the optic nerve of Anurans—an electron microscope study. *J. Biophys. Biochem. Cytol.*, 7:107–120.

90. Maxwell, D. S., Kruger, L., and Pineda, A. (1969): The trigeminal nerve root with special reference to the central-peripheral transition zone: An electron microscopic study in the macaque. *Anat. Rec.*, 164:113–126.

91. McDonald, W. I. (1974): Remyelination in relation to clinical lesions of the central nervous system. *Br. Med. Bull.*, 30:186–189.

92. McDonald, W. J., and Ohrlich, G. D. (1971): Quantitative anatomical measurements on simple isolated fibres from the cat spinal cord. *J. Anat.*, 110:191–202.

93. McFarland, D. E., and Friede, R. L. (1971): Number of fibres per sheath cell and internodal length in cat cranial nerves. *J. Anat.*, 109:169–176.

94. Mokrasch, L. C., Bear, R. S., and Schmitt, F. O. (1971): Myelin. *Neurosci. Res. Program Bull.*, 9:440–598.

95. Mugnaini, E. (1972): The histology and cytology of the cerebellar cortex. In: *The Comparative Anatomy and Histology of the Cerebellum: The Human Cerebellum, Cerebellar Connections and Cerebellar Cortex*, edited by O. Larsell and J. Jansen, pp. 201–262. University of Minnesota Press, Minneapolis.

96. Mugnaini, E., and Schnapp, B. (1974): Possible role of zonula occludens of the myelin sheath in demyelinating conditions. *Nature (Lond)*, 251:725–726.

97. Narang, H. K., and Wisniewski, H. M. (1977): The sequence of myelination in the epiretinal portion of the optic nerve in the rabbit. *Neuropathol. Appl. Neurobiol.*, 3.15–27.

98. Němeček, S., Pařizek, J., Spaček, J., and

Němečkova, J. (1969): Histological, histochemical and ultrastructural appearance of the transitional zone of the cranial and spinal nerve roots. *Folia Morphol. (Praha)*, 17: 171–181.

99. Ochs, S. (1975): A unitary concept of axoplasmic transport based on the transport filament hypothesis. In: *Recent Advances in Myology*, edited by W. G. Bradley, D. Gardner-Medwin, and J. N. Walton, pp. 189–194. Excerpta Medica/American Elsevier, New York.

100. Palay, S. L., and Chan-Palay, V. (1974): *Cerebellar Cortex. Cytology and Organization*. Springer-Verlag, New York.

101. Palay, S. L., Sotelo, O., Peters, A., and Orkand, P. M. (1968): The axon hillock and the initial segment. *J. Cell Biol.*, 38: 193–201.

102. Pappas, G. D., and Waxman, S. G. (1972): Synaptic fine structure: Morphological correlates of chemical and electrotonic transmission. In: *Structure and Function of Synapses*, edited by D. P. Purpura and G. D. Pappas, pp. 1–47. Raven Press, New York.

103. Peracchia, C. (1970): A system of parallel septa in crayfish nerve fibers. *J. Cell Biol.*, 44:125–133.

104. Peracchia, C., and Robertson, J. D. (1971): Increase in osmiophilia of axonal membranes of crayfish as a result of electrical stimulation, asphyxia, or treatment with reducing agents. *J. Cell Biol.*, 51:223–239.

105. Peters, A. (1960): The structure of myelin sheaths in the central nervous system of Xenopus laevis (Daudin). *J. Biophys. Biochem. Cytol.*, 7:121–126.

106. Peters, A. (1964): Further observations on the structure of myelin sheaths in the central nervous system. *J. Cell Biol.*, 20:281–296.

107. Peters, A. (1964): Observations on the connexions between myelin sheaths and glial cells in the optic nerves of young rats. *J. Anat.*, 98:125–134.

108. Peters, A. (1966): The node of Ranvier in the central nervous system. *Q. J. Exp. Physiol.*, 51:229–236.

109. Peters, A. (1968): The morphology of axons of the central nervous system. In: *The Structure and Function of Nervous Tissue*, Vol. 1, edited by G. H. Bourne, pp. 141–186. Academic Press, New York.

110. Peters, A., Palay, S. L., and Webster, H. de F. (1976): *The Fine Structure of the Nervous System. The Neurons and Supporting Cells*. Saunders, Philadelphia.

111. Peters, A., and Proskauer, C. C. (1969): The ratio between myelin segments and oligodendrocytes in the optic nerve of the adult rat. *Anat. Rec.*, 163:243 (abstract).

112. Peters, A., Proskauer, C. C., and Kaiserman-Abramoff, I. R. (1968): The small pyramidal neuron of the cat cerebral cortex: The axon hillock and the initial segment. *J. Cell Biol.*, 39:604–619.

113. Peters, A., and Vaughn, J. E. (1970): Morphology and development of the myelin sheath. In: *Myelination*, edited by A. N. Davison and A. Peters, pp. 3–79. Charles C Thomas, Springfield, Ill.

114. Phillips, D. D., Hibbs, R. G., Ellison, J. P., and Shapiro, H. (1972): An electron microscopic study of central and peripheral nodes of Ranvier. *J. Anat.*, 111:229–238.

115. Pinching, A. J. (1971): Myelinated dendritic segments in the monkey olfactory bulb. *Brain Res.*, 29:133–138.

116. Raine, C. S. (1976): Experimental allergic encephalomyelitis and related conditions. In: *Progress in Neuropathology*, Vol. III, edited by H. M. Zimmerman, pp. 225–251. Grune & Stratton, New York.

117. Raine, C. S., Ghetti, B., and Shelanski, M. L. (1971): On the association between microtubules and mitochondria within axons. *Brain Res.*, 34:389–393.

118. Reale, E., Luciano, L., and Spitznas, M. (1975): Zonulae occludentes of the myelin lamellae in the nerve fibre layer of the retina and in the optic nerve of the rabbit: A demonstration by the freeze-fracture method. *J. Neurocytol.*, 4:131–140.

119. Reiser, P. J., and Webster, H. de F. (1974): Regeneration and remyelination of Xenopus tadpole optic nerve fibres following transection or crush. *J. Neurocytol.*, 3:591–618.

120. Rosenbluth, J. (1966): Redundant myelin sheaths and other ultrastructural features of the toad cerebellum. *J. Cell Biol.*, 28: 73–93.

121. Rosenbluth, J. (1976): Intramembranous particle distribution at the node of Ranvier and adjacent axolemma in myelinated axons of the frog brain. *J. Neurocytol.*, 5:731–745.

122. Samorajski, T., and Friede, R. L. (1968): A quantitative electron microscopic study of myelination in the pyramidal tract of rat. *J. Comp. Neurol.*, 134:323–338.

123. Schnapp, B., and Mugnaini, E. (1975): The myelin sheath: electron microscopic studies with thin sections and freeze-fracture: In: *Golgi Centennial Symposium: Perspectives in Neurobiology*, edited by M. Santini, pp. 209–233. Raven Press, New York.

124. Schnapp, B., Peracchia, C., and Mugnaini, E. (1976): The paranodal axo-glial junction in the central nervous system studied with thin sections and freeze-fracture. *Neuroscience*, 1:181–190.

125. Schröder, J. M. (1974): Two-dimensional reconstruction of Schwann cell changes following remyelination of regenerated nerve fibers. In: *Proceedings of the Symposium on Structure and Function of Normal and Diseased Muscle and Peripheral Nerve*, edited by I. Hausmanowa-Petrusewicz and H.

Jedrzejowska, pp. 299–304. Polish Medical Publishers, Poland.

126. Singer, M., and Steinberg, M. C. (1972): Wallerian degeneration: A reevaluation based on transected and colchicine-poisoned nerves in the amphibian, Triturus. *Am. J. Anat.*, 133:51–84.

127. Sloper, J. J., and Powell, T. P. S. (1973): Observations in the axon initial segment and other structures in the neocortex using conventional staining and ethanolic phosphotungstic acid. *Brain Res.*, 50:163–169.

128. Smart, I. (1965): Reconstruction of myelinated Schwann cells by unrolling. *J. Anat.*, 99:212–213.

129. Smith, D. S., Järlfors, U., and Beránek, R. (1970): The organization of synaptic axoplasm in the lamprey (Petromyzon marinus) central nervous system. *J. Cell Biol.*, 46:199–219.

130. Soifer, D., editor (1975): The biology of cytoplasmic microtubules. *Ann. NY Acad. Sci.*, 253:1–848.

131. Sotelo, C., and Palay, S. L. (1970): The fine structure of the lateral vestibular nucleus in the rat. II. Synaptic organization. *Brain Res.*, 18:93–115.

132. Sotelo, C., and Palay, S. L. (1971): Altered axons and axon terminals in the lateral vestibular nucleus of the rat: Possible example of axonal remodeling. *Lab. Invest.*, 25:653–671.

133. Suzuki, K., and Grover, W. D. (1970): Ultrastructural and biochemical studies of Schilder's disease. *J. Neuropathol. Exp. Neurol.*, 29:392–404.

134. Tani, E., Ikeda, K., and Nishiura, M. (1973): Freeze-etching images of central myelinated nerve fibers. *J. Neurocytol.*, 2:305–314.

135. Terry, R. D., and Penã, C. (1965): Experimental production of neurofibrillary degeneration. *J. Neuropathol. Exp. Neurol.*, 24:200–210.

136. Tilney, L. G., Bryan, J., Bush, D. J., Fujiwara, K., Mooseker, M. S., Murphy, D. B., and Snyder, D. H. (1975): Microtubules: Evidence for 13 protofilaments. *J. Cell Biol.*, 59:267–275.

137. Uchizono, K. (1975): *Excitation and Inhibition*. Igaku Shoin Ltd., Tokyo.

138. Waxman, S. G. (1970): Closely spaced nodes of Ranvier in the teleost brain. *Nature (Lond)*, 227:283–284.

139. Waxman, S. G. (1971): An ultrastructural study of patterns of myelination in preterminal fiber in teleost oculomotor nuclei, electromotor nuclei, and spinal cord. *Brain Res.*, 27:189–201.

140. Waxman, S. G. (1972): Regional differentiation of the axon: A review with special reference to the concept of multiplex neurons. *Brain Res.*, 47:269–288.

141. Waxman, S. G. (1974): Ultrastructural differentiation of the axon membrane at synaptic and non-synaptic central nodes of Ranvier. *Brain Res.*, 65:338–342.

142. Waxman, S. G. (1975): Integrative properties and design principles of axons. *Int. Rev. Neurobiol.*, 18:1–40.

143. Waxman, S. G. (1975): Electron-microscopic observations on preterminal fibers in the oculomotor nucleus of the cat: With special reference to the relation between axon diameter and myelin thickness in mammalian gray matter. *J. Neurol. Sci.*, 26:395–400.

144. Waxman, S. G. (1975): Ultrastructural observations on branching patterns of central axons. *Neurosci. Lett.*, 1:251–256.

145. Waxman, S. G., and Bennett, M. V. L. (1972): Relative conduction velocities of small myelinated and non-myelinated fibres in the central nervous system. *Nature [New Biol.]*, 238:217–219.

146. Waxman, S. G., and Melker, R. J. (1971): Closely spaced nodes of Ranvier in the mammalian brain. *Brain Res.*, 32:445–448.

147. Waxman, S. G., Pappas, G. D., and Bennett, M. V. L. (1972): Morphological correlates of functional differentiation of nodes of Ranvier along single fibers in the neurogenic electric organ of the knife fish Sternarchus. *J. Cell Biol.*, 53:210–224.

148. Waxman, S. G., and Swadlow, H. A. (1976): Morphology and physiology of visual callosal axons: Evidence for a supernormal period in central myelinated axons. *Brain Res.*, 113:179–187.

149. Webster, H. de F. (1971): The geometry of peripheral myelin sheaths during their formation and growth in rat sciatic nerves. *J. Cell Biol.*, 48:348–367.

150. Wendell-Smith, C. P., Blunt, M. J., and Baldwin, F. (1966): The ultrastructural characterization of macroglial cell types. *J. Comp. Neurol.*, 127:219–239.

151. Westrum, L. E. (1970): Observations on initial segments of axons in the prepyriform cortex of the rat. *J. Comp. Neurol.*, 139:337–353.

152. Westrum, L. E., and Gray, E. G. (1976): Microtubules and membrane specializations. *Brain Res.*, 105:547–550.

153. Willey, T. J. (1973): The ultrastructure of the cat olfactory bulb. *J. Comp. Neurol.*, 152:211–232.

154. Wisniewski, H., and Raine, C. S. (1971): An ultrastructural study of experimental demyelination and remyelination. V. Central and peripheral nervous system lesions caused by diphtheria toxin. *Lab. Invest.*, 25:73–80.

155. Wisniewski, H., Shelanski, M. L., and Terry, R. D. (1968): Effects of mitotic spindle inhibitors on neurotubules and neurofilaments in anterior horn cells. *J. Cell Biol.*, 38:224–229.

156. Wuerker, R. B. (1970): Neurofilaments and glial filaments. *Tissue Cell,* 2:1–10.

157. Wuerker, R. B., and Palay, S. L. (1969): Neurofilaments and microtubules in anterior horn cells of the rat. *Tissue Cell,* 1:387–402.

158. Yu, R. C-P., and Bunge, R. P. (1975): Damage and repair of the peripheral myelin sheath and node of Ranvier after treatment with trypsin. *J. Cell Biol.,* 64:1–14.

159. Zelená, J. (1970): Ribosome-like particles in myelinated axons of the rat. *Brain Res.,* 24:359–363.

160. Zelená, J .(1972): Ribosomes in myelinated axons of dorsal root ganglia. *Z. Zellforsch.,* 124:217–229.

161. Zenker, W., and Hohberg, E. (1973): A-α-nerve fiber: number of neurotubules in the stem fibre and in the terminal branches. *J. Neurocytol.,* 2:143–148.

Physiology and Pathobiology of Axons, edited by
S. G. Waxman. Raven Press, New York © 1978.

Membrane Architecture of Myelinated Fibers as Seen by Freeze-Fracture

Bruce Schnapp and Enrico Mugnaini

Laboratory of Neuromorphology, Department of Biobehavioral Sciences, University of Connecticut, Storrs, Connecticut 06268

Within the relatively brief time since its development, the freeze-fracture (or freeze-etching) method (57) has made a substantial contribution to our present concept of biological membrane organization. The method is characterized by the remarkable fact that when a sample of frozen tissue is cleaved the fracture process tends to split cell membranes through the center of their lipid bilayer (9). Cleavage along this plane generates two fracture surfaces (referred to as "faces") which complement each other within the interior of the membrane (Fig. 1). Each fracture face is the internal surface of a half-membrane. The surface associated with the exoplasmic half of the membrane is called E-face, and the surface associated with the protoplasmic half of the membrane the P-face (11). The cleavage process is carried out under vacuum; the exposed fracture surface is shadowed with platinum; and the replica is reinforced with a carbon film. The metal replica is dissociated from the underlying tissue, collected on a grid, and viewed in the transmission electron microscope (15).

It is common practice to fix tissue samples in aldehydes, as for thin-section electron microscopy, and to equilibrate small blocks of tissue with 20–30% glycerol prior to rapid freezing in Freon 22 cooled to the temperature of liquid nitrogen. The glycerol acts as a cryoprotectant to prevent ice crystal formation; if used without prior fixation, however, glycerol often introduces its own artifacts (54). Nevertheless, freeze-fracture of unfixed, glycerinated specimens can provide useful information (22,94). A recent and promising development is the use of rapid freezing devices to prepare tissues without prior fixation or cryoprotection (39,101). Extensive evaluations of the methods have been published (3,15).

Freeze-fractured biological membranes usually appear as particle-laden surfaces. It is now accepted that the homogeneous, background surface represents the lipid moieties of the membrane half (20), whereas the particles correspond to membrane proteins at least partially situated within the bilayer (29,91). In most cases the particles are distributed randomly over the fracture surface, although they can assume very regular and characteristic arrays in specialized membranes or membrane regions. For example, the different classes of intercellular junctions (e.g., gap, tight, and septate junctions) are each characterized by the presence of a distinct, orderly array of particles within the junctional membranes (95).

It is the purpose of this account to review how the freeze-fracture method has contributed to our present insight into the structural organization of myelinated axons. Following a brief survey of the organization of myelin sheaths, we discuss: (a) the fracture properties and membrane organization of the compact myelin; (b) the cell junctions occurring between adjoining turns of the myelin sheath (reflexive junctions) in different regions of the internode; (c) the paranodal axoglial junction; (d) the organization of the internodal and nodal axon membrane; and (e) features associated with the surface of peripheral myelin sheaths. We also attempt to outline the nu-

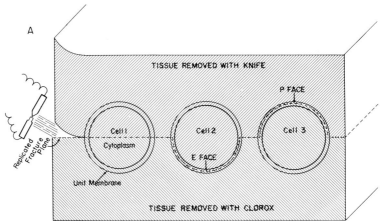

Freeze—Fracturing of Tissue Block and Replication

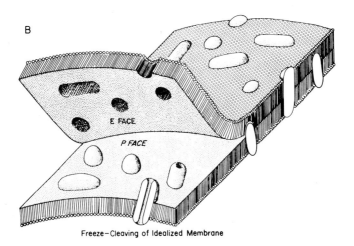

Freeze—Cleaving of Idealized Membrane

FIG. 1. Freeze-fracture method. **A:** Fracturing of a tissue block is represented. Cell 1 is cut across in the fracture process, whereas in cells 2 and 3 the plasmalemma is cleaved in the middle, creating a fracture face E (cell 2) and a fracture face P (cell 3). When the replica is photographed, the membrane vista of cell 2 appears concave and that of cell 3 convex. **B:** The cleaving process of a cell membrane produces two fracture surfaces. The E face is the internal membrane surface associated with the exoplasmic half of the membrane, and the P face the internal membrane surface associated with the protoplasmic half. The intact membrane is composed of a lipid bilayer within which globular proteins are situated. The lipid moieties have polar head groups oriented toward the aqueous interfaces and hydrophobic fatty acid tails directed toward the center of the bilayer. Freeze-cleavage splits the bilayer through the center of the hydrophobic region and thus generates two complementary fracture surfaces, or "faces." The membrane proteins remain intact and cleave with one of the half-membranes, leaving a pit on the complementary fracture surface. The proteins thus appear as particles protruding from the homogeneous background of the fractured lipid bilayer. Two of the idealized protein particles are represented with a channel, or pore, through which ions and small solutes may pass.

merous pitfalls which will be encountered when freeze-fracture studies of myelinated fibers are expanded to the experimental physiological and neuropathological domains after surpassing the normative stage to which they are now largely confined.

ORGANIZATION OF MYELIN SHEATHS

For many years now it has been recognized that central and peripheral myelin sheaths are structured according to analogous principles. Our studies have reaffirmed this notion. In this account we consider central and peripheral myelin together, emphasizing essential differences when appropriate.

The basic organization of myelinated axons in thin section electron microscopy is discussed elsewhere in this volume as well as in recent reviews (69,71,77). These reports should be consulted as an introduction to our survey, in which we dwell only on those features of the myelin architecture that are particularly relevant to the interpretation of freeze-fracture images.

The x-ray and neutron diffraction studies of central nervous system (CNS) and peripheral nervous system (PNS) myelin were critically re-evaluated by Kirschner and Caspar (47). They furnished measurements on various species, developing animals, and mice mutants with myelin deficits. Myelin biochemistry was also reviewed recently (33,58). Tentative molecular models of the myelin membrane have been proposed, taking into account the results of recent freeze-fracture studies (12,47).

Figure 2 represents our conception of the myelin sheath in the central and peripheral nervous systems. In both cases the myelin is derived from a glial cell process shaped like a flattened trapezoid. Cytoplasm is excluded from within the central region of the flap to form compact myelin. Cytoplasm is invariably present as a border, or belt (the *marginal cytoplasmic belt*), around the perimeter of the sheath; the sides of this peripheral rim of cytoplasm are designated the *outer, inner,* and *lateral* (paranodal) *belts*. The more conventional terminology—outer, inner, and lateral *loops*—is appropriate for thin sections through these regions but not for the three-dimensional vistas which freeze-fracture replicas afford.

Within the otherwise compact domain, cytoplasm is present in a few restricted areas, known as cytoplasmic incisures, which are distributed irregularly along the internode. These can be oriented longitudinally, circumferentially (as in Schmidt–Lanterman incisures), or obliquely with respect to the long axis of the fiber (59,83,88). In cross sections of peripheral fibers, several longitudinal incisures are often seen in register between adjacent lamellae; these are frequently misinterpreted as Schmidt–Lanterman incisures, which are evident as repeating structures only in longitudinally sectioned fibers. Incisures may be complete (i.e., connecting two sides of the cytoplasmic belt), incomplete, and perhaps even temporarily isolated from the marginal belt. One incisure can join or anastomose with another (59). The idea, then, is of a network of cytoplasm within the central, compact domain. Incisures are much more frequent and regular in peripheral myelinated fibers than in central fibers (41,83). Our combined thin-sec-

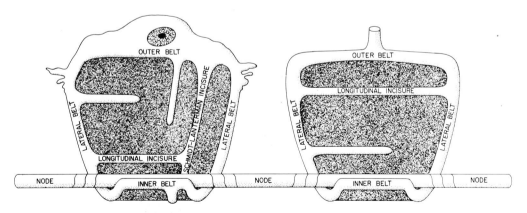

FIG. 2. Diagram showing, with exaggerated proportions, the distribution of cytoplasm in peripheral (*left*) and central (*right*) myelin sheaths. In both cases the sheath is derived from a glial cell process shaped like a trapezoid, with the shorter base apposed to the axon. Cytoplasm is excluded from most of the central region of the sheath to form the compact myelin (*shaded*). Cytoplasm is present as a belt around the perimeter of the sheath. The sides of the cytoplasmic border are termed inner, outer, and lateral (paranodal) belts. Cytoplasm can occur within the otherwise compact domain of the sheath as complete and incomplete longitudinal or circumferential (Schmidt–Lanterman) incisures. Incisures are more frequent and regular in the PNS than in the CNS.

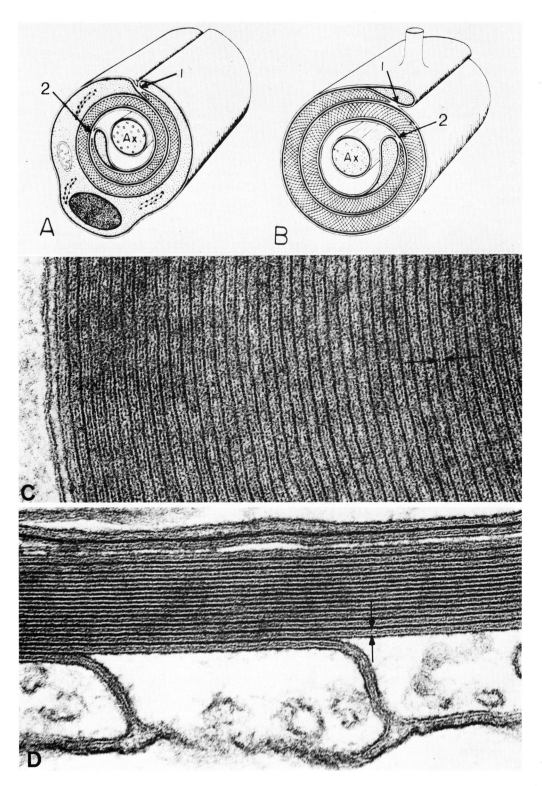

FIG. 3. A and **B:** Peripheral **(A)** and central **(B)** myelin sheaths emphasizing the extent (exaggerated) of the intramyelinic extracellular space (*cross-hatched*), bordered by tight junctions at the outer (1) and inner (2) mesaxons. (Ax) Axon. The periaxonal space is white and unmarked. **C** and **D:** Peripheral **(C)** and central **(D)** myelin sheaths in thin section. Note the paired minor dense lines (*arrows*) delineating a thin extracellular cleft. ×200,000.

tion and freeze-fracture studies (88) have shown that small, longitudinal incisures are more frequent in the CNS than has been appreciated in previous investigations (however, see ref. 41). An improved and detailed account of the distribution of the cytoplasm in the peripheral myelin sheath was recently published (59).

It is now well established that there is a narrow extracellular space maintained between adjacent myelin lamellae in both peripheral and central myelin sheaths. The space extends from the periaxonal space, through the myelin spiral, to the extracellular compartment of the brain or nerve (Fig. 3A and B). In thin sections the intramyelinic space is evident between paired minor dense lines (Fig. 3C and D). On the basis of x-ray diffraction data from fresh frog preparations, this space measures 15 Å in PNS myelin and 6 Å in CNS myelin (106). The intramyelinic space has been repeatedly demonstrated in the PNS with conventional thin section electron microscopy (56,62,88), tracers (80), and glutaraldehyde embedment (37,72). The space within the central myelin has been recognized electron microscopically in edematous brain tissue (44) and in specimens fixed directly in a ferrocyanide-reduced osmium fixative (46,83). In our thin-sectioned material, the intramyelinic space measures 20–30 Å in the PNS and 10–15 Å in the CNS.

FREEZE-FRACTURE PROPERTIES OF THE COMPACT MYELIN MEMBRANE

Freeze cleavage of the compact myelin always produces two kinds of fracture surface (Figs. 4–6). The P-face represents the half-membrane bound to the major dense line (or glial cytoplasm in the case of an incisure); the half-membrane associated with the E-face remains bound to the intramyelinic space (89). Thus, in spite of the close apposition of successive turns of the myelin lamella and the coming together of the cytoplasmic membrane leaflets, the fracture properties of myelin resemble those of other biological membranes.

Initially it was thought that the freeze-fractured myelin membrane was particle-free (6,7, 10,23,51,98) and in this way distinct from most other biological membranes. In fact, this observation seemed consistent with the low protein/lipid ratio of purified myelin (0.2 in the CNS) (63,64,65) relative to other membrane preparations, e.g., 0.52 in isolated erythrocyte membranes (96). Our observations (88,89) and those of others (74,86) indicate that, on the contrary, both central and peripheral myelin contain more than 1,000 particles/ μm^2 of membrane surface. It is probable that differences in preparation of the myelin, most likely fixation, can account for the discrepancy between the recent and the initial findings.

The fracture properties of the intramembrane particles associated with central and peripheral myelin fixed in aldehydes are different in some respects. This is to be expected, of course, given the distinct biochemistry of myelin in the PNS and CNS. In the CNS there is a very definite distribution of particle shapes between rounded and ellipsoidal (Fig. 6a). The ellipsoidal particles are further distinguished by the fact that they cast a small shadow and hence protrude only slightly from the face of the fractured membrane. Each class of particles shows some variation in size, although more variation is seen among the rounded particles. Such a well-defined divergence of particle shape does not ordinarily occur in the randomly distributed particles of other membranes, e.g., the internodal axolemma (Figs. 5 and 21, below). As in most other biological membranes, in CNS myelin the particles fracture almost exclusively with the P-face. In high-resolution replicas, the E-face presents a complementary image in that both elongated and rounded pits can be identified in numbers approaching the distribution of particles on the P-face (89).

In peripheral myelin, ellipsoidal and rounded particles can also be recognized (Fig. 6b). Although most of the particles fracture with the P-face, a large number (many more than in the CNS) of predominantly small particles cleave with the E-face. Pits are generally more difficult to identify. These features of the compact myelin membrane have been found in several warm- and cold-blooded species (88).

It should be made clear that the relationship between the randomly distributed freeze-fracture particles and membrane associated proteins is only superficially understood for even

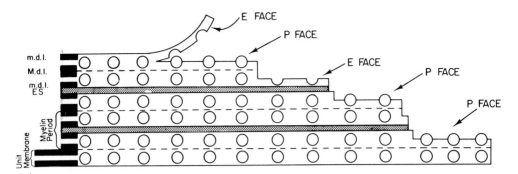

FIG. 4. Fracture properties of the compact myelin in the CNS. The intramyelinic extracellular space (ES) between adjacent lamellae is stippled. The major dense line (M.d.l.) is represented by the dashed line, and the minor dense lines are labeled m.d.l. The P-face of the fractured myelin membrane remains bound to the major dense line, and the E-face to the extracellular space. In central myelin most of the particles remain associated with the P-face, and pits are seen on the E-face. In peripheral myelin, many particles also cleave with the E-face.

the most well characterized membranes. Although certain known integral membrane proteins can be identified with some freeze-fracture particles (13,29,99), many essential relationships are simply not known. For example, it is not known to what extent a protein must interact with the bilayer to be evident as a freeze-fracture particle. It is not known whether all integral membrane proteins can be identified as freeze-fracture particles. It is not known how to distinguish between particles representing monomeric species, protein aggregates, or lipid-protein complexes. Until these uncertainties are clarified, it is difficult to discuss the relationship of the particles associated with the freeze-fractured compact myelin and the proteins characterized in myelin fractions (63). The likelihood of certain relationships, however, should be pointed out. The proteolipid protein in the central myelin and the major glycoprotein in the peripheral myelin have the biochemical properties of integral membrane proteins (12, 91) and, therefore, are expected to be evident in freeze-fractured myelin, although peripheral glycoproteins related to particle free membranes have been seen in certain cells (73). The basic proteins, on the other hand, have the properties of peripheral membrane proteins (12, 91) and would be less likely to appear as a freeze-fracture particle (89). Interestingly, Mateu et al. (53) found that when central or peripheral basic proteins were incorporated into artificial lamellar phase lipid bilayers the preparations assumed the repeat periods corresponding to central and

peripheral myelin, respectively. Freeze-fracture faces of these preparations did not have particles.

Although meaningful correlations between the freeze-fracture particles and the myelin proteins are at this time impossible, the selective extraction of some of the protein components from myelin fractions together with freeze-fracture analysis, or the incorporation of purified myelin proteins into artificial membrane preparations, as Mateu and his coworkers have already attempted, are likely to provide some of the information necessary to establish valid relationships. For this reason, detailed analysis of the different particle types associated with the freeze-cleaved myelin membrane is important. Furthermore, such information is useful by itself in drawing relationships between different types of myelin. For example, the difference in the appearance of the fracture faces of central and peripheral myelin must be related to their distinct protein compositions. Interaction between proteins of neighboring lamellae may be involved in maintaining interlamellar adhesion (12,74,89). The larger amount of glycoproteins in peripheral sheaths may be reflected by the larger extracellular spaces and the numerous E face particles demonstrable in our replicas. Before compaction of the sheath, immature myelin membranes (Fig. 10) have few intramembrane particles in accordance with developmental biochemical data on protein composition of myelin fractions (104). Perhaps extensive studies of abnormal and normal myelin will

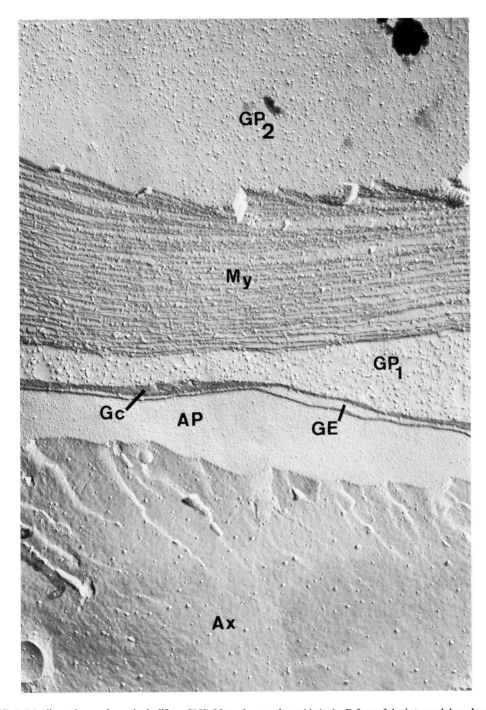

FIG. 5. Myelinated axon from the bullfrog CNS. Note the axoplasm (Ax), the P-face of the internodal axolemma (AP), the E-face of the first glial membrane (GE), the inner belt of glial cytoplasm (Gc), the P-face of the second glial membrane (GP₁), several obliquely fractured myelin lamellae (My), and a particle-studded fracture face (GP₂) similar in appearance to GP₁. Note that the particles distributed on the axonal P-face are different from those on the myelinic P-face. ×55,125.

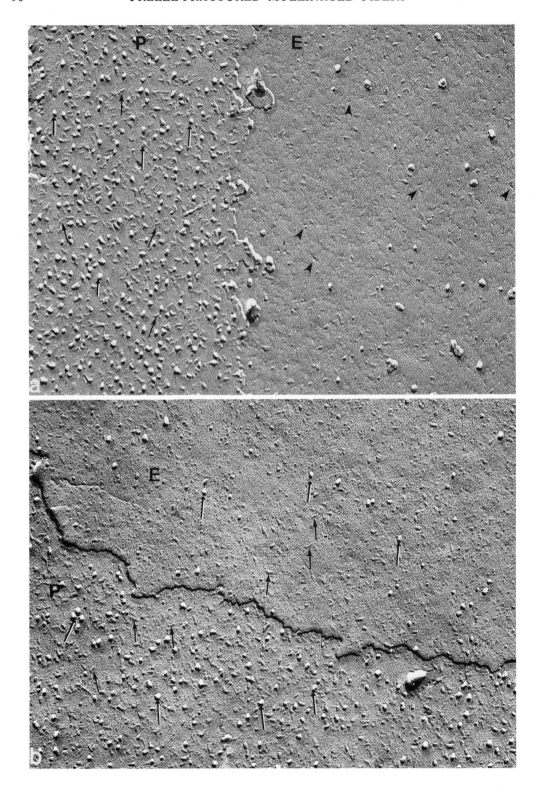

reveal differences in particle populations. Comparisons should be made between specimens treated in identical ways. This is a very important point since we are well aware that the structural details, such as particle shape, size and distribution, are dependent on factors such as whether or not the tissue has been fixed prior to glycerination.

INTRAMYELINIC JUNCTIONS

Myelinic Zonula Occludens

In thin sections of well-preserved myelinated fibers, spots of membrane fusion (indicating the presence of a tight junction) are found in the CNS and PNS at the following sites (60, 88): (a) the inner and outer mesaxons of peripheral myelin and the corresponding sites in central fibers; (b) between adjacent paranodal loops; and (c) between membranes enclosing cytoplasmic incisures. It is interesting that in his pioneering studies Robertson (84) noticed the existence of spots of membrane fusion at the external mesaxon, although at that time their identification as tight junctions was not appreciated.

Freeze-fracture shows (60,88) that each of these tight junctional sites is part of a continuous zonula occludens, which follows the entire cytoplasm-containing perimeter of the myelin sheath and extends into the cytoplasmic incisures (Figs. 7–11). Like tight junctions in many other tissues, the junctional subunit consists of a strand or sometimes a row of particles; the strands are apparently shared by the adjoined membranes and, in general, fracture as a single unit with the P-face of one membrane, leaving a groove on the complementary E-face (94,103). Occasionally, small fragments of the strand remain attached to the E-face, leaving a space in the otherwise continuous strand on the P-face (Figs. 8 and 9).

In the myelin the strands assume a parallel array and do not anastomose. There can be anywhere from a single to a dozen parallel strands at a given location. In fortunate fractures, it can be seen that one tight junctional strand can continue, uninterrupted, around the corners of the glial trapezoid (88), e.g., from the outer mesaxon through the paranodal region. On the other hand, within a single fiber the number of tight junctions may vary at the different sides of the trapezoid; for example, in Fig. 9 two strands are present along a portion of the external mesaxon and three strands are evident at the paranodal border. Occasionally, strands end abruptly (Fig. 9b, arrow).

The parallel array of the tight junctional strands in the myelin is somewhat unusual; in most other tissues, the strands anastomose extensively (18,27,94,102). Other exceptions, where the strands can have a parallel arrangement, are the Sertoli cell tight junctions in the seminiferous epithelium (31), tight junctions between hair and supporting cells in the reticular lamina of the organ of Corti (34), in the epithelium of the choroid plexus (14), and in certain regions of the snake nephron (67).

Claude and Goodenough (18) have examined a variety of epithelial tissues with the freeze-fracture method to see if the structure of the tight junction was different in tight and leaky epithelia. Their findings showed that, in general, a correlation did exist between the width and complexity of the junctional network and the tightness of the epithelium. According to their criteria the myelinic zonula occludens might be classified as moderately leaky.[1]

---

[1] Other investigators, however, have denied a strict correlation between the extensiveness of the tight junctional network and the permeability of the extracellular pathway across the epithelium (Martinez-Palomo, A. and Erleij, D.: *PNAS, 72:* 4487–91, 1975.; Mollgard, K., Malinowska, D. H., and Saunders, N. R.: *Nature* 264:293–4, 1976.) and suggested that the permeability properties of the tight junction reside in an aspect of their molecular structure not evident in the electron microscope.

←

FIG. 6. P- and E-faces of the central (**a**) and peripheral (**b**) compact myelin membranes in the bullfrog. Elliptical (*black arrows*) and rounded (*black and white arrows*) particles are evident in central and peripheral myelin. Compared to the rounded particles, the elongated ones protrude only slightly from the fracture surface. In the CNS almost all of the particles cleave with the P-face, leaving rounded and elongated pits (*arrowheads*) on the E-face. In the PNS, numerous particles, many of which are smaller than the round particles of central myelin, remain bound to the E-face. ×120,000.

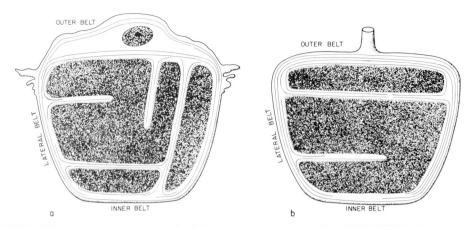

FIG. 7. Localization of the zonula occludens with respect to the cytoplasmic domains of the peripheral (*left*) and central (*right*) myelin sheaths. Individual strands are represented by the lines. The strands run in parallel array in the plasmalemma along the cytoplasmic border and continue into that of the incisures. Some strands continue uninterrupted around the corners of the sheath, whereas others end blindly. Thus within a given fiber the number of tight junctional strands can vary at different sites within the sheath. To simplify the presentation of this scheme, the paranodal tight junction is represented on the face of the lateral belt. In reality, this aspect of the glial membrane is junctionally apposed to the paranodal axon membrane; the tight junction is located on the side of the lateral belt.

The functional significance of the intramyelinic tight junction is still largely a matter of speculation. As in other tissues, where the zonulae occludentes apparently provide a barrier to intercellular diffusion (95), electron dense tracers (e.g., peroxidase, microperoxidase, and ferritin) are excluded from the intramyelinic compartment when these substances are applied to a live preparation (26,68,60, 100). Lanthanum has been found to penetrate the intramyelinic space, apparently passing through the zonula occludens (35,62,80). This result is difficult to interpret, however, since the lanthanum is usually applied with a fixative, and this could change the properties of the tight junctions; it is a fact that glutaraldehyde–lanthanum alters the permeability of gap junctions (5). Even when a live preparation is exposed to this tracer (42), the interpretation is not straightforward since lanthanum itself can provoke tissue necrosis (see, however, ref. 97). The extent to which the myelinic zonula occludens provides a permeability barrier thus remains to be measured. Clearly the matter deserves further attention.

Besides isolating an intramyelinic extracellular compartment and thus reducing radial diffusion in the internodal region of the sheath, the tight junction may help in several ways to maintain the compact wrapping of the myelin

$\longrightarrow$

FIG. 8. Zonula occludens at the external mesaxon in the PNS (**b**) and at the corresponding site in the CNS (**a**). **a:** The axoplasm (ax) and several compact myelin lamellae (m) of this fiber have been cross-fractured (*top*). An unrelated glial membrane (gl), probably from an astrocytic process, passes above the myelinated axon. The outer belt of glial cytoplasm is indicated between the arrows. The parallel, tight junctional strands (*arrowhead*) have remained bound to the P-face (P) of the lamella underlying the outer belt. In the lower portion of the figure, the fracture plane passes through the membrane of the outer belt, exposing its E-face (E). Parallel furrows can be seen at the asterisk, where the strands have fractured with the discarded half of the outer belt membrane. ×30,000. **b:** The axoplasm (ax) and compact myelin (m) have been cross-fractured (*bottom*). The outer belt of Schwann cell cytoplasm is marked by the asterisk. The P-faces of the Schwann cell surface (PS) and the first myelin lamella (P_1) underlying the outer belt are exposed. The tight junctional strands bound to the latter membrane face are indicated by the arrows. Note the stomata of caveolae on the outer surface of the Schwann cell surface (*arrowheads*). Their distribution and functional significance is treated in a separate account (59). ×37,-000.

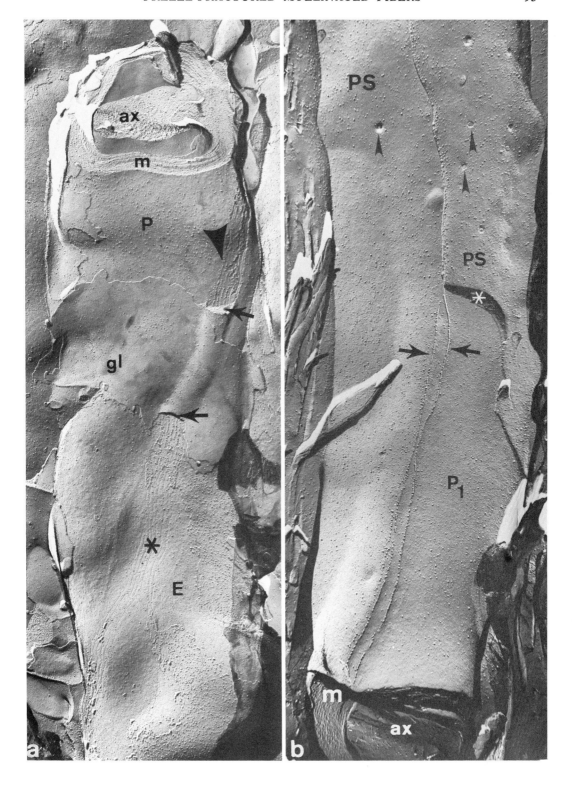

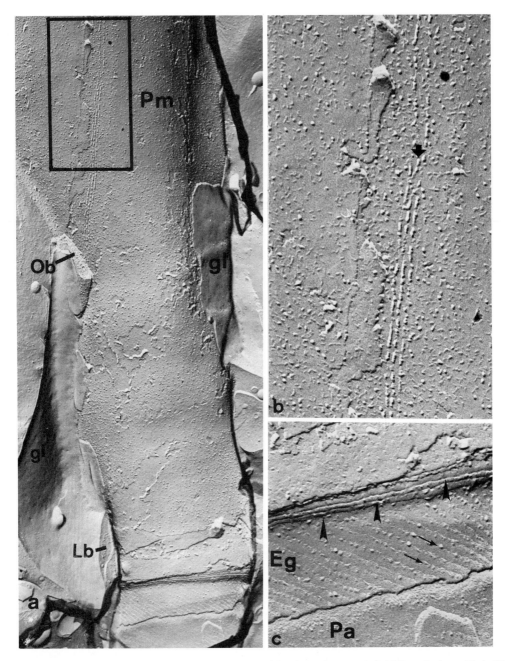

FIG. 9. a: Myelinic zonula occludens in the region of transition from the outer belt (Ob) to the lateral belt (Lb) in a central fiber from the bullfrog. The membrane of a separate glial cell process (gl) lies over the surface of this particular fiber. At the bottom of the figure, the fracture process exposed the E-face of the paranodal glial membrane (i.e., the lateral belt) and the junctionally apposed axonal P-face. These are shown, labeled, at higher magnification in **c.** At the top of the figure, the P-face (Pm) of the first myelin lamella subjacent to the outer belt is shown. The area enclosed within the rectangle is shown at higher magnification in **b.** ×37,000. **b:** The tight junctional strands are bound to the P-face of the first myelin lamella underlying the outer belt. Three parallel strands are evident at the bottom of the figure. One ends blindly (*arrow*) whereas the other two continue. ×95,-000. **c:** The portion of the glial E-face (Eg), which is junctionally apposed to the axolemma (Pa), has coinciding undulations and chains of globules (*arrows*). Three tight junctional furrows (*arrowheads*) are present on that aspect of the glial membrane which turns away from the axolemma and faces the adjacent turn of the lateral belt. ×95,000.

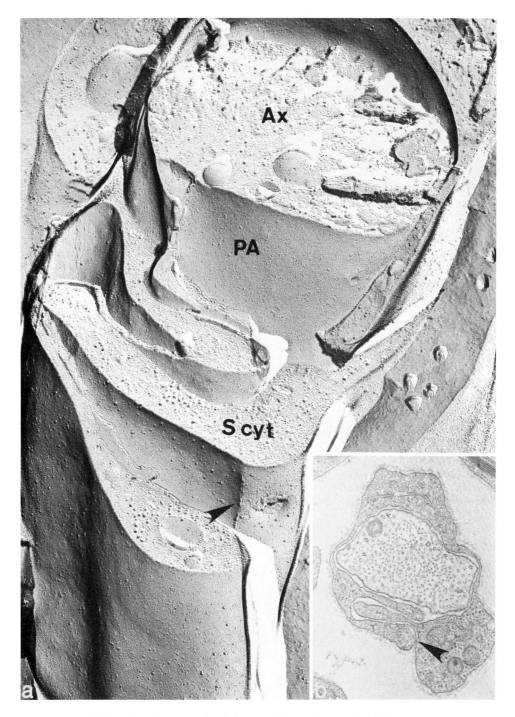

FIG. 10. Zonula occludens in an immature sheath from the developing rat trigeminal nerve. The axoplasm (Ax) has been cross-fractured and the axonal P-face (Pa) exposed. The axon is enveloped within a loose spiral of Schwann cell cytoplasm (S cyt). The strand of a tight junction is evident on the P-face of the Schwann cell process at the outer aspect of the spiral (*arrowhead*) corresponding to the outer mesaxon. Note that there are fewer P-face particles than in mature fibers. ×66,000. **Inset:** Matching thin section of a rat trigeminal fiber at a similar stage of myelination. The arrowhead marks a point of membrane contact indicating the occurrence of the tight junction. ×32,000.

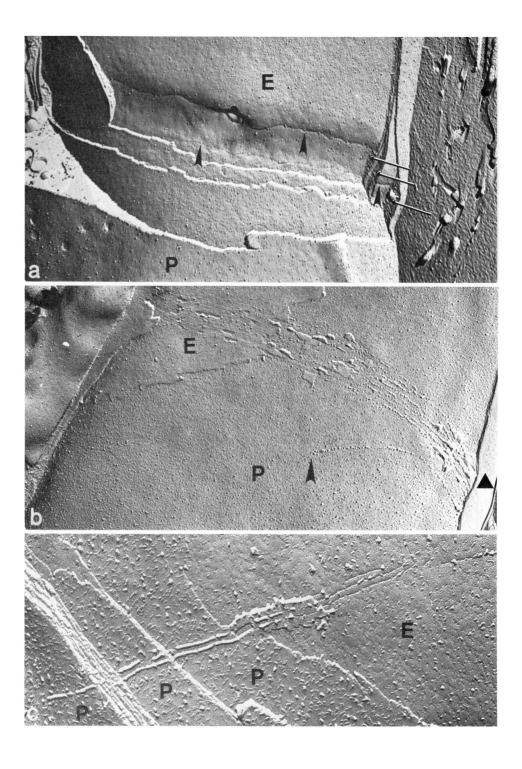

sheath. There is good evidence that, in certain epithelia the zonula occludens also provides a site for cell-to-cell attachment as well as a barrier to extracellular diffusion (103). Other consequences of the myelinic zonula occludens may be a restriction on lateral diffusion of proteins between compact and cytoplasmic domains of the myelin sheath[2] and the sequestration of autoantigenic components (60) within an isolated extracellular compartment.

We noticed that the myelinic tight junction is at least partially established at a very early stage of myelination, well before compaction takes place (Fig. 10). It is therefore possible that this junction contributes to the myelination process itself. A detailed study of myelination with thin sections and freeze-fracture is in progress.

An interesting observation, related to the presence of the zonula occludens along the cytoplasmic incisures, is the existence of tight junctions within the compact myelin, apparently in the absence of an incisure (Fig. 11b and c). Frequently these strands are seen in register between successive lamellae (23,79, 89). In these cases the arrangement and orientation of the tight junctions resemble the arrangement and orientation of the various incisures that can occur in central and peripheral sheaths. Focal, disoriented arrays of tight junctional strands within a single lamella are also

---

[2] One may expect that the distribution of intramembrane particles at the outer surface of the sheath is different from that in the inner turns of the myelin lamella. In fact, we obtained some replicas from peripheral nerves where there is a difference in the density of particles on the two sides of the zonula occludens. However, this has not yet been documented definitely.

seen on occasion (89). These observations, taken together, have led us to speculate that the formation of a tight junction might precede the intrusion of cytoplasm during the genesis of an incisure and/or that the tight junction remains following involution of an incisure. It has also been suggested (23,79) that the tight junctions within the compact myelin represent the so-called radial component (70). This conclusion is debatable (89), especially since staining of the tight junctional fibril—whether single or double (16,103)—has not been demonstrated in other epithelia.

The variations in the number and patterns of tight junctional strands in different myelin sheaths, and in different portions of the same internode, may render it difficult to recognize pathological alterations of the myelinic zonula occludens.

Gap Junctions and Adherent Junctions

Besides the zonula occludens, which is a regular feature at the periphery of the central and peripheral myelin sheath, other intramyelinic junctions are less consistently observed. Our own unpublished observations and those of others (36,55) demonstrated, in thin sections, the frequent occurrence of isolated and serial adherent junctions at the sites where we now know the tight junction to be located. As is often the case with intermediate junctions in other tissues (95), those in the myelin are apparently not associated with an intramembrane structure identifiable in freeze-fracture replicas.

We and others (86) also noted a few cases in which gap junctions are associated with the myelinic zonula occludens in the regions of the

---

←

FIG. 11. a: Tight junctions associated with a Schmidt–Lanterman incisure in a peripheral myelinated fiber. The incisure is successively cross-fractured (*arrows*) as it follows a circumferential path around the axon. The arrowheads point to furrows left by the tight junctional strands which adjoin adjacent levels of the incisure. The E-face (E) of a myelin lamella containing the tight junction and the P-face of the Schwann cell surface (P) have been exposed. ×45,000. b: Circumferential tight junctions in a myelinated axon from the turtle CNS. The P-face (P) of one myelin lamella contains a group of tight junctional strands, and the E-face (E) of the junctionally apposed myelin lamella has parallel furrows. The arrowhead points to a strand which diverges from the group and ends abruptly. Whether these tight junctions are associated with a cytoplasmic incisure is not clear. If present, cytoplasm should have been apparent at the triangle. ×43,800. c: Central myelin in the bullfrog showing longitudinally oriented tight junctions in register between successive compact lamellae. The fracture properties of these junctions are identical to those associated with the cytoplasmic incisures; the fibrils cleave with the P-face (P), leaving furrows on the E-face (E). ×75,000.

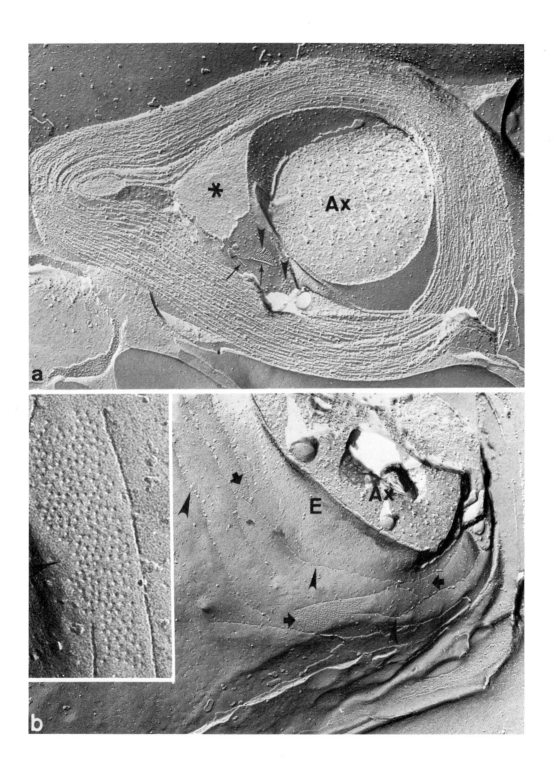

outer, inner, and lateral belts (Fig. 12). In our material these are very rare, but this may, in part, be a sampling problem since the gap junction may occupy only a very small fraction of the total membrane surface in a given fiber. The vertebrate gap junctions are recognized on the P-face by closely packed (only sometimes in hexagonal array) particles with a definite subunit structure (32). The complementary E-face has well-defined and similarly spaced pits. As illustrated, the myelin gap junctions are relatively small and are always closely associated with the tight junctional strands. There is good evidence that gap junctions provide a system of channels which allow ions and small molecules to flow between adjoining cells (4,30,32,52,68,95). Considering this as their primary function, it is not apparent why gap junctions exist between different parts of the same cell, already connected by a large cytoplasmic channel and only a few micrometers apart. Reflexive gap junctions have been observed in other types of cells (38,45, 75).

In some of our pictures there seems to be a noteworthy correlation between the presence of the gap junction and a subtle alteration in the arrangement of the associated zonula occludens. Instead of the usual continuous and parallel strands, there is a marked tendency for some strands to be short, discontinuous, and disoriented. The small gap junctions are very closely associated with these discontinuous strands (Fig. 12a and b). Very similar configurations were found to accompany the reorganization of the cell junctions between neuroepithelial cells during neurulation (21). Thus we wonder whether the expression of the gap junction, the tight junction, and desmosomoid

attachments are somehow regulated together, e.g., at the level of protein synthesis of the junctional subunits or at the level of their incorporation and assembly within the membrane. In support of this idea is the very general coincidence of these structures in many types of tissue. The formation of a complex of junctions rather than of the tight junction alone may be related in some way to the presence of interruptions of the tight junctional strands. A remote possibility is that the junctional complexes are the result of a partially successful repair process following focal pathology.

Gap junctions may also exist at the surface of myelin sheaths (86) and perhaps also between oligodendrocytic cell bodies (61,69,92).

PARANODAL AXOGLIAL JUNCTION

The myelin sheath has the shape of a trapezoid, positioned so that its shorter base is apposed to the axon (Fig. 2). Consequently, the lateral belts of the sheath follow a tight, helical path toward the node as the myelin winds around the axon. The area of apposition between the lateral belt and the axon, designated the paranodal region, is a transitional zone separating the internodal region proper from the node of Ranvier.

The paranodal region is of great interest to the neurocytologist. By virtue of the path followed by the lateral belt, each myelin lamella is brought into direct contact with the paranodal axolemma. Actually, the lateral belt leaves an imprint on the axon surface (Figs. 13 and 14). With the exception of a narrow spiral band, which continues from the internodal to the nodal portion, the paranodal axolemma presents special features. Here is

←

FIG. 12. Gap junctions associated with the myelin sheath. **a**: Myelinated fiber from the bullfrog CNS. The fiber has been cross-fractured, exposing the axoplasm (Ax) and the inner belt of glial cytoplasm (*). The myelin sheath surrounding the axon is redundant (*left side*). Tight junctional strands (*arrows*) and two focal gap junctions (*arrowheads*) can be identified on the P-face of the inner belt. Note that the upper of the two gap junctions is associated with a short, discontinuous strand of the zonula occludens. ×45,000. **b**: Myelinated fiber axon from the bullfrog CNS in the paranodal region. The axoplasm (Ax) has been cross-fractured and a portion of the glial E-face (E) participating in the axoglial junction exposed. Tight junctional furrows (*arrowheads*) are seen where the glial membrane turns away from the axolemma to face the neighboring turn of the lateral belt. Notice that the furrows are discontinuous and end abruptly (compare this with the usual, continuous parallel array in Figs. 8 and 9). The location of three gap junctions (*arrows*) is marked by the presence of closely packed pits. ×80,000. **Inset**: Gap junction at higher magnification. Pits are distinguished from particles by their inverted shadow. The direction of platinum shadowing in the inset points from left to right (*arrowhead*). ×210,000.

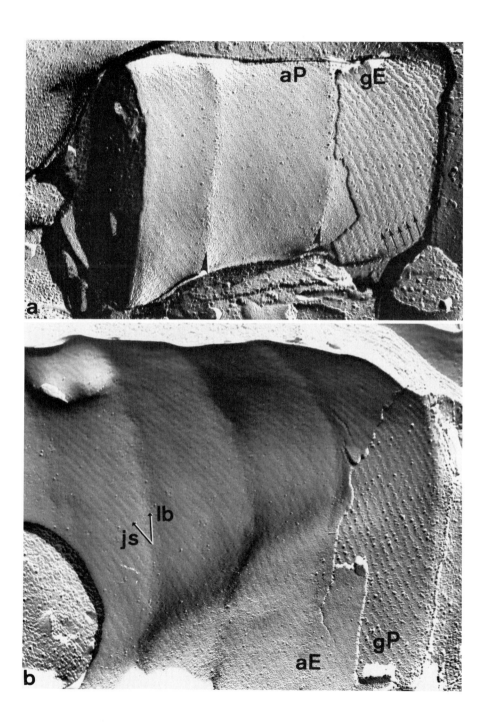

formed an extensive and unusual intercellular junction between the axon and the glial cell which ensheaths it. In fact, this is the only specialized zone of contact between these two cells. A second noteworthy feature is that each node of Ranvier is bordered on either side by the paranodes of two successive myelin segments (Fig. 15). The Ranvier nodes, of course, are specialized domains of the axon involved in generating the action potential (Cahalan, *this volume*). One might expect, therefore, that the structural integrity of the paranodal regions is critical for maintenance of the nodal physiology. In fact, this seems to be the case. In an elegant study of diphtheria toxin-induced demyelination in ventral roots, Rasminsky and Sears (78) clearly showed that slowing of conduction in single nerve fibers (prior to conduction block) is accompanied by changes in the passive electrical characteristics of the paranodal regions. Moreover, their findings suggest that these zones of the fiber are a primary locus for action of the toxin. The reader is referred to Rasminsky (*this volume*) for further discussion of the physiology of demyelination.

Several descriptions of the paranodal axoglial junction have been published (24,51,86, 90). What follows is a discussion of the junctional organization as we understand it. A detailed discussion on the diversity of opinion concerning the structure of the axoglial junction is available elsewhere (90). The emphasis in this account is on the morphology of the junction in the CNS. The corresponding junction in the PNS is similar (90).

The axoglial junction does not immediately conform to any known class of intercellular junction, although some aspects of its organization are reminiscent of septate junctions (95). Where the paranodal glial and axonal membranes are junctionally apposed (Figs. 15 and 16), the intercellular space is reduced to approximately 30 Å and is interrupted by regularly repeating septa (Fig. 15a)—the "transverse bands" (Hirano and Dembitzer, *this volume*). These septa have a diagonal orientation with respect to the long axis of the lateral belt. Within the region of junctional contact the glial and axonal membranes are undulated in a regular manner such that the crests of the undulations coincide with the intercellular septa (Fig. 16b). Finally, within both junctional membranes there are chains of globules that are in register with the undulations and therefore with the intercellular septa (Figs. 13–18). The angle at which the undulations and chains of particles (and most likely the septa) are oriented with respect to the lateral belt varies between species. In birds and cold-blooded vertebrates, the acute angle between the junctional components and the long axis of the lateral belt is approximately 30°. In mammals this angle is considerably less and may approach 0°, in which case the junctional features would follow the lateral belt (24,42,86). This variation accounts for some of the divergence of opinion concerning the organization of this junction.

Although the axoglial junction has symmetrical features (i.e., both membranes have undulations and chains of particles that coincide with the intercellular septa), there is a striking and undeniably asymmetrical character to the junction. This is evident in the

←

FIG. 13. The four fracture faces associated with the axoglial junction in central myelinated axons in the turtle. **a:** The glial E-face (gE) and axonal P-face (aP) have been exposed. The junctional specializations associated with the glial membrane are more obvious and regular than those of the axonal membrane. The glial membrane is undulated and contains parallel chains of particles in register with shallow grooves (*arrows*). These particles cleave with either fracture face. The axonal P-face is also undulated and contains chains of particles in register with those of the glial membrane (Fig. 17). These features are not obvious in this particular micrograph. The arrowheads point to the aspect of the axolemma which faces the space between the paranodal loops. This nonjunctional spiral band of the membrane is covered with randomly distributed particles. ×75,000. **b:** View of the axoglial junction complementary to that shown in **a.** The axonal E-face (aE) appears above the glial P-face (gP). The undulations of the axonal membrane are much more obvious in this figure. Their coincidence with the undulations and chains of particles in the glial membrane are most clearly seen at the top right-hand side of the figure. Note that the chains of the particles within the glial P-face are situated on narrow ridges. On the left side of the figure, the long axis of the lateral belt (lb) and the axis of the junctional specializations (js) are indicated together. The acute angle between them is usually 30° in submammalian species. ×62,000.

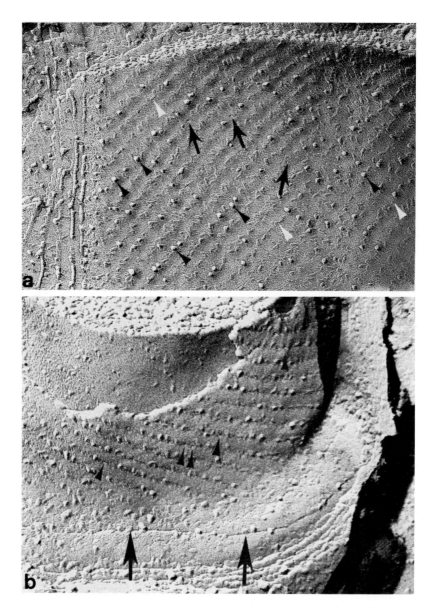

FIG. 14. The glial membrane shows very little variation in its fracture properties. **a**: P-face. The chains of particles (*black arrowheads*) are situated on the ridges of the undulations. Where a particle has cleaved with the E-face, a pit (*black arrow*) or a small protrusion (*white arrowhead*) is evident. **b**: E-face. The particles are situated in shallow grooves. Pits (*arrowheads*) are recognized where a particle has cleaved with the P-face. The paranodal tight junction is marked by arrows. ×95,000.

very different fracture properties of the two membranes. In fixed or unfixed specimens, the glial membrane fractures such that the junctional particles remain attached to either membrane half with approximately equal frequency. The particles are always rigidly aligned in rows and the undulations are always evident (Figs. 13–15). In the axonal membrane, the undulations and the chains of particles are usually less obvious (Figs. 13, 15, and 17). When the particles are apparent, they remain strictly with the P-face. The most striking and distinctive characteristic of the axonal membrane, however, is the variability in the appearance of its fracture faces. For example, the P-face can be completely flat with no particles (Fig. 17a), flat with chains of particles (Fig. 17b), undulated with no particles (Fig. 17c), or undulated with chains of particles (Fig. 17d). Furthermore, the extracellular half of the membrane (face E) sometimes contains a unique crystalline array of tiny subunits superimposed on its usual features (Fig. 18). The morphology of this array varies in the extent to which the tiny subunits are resolved. When present, the array is usually recognized as a series of diagonal striations situated on the junctional ridges of the E-face (Figs. 18a and 19b). Only in a very small fraction of cases were we able to distinguish the individual subunits; Fig. 18a is by far the clearest example we have encountered. Also the E-face appears flat in some replicas (Fig. 18b).

The elusiveness of the junctional components associated with the axolemma also distinguishes this junction from other intercellular junctions. By contrast, the fracture properties and appearance of gap, tight, and septate junctions are perhaps the most stable and invariant features associated with freeze-fractured cell membranes.

The source of the variability and whether it has a functional significance are important questions. At present, we believe that all of the variations are, for the most part, independent of the resolution of the replica. It is probable that the fixation procedure, which generally varies among animals owing to the difficulties in preparing nervous tissue for electron microscopy, accounts for some of the variation; for instance, the undulations of the axolemma are usually most obvious in unfixed specimens (Figs. 17b, 18c, and 19b). Since the junctional axolemma appears discontinuous in standard thin sections (90), one may also consider the possibility that it contains saturated lipids with a crystalline packing or that it is occasionally split off-center by freeze-fracturing. Whatever the complete explanation, the fracture properties of the axolemma make it difficult to construct even a supramolecular model for the junctional organization. Our schema presented in Fig. 16b is therefore only tentative.

If the variations of the freeze-fractured junctional membrane appear independently of

the conditions of the tissue under investigation, neuropathological evaluation of the paranodal structure may be very difficult. Assuming that our observations are valid across the species, the integrity of the axoglial junction can be evaluated more reliably by studying the glial than the axolemmal fracture faces.

In evaluating pathological material one should also keep in mind that several kinds of irregularity in the arrangement of the junctional features on the axonal membrane occur in normal material. Some of these were illustrated by Schnapp et al. (90). Others are presented here in Figs. 19 and 20. Large patches of randomly distributed particles may interrupt the otherwise continuous, junctionally specialized membrane (Fig. 19a). These patches may correspond to an area of the paranodal axolemma apposed to a localized area of compact myelin or to an unattached or partially attached loop, features which have been observed in thin sections. Disoriented patches of junctional membrane may exist within the otherwise regularly arranged membrane (Fig. 19b). In the latter case, the patches tend to be localized at the border of the internodal and paranodal regions. Cases where not all the turns of the lateral belt make contact with the axolemma (Fig. 20) may create difficulties of interpretation.

Despite the greater insight into the structural organization of the axoglial junction provided by the freeze-fracture method, its functional significance remains an imposing question. It has been suggested that the junction serves to impede the flow of ions between the nodal and periaxonal extracellular compartments (17), an assumption that is consistent with the conduction properties of myelinated axons. This notion receives some support from tracer experiments. When peroxidase is applied to a live preparation, it is generally excluded from the periaxonal space (43), apparently by virtue of the axoglial junction. Microperoxidase (26) and lanthanum (42) can pass, at least to some extent, through the paranodal extracellular space. The narrow spiral channel between the apposing turns of the lateral belt and the fractionated extracellular space between the septa may account for some degree of diffusion, although the labyrinthine nature of the space may be sufficient to slow

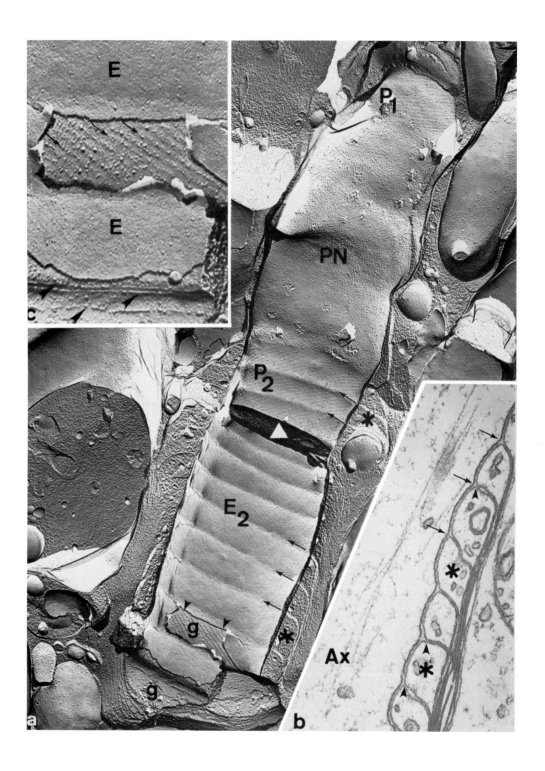

substantially the movement of even small solutes and ions.

Contribution of cation binding materials to the electric phenomena at peripheral nodes has been suggested (49,50). A possible direct role of the axoglial junction in saltatory conduction was considered by Livingston et al. (51). It has been shown that the axoglial junction serves to attach the myelin sheath to the axon and that it can be split in tissue-cultured peripheral nerves by exposure to low calcium (8) or small amounts of trypsin (107). In both cases, the paranodal loops retract, with consequent widening of the nodal region.

Telescoping of the myelin sheath *in vivo* in several pathological conditions (2) also involves an alteration to the axoglial junction. Excessive pressure is one of the conditions provoking telescoping (66). Evidently, the axoglial junction is of primary biomechanical importance.

Beyond this, there are very few data bearing directly on the functional significance of the axoglial junction. We are intrigued by the curious relationship of the neuron and the myelinating glial cell. During development, the axons of only certain neurons are "identified" by the glial cell and myelinated. Once initiated, myelin formation is coupled to the growth of the axon (27). After myelination is complete, if the axon is cut, glial cells associated with myelin segments removed from the site of the lesion react to the axonal degeneration. Of course, one wonders whether these activities are mediated through the paranodal junction.

INTERNODAL AND NODAL AXOLEMMA

The freeze-fractured internodal axolemma is unspecialized in the sense that it is generally devoid of any regular array of membrane particles. Livingston et al. (51) and Sandri et al. (86) indicated that the axoglial junction continues through the internodal region between the inner belt of glial cytoplasm and the axolemma. Our own observations indicate that the junction is restricted to the paranodal region; rarely, however, a small focal spot of junctional membrane can be observed on the E- or P-face of the internodal axon (90).

The P-face of the internodal axolemma has $\sim$ 1,600 particles/μm^2 distributed at random over the fracture surface. Morphologically, they seem to constitute a relatively homogeneous population; virtually all of the particles are rounded and measure 70–120 Å (Figs. 5 and 21). In poorly fixed specimens (Fig. 25b,

←

FIG. 15. Paranodal axoglial junction in the CNS. **a**: Starting from the top of the figure, the fracture process has exposed the axonal P-face (P$_1$) at the very end of one paranodal region, at the node of Ranvier (PN), and at the next paranodal region (P$_2$). At the triangle, the fracture plane cuts across the axoplasm and then cleaves to the paranodal axolemma, now exposing its E-face (E$_2$). At the arrowheads the fracture plane jumps across the intercellular space and continues through the junctionally apposed glial membrane, exposing its P-face (g). Another portion of the same glial P-face can be seen at the bottom. This region of the replica is shown at higher magnification in **c**. The axon surface at the paranode is regularly indented by the lateral belt as the latter winds in a tight helical path around the axon. The lateral belt has been cross-fractured and appears as a series of paranodal loops (*) in register with the indentations. The arrows point along several portions of the narrow band between the indentations which face the extracellular space between paranodal loops. The corresponding points in thin sections are also indicated by arrows in **b**. Within the region of the indentations, the glial and axonal membranes are junctionally apposed. The indentations of the axonal P-faces contain diagonally oriented components, which are illustrated at higher magnification and in more detail in **B** and **C**. The corresponding junctional specializations in the glial membrane are more obvious. ×31,200. **b**. Matching thin section through the paranodal region. The paranodal loops (*) and the axoplasm (Ax) are labeled. The arrows point to the space between neighboring loops. Between the arrows the lateral belt indents the surface of the axon as their membranes become junctionally apposed. This specimen was fixed with ferrocyanide–osmium; note that in the region of junctional apposition between the arrows, the membranes are regularly undulated. The transverse bands (intercellular septa) are just barely evident at this magnification. At the arrowheads the tight junctions between paranodal loops are well resolved. ×60,000. **c**. High magnification of the lower portion of **a**. The chains of particles within the glial P-face (*arrows*) are oriented at an angle of approximately 30° with respect to the long axis of the lateral belt. The axonal E-face (E) in this fiber appears flat. The arrowheads point to the strands of the tight junction on that portion of the glial membrane which turns away from the axolemma and faces the adjacent turn of the lateral belt. ×81,000.

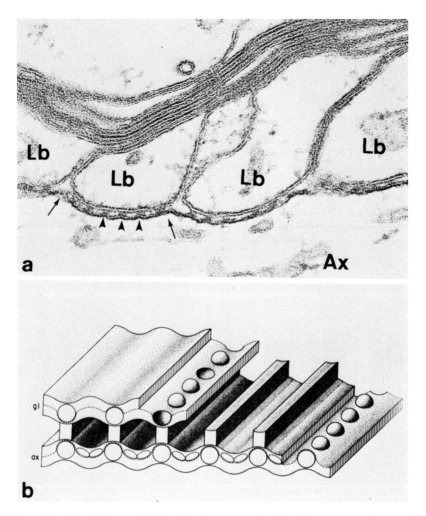

FIG. 16. a: Thin section through the axoglial junction from a specimen fixed in potassium ferrocyanide–osmium. This fixative preserves the trilaminar appearance of both junctional membranes, the intercellular septa, and the undulations. The septa appear to be in register with the crests of the undulations of the axolemma (*arrowheads*). (Lb) Lateral belt. (Ax) Axoplasm. ×240,000. **B:** A segment of the junction, equivalent to that represented between the two arrows in **A,** is represented. This shows a tentative model of the junction and attempts to combine features seen in thin sections and in freeze-fracture replicas. The glial (gl) and axonal (ax) membranes are undulated such that the crests of the undulations coincide with the intercellular septa (transverse bands). The dashed line indicates the fracture plane; only the glial E-face and the axonal P-face are shown. The chains of particles in the glial membrane cleave with either fracture face. The corresponding particles in the axonal membrane, when they are apparent, fracture exclusively with the P-face. The crystalline array occasionally encountered on the axonal E-face is represented by paired subunits. The location of the latter within the outer half of the axolemma, lateral to the septa, is tentative.

below) the particles clump in the plane of the membrane. The internodal E-face has only ~ 200 particles/μm²; pits are difficult to demonstrate (Fig. 21).

The axolemma at the node of Ranvier is of special interest since it is here that the voltage-sensitive ion channels responsible for the generation of the action potential are known to reside. Although this region does not contain any regular array of freeze-fracture particles, it is noteworthy that the nodal E-face as well as the P-face contain a large number of par-

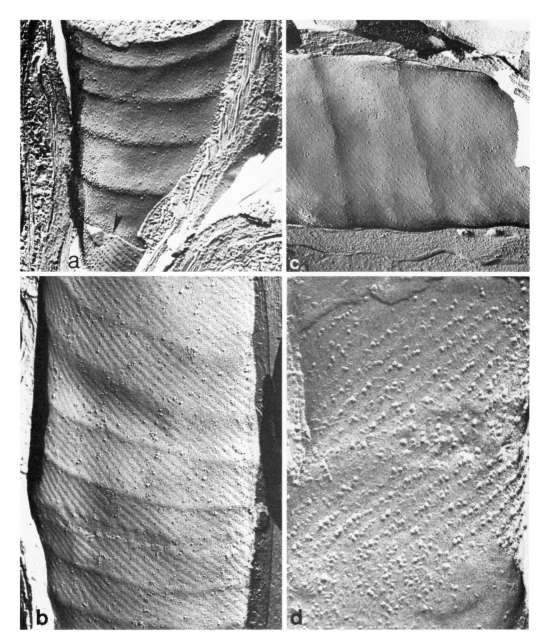

FIG. 17. Variations in the appearance of the paranodal axonal P-face. **a.** The junctional membrane is flat with very few particles. The glial E-face is evident at the arrowhead. ×49,300. **b:** The undulations are very obvious, and the particles are few and variously distributed. This figure is from an unfixed specimen. ×60,000. **c:** The junctional membrane is flat with chains of particles. ×36,000. **d:** The junctional membrane is undulated and contains chains of particles in register with the undulations. ×120,000.

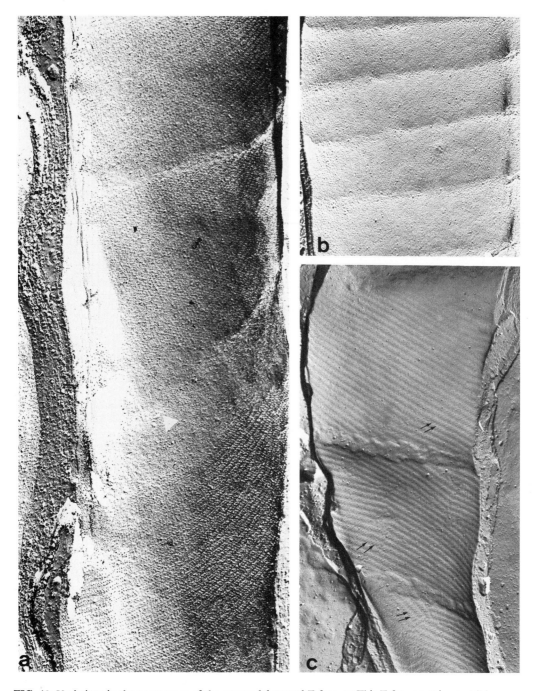

FIG. 18. Variations in the appearance of the paranodal axonal E-face. **a**: This E-face contains a striking crystalline array of tiny subunits. The relationship of this array to the junction is obvious by virtue of the arrangement and orientation of the subunits comprising the array. The appearance of the lattice differs between the two regions separated by the segment which is flat (*triangle*). ×60,000. **b**: On this fiber the junctional membrane is nearly flat. ×50,000. **c**: Paranodal E-face from an unfixed specimen. The undulations are especially obvious. In some areas a diagonal axis (oriented with the arrows) can be recognized which is apparently related to the lattice structure illustrated in **a**. ×50,000.

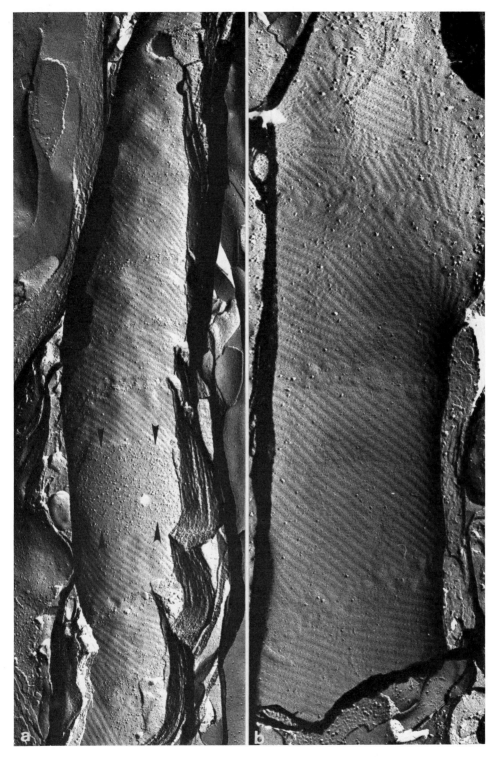

FIG. 19. Irregularities associated with the junctional features on the axonal fracture faces. **a:** P-face of the para-nodal axolemma from an unfixed specimen. The undulations are very obvious. At the arrowheads, the junctional membrane is interrupted by a segment of unspecialized membrane where undulations are not evident and numerous particles are distributed at random. ×48,000. **b:** E-face of the paranodal axolemma from an unfixed specimen. Patches of disoriented junctional membrane, recognized by the parallel undulations, are evident at the border of the internodal (*top*) and paranodal regions. ×68,000.

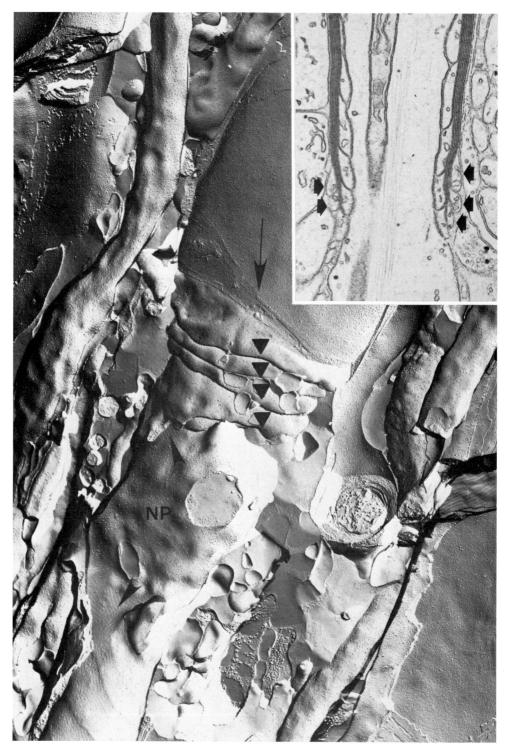

FIG. 20. The fracture process has exposed the nodal (NP) and paranodal (*arrowheads*) P-face of a myelinated axon. The paranodal axolemma presents the characteristic undulations. The upper paranode is irregular. The fracture process has exposed the P-face of a series of turns of the lateral belt (*triangles*) which are not in contact with the axon. The arrow shows tight junctional strands of the lateral belt. ×26,100. **Inset:** Matching electron micrographs from a thin section. The arrows indicate paranodal loops unattached to the axon; this is a rather common winding defect corresponding almost exactly to that shown tridimensionally on the replica.

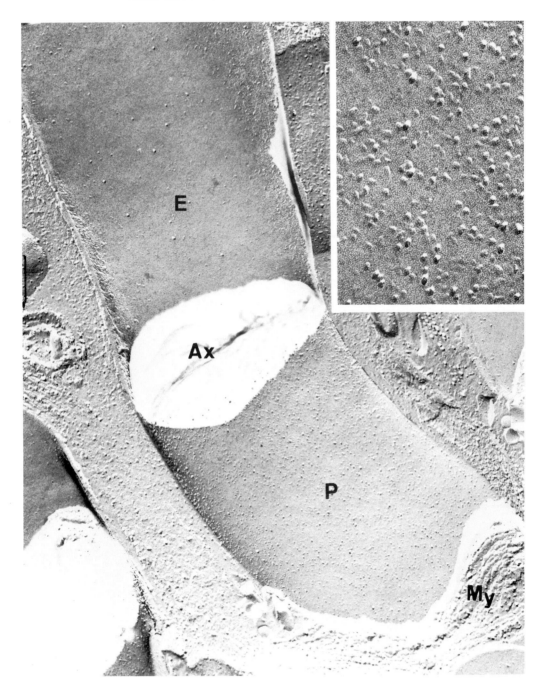

FIG. 21. Internodal axolemma in a fiber from the turtle optic nerve. The P- and E-faces of a single fiber have been exposed. (My) Compact myelin. (Ax) Axoplasm. The P-face contains numerous particles distributed at random. The E-face has few particles. ×62,500. **Inset:** At higher magnification the P-face particles appear relatively homogeneous in size and shape when compared with the particles which fracture with the nodal P- and E-faces. ×200,000.

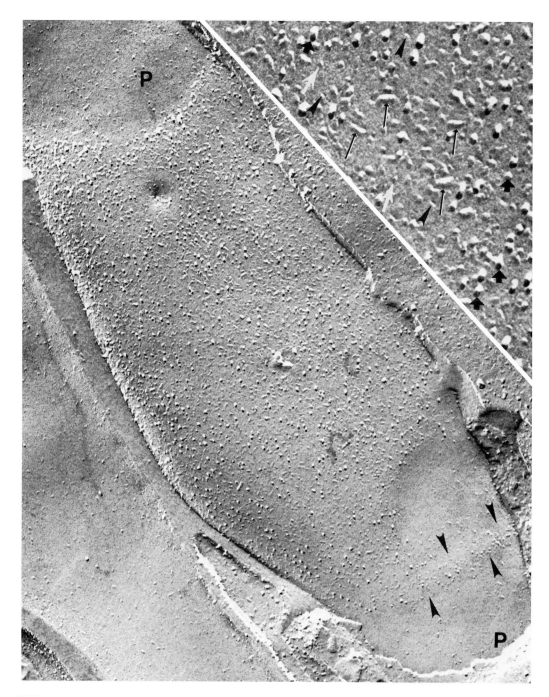

FIG. 22. P-face of the nodal axolemma from the turtle optic nerve. The two paranodal regions on either side of the node are labeled. The nodal P-face itself contains a great many particles distributed at random. At the bottom, note that the nodal region merges with the particle-laden narrow ridge (*arrowheads*), which faces the space between paranodal loops. ×75,000. **Inset:** Portion of the nodal P-face at higher magnification. There is a striking variation in particle shapes and sizes. Large, rounded particles (*black arrows*); small, rounded particles (*white arrows*); large, elongated particles (*black* and *white arrows*); and many pits (*black arrowheads*) are evident. ×240,000.

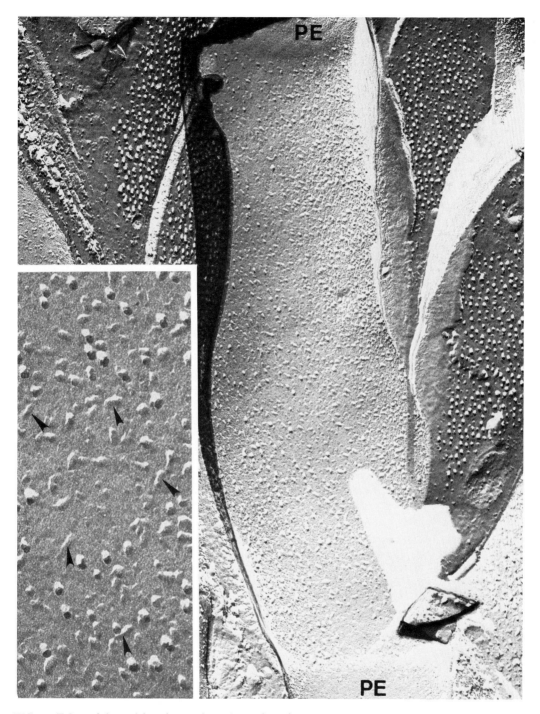

FIG. 23. E-face of the nodal axolemma from the turtle optic nerve. (PE) The two paranodal regions on either side of the node. In contrast to the internodal E-face, the nodal E-face contains many particles distributed at random. ×75,000. **Inset:** At a higher magnification, the E-face particles are seen to vary in size and shape as do those on the nodal P-face (Fig. 22). Many rounded and some large, elongated (*arrowheads*) particles are evident. ×200,000.

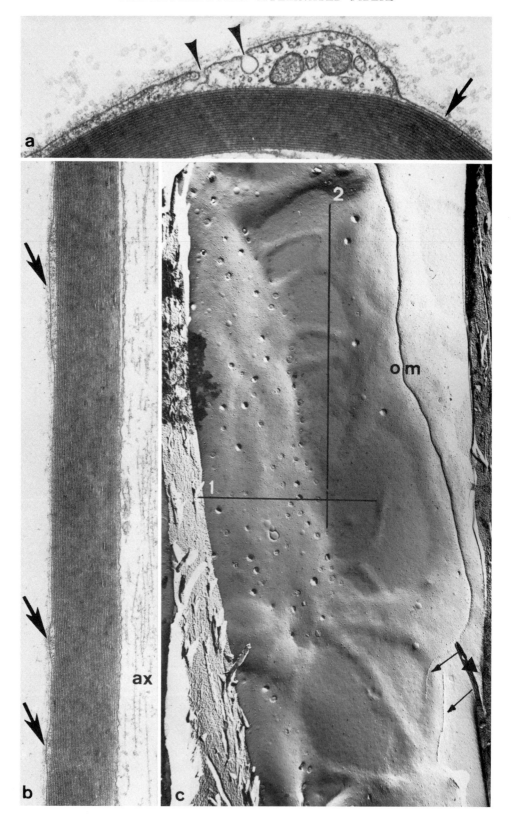

ticles (85,86,90). This is in contrast to the internodal axolemma, where accumulations of E-face particles are not evident. Hence, one concludes that the node of Ranvier is a specialized domain of axon membrane as expected from its physiological significance (see chapters by Waxman, *this volume;* Rasminsky, *this volume*).

In our turtle material, the P-face contains ~ 1,600 particles/μm²; these are randomly distributed like those in the internodal axolemma, but there is a much greater variation in particle shape and size on the nodal P-face (compare Figs. 21 and 22). These particles measure 60–230 Å, with a large number of elongated particles being over 200 Å. Pits, apparently left by particles cleaving with the E-face, can also be seen (Fig. 22, inset).

In the turtle optic nerve where we have obtained consistent measurements, the nodal E-face contains ~ 1,500 particles/μm² (Fig. 23); these vary in shape and range in size from 35 to 220 Å, with most between 100 and 150 Å. Rosenbluth (85), in the frog CNS, considers these particles as a homogeneous population and suggests that they represent the voltage-sensitive ion channels since: (a) their density, although not sufficiently well correlated (1,19,82), is in the same order of magnitude as that of the estimated channel density in peripheral nodes, and (b) they are distinct from most freeze-fracture particles since they fracture with the E-face. He further supposes that the P-face particles represent, in part, the Na,K ion pumps. Rosenbluth also suggested that the particles of the narrow helical pathway representing the nonjunctional portion of the paranodal axolemma may represent iono-

phores in transit to and from the node, and that the paranodal junction may be involved in localizing and concentrating functionally important particles in the nodal axolemma.

Future experimental studies on freeze-fractured nodal membranes may shed light on the nature and dynamic properties of the nodal axolemma particles. Although technically demanding, a useful approach may require freeze-fracturing of single fibers that have been tested and changed electrophysiologically, chemically, or pharmacologically.

At present, the most striking finding on the freeze-fracture features of the nodal axolemma is that of Kristol et al. (48). They noted in the knifefish electric organ that wide nodes which do not show an action potential and lack electron-dense material undercoating attached to the cytoplasmic aspect of the axolemma have few nodal face E-particles, whereas the narrow nodes that show an action potential and have an undercoating of the axolemma show a high number of E-face particles.

SURFACE OF THE PERIPHERAL MYELIN SHEATH

Although it is generally accepted that the surface of the peripheral myelin sheath is filled with cytoplasm, this concept should be limited only to the perinuclear region (59). Actually the inner turn and most of the outer internodal surface of the sheath consist of a delicate cytoplasmic reticulum that communicates with the marginal belt and the incisures (59). Although this can be demonstrated in thin sections, the idea is most easily grasped by viewing fracture faces of this region of the

←

FIG. 24. Outer surface of the peripheral myelin sheath. **a:** Cross-cut myelinated fiber in thin section. Note the organelle-rich cytoplasmic region bulging from the perimeter of the sheath. On the right side the cytoplasmic layer becomes extremely thin and the outer turn of the sheath appears semicompact (*arrow*). Arrowheads indicate two caveolae. ×50,430. **b:** Longitudinally cut myelinated fiber in thin section. The plane of section passes through three thin cytoplasmic regions (*arrows*) devoid of large organelles and protruding slightly from the perimeter of the fiber. Between the cytoplasmic regions the outer turn of the sheath is semicompact. ax-Axon ×39,600. **c:** Outer surface of a freeze-fractured sheath. The P-face of the Schwann cell membrane has been exposed. Thus (Fig. 1, cell 3) the convex areas represent regions of the outer turn bulging from the contour of the sheath. Conspicuous convexities of the fracture face studded with caveolar stomata correspond to organelle-rich cytoplasmic regions such as is represented in **a.** The finger-like elevations correspond to organelle-poor cytoplasmic regions shown in **b.** The flat portions in between correspond to semicompact regions. Lines 1 and 2 demarcate planes corresponding approximately to those shown in thin section in **a** and **b,** respectively. (om) Outer mesaxonal furrow. The triangle indicates the cross-fractured mesaxonal cytoplasm; and the arrow, the mesaxonal tight junctional strands. ×21,600.

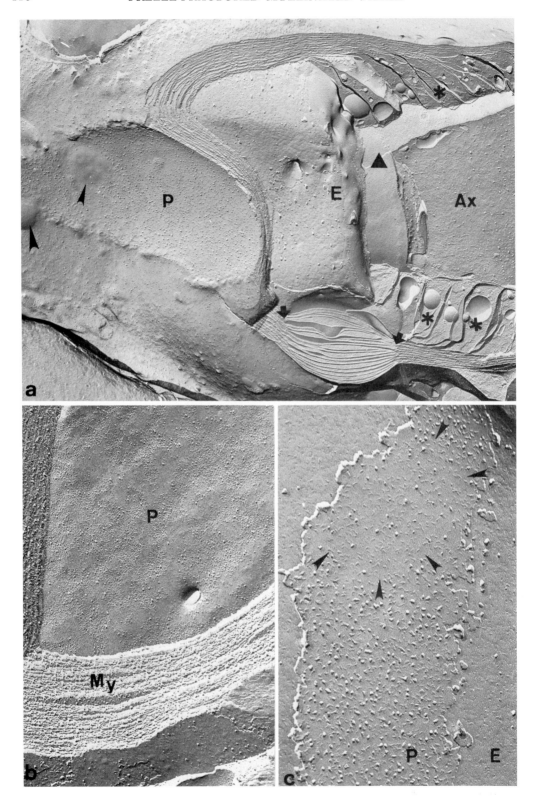

sheath (Fig. 24c). From thin sections it can be seen that large (Fig. 24a) and small (Fig. 24b) cytoplasmic zones are separated by areas where the outermost lamella is "semicompact," i.e., where the cytoplasmic surfaces of the apposed Schwann cell membrane approach to within 50 Å of each other. A major dense line, however, is not formed (hence the term semicompact). "Caveolae" (Fig. 24a and c) are associated with the plasmalemma of the perinuclear region and the larger pockets of cytoplasm constituting the reticulum (see also ref. 86). The caveolae are distinct from pinocytotic vesicles since they do not move into the cytoplasm although they become filled with tracers such as horseradish peroxidase (59). They may serve to increase the surface area of the fiber during movement related stretching of the nerve.

In peripheral fibers larger than 3–5 μm, the outer turn of the lateral belt usually forms a conspicuous system of nodal villi, suggesting secretory activity. The villi are represented in Fig. 2. Their function remains unknown (49). Freeze-fractured nodal villi have been illustrated by Sandri et al. (86). No special features were noted.

DIFFICULTIES AND PITFALLS ASSOCIATED WITH THE FREEZE-FRACTURE METHOD

Currently the freeze-fracture method is a routine procedure accessible to most laboratories equipped for electron microscopy. With the exception of a few recent improvements, the methodology has not changed dramatically during the last few years. Nevertheless, the nature of the technique presents some significant obstacles to those of us interested in studying the membrane structure of myelinated axons under experimental or pathological conditions. A primary difficulty lies in the inherent randomness of the fracture process. Although the experimenter can initiate the cleavage at a particular level of a block of peripheral nerve or central nerve tract, he cannot dictate which membranes within a given fiber will be fractured. The fact is that the interesting features associated with myelinated axons (i.e., the zonula occludens, the axoglial junction, and the nodal and internodal axolemma) occupy a very small fraction of the total membrane surface in any preparation. Thus a great number of replicas must be scanned before a meaningful and informative fracture surface is encountered. This fact renders even simple observations on normal preparations a laborious and time-consuming affair.

It is likely that freeze-fractured degenerating or pathologically affected fibers assume configurations similar to those seen in normal, poorly preserved fibers. Since some preservation artifacts may be present even in carefully prepared specimens, it will be difficult to distinguish these from meaningful alterations (e.g., ref. 81). We already encountered this problem in ongoing investigations of Wallerian degeneration and on the myelin-deficient mouse mutant "quaking" (87).

In all the animal species studied so far, we noticed a marked tendency of the myelin and the axolemmal particles to separate within the plane of the membrane, leaving large areas of

FIG. 25. Artifacts associated with freeze-fractured myelinated fibers. a: Myelinated fiber from the bullfrog CNS at the transition between internode (*left side*) and paranode (*right side*). Several paranodal loops (*) have been cross-fractured. A small portion of the paranodal axonal P-face (*triangle*) has remained bound to the axoplasm (Ax). The E-face of the first paranodal loop (E) and the P-face (P) of a compact myelin lamella in the internodal region are shown. Several artifacts are evident in this micrograph: First, between the arrows, the myelin lamellae have separated and the corresponding fracture faces appear free of particles; second, particle-free areas (*arrowheads*), or "blebs," occur on the otherwise particulate myelinic P-face; third, the contour of the sheath is irregular owing to partial collapse of the sheath (P); and fourth, the endoplasmic reticulum in the paranodal loops is swollen. ×27,000. b: Central myelinated axon from the turtle. The compact myelin (My) has been fractured obliquely and the internodal axonal P-face exposed (P). In well-preserved fibers the particles on this face are randomly distributed (Figs. 5 and 21). In this case the particles are clumped, leaving discrete areas of the fracture surface smooth. ×50,000. c: P- and E-faces of the compact myelin from the bullfrog CNS. The region of the P-face demarcated by the arrowheads is almost devoid of rounded particles, although the elongated particles remain. This may reflect a movement of particles within the plane of the membrane and probably precedes formation of the blebs illustrated in a. ×80,000.

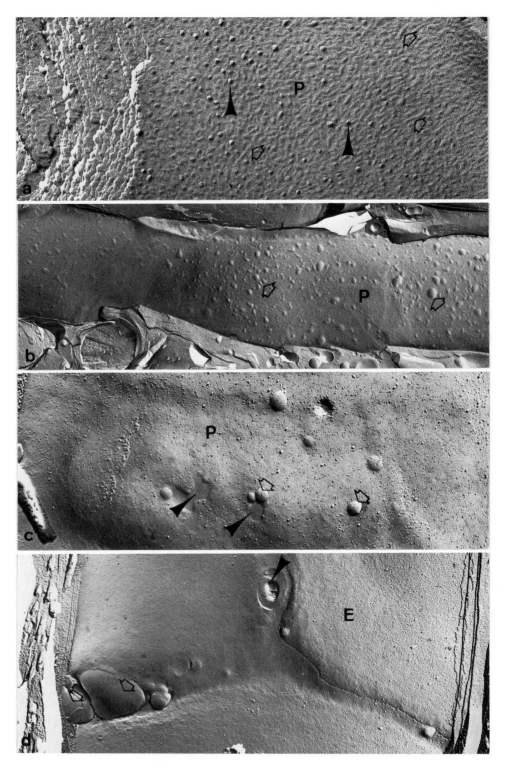

FIG. 26. Various kinds of gross artifacts in freeze-fractured myelin sheaths from healthy animals. **a:** "Orange peel" configuration of the myelinic P face. Note the irregular elevations (*arrows*) different from normal particles (*arrowheads*). ×100,800. **b:** Myelinic P-face covered with multiple, particle-free blebs (*arrows*) of varying size. ×9,600. **c:** Isolated small blebs (*arrows*) and depressions (*arrowheads*) of the myelinic P-face. ×48,000. **d:** Larger blebs (*arrows*) and invaginations (*arrowhead*) may involve several myelin lamellae, as seen in this poorly fixed peripheral sheath where the E-face particles have a patchy distribution. ×28,800.

membrane surface devoid of particles (Fig. 25). This is usually associated with other characteristics of poorly preserved tissue, e.g., irregular packing and splitting of the myelin, swollen endoplasmic reticulum, and clumping of axoplasmic organelles.

Collapse of the myelin sheath (Fig. 25a) and the axolemma (not illustrated) is also quite common. A diffuse orange-peel deformation of the myelin fracture faces is often present in specimens with freezing artifacts (Fig. 26a) (93). In addition, focal deformations of the fractured myelin (Fig. 26b–d) (attributable primarily to insufficient stabilization at the moment of freezing) are also common in replicas in blocks from perfused animals.

CONCLUSIONS

In conclusion, the advantageous condition represented by saltatory conduction of nerve fibers rests on an astoundingly complex bio-architectural marvel, which is perhaps the most unique cytological feature in the animal kingdom. Yet this vital association between axons and glial cells is very labile.

The basic principles of architecture of myelin sheaths can be summarized as follows:

1. Each myelin segment is formed by a single myelinating cell and consists of a trapezoidal cellular flap wrapped around the axon.

2. The cellular flap contains little cytoplasm, confined to the periphery (marginal cytoplasmic belt) and to longitudinally and circumferentially oriented clefts (incisures), and forms a myelin membrane where the cytoplasmic leaflets appear united to form the "major dense line."

3. The regular apposition of the turns of the spiraled myelin membrane gives rise to a periodic structure where the intercellular cleft remains thinner than in any other unspecialized cell-to-cell apposition. This is possible in spite of the relatively low protein/lipid ratio and the random distribution of nonjunctional intramembrane proteins.

4. In spite of the close apposition of its exoplasmic and cytoplasmic leaflets, the freeze-fracture properties of the myelin lamella resemble those of other membranes, and the nonjunctional intramembrane particles do not show a lateral order.

5. The borders of each myelin segment are sealed by a system of tight junctions (zonula occludens), which also accompany the cytoplasmic incisures.

6. Each myelin segment adheres to the axon, bound at both ends by virtue of an extensive cell junction (the septate-like paranodal axoglial junction), with an oriented extracellular matrix and aligned intramembrane particles.

ACKNOWLEDGMENTS

This work was supported by NIH grant NS–09904–07.

REFERENCES

1. Armstrong, C. M. (1975): Ionic pores, gates and gating currents. *Q. Rev. Biophys.*, 7:179–210.
2. Asbury, A. K., Gale, M. K., Cox, S. C., Baringer, J. R., and Berg, B. O. (1972): Giant axonal neuropathy: A unique case with segmental neurofilamentous masses. *Acta Neuropathol.*, 20:237–247.
3. Benedetti, E. L., and Favard, P. (1973): *Freeze-Etching Techniques and Applications.* Societe Francaise de Microscopie Electronique, Paris.
4. Bennett, M. V. L. (1973): Function of electrotonic junctions in embryonic and adult tissues. *Fed. Proc.*, 32:65–75.
5. Bennett, M. V. L., and Spira, M. (1973): Effects of fixatives for electron microscopy on electrical coupling and tracer movement between embryonic cells. *J. Cell Biol.*, 59: 22A.
6. Bischoff, A., and Moor, H. (1967): Ultrastructural differences between the myelin sheaths of peripheral nerve fibers and CNS white matter. *Z. Zellforsch.*, 81:303–310.
7. Bischoff, A., and Moor, H. (1967): The ultrastructure of the difference "factor" in the myelin. *Z. Zellforsch.*, 81:571–580.
8. Blank, W. F., Bunge, M. P., and Bunge, R. P. (1974): Sensitivity of the myelin sheath, particularly the Schwann cell-axolemmal junction, to lowered calcium levels in cultured sensory ganglia. *Brain Res.*, 67: 503–518.
9. Branton, D. (1966): Fracture faces of frozen membranes. *Proc. Natl. Acad. Sci. USA*, 55:1048–1056.
10. Branton, D. (1967): Fracture faces of frozen myelin. *Exp. Cell Res.*, 45:703–707.
11. Branton, D., Bullivant, S., Gilula, N. B., Karnovsky, M. J., Moor, H., Mühlethaler, K., Northcote, D. H., Packer, L., Satir, B., Satir, P., Speth, V., Staehelin, L. A., Steere,

R. L., and Weinstein, R. S. (1975): Freeze-etching nomenclature. *Science,* 190:54–56.

12. Braun, P. (1977): Molecular architecture of myelin. In: *Myelin,* edited by P. Morrel, pp. 91–115. Plenum Press, New York.

13. Bretsher, M. S. (1971): A major protein which spans the human erythrocyte membrane. *J. Mol. Biol.,* 59:351–357.

14. Brightman, M. W., Prescott, L., and Reese, T. S. (1975): Intercellular junctions of special ependyma. In: *Brain Endocrine Interaction, Vol. II: The Ventricular System in Neuroendocrine Mechanisms,* edited by K. M. Knigge, D. E. Scott, and H. Kobayashi, pp. 146–165. Karger, Basel.

15. Bullivant, S. (1973): Freeze-etching and freeze-fracturing. In: *Advanced Techniques in Biological Electron Microscopy,* edited by J. K. Koehler, pp. 67–112. Springer-Verlag, Berlin.

16. Bullivant, S. (1976): Evidence that the tight junction sealing element consists of two side-by-side fibrils. *J. Cell Biol.,* 70:35a.

17. Bunge, R. P. (1968): Glial cells and the central myelin sheath. *Physiol. Rev.,* 48: 197–251.

18. Claude, P., and Goodenough, D. A. (1973): Fracture faces of zonulae occludentes from "tight and leaky" epithelia. *J. Cell Biol.,* 58:390–400.

19. Conti, F., Hille, B., Neumcke, B., Nonner, W., and Staempfli, R. (1976): Conductance of the sodium channel in myelinated nerve fibers with modified sodium inactivation. *J. Physiol. (Lond),* 262:729–742.

20. Deamer, D. W., Leonard, R., Tardieu, A., and Branton, D. (1970): Lamellar and hexagonal lipid phases visualized by freeze-etching. *Biochim. Biophys. Acta,* 219:47–60.

21. Decker, R. S., and Friend, D. S. (1974): Assembly of gap junctions during amphibian neurulation. *J. Cell Biol.,* 62:32–47.

22. Dempsey, G. P., Bullivant, S., and Watkins, W. B. (1973): Endothelial cell membranes: Polarity of particles as seen by freeze-fracturing. *Science,* 179:190–192.

23. Dermietzel, R. (1974): Junctions in the central nervous system of the cat. I. Membrane fusion in central myelin. *Cell Tissue Res.,* 148:565–576.

24. Dermietzel, R. (1974): Junctions in the central nervous system of the cat. II. A contribution to the tertiary structure of the axonal-glial junctions in the paranodal region of the node of Ranvier. *Cell Tissue Res.,* 148:577–586.

25. Epand, R. M., Moscarello, M. A., Zierenberg, B., and Vail, W. J. (1974): The folded conformation of the encephalitogenic protein of the human brain. *Biochemistry,* 13: 1264–1267.

26. Feder, N., Reese, T. S., and Brightman, M. W. (1969): Microperoxidase, a new tracer of low molecular weight: A study of the interstitial compartments of the mouse brain. *J. Cell Biol.,* 43:35A–36A.

27. Friede, R. L. (1972): Control of myelin formation by axon caliber (with a model of the control mechanism). *J. Comp. Neurol.,* 144:233–252.

28. Friend, D., and Gilula, N. B. (1972): Variations in tight and gap junctions in mammalian tissues. *J. Cell Biol.,* 53:758–776.

29. Grant, C. W. M., and McConnell, H. M. (1974): Glycophorin in lipid bilayers. *Proc. Natl. Acad. Sci. USA,* 71:4653–4657.

30. Gilula, N. B., Reeves, O. R., and Steinbach, A. (1973): Metabolic coupling, ionic coupling, and cell contacts. *Nature (Lond),* 235:262–265.

31. Gilula, N. B., Fawcett, D. W., and Aoki, A. (1976): The Sertoli cell occluding junctions and gap junctions in mature and developing mammalian testis. *Dev. Biol.,* 50:142–168.

32. Goodenough, D. A. (1976): The structure and permeability of isolated hepatocyte gap junctions. *Cold Spring Harbor Symp. Quant. Biol.,* 40:37–43.

33. Gregson, N. A. (1976): The chemistry and structure of myelin. In: *The Peripheral Nerve,* edited by D. N. Landon, pp. 512–604. Chapman and Hall, London.

34. Gulley, R. L., and Reese, T. S. (1976): Intercellular junctions in the reticular lamina of the organ of Corti. *J. Neurocytol.,* 5:479–507.

35. Hall, S. M., and Williams, P. L. (1971): The distribution of electron-dense tracers in peripheral nerve fibers. *J. Cell Sci.,* 8:541–555.

36. Harkin, J. C. (1964): A series of desmosomal attachments in the Schwann sheath of myelinated mammalian nerves. *Z. Zellforsch.,* 64:189–195.

37. Hedley-White, E. T., and Kirschner, D. A. (1976): Morphological evidence of alteration in myelin structure with maturation. *Brain Res.,* 113:487–497.

38. Herr, J. C. (1976): Reflexive gap junctions. *J. Cell Biol.,* 69:495–501.

39. Heuser, J. E., Reese, T. S., and Landis, D. M. D. (1976): Preservation of synaptic structure by rapid freezing. *Cold Spring Harbor Symp. Quant. Biol.,* 40:17–24.

40. Hirano, A., Becker, M. H., and Zimmerman, H. M. (1969): Isolation of the periaxonal space of the central myelinated nerve fiber with regard to the diffusion of peroxidase. *J. Histochem. Cytochem.,* 17:512–516.

41. Hirano, A., and Dembitzer, H. M. (1967): A structural analysis of the myelin sheath in the central nervous system. *J. Cell Biol.,* 34:555–567.

42. Hirano, A., and Dembitzer, H. M. (1969): The transverse bands as a means of access to the periaxonal space of the central myelinated fiber. *J. Ultrastruct. Res.,* 28:141–149.

43. Hirano, A., Dembitzer, H. M., Becker, N. H.,

and Zimmerman, H. M. (1969): The distribution of peroxidase in the triethylin-intoxicated rat brain. *J. Neuropathol. Exp. Neurol.*, 28:507–511.

44. Hirano, A., Zimmerman, H. M., and Levine, S. (1966): Myelin in the central nervous system as observed in experimentally induced edema in the rat. *J. Cell Biol.*, 31:397–411.

45. Iwayama, T. (1971): Nexuses between areas of the surface membrane of the same arterial smooth muscle cell. *J. Cell Biol.*, 49:521–525.

46. Karnovsky, M. J. (1971): The use of ferrocyanide-reduced osmium tetroxide in electron microscopy. In: *Abstracts of Papers Eleventh Annual Meeting, American Society of Cell Biology*, p. 146.

47. Kirschner, D. A., and Casper, D. L. D. (1977): Diffraction studies of molecular organization in myelin. In: *Myelin*, edited by P. Morell, pp. 51–89. Plenum Press, New York.

48. Kristol, C., Akert, K., Sandri, C., Wyss, U. R., Bennett, M. V. L., and Moor, H. (1977): The Ranvier nodes in the neurogenic electric organ of the knifefish Sternarchus: A freeze-etching study on the distribution. *Brain Res.* 125:197–212.

49. Landon, D. N., and Hall, S. (1976): The myelinated nerve fiber. In: *The Peripheral Nerve*, edited by D. N. Landon, pp. 1–105. Chapman and Hall, London.

50. Langley, O. K., and Landon, D. N. (1967): A light and electron histochemical approach to the nodes of Ranvier and myelin of peripheral nerve fibers. *J. Histochem. Cytochem.*, 15:722–731.

51. Livingston, R. B., Pfenninger, K., Moor, H., and Akert, K. (1973): Specialized paranodal and interparanodal glial-axonal junctions in the peripheral and central nervous system: A freeze-etching study. *Brain Res.*, 58:1–24.

52. Lowenstein, W. R. (1976): Permeable junctions. *Cold Spring Harbor Symp. Quant. Biol.*, 40:49–63.

53. Mateu, L., Luzzati, V., London, Y., Gould, R. M., Vossenberg, F. G. A., and Olive, J., Jr. (1973): X-ray diffraction and electron microscope study of the interactions of myelin components: The structure of a lamellar phase with a 150 to 180 Å repeat distance containing basic proteins and acidic lipids. *J. Mol. Biol.*, 75:697–709.

54. McIntyre, J. A., Gilula, N. B., and Karnovsky, M. S. (1974): Cryoprotectant-induced redistribution of intramembranous particles in mouse lymphocytes. *J. Cell Biol.*, 60:192–203.

55. Metuzals, J. (1962): Ultrastructure of Ranviers node in central fibers, analyzed in serial secions. In: *Fifth International Congress of Electron Microscopy*, Vol. 2, edited by S. Breese, Jr., p. 9. Academic Press, New York.

56. Mizuhira, V., and Ozawa, H. (1967): On the fine structure of nerve myelin by means of glutaraldehyde fiaxtion. *J. Electron Microsc.*, 16:169–177.

57. Moor, H., and Mühlethaler, K. (1963): Fine structure in frozen-etched yeast cells. *J. Cell Biol.*, 17:609–628.

58. Morell, P. (1977): *Myelin*, edited by P. Morell. Plenum Press, New York.

59. Mugnaini, E., Osen, K. K., Schnapp, B., and Friedrich, V. L., Jr. (1977): Distribution of Schwann cell cytoplasm and plasmalemmal vesicles (caveolae) in peripheral myelin sheaths: An electron microscopic study with thin sections and freeze-fracturing. *J. Neurocytol. (in press)*.

60. Mugnaini, E., and Schnapp, B. (1974): The zonula occludens of the myelin sheath: Its possible role in demyelinating conditions. *Nature (Lond)*, 251:725–726.

61. Mugnaini, E., and Walberg, F. (1964): Ultrastructure of neuroglia. *Ergeb. Anat. Entwicklungsgesch.*, 37:193–236.

62. Napolitano, L. M., and Scallen, T. J. (1969): Observations on the fine structure of peripheral nerve myelin. *Anat. Rec.*, 163:1–6.

63. Norton, W. T. (1977): Isolation and characterization of myelin. In: *Myelin*, edited by P. Morell, pp. 161–199. Plenum Press, New York.

64. Norton, W. T. (1977): Chemical pathology of diseases involving myelin. In: *Myelin*, edited by P. Morell, pp. 383–413. Plenum Press, New York.

65. Norton, W. T. (1975): Myelin: Structure and biochemistry. In: *The Nervous System*, edited by D. B. Tower, Vol. I, pp. 467–481. Raven Press, New York.

66. Ochoa, J., Fowler, T. J., and Gilliat, R. W. (1972): Anatomical changes in peripheral nerves compressed by a pneumatic tourniquet. *J. Anat.*, 113:433–455.

67. Peek, W. D., Shivers, R. R., and McMillan, D. D. (1977): Freeze-fracture analysis of junctional complexes in the nephron of the garter snake Thamnophis sirtalis. *Cell Tissue Res.*, 179:441–452.

68. Peracchia, C. (1973): Low resistance junctions in crayfish. II. Structural details and further evidence for intercellular channels by freeze-fracture and negative staining. *J. Cell Biol.*, 57:66–76.

69. Peters, A. (1962): Plasma membrane contacts in the central nervous system. *J. Anat.*, 96:237–248.

70. Peters, A. (1964): Further observations on the structure of myelin sheaths in the central nervous system. *J. Cell Biol.*, 20:281–296.

71. Peters, A., Palay, S. L., and Webster, H. de F. (1976): *The Fine Structure of the Nervous System*. Saunders, Philadelphia.

72. Peterson, R. G., and Pease, D. C. (1972):

Myelin embedded in polymerized glutaralde-hyde-urea. *J. Ultrastruct. Res.,* 41:115–132.

73. Pinto Da Silva, P., Martinez-Palomo, A., and Gonzalez-Robles, A. (1975): Membrane structure and surface coat of Entamoeba histolytica. *J. Cell Biol.,* 64:538–550.

74. Pinto Da Silva, P., and Miller, R. G. (1975): Membrane particles on fracture faces of frozen myelin. *Proc. Natl. Acad. Sci. USA,* 72:4046–4050.

75. Pricam, C., Humbart, F., Perrelet, A., and Orci, L. (1974): Gap junctions in mesangial and lacis cells. *J. Cell Biol.,* 63:349–354.

76. Quarles, R. H., Everly, J. L., and Brady, R. O. (1973): Evidence for the close association of a glycoprotein with myelin rat brain. *J. Neurochem.,* 21:1177–1191.

77. Raine, C. S. (1977): Morphological aspects of myelin and myelination. In: *Myelin,* edited by P. Morell, pp. 1–49. Plenum Press, New York.

78. Rasminsky, M., and Sears, T. A. (1972): Internodal conduction in undissected demyelinated nerve fibers. *J. Physiol. (Lond),* 227:323–350.

79. Reale, E., Luciano, L., and Spitznas, M. (1975): Zonulae occludentes of the myelin lamellae in the nerve fiber layer of the retina and in the optic nerve of the rabbit: A demonstration by the freeze-fracture method. *J. Neurocytol.,* 4:131–140.

80. Revel, J. P., and Hamilton, D. W. (1969): The double nature of the intermediate dense line in peripheral nerve myelin. *Anat. Rec.,*

81. Reier, P. J., Tabira, T., and Webster, H. deF. (1976): Hexachlorophene (HCP) induced CNS myelin lesions studied with freeze-fracture and electron-dense tracer techniques. *Neurosci. Abstr.,* 2:745. 163:7–16.

82. Ritchie, J. M., and Rogart, R. B. (1977): Density of sodium channels in mammalian myelinated nerve fibers and the nature of the axonal membrane under the myelin sheath. *Proc. Natl. Acad. Sci. USA,* 74:211–215.

83. Robertson, J. D. (1958): The ultrastructure of Schmidt-Lanterman clefts and related shearing defects of the myelin sheath. *J. Biophys. Biochem. Cytol.,* 4:39–46.

84. Robertson, J. D. (1958): Structural alterations in nerve fibers produced by hypertonic solutions. *J. Biophys. Biochem. Cytol.,* 4:349–364.

85. Rosenbuth, J. (1976): Intramembranous particle distribution at the node of Ranvier and adjacent axolemma in myelinated axons of the frog brain. *J. Neurocytol.,* 5:731–745.

86. Sandri, C., Van Buren, J. M., and Akert, K. (1977): Membrane morphology of the vertebrate nervous system. *Prog. Brain Res. (in press).*

87. Schnapp, B., and Friedrich, V. L., Jr. (1977): Unpublished observations.

88. Schnapp, B., and Mugnaini, E. (1975): The myelin sheath: electron microscopic studies with thin sections and freeze-fracture. In: *Golgi Centennial Symposium: Proceedings,* edited by M. Santini, pp. 209–233. Raven Press, New York.

89. Schnapp, B., and Mugnaini, E. (1977): Freeze-fracture properties of central myelin in the bullfrog. *Neuroscience,* 1:459–467.

90. Schnapp, B., Peracchia, C., and Mugnaini, E. (1976): The paranodal axo-glial junction in the central nervous system studied with thin sections and freeze-fracture. *Neuroscience,* 1:181–190.

91. Singer, S. J. (1971): The molecular organization of biological membranes. In: *Membrane Structure and Function,* edited by L. I. Rothfield, pp. 146–222. Academic Press, New York.

92. Sotelo, C., and Angaut, P. (1973): The fine structure of the cerebellar central myelin in the cat. I. Neurons and neuroglial cells. *Exp. Brain Res.,* 16:410–430.

93. Staehelin, L. A. (1968): The interpretation of freeze-etched artificial and biological membranes. *J. Ultrastruct. Res.,* 22:326–347.

94. Staehelin, L. A. (1973): Further observations on the fine structure of freeze-cleaved tight junctions. *J. Cell Sci.,* 13:763–786.

95. Staehelin, L. A. (1975): Structure and function of intercellular junctions. *Int. Rev. Cytol.,* 39:191–284.

96. Steck, T. L. (1974): The organization of proteins in the human red blood cell membrane. *J. Cell Biol.,* 62:1–19.

97. Strum, J. M. (1977): Lanthanum "staining" of the lateral and basal membranes of the mitochondria-rich cell in toad bladder epithelium. *J. Ultrastruct. Res.* 59:126–139.

98. Tani, E., Ikeda, K., and Nishiura, M. (1973): Freeze-etching images of central myelinated nerve fibers. *J. Neurocytol.,* 2:305–314.

99. Tillack, T. W., Scott, R. E., and Marchesi, V. T. (1972): The structure of erythrocyte membranes studied by freeze-etching. *J. Exp. Med.,* 135:1209–1227.

100. Towfighi, J., and Gonatas, N. (1977): The distribution of peroxidases in the sciatic nerves of normal and hexachlorophene intoxicated developing rats. *J. Neurocytol.,* 6:39–47.

101. Van Harraveld, A., and Crowell, J. (1964): Electron microscopy after rapid freezing on a metal surface and substitution fixation. *Anat. Rec.,* 149:381–386.

102. Wade, J. B., and Karnovsky, M. J. (1974): The structure of the zonula occludens: A single fibril model based on freeze-fracture. *J. Cell Biol.,* 60:168–180.

103. Wade, J. B., and Karnovsky, M. J. (1974): Fracture faces of osmotically disrupted zonulae occludentes. *J. Cell Biol.,* 62:344–350.

104. Wiggins, R. C., Benjamins, J. A., and Morell, P. (1975): Appearance of myelin proteins in rat sciatic nerve during development. *Brain Res.,* 89:99–106.

105. Wood, J. G., and Dawson, R. M. C. (1974): Some properties of a major structural glycoprotein of sciatic nerve. *J. Neurochem.,* 22: 627–630.

106. Worthington, C. R. (1971): X-ray analysis of nerve myelin. In: *Biophysics and Physiology of Excitable Membranes,* edited by W. J. Adelman, pp. 1–46. Van Nostrand Reinhold, New York.

107. Yu, R., and Bunge, R. P. (1975): Damage and repair of the peripheral myelin sheath and node of Ranvier after treatment with trypsin. *J. Cell Biol.,* 64:1–14.

Physiology and Pathobiology of Axons, edited by
S. G. Waxman. Raven Press, New York © 1978.

Functional Architecture of the Initial Segment

Stephen G. Waxman and Donald C. Quick

Department of Neurology, Harvard Medical School, Beth Israel Hospital, Boston, Massachusetts 02215; and Harvard–MIT Program in Health Sciences and Technology, Massachusetts Institute of Technology, Cambridge, Massachusetts 02139

The axonal initial segment, where the axon takes origin from the perikaryon and hillock region, is specialized morphologically and physiologically. Morphologically this region serves as the junction between perikaryon and axon and thus occupies a crucial position with respect to the metabolic interplay between these two components of the neuron. Physiologically, it is at the initial segment that impulses are generated in most neurons, prior to their propagation along the axon and into the teledendron (Raymond and Lettvin, *this volume*). The initial segment therefore serves as a "trigger zone," or encoder region, where the temporal patterning of the impulses in a series, prior to transmission along the axon, is established.

The early neuroanatomists recognized, even at the light microscopic level, morphological specialization of the initial segment. Diameter was often reduced from that of the conical axon hillock and in some cases was less than that of more distal parts of the axon. Spinous processes were sometimes present; and the initial segment, like the axon hillock, was noted to be relatively devoid of Nissl substance. In dorsal root ganglion cells (e.g., ref. 18), the initial part of the axon was elaborated to form a winding glomerulus.

PHYSIOLOGICAL DIFFERENTIATION OF THE INITIAL SEGMENT

Physiological evidence derived from both synaptic and antidromic activation of spinal motor neurons indicates that the impulse is initiated at the axon hillock–initial segment and secondarily invades the somadendritic component of the neuron and the axon trunk (2,5,6). Eccles (4) postulated a lower threshold for the initial segment than for the soma or dendrites. This mode of impulse initiation is manifested by an inflection (particularly evident after electrical differentiation of the records) in the rising phase of the motor neuron spike (Fig. 1). This inflection reflects the double composition of the motor neuron action potential, in which the initial segment (IS) spike arises at a lower threshold than the somadendrite (SD) spike.

On the basis of computer simulation studies of the generation of motor neuron action potentials, Dodge and Cooley (3) predicted that there would be sharp spatial gradients of sodium channel density over the surface of motor neurons, ranging from very low channel density values in the dendrites, to a minimally excitable density in the soma, and to high values in the spike initiation region in the initial segment. Their data suggested that, in order for the initial segment trigger zone to excite the axon reliably, in spite of the electrical load imposed by the soma and dendrites, sodium channel density at the initial segment should approach that at the node of Ranvier. From a physiological point of view, then, it would be expected that the membrane at the initial segment represents a highly specialized part of the neuronal surface.

STRUCTURAL CORRELATES OF INITIAL SEGMENT DIFFERENTIATION

The ultrastructure of the initial segment, as determined by transmission electron microscopy following staining with lead and uranyl

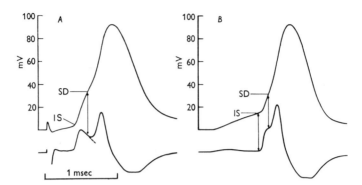

FIG. 1. Tracings of intracellularly recorded spike potentials evoked by antidromic (**A**) and synaptic (**B**) stimulation of a motoneuron. The lower traces show electrically differentiated records. Origins of the IS and SD spikes are indicated. The IS spike arises at a lower threshold. (Modified from ref. 2.)

salts, was carefully described by Palay et al. (11), Peters et al. (12), and Conradi (1), and is only briefly reviewed here. As at the node of Ranvier (Berthold, *this volume;* Waxman, *this volume*), there is an electron-dense cytoplasmic undercoating approximately 200 Å thick subjacent to the axolemma. Palay et al. (11) suggested that this dense material represents a structural modification of the cell surface related to specific membrane properties. The undercoating is, in fact, absent in internodal regions of the myelinated fiber, where sodium channel density is so low (see below) that the membrane is essentially inexcitable. A second morphological specialization of the initial segment is the appearance of microtubules clustered into distinct fascicles. This feature is not consistently observed at nodes of Ranvier.

Are there any other distinctive cytological characteristics of the functionally specialized initial segment? It is known that, when peripheral or central myelinated fibers are fixed in cacodylate-buffered aldehydes and osmium tetroxide and subsequently exposed to ferric ion and ferrocyanide,[1] aggregates of stain are localized specifically on the cytoplasmic surface of the unmyelinated axolemma at the nodes; internodal and paranodal regions of the axolemma are not stained (14,20; Waxman, *this volume*). The absence of staining of internodal and paranodal regions of the axon

membrane is not due to inaccessibility to the ferric ion or ferrocyanide, since these regions are unstained even in experiments in which the stain was permitted direct access to the axoplasm and where diffusion through the axoplasm was clearly demonstrated (14). Several lines of reasoning suggest that this mode of staining may selectively mark regions of physiological differentiation of the axon membrane.

The first derives from a comparison of the spatial distribution of stain, with pharmacological data on sodium channel density in peripheral nerves. From measurements of the binding of radioactive saxitoxin, Ritchie and Rogart (16) estimated the sodium channel density at nodes of Ranvier as $12,000/\mu m^2$. Nonner et al. (10), on the basis of voltage clamp data, estimated nodal sodium channel density as 5,000 channels/μm^2. In contrast to the high sodium channel density at nodes, the density of sodium channels is relatively low in the internodes beneath the myelin (less than 25 channels/μm^2) (16) and for the membrane of unmyelinated C-fibers (110 channels/μm^2) (17). As noted above, the internodal membrane of myelinated fibers does not stain with the ferric ion–ferrocyanide technique. In addition, the membranes of C-fibers, even where directly exposed to the extracellular milieu, do not stain (19).

A second line of evidence derives from studies on the electrocyte axons in the gymnotid *Sternarchus,* in which there are both excitable and inexcitable nodes (21). Kristol et al. (9) studied these axons using freeze-fracture tech-

---

[1] The method used here is different from that used to stain the nodal "gap substance" and is described in detail by Quick and Waxman (15).

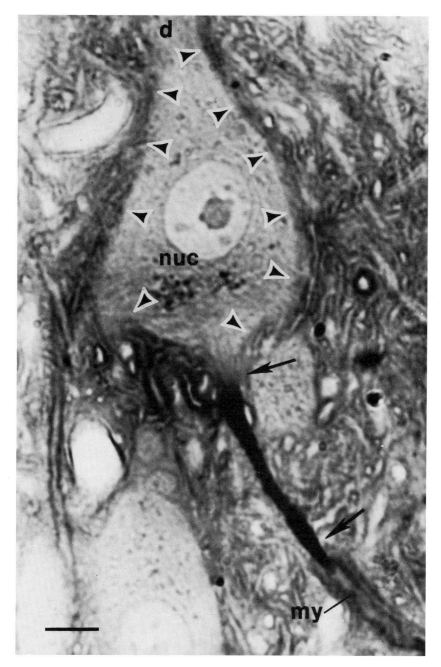

FIG. 2. Light micrograph showing staining of the entire initial segment (between *arrows*) of a rat spinal motor neuron exposed to ferric ion and ferrocyanide. The surface of the dendrites (d) and perikaryon are unstained (*arrowheads*). (d) Dendrite. (my) Myelin sheath of first internode. Scale = 10 μm.

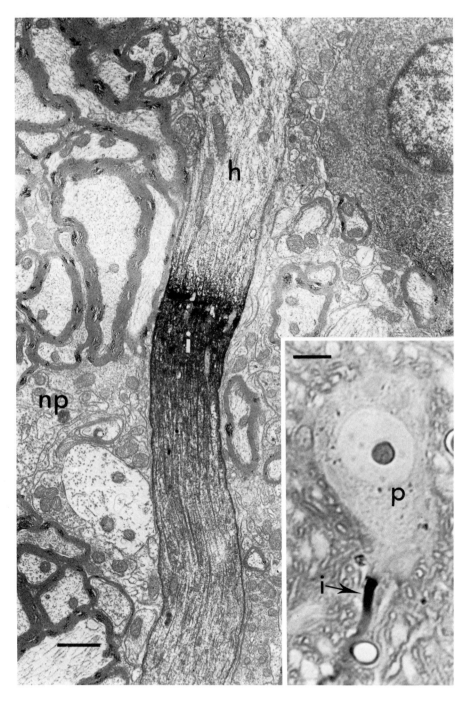

FIG. 3. Inset: Light micrograph of a rat spinal neuron stained with ferric ion-ferrocyanide. The initial segment (i) is densely stained, but there is no visible staining of the perikaryon (p). Scale = 10 μm. Electron micrograph of the axon hillock (h) and initial segment (i) from the same section, after reembedding and ultrathin sectioning. Note the intra-axonal location of the stain. The adjacent neuropil (np) is not stained. Scale = 1 μm.

niques. They found a higher density of external face membrane particles at the excitable nodes than at the inexcitable nodes, which exhibited particle density profiles similar to those of the internodes, and they suggested that these particles might be related to ionic channel or pump sites. When the *Sternarchus* electrocyte axons were examined with the ferric ion–ferrocyanide technique, it was evident in sectioned material and in dissected single fibers that only the small excitable nodes were sites of deposition of the stain (14).

Since it appeared that this technique may provide a cytochemical marker for regions of the myelinated axon membrane engaged in impulse initiation or propagation, we examined initial segments using this technique (20). Figure 2 shows a spinal motor neuron from an adult rat perfused with Karnovsky's (7) aldehyde mixture in cacodylate buffer, postfixed in osmium tetroxide in cacodylate buffer, teased, and then stained in $FeCl_3$ followed by $K_4Fe(CN)_6 \cdot 3H_2O$. As shown in Fig. 2, the initial segment (between the arrows) can be specifically visualized at the light microscopic level using this technique. The length of the initial segment shown in Fig. 2 is 36 μm; the diameter varies somewhat along the course of the initial segment but is approximately 2.6 μm (mean of eight equidistant measurements). These values correspond well with those deduced by Conradi (1) from ultrastructural serial section analysis of cat spinal motor neurons.

Figure 3 shows a light micrograph of a 3-μm section of another initial segment (inset) and an electron micrograph of the same cell following resectioning for electron microscopy. Note that in Figs. 2 and 3 the initial segments are densely stained but that no stain is present in the cell body or dendrites. Similarly, synapses were not stained. Within the initial segment, the ferric ion–ferrocyanide is localized inside the unmyelinated axon. As at the nodes of Ranvier, the densest deposits are usually located subjacent to the inner surface of the axolemma, but some stain does diffuse into the axoplasm, where microtubules appear to have a special affinity for the stain.

The essential point illustrated by these micrographs is that the axon initial segment, in contrast to the perikaryon and dendrites, is specifically stained by this specialized technique. We interpret the specific staining of the initial segment as a reflection of its physiological specialization and perhaps as a cytochemical correlate of a high density of ionic channels. It should be emphasized in this regard that for some specialized neurons the impulse initiation site may not be fixed but may shift, depending on the physiological state of the cell (e.g., ref. 8). Such shifting of the spike initiation zone does not, however, necessarily imply rapid changes in the density of sodium channels but may rather reflect changing distributions of synaptic conductances and current flows (13). It is possible, of course, that some plasticity in ionic channel distribution may exist at the initial segment. Regardless of whether such plasticity exists, we are led to conclude that structure–function relations at the initial segment play an important role in the specification of neuronal integrative properties and, in particular, in the determination of the functional characteristics of the "encoder" region of the neuron.

ACKNOWLEDGMENTS

This work was supported in part by grants NS-12307 and RR-05479 and Research Career Development Award KO4-NS-00010 from the National Institutes of Health, and by grant RG-1133A1 from the National Multiple Sclerosis Society.

REFERENCES

1. Conradi, S. (1969): Observations on the ultrastructure of the axon hillock and initial axon segment in lumbosacral motoneurons in the cat. *Acta Physiol. Scand. [Suppl.]*, 332:65–84.
2. Coombs, J. S., Curtis, D. R., and Eccles, J. C. (1957): The generation of impulses in motoneurons. *J. Physiol. (Lond)*, 139:232–249.
3. Dodge, F. A., Jr., and Cooley, J. W. (1973): Action potential of the motoneuron. *IBM J. Res. Dev.*, 17:219–229.
4. Eccles, J. C. (1964): *The Physiology of Synapses*, Springer-Verlag, New York.
5. Fatt, P. (1957): Sequence of events in synaptic activation of a motoneurone. *J. Neurophysiol.*, 20:61–80.
6. Fuortes, M. G. F., Frank, K., and Becker, M. C. (1957): Steps in the production of motoneuron spikes. *J. Gen. Physiol.*, 40:735–752.
7. Karnovsky, M. J. (1967): The ultrastructural basis of capillary permeability studied with

peroxidase as a tracer. *J. Cell Biol.,* 35:213–236.

8. Kriebel, M. E., Bennett, M. V. L., Waxman, S. G., and Pappas, G. D. (1969): Oculomotor neurons in fish: Electrotonic coupling and multiple sites of impulse initiation. *Science,* 166:520–524.

9. Kristol, C., Akert, K., Sandri, C., Wyss, U., Bennett, M. V. L., and Moor, H. (1977): The Ranvier nodes in the neurogenic electric organ of the knife fish *Sternarchus:* A freeze-etching study on the distribution of membrane-associated particles. *Brain Res.,* 125:197–212.

10. Nonner, W., Rojas, E., and Stämpfli, R., (1975): Gating currents in the node of Ranvier: Voltage and time dependence. *Philos. Trans. R. Soc. B.,* 270:483–492.

11. Palay, S. L., Sotelo, C., Peters, A., and Orkand, P. M. (1968): The axon hillock and the initial segment. *J. Cell Biol.,* 38:193–201.

12. Peters, A., Proskauer, C. C., and Kaiserman-Abramof, I. R. (1968): The small pyramidal neuron of the rat cerebral cortex: The axon hillock and initial segment. *J. Cell Biol.,* 39:604–619.

13. Purpura, D. P. (1967): Comparative physiology of dendrites. In: *The Neurosciences. A Study Program,* edited by G. C. Quarton, T. Melnechuk, and F. O. Schmitt. Rockefeller University Press, New York.

14. Quick, D. C., and Waxman, S. G. (1977): Specific staining of the axon membrane at nodes of Ranvier with ferric ion and ferrocyanide. *J. Neurol. Sci.,* 31:1–11.

15. Quick, D. C., and Waxman, S. G. (1977): Ferric ion, ferrocyanide, and inorganic phosphate as cytochemical reactants at peripheral nodes of Ranvier. *J. Neurocytol.* 6:555–570.

16. Ritchie, J. M., and Rogart, R. B. (1977): Density of sodium channels in mammalian myelinated nerve fibers and nature of the axonal membrane under the myelin sheath. *Proc. Natl. Acad. Sci. USA,* 74:211–215.

17. Ritchie, J. M., Rogart, R. B., and Strichartz, G. (1976): A new method for labeling saxitoxin and its binding to non-myelinated fibers of the rabbit vagus, lobster walking, and garfish olfactory nerves. *J. Physiol. (Lond),* 261:477–494.

18. Spencer, P. S., Raine, C., and Wisniewski, H. (1973): Axon diameter and myelin thickness —unusual relationships in dorsal root ganglia. *Anat. Rec.,* 176:224–245.

19. Waxman, S. G., and Quick, D. C. (1977): Cytochemical differentiation of the axon membrane in A- and C-fibers. *J. Neurol. Neurosurg. Psychiatry,* 40:379–386.

20. Waxman, S. G., and Quick, D. C. (1977b): Intra-axonal ferric ion-ferrocyanide staining of nodes of Ranvier and initial segments in central myelinated fibers. *Brain Res. (in press).*

21. Waxman, S. G., Pappas, G. D., and Bennett, M. V. (1972): Morphological correlates of functional differentiation of nodes of Ranvier along single fibers in the neurogenic electric organ of the knife fish *Sternarchus. J. Cell Biol.,* 53:210–224.

Physiology and Pathobiology of Axons, edited by
S. G. Waxman. Raven Press, New York © 1978.

Conduction Properties of Normal Peripheral Mammalian Axons

A. S. Paintal

Department of Physiology, Vallabhbhai Patel Chest Institute, Delhi University, Delhi 110007, India

The two main properties of a nerve fiber that are of primary functional importance are its conduction velocity (CV) and the maximum frequency of discharge it can propagate. The conduction velocity of the nerve fiber depends mainly on its diameter (D), which determines the electrical properties of the conducting system. In the case of medullated fibers, conduction velocity is also determined by the length of the internodes (L) across which the nerve impulse jumps. Of the three variables (CV, D, and L) the only one that can be measured with reproducible precision is the conduction velocity of the fiber; the other two variables are subject to errors due to variable shrinkage of the fiber, measurement of internodal length, etc.

Two important morphological relations of nerve fibers to conduction velocity are the conduction velocity/fiber diameter ratio (CV/D) and the relation of internodal length to conduction velocity, which gives a measure of internodal conduction time. The former ratio, which is extensively used, has been determined by relatively direct measurements of diameter and conduction velocity; the latter (apart from electrophysiological methods used; see below) is deduced from measurements of diameter and internodal length.

CONDUCTION VELOCITY/DIAMETER RATIO

Unlike a direct correlation between the diameter of fibers of invertebrates with their conduction velocities (17,40,41), no such correlation has yet been made in the case of mammalian medullated nerve fibers because it has not been possible to measure the diameter of a particular fiber and determine its conduction velocity. However, in the case of the frog, Tasaki made direct measurements of both in the same fiber and obtained a CV/D ratio of 2.05, with a large scatter of points which he attributed to nonuniformity of the diameter of the fiber along its course (49). Tasaki observed an even greater scatter of points relating fiber diameter and internodal length (49); the question that therefore arises is if this scatter is due to errors in measuring the diameter or internodal length, or if the variation in internodal length and diameter is real. It is a question that arises repeatedly when considering the measurements relating to mammalian nerve fibers (see below), and it is important that it be answered.

In the case of mammalian fibers, the correlation between conduction velocity and fiber diameter has been indirect. Hursh (21) based his conclusions on the assumption that the fastest conducting fibers in the compound action potential are those corresponding to fibers with the largest diameters. A similar indirect correlation was made by Boyd and Davey (2,3) based on mean values of fiber diameters and conduction velocities. These investigators (3) pointed out that there are uncertainties in estimates of mean conduction velocities. An important conclusion of Boyd is that the ratio in the case of small-diameter fibers (ca. 2 to 6 μm) is less than that in the large-diameter fibers. In the small fibers the ratio was 4.5, compared to 5.7 in the large-diameter fibers (2,3).

TABLE 1. *Properties of mammalian medullated and nonmedullated fibers*

Measurements at 37°C	A fibers (20–1 μm)	C fibers
Conduction velocity (meters sec)	120–4.5	3.0–0.5
Spike duration (msec)	0.3 –1.6	1.1–2.8
Rise time (msec)	0.07–0.4	0.2–0.52
Fall time (msec)	0.23–1.2	0.8–2.4
ARP (msec)	0.45–3.2	1.1–2.8
Mean blocking temperature (°C)	7.6	4.3–2.7
Q_{10} Conduction velocity		
27°–37°C	+1.6	+1.5
18°–28°C	+2.5	+2.1
8°–18°C	+4.8	+3.0
Q_{10} Spike duration 27°–37°C	−3.5	
Q_{10} Rise time 27°–37°C	−2.5	
Q_{10} Fall time 27°–37°C	−3.5	
Q_{10} ARP		
27°–37°C	−3.2	
18°–28°C	−3.6	
8°–18°C	−12.2	

Data obtained from refs. 23,32–34,36.

EFFECT OF TEMPERATURE ON CV/D RATIO

The ratios obtained by Boyd and Davey (2,3) and by Hursh (21) are approximately the same in the large fibers when the difference in the temperature at which the conduction velocity measurements were made is taken into account (38), keeping in mind that the Q_{10} (temperature coefficient) for the CV/D ratio is 1.6 since the Q_{10} for the conduction velocity is 1.6 (Table 1). This aspect was dealt with earlier (38). Thus at 37°C—particularly in view of the observations of Waxman and Bennett (54)—one can justifiably use the ratio of 5.7 instead of the ratio of 6 obtained by Hursh, who made his measurements at 37.5°C. On the other hand, the classic relation of conduction velocity to fiber diameter (21) is valid at 37.5°C, certainly for the large-diameter fibers.

RELATION OF INTERNODAL LENGTH TO DIAMETER

It is well known that the internodal length of nerve fibers increases with their diameter. It is also recognized that, for practical purposes, the relation between the two is linear. However, the L/D ratio varies in different animals: in cats it is 90 (21), rabbits 59 (53)

to 72 (5), rats 175 (12), frogs 146 (49), and man 100 (27). An important aspect that has not received adequate attention is the fact that there are wide variations in internodal length for the same fiber diameter. This feature is striking in the nerve fibers of elderly human subjects (27) and in regenerating nerves (5). However, wide scatters have also been seen in normal cat (21), frog (49), and rat (12) nerves. To some extent these variations may be due to variations in the diameter of the fiber (49). Errors due to sampling must therefore be considered. There may also be variations in measurement of internodal length due to differences in technique. The possible role of errors is highlighted by the fact that the results of different investigators reveal widely different L/D ratios in the same animal. For example, Schnepp and Schnepp (45) reported a ratio of 75 in cat nerve fibers, whereas the ratio from Hursh's data indicate a value of 90. Similarly, in the rat, Schnepp and Schnepp (45) report a ratio of 79, whereas the results of Fullerton and Barnes (12) indicate a ratio of 175. Are these differences due to variations in the value for internodal length? These doubts have raised the need for reinvestigation of these values and for examining the electrophysiological methods for measuring internodal distance described below.

ELECTROPHYSIOLOGICAL METHOD OF MEASURING INTERNODAL LENGTH

Recently two techniques have been used for measuring internodal length electrophysiologically. The first is the technique used by Rasminsky and Sears (42) based on the approach used by Huxley and Stämpfli (22). In this technique Rasminsky and Sears (42) used a pair of electrodes 100 μm in diameter placed approximately 400–600 μm apart on filaments of the ventral root. The two electrodes were moved along the ventral root filament, and the variation in the latency of the evoked potential (with respect to a fixed point of stimulation) was recorded. The points where the latency suddenly changed were assumed to represent the nodes. Figure 1A shows the internodal conduction time recorded by Rasminsky and Sears in the different fibers. They found that at 37°C this amounted to 19.7 μsec in fibers with internodal lengths ranging from 0.75 to 1.45 mm. The conduction velocity of these fibers would therefore be 38 to 74 meters/sec.

If one were to use the observations of Fullerton and Barnes (12), assuming an L/D ratio of 175, it would follow that the diameter of the fibers corresponding to internodal lengths

of 750 and 1,450 μm would be 4.3 and 8.3 μm. This would give a CV/D ratio of approximately 9. Such a large ratio has not been reported so far. Thus it is not possible to reconcile the observations of Fullerton and Barnes (12) with those of Rasminsky and Sears (42). On the other hand, Schnepp et al., who obtained a CV/D ratio of 6.1 in the rat (46), reported an L/D ratio of 79 (45), i.e., approximately half that indicated by Fullerton and Barnes (12). With such large differences in values reported by various investigators, it is difficult to draw firm conclusions. However, it seems that the L/D ratio obtained by Schnepp and Schnepp (45) is perhaps uniformly lower than those of other investigators; they reported a ratio of 75 in the cat, which is obviously lower than the ratio reported by Hursh (21). One is therefore in a dilemma in choosing between the observations of Fullerton and Barnes (12) and those of Schnepp and Schnepp (45) for establishing the value of the technique used by Rasminsky and Sears (42) for measuring internodal length by electrophysiological methods.

The observations of Rasminsky and Sears (42) also cannot be reconciled with those of Boyd and Davey (2,3); the results of the former indicate that the CV/D ratio is maxi-

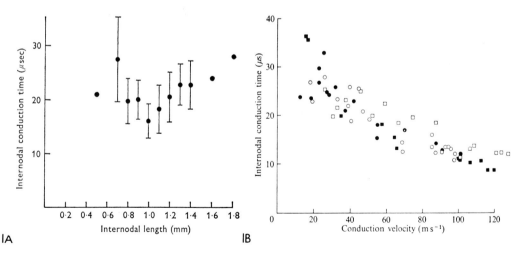

IA   IB

FIG. 1. **A:** Relationship between internodal conduction time and internodal length for normal oxygenated ventral root fibers of the rat at 37°C. The data is plotted with average internodal conduction times calculated for fibers grouped by internodal length in increments of 0.1 mm. Vertical bars represent 1 SD. (From ref. 42.) **B:** Observed variation of internodal conduction time with conduction velocity in fibers of the cat. (From ref. 25.)

mum for fibers with internodal lengths of 750–1,450 μm and that the ratio decreases for shorter or longer fibers. Boyd and Davey (2,3), on the other hand, found the ratio to be approximately 5.7 for large fibers and 4.5 for small ones. The observations of Coppin and Jack (4) also indicate that the ratio falls with a reduction in fiber diameter. Another noteworthy result from the observations of Rasminsky and Sears (42) is that there is a large variation in the conduction velocity of fibers with the same internodal length (Fig. 1A). For example, at an internodal length of 1,200 μm the conduction velocity is 39–82 meters/sec, and at an internodal length of 800 μm the velocity is 27–49 meters/sec. Such large variations, although striking, are not unexpected; Hursh (21) found that in the cat there is considerable variation in diameter at any internodal length. Moreover, the large variation can be fully accounted for if it is assumed that age influences internodal length in the fibers of the rat, as it does in man. Lascelles and Thomas (27) showed that the variation is indeed large. For example, at an internodal length of approximately 500 μm the diameter of fibers may vary from 3 to 11 μm. An even greater variation of diameter with regard to internodal length is seen in regenerating nerve fibers (5).

The second method of determining internodal conduction distance electrophysiologically is that used by Coppin and Jack (4), which was originally reported by Lussier and Rushton (28). Some implications of the results obtained by this technique are discussed elsewhere (38). Coppin and Jack (25) used this technique to estimate internodal conduction time (Fig. 1B), an important factor in the process of impulse conduction.

INTERNODAL CONDUCTION TIME

Since internodal length and diameter vary linearly throughout the range of fiber diameters in the cat (21), rabbit (5), and man (27), and since the conduction velocity/fiber diameter ratio is fixed (at least over a certain range of fiber diameters) (2,3), it follows that over the same range of fiber diameters (or CV) the internodal conduction time should be the same in fibers of different diameters. Assuming a

CV/D ratio of 5.7, the internodal conduction time should be approximately 16 μsec in fibers larger than 6 μm at 37°C in the cat (L/D ratio = 90). If one uses Boyd's ratio of 4.5 for the small-diameter fibers, the internodal conduction time is 20 μsec in (cat) fibers below 6 μm in diameter, corresponding roughly to a conduction velocity of 30 meters/sec. These values for internodal conduction time are consistent with only a few of the observations of Coppin and Jack (Fig. 1B) since the majority of their values are either much larger or smaller than 16 μsec—ranging from 9 μsec for fibers with conduction velocities of 120 meters/sec to 36 μsec for fibers with velocities of 20 meters/sec (Fig. 1b). The mean conduction time for the six fibers at 100 meters/sec in Fig. 1B (i.e., corresponding to $D = 17.5$ μm using a ratio of 5.7) is approximately 11 μsec (Fig. 1B).

On the basis of an L/D ratio of 90, the internodal length corresponds to approximately 1,500 μm. It follows, then, that the conduction velocity of the fiber corresponding to an internodal conduction time of 11 μsec and internodal length of 1,500 μm should be 136 meters/sec. There is thus a discrepancy of 36%, part of which may be due to variations in internodal length for the same diameter (21). On the other hand, the results of Coppin and Jack are compatible with the L/D ratio of 75 obtained by Schnepp and Schnepp (45). Thus again there is uncertainty.

RATIO g (AXON DIAMETER/FIBER DIAMETER)

The ratio of axon diameter to fiber diameter g in medullated fibers was a subject of debate in the past because of the relatively small value reported by some investigators for small-diameter fibers (44). From theoretical considerations, Rushton concluded that the optimal ratio of g should be 0.6, although a variation of g between 0.47 and 0.74 theoretically made a difference of only 5% in the conduction velocity. Hodgkin (19) carried the argument further and concluded that the optimal ratio should be 0.7. Subsequently, from digital computer solutions, Goldman and Albus (15) confirmed these conclusions, finding that the conduction velocity changed only a small amount between *g* values of 0.6 and 0.7. This point has been discussed by Jack et al. (25). More recent ultrastructural studies amply confirmed in the cat that the ratio is practically the same (~0.6) in fibers of different diameters. For example, Friede and Samorajski (11) found that the critical diameter above which the fibers of the vagus and sciatic nerves of the mouse became myelinated was 1.1 μm —thus confirming the observations of Duncan (7)—and that the ratio *g*, which varied between 0.5 and 0.9, was not related to fiber diameter. Indeed Fig. 4 of their report (11) shows the scatter of the points around a ratio of 0.7–0.75 in fibers with diameters between 1 and 4 μm. Subsequently Schnepp and Schnepp (45) found that the ratio (0.6) was practically constant over a wide range of fiber diameters in various mammals (mouse, rat, guinea pig, cat, and dog).

ACCOMMODATION

One of the intriguing features of peripheral neural activity is the way in which repetitive activity can be generated at sensory receptors when it is well known that, as a rule, a rectangular pulse produces only one impulse in nerve fibers. Fundamental differences in the properties of motor and sensory fibers have therefore been sought. Erlanger and Blair (8) and Skoglund (47) found some evidence to show that the critical slope for linearly rising currents for stimulation of sensory fibers was less than that for motor fibers; i.e., the accommodation was greater in motor fibers than in sensory ones. Differences between skin and muscle sensory fibers were reported by Granit and Skoglund (16), the accommodation in sensory fibers of the skin being less. This question was reinvestigated by Vallbo (52), who studied the accommodation of fibers of slowly and rapidly adapting receptors running in the same nerves, thereby excluding possible errors in the earlier procedures followed. He found that although the accommodation in sensory fibers was a little less than in motor fibers, the accommodation in the fibers of slowly adapting receptors was approximately the same as that in the fibers of rapidly adapting sensory receptors. Thus there were no basic differences in the properties of the nerve fibers

that could be invoked to account for the greater degree of repetitive firing in slowly adapting receptors. It follows that the properties of the first node, where the impulse is initiated at sensory receptors (6), must be different from that of the more central nodes. Use of more advanced techniques might help to resolve the differences in the accommodation of different sensory fibers at the periphery. Here it is noteworthy that Bergman and Stämpfli (1), in voltage clamp studies, reported differences in the nodal characteristics of motor and sensory fibers.

When considering the differences in the accommodation of the first node from the more central parts of the sensory fiber, one must keep in mind that the diffusion barrier in this region is much less than that in the main nerve trunk, this being the reason for action of several chemical substances that produce excitatory effects (31). It is therefore conceivable that certain ionic differences may be of importance in relation to accommodation. Such differences, if found at the first node, are also applicable to the juxtareceptor regions in the case of nonmedullated fibers, which are in fact even more susceptible to the action of chemical substances (31,37).

SPIKE DURATION AND RISE TIME IN MEDULLATED FIBERS

Until recently it was generally assumed that the duration of the spike is the same in all medullated nerve fibers, i.e., approximately 0.4–0.5 msec. This view arose from the observations of Gasser and Grundfest (14) who, largely from extrapolations of the compound action potential of the entire saphenous nerve down to zero conduction distance, concluded that the spike duration of the fibers with velocities between 40 and 10 meters/sec had the same spike duration (approximately 0.5 msec). This conclusion was supplemented by measurements of the spike duration of individual fibers. The spikes used for these measurements were recorded in different experiments and from a variety of preparations, e.g., rabbit cervical sympathetic, cat hypogastric, rabbit depressor, and rabbit saphenous nerves (14). Even so, their measurements of the spikes show an inverse relation between

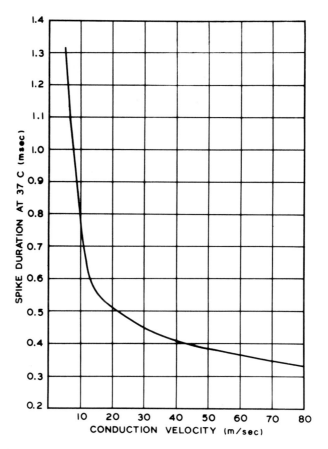

FIG. 2. Relation of spike duration (at 37°C) of medullated fibers to their conduction velocities ranging from 5 to 80 meters/sec. The curve approximates the mean spike duration at various conduction velocities. There is usually a wide scatter of the values at any particular conduction velocity, e.g., see Fig. 4. (From ref. 34.)

spike duration and conduction velocity. Apparently, Gasser and Grundfest (14) did not notice the relationship because they measured spike durations to the first decimal place (34).

It is now certain that spike duration varies inversely with conduction velocity. As shown in Fig. 2 and Table 1, at 37°C it ranges from 0.3 msec in the fastest fibers to approximately 1.6 msec in the slowest medullated fibers. These observations on medullated nerve fibers apply in general to both sensory and motor fibers as the impulses were recorded in fibers of the vagus and saphenous nerves. They also apply to preganglionic sympathetic fibers which had so far been described as a separate group (38). There is therefore no longer any need to group them separately (34). The inverse relation between spike duration and conduction velocity was confirmed by Coppin in peripheral nerve fibers (24).

The increase in spike duration with a fall in conduction velocity is due largely to an increase in the fall time, but is also due to an increase in the rise time of the impulse. This important point, which came to light recently (34), had not been taken into account in important theoretical treatments of this subject (e.g., ref. 44). In fact, it was tacitly assumed that it is the same in all fibers (see below). At 37°C the rise time varies from 70 μsec in the fastest fibers to approximately 400 μsec in the slowest fibers (Fig. 3; Table 1). It is clear that the rise time must influence the conduction velocity of the fiber—the slower the rate of rise of the impulse, the slower the conduction velocity, as it will take longer for the impulse to excite the neighboring node. If the internodal length of fibers of different diameters had been the same, then this factor (i.e., rise time) would have had a profound influ-

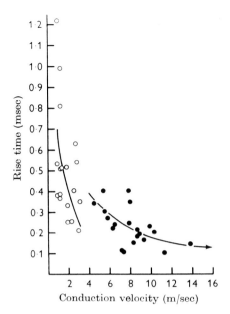

FIG. 3. Relation of rise time to conduction velocity at 37°C in medullated (*filled circles*) and nonmedullated (*open circles*) fibers of the aortic nerve of cats. (From ref. 36.)

ence on the conduction velocity, because the time to reach threshold excitation of the neighboring node would have been much longer in the small-diameter fibers with a longer rise time. However, nature seems to have dealt with this aspect by ensuring that the small-diameter fibers with slow rates of rise of the impulse have a short internodal length. The internodal conduction time is the same for a particular range of fiber diameters because of the linear relation between fiber diameter and conduction velocity on the one hand and fiber diameter and internodal length on the other. In the large-diameter fibers of the cat, the internodal conduction time is approximately 16 μsec at 37°C, assuming a CV/D ratio of 5.7 and an L/D ratio of 90 (see above). Thus the neighboring node is excited when the impulse rises to approximately 21% of its full amplitude in the large-diameter fibers. This is in agreement with the generally accepted safety factor of 5 (49). In the small-diameter fibers—e.g., those conducting at approximately 16 meters/sec ($D = 3.3$ μm; $L = 300$ μm; CV/D ratio = 4.5)—the internodal conduction time is 20 μsec and the impulse approximately 14% of its full amplitude by the time

the next node is excited. This gives a safety factor of approximately 7. If the safety factor is assumed to be the same in all fibers of different diameters, the observations of Coppin and Jack (25) (Fig. 1B), which show that the conduction time is greater in the small-diameter fibers, are significant. Indeed their observations extrapolated to fibers of 15 meters/sec, yielding an internodal conduction time of 30 μsec, indicate that the impulse will have reached 21% of its full amplitude when it has excited the next node. This is the same as that for the largest fibers; i.e., there is a safety factor of 5. It should be pointed out that the observations of Coppin and Jack (4) give a CV/D ratio of 7 for fibers with a diameter of 20 μm, a ratio of 2.6 for a 3-μm fiber, and a ratio of 1.5 for 1-μm fibers. According to these investigators, $CV = 1.5$ $D^{1.5}$. As has been pointed out (38), these conclusions differ from the generally accepted ones.

It appears that a reduction in temperature increases the safety factor: Although the Q_{10} for conduction velocity is 1.6 in all medullated fibers (33), the Q_{10} for the rise time is approximately 2.5 (Table 1) between 27° and 37°C. This value is similar to that obtained in the squid axon (20) and to that recorded by Inman and Peruzzi (23) in the sensory fiber of the mammalian Pacinian corpuscle. The Q_{10} for spike duration is higher than that for the rise time, i.e., 3.4 between 37° and 27°C. Again this is similar to the value obtained by Hodgkin and Katz (20) in the squid axon. Tasaki and Fugita (51) reported a similar value in the frog.

SPIKE DURATION AND RISE TIME IN NONMEDULLATED FIBERS

As in the case of medullated fibers, the spike duration and rise time vary inversely with the conduction velocity of the fibers (Fig. 4). This was confirmed by Pearson et al. (40). The most noteworthy point is that the relation of conduction velocity to spike duration and rise time is such as to provide no distinction between medullated and nonmedullated fibers in this range of conduction velocities i.e., from 0.9 to 14 meters/sec at 37°C. If it is assumed that peripheral nerve fibers become nonmedullated at diameters below 1 μm (7), the lowest conduction velocity

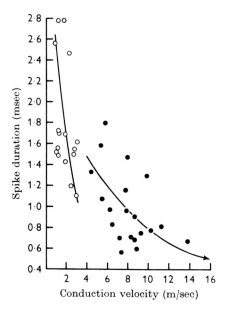

FIG. 4. Relation of spike duration to conduction velocity at 37°C in medullated (*filled circles*) and nonmedullated (*open circles*) fibers of aortic nerves of cats. (From ref. 36.)

for medullated nerve fibers would be 4.5 meters/sec [using Boyd's ratio (2,3)]. According to Gasser (13), the maximum conduction velocities of nonmedullated fibers is 2.5 meters/sec. The validity of these figures is supported by the fact that relatively few fibers are found in the range 2.5–4.5 meters/sec (Figs. 3 and 4). This is particularly noteworthy because the sample of nerve fibers in Figs. 3 and 4 were obtained from the aortic nerve of the cat, which has medullated and nonmedullated fibers. Moreover, all the fibers are sensory and carry impulses from aortic chemoreceptors (39). Keep in mind that in the central nervous system the position is different; here, Waxman and colleagues (48,54) showed that there are many medullated fibers between 0.25 and 1.0 μm in the reptile oculomotor nucleus and the splenium of the corpus callosum of the rabbit. An interesting feature is that the ratio g is 0.6 in the small-diameter fibers, which confirms the predictions of Rushton (44) and Hodgkin (19) relating to the optimal relative thickness of myelin sheath (capacity) and axon diameter (resistance) for ensuring maximum conduction velocity.

The presence of relatively few fibers with conduction velocities between 2.5 and 4.5 meters/sec would support Rushton's conclusion (44) that 1 μm is the critical diameter above which myelin increases conduction velocity and below which conduction is faster without myelination. This consideration becomes particularly significant if it is assumed (quite justifiably) that the distribution of fiber diameter in the aortic nerve will be similar to that in the carotid nerve in which Eyzaguirre and Uchizono (9) found only 12 of approximately 2,000 nonmedullated fibers with diameters between 1 and 1.3 μm; they found none larger than 1.3 μm. Moreover, out of 570 medullated fibers less than 7 μm in diameter, they found no fiber under 1 μm. These values are in agreement with those of Duncan (7). Thus there is a large difference between the relative number of small medullated and nonmedullated fibers in peripheral nerves on the one hand and in the central nervous system [e.g., the splenium of the corpus collosum (55)] on the other.

It is therefore possible that the nature of conduction in the two groups is different, and that in peripheral nerves Rushton's conclusion (44) is valid. As argued by Waxman and Bennett (54), it may not hold true in the fibers of the central nervous system. In this connection it must be pointed out that the role of the rise time was not taken into consideration by Rushton when accounting for the differences in the conduction velocities of different-diameter fibers. In fact, he assumed that the rate of rise of the impulse was the same in all fibers. However, it is clear that this factor (i.e., rise time) by itself cannot account for the fact that the conduction velocity of the medullated fibers of 1 μm (4.5 meters/sec) is nearly twice as great as the conduction velocity of the nonmedullated fibers of the same diameter (2.5 μm) since the rise time is approximately the same in both groups (Fig. 3). This increased velocity in the medullated fibers must therefore be attributed to saltatory conduction.

Several important points emerge from the relation between conduction velocity and rise time in the slowest conducting medullated fibers and nonmedullated fibers shown in Fig. 3. For instance, if the curve for the medullated fibers is extrapolated to lower velocities (e.g., 3 meters/sec), it follows that the expected rise times in such hypothetical fibers would be 1.5–2 times the rise time in nonmedullated fibers of the same conduction velocity (36). Thus from this point of view, there would be a distinct disadvantage in terms of conduction velocity for fibers to be medullated in this diameter range. Presumably the rate of rise of the impulse is determined primarily by the number of sodium channels available, and these might be relatively few in the small-diameter fibers even though the surface area increases relative to volume; thus it is important to determine the role these play with respect to the advantages gained by saltatory conduction. In this connection, according to the computation of Marks and Loeb (29), the nodal current varies linearly with the conduction velocity of medullated fibers.

RELATION OF CONDUCTION VELOCITY TO DIAMETER IN NONMEDULLATED FIBERS

One of the important conclusions flowing from the observation that the rise time of nonmedullated fibers varies inversely with conduction velocity (Fig. 3) was that this factor should influence the conduction velocity of nonmedullated fibers also—making it faster

in the larger nonmedullated fibers owing to the faster rate of rise of the impulse in them (and vice versa). Indeed it was suggested (36) that in view of this the conduction velocity should tend to vary linearly with diameter rather than as the square root of fiber diameter, as had been assumed from the observations of Pumphrey and Young (41). It is therefore noteworthy that Pearson et al. (40) found conduction velocity to vary as the 0.78 power of diameter of nonmedullated nerve fibers of the cockroach. The actual relationship varies in different species, being different in the locust; it is therefore important that CV/D relations should be established in nerve fibers of the same animal.

ABSOLUTE REFRACTORY PERIOD

One of the important facts that emerged from recent studies is that the absolute refractory period (ARP) for the propagation of the impulse is always longer than the ARP for the initiation of the impulse (ARP$_i$) (Fig. 5) (34,38). This is not generally recognized. In fact, the difference can be quite large, and it becomes particularly obvious when the temperature of the nerve fibers is lowered. Figure 6 shows the relation between conduction ve-

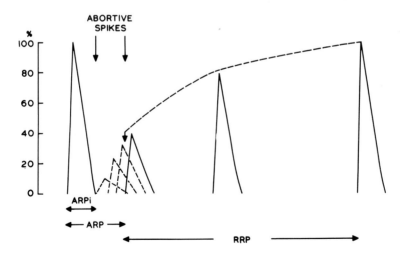

FIG. 5. Relative proportions of various parts of refractory period in a slow fiber. ARP is twice the spike duration (Fig. 6). RRP (relative refractory period) is four times the ARP. (ARP$_i$) Absolute refractory period for spike initiation. Note that only abortive spikes are initiated during the interval between the end of the first spike and the end of the ARP. In a fast fiber the ARP would be approximately 1.5 times the spike duration. Interrupted curve indicates the recovery of excitability. This becomes discontinuous at the ARP (*arrow*). No time scale is given because spike duration has been used as a unit of time. (From ref. 38.)

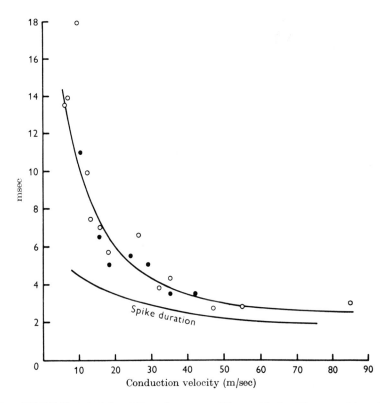

FIG. 6. Relation of ARP (*filled circles*) and time of recovery of the amplitude of the second impulse (*open circles*) to 40% of normal following a preceding impulse to the normal conduction velocity of the fibers at 20°C. The lower curve shows the relation of spike duration at 20°C to normal (i.e., 37°C) conduction velocity. Note the identity of the ARP with the interval for 40% recovery of spike amplitude and the marked disparity between spike duration and ARP at the lower levels of conduction velocity. (From ref. 34.)

locity and the ARP at 20°C, and the relation between spike duration and conduction velocity, which is less than the ARP at all levels of conduction velocity, especially at the lower levels. This difference is due to the fact that, although an impulse can be initiated after the end of the spike, such impulses are in fact abortive because they are unable to propagate until they attain propagating amplitude, which is approximately 40% the spike height (34) (Fig. 5). The fact that the time for 40% recovery of the spike height is similar to that of the ARP supports this conclusion (Fig. 6).

The above observations pertain to medullated fibers in peripheral nerves (vagus and saphenous) (34). Recently Swadlow and Waxman (48) confirmed them in the callosal fibers of the rabbit's brain. The inverse relation between conduction velocity and ARP also applies to nonmedullated fibers; however, in this case one does not know if there is any difference between ARP and ARP$_1$, although judging by the relative values for spike duration at 37°C and assuming a Q_{10} of 3.5 there does not seem to be an obvious difference between the two. For example, the ARP of fibers conducting at approximately 1.5 meters/sec at 17°C is approximately 27 msec (36). The spike duration of such fibers is 1.8–2.0 msec at 37°C (Fig. 4). Using a Q_{10} of 3.5, this would give a value of 22–24 msec at 17°C for spike duration at 17°C. It thus appears that there is not much of a difference between ARP and ARP$_1$, but this point needs direct confirmation.

In view of the obvious inverse relation between conduction velocity and the ARP, it is curious that this clear relation was not recognized until recently (33). The reasons for this are briefly recounted elsewhere (38).

MAXIMUM TRANSMISSIBLE FREQUENCIES

The maximum frequency of discharge that can be transmitted in nerve fibers depends on their conduction velocities (Figs. 7 and 8). This is not surprising since the ARP of the fibers, as well as the relative ARP (33), varies inversely with the conduction velocity of the fibers (Fig. 6). However, other factors are also involved, and there is a difference between the least interval between the first two impulses of a train and the least interimpulse intervals of the rest of the train.

The relation between conduction velocity and the reciprocal of the least interval between two impulses at 37°C is shown in Fig. 7. Clearly this frequency is much less than the frequency that would be expected from the absolute refractory period of the fibers (Table 1), according to which in the fastest fibers the maximum frequency should be approximately 2,000 impulses/sec. Such frequencies have indeed been recorded, but this is possible only when there is a negligible conducting distance between the recording and stimulating electrodes. On the other hand, when there is a certain conduction distance the second impulse lags behind the first more and more with an increase in conduction distance; this is be-

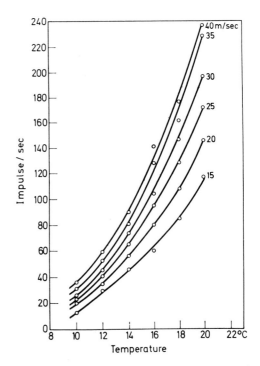

FIG. 8. Relation between maximum frequency of discharge of a brief train of impulses that can pass unblocked between 10° and 20°C in fibers of different conduction velocities. (From ref. 35.)

cause the conduction velocity of the second impulse traveling in the relative refractory period of the first is much less than the conduction velocity of the first impulse (49,50). The amount of lag therefore depends on the conduction velocity of the fiber itself even if the percentage recovery of conduction velocity at a fixed time after the first impulse is the same in all fibers. However, as has been shown (33), the rate of recovery of conduction velocity of the second impulse is not the same in all fibers: it varies with the conduction velocity of the fiber, being much slower in fibers of slow conduction velocity. This further increases the interval between the impulses. It follows that the least interval increases more and more with increasing conduction distance until the conduction velocity of the second impulse becomes 100% of normal (49,50). The conduction distance at which this happens has not been determined, but judging by the rate of recovery of conduction velocity in slow and fast fibers (33), it is obvious that

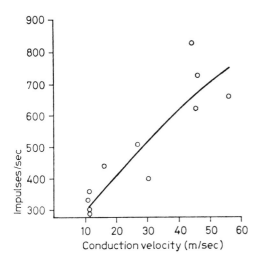

FIG. 7. Relation of peak frequency of discharge (i.e., reciprocal of smallest interval between first two impulses) at 37°C to conduction velocity of vagal nerve fibers. (From ref. 33.)

the conduction distance is much greater in faster conducting fibers.

It is important to appreciate that the ARP after the second impulse is the same as that after the first (18) in fibers of different conduction velocities (36). However, the least interval between the second and third impulses is less than that after the first and second. This is because the conduction velocity of the third impulse (and subsequent impulses) traveling in the relative refractory period of the second impulse is the same as that of the second impulse. This interval is what determines the maximal transmissible frequency in nerve fibers and, as is to be expected, it varies with the conduction velocity of the fibers (Fig. 8).

Lowering the temperature reduces the maximum transmissible frequency, again because of an increase in the refractory period (Q_{10} of 3.2–3.6 between 18° and 37°C; Table 1). Figure 8 shows the variation of the maximal transmissible frequency with conduction velocity at 10°–20°C. It must be pointed out that the maximum transmissible frequency shown in Fig. 8 is much greater than the frequency of discharge generated in efferent or sensory fibers normally *in vivo*. Indeed the normal activity at 37°C in motoneurons or sensory receptors is much less than the maximal transmissible frequency at 20°C. The main utility of Fig. 8 is that it provides information about the frequencies of discharge that emerge through a region of cold block, a procedure commonly used for producing so-called differential block of sensory nerve fibers, e.g., of the vagus (30). There is actually no differential block by cold because it has been shown conclusively that conduction in medullated nerve fibers of different conduction velocities is blocked at approximately 7.6°C (10,32). Conduction in nonmedullated fibers is blocked at a slightly lower temperature, i.e., approximately 4.3°C (36) or 2.7°C (10; see ref. 38 for details). What actually happens when a region of the nerve is cooled with a thermode is that at the appropriate temperatures the high-frequency discharges generated in sensory fibers are blocked, leaving the low-frequency discharges to pass through; thus the resulting reflex effects are not due to blocked conduction in the fibers but to blocked discharges with frequencies that are higher

than the maximum transmissible frequencies for that temperature. The actual frequency of the discharge emerging from the cooled region depends on the frequency of the discharge entering it, as well as on certain local conditions existing in the cooled region (33). When the input frequency slightly exceeds the maximum transmissible frequency, the discharge (except for the first impulse) is totally blocked. This, as pointed out, is presumably because each succeeding impulse that arrives during the ARP (not the ARP_1) of the preceding impulse produces an abortive impulse; this impulse does not propagate but nevertheless leaves behind a state of refractoriness so that the succeeding impulse is influenced in the same way (34).

This information has been of considerable value for explaining the mechanism underlying Head's paradoxical reflex (35). Moreover, it was utilized recently by Kappagoda et al. (26) to account for the reflex effects of certain atrial receptors on the heart rate.

REFERENCES

1. Bergman, C., and Stämpfli, R. (1966): Différence de perméabilité des fibres nerveuses nyelinisées sensorielles et motrices a l'ion potassium. *Helv. Physiol. Pharmacol. Acta*, 24: 247–298.
2. Boyd, I. A. (1964): The relation between conduction velocity and diameter for the three groups of efferent fibres in nerves to mammalian skeletal muscle. *J. Physiol. (Lond)*, 175:33–35P.
3. Boyd, I. A., and Davey, M. R. (1968): *Composition of Peripheral Nerves*, pp. 1–57. Livingstone, Edinburgh.
4. Coppin, C. M. L., and Jack, J. J. B. (1972): Internodal length and conduction velocity of cat muscle afferent nerve fibres. *J. Physiol., (Lond)*, 222:91–93P.
5. Cragg, B. G., and Thomas, P. K. (1964): The conduction velocity of regenerated peripheral nerve fibres. *J. Physiol. (Lond)*, 171:164–175.
6. Diamond, J., Gray, J. A. B., and Sato, M. (1956): The site of initiation of impulses in Pacinian corpuscles. *J. Physiol. (Lond)*, 113: 54–67.
7. Duncan, D. (1934): A relation between axon diameter and myelination determined by measurement of myelinated spinal root fibres. *J. Comp. Neurol.*, 60:437–462.
8. Erlanger, J., and Blair, E. A. (1938): Comparative observation of motor and sensory fibers with special reference to the repetitiousness. *Am. J. Physiol.*, 121:431–453.

9. Eyzaguirre, C., and Uchizono, K. (1961): Observations on the fibre content of nerves reaching the carotid body of the cat. *J. Physiol. (Lond)*, 159:268–281.

10. Franz, D. N., and Iggo, A. (1968): Conduction failure in myelinated and non-myelinated axons at low temperatures. *J. Physiol. (Lond)*, 199:319–345.

11. Friede, R. L., and Samorajski, T. (1967): Relation between the number of myelin lamallae and axon circumference in fibers of vagus and sciatic nerves of mice. *J. Comp. Neurol.*, 130:223–232.

12. Fullerton, P. M., and Barnes, J. M. (1966): Peripheral neuropathy in rats produced by acrylamide. *Br. J. Ind. Med.*, 23:210–221.

13. Gasser, H. S. (1950): Unmedullated fibers originating in dorsal root ganglia. *J. Gen. Physiol.*, 33:651–690.

14. Gasser, H. S., and Grundfest, H. (1939): Axon diameters in relation to the spike dimensions and the conduction velocity in mammalian A fibers. *Am. J. Physiol.*, 127:393–414.

15. Goldman, L., and Albus, J. S. (1968): Computation of impulse conduction in myelinated fibres: Theoretical basis of the velocity-diameter relation. *Biophys. J.*, 8:596–607.

16. Granit, R., and Skoglund, C. R. (1943): Accommodation and autorhythmic mechanism in single sensory fibers. *J. Neurophysiol.*, 6:337–348.

17. Hodes, R. (1953): Linear relationship between fiber diameter and velocity of conduction in giant axon of squid. *J. Neurophysiol.*, 16:145–154.

18. Hodgkin, A. L. (1938): The subthreshold potentials in a crustacean nerve fibre. *Proc. R. Soc. B.*, 126:87–121.

19. Hodgkin, A. L. (1964): *The Conduction of the Nervous Impulse*, pp. 52–53. University Press, Liverpool.

20. Hodgkin, A. L., and Katz, B. (1949): The effect of temperature on the electrical activity of the giant axon of the squid. *J. Physiol. (Lond)*, 109:240–249.

21. Hursh, J. B. (1939): Conduction velocity and diameter of nerve fibers. *Am. J. Physiol.*, 127:131–139.

22. Huxley, A. F., and Stämpfli, R. (1949): Evidence for saltatory conduction in peripheral myelinated nerve fibres. *J. Physiol. (Lond)*, 108:315–339.

23. Inman, D. R., and Peruzzi, P. (1961): The effects of temperature on the responses of Pacinian corpuscles. *J. Physiol. (Lond)*, 155:280–301.

24. Jack, J. J. B. (1975): Physiology of peripheral nerve fibres in relation to their size. *Br. J. Anaesth.*, 47:173–182.

25. Jack, J. J. B., Noble, D., and Tsien, R. W. (1975): *Electric Current Flow in Excitable Cells*. Clarendon Press, Oxford.

26. Kappagoda, C. T., Linden, R. J., and Sivana-

than, N. (1977): The receptors which mediate a reflex increase in heart rate. *J. Physiol. (Lond)*, 266:89–90P.

27. Lascelles, R. G., and Thomas, P. K. (1966): Changes due to age in internodal length in the sural nerve in man. *J. Neurol. Neurosurg. Psychiatry*, 29:40–44.

28. Lussier, J. J., and Rushton, W. A. H. (1952): The excitability of a single fibre in a nerve trunk. *J. Physiol. (Lond)*, 117:87–108.

29. Marks, W. B., and Loeb, G. E. (1976): Action currents, internodal potentials, and extracellular records of myelinated mammalian nerve fibers derived from node potentials. *Biophys. J.*, 16:655–668.

30. Paintal, A. S. (1963): Vagal afferent fibres. *Ergeb. Physiol.*, 52:74–156.

31. Paintal, A. S. (1964): Effects of drugs on vertebrate mechanoreceptors. *Pharmacol. Rev.*, 16:341–380.

32. Paintal, A. S. (1965): Block of conduction in mammalian myelinated nerve fibres by low temperatures. *J. Physiol. (Lond)*, 180:1–19.

33. Paintal, A. S. (1965): Effects of temperature on conduction in single vagal and saphenous myelinated nerve fibres of the cat. *J. Physiol. (Lond)*, 180:20–49.

34. Paintal, A. S. (1966): The influence of diameter of medullated nerve fibres of cats on the rising and falling phases of the spike and its recovery. *J. Physiol. (Lond)*, 184:791–811.

35. Paintal, A. S. (1966): Re-evaluation of respiratory reflexes *Q. J. Exp. Physiol.*, 51:151–163.

36. Paintal, A. S. (1967): A comparison of the nerve impulses of mammalian non-medullated nerve fibres with those of the smallest diameter medullated fibres. *J. Physiol. (Lond)*, 193:523–533.

37. Paintal, A. S. (1971): Action of drugs on sensory nerve endings. *Annu. Rev. Pharmacol.*, 11:231–240.

38. Paintal, A. S. (1973): Conduction in mammalian nerve fibres. In: *New Developments in Electromyography and Clinical Neurophysiology*, Vol. 2, edited by J. E. Desmedt, pp. 19–41. Karger, Basel.

39. Paintal, A. S., and Riley, R. L. (1966): Responses of aortic chemoreceptors. *J. Appl. Physiol.*, 21:543–548.

40. Pearson, K. G., Stein, R. B., and Malhotra, S. K. (1970): Properties of action potentials from insect motor nerve fibres. *J. Exp. Biol.*, 53:299–316.

41. Pumphrey, R. J., and Young, J. Z. (1938): Rates of conduction of nerve fibres of various diameters in cephalopods. *J. Exp. Biol.*, 15:453.

42. Rasminsky, M., and Sears, T. A. (1972): Internodal conduction in undissected demyelinated nerve fibres. *J. Physiol. (Lond)*, 227:323–350.

43. Rushton, W. A. H. (1937): Initiation of the

propagated disturbance. *Proc. R. Soc. B.,* 124:210.

44. Rushton, W. A. H. (1951): A theory of the effects of fibre size in medullated nerve. *J. Physiol. (Lond),* 115:101–122.
45. Schnepp, P., and Schnepp, G. (1971): Faseranalytische Untersuchungen an peripheren Nerven bei Tieren verschiedener Grösse. II. Verhältnis Axondurchmesser/gesamtdurchmesser und Internodallänge. *Z. Zellforsch.,* 119:99–114.
46. Schnepp, G., Schnepp, P., and Spaan, G. (1971): Faseranalytische Untersuchungen an peripheren Nerven bei Tieren verschiedener Grösse. I. Fasergesamtzahl, Faserkaliber und Nervenleitungsgeschwindigkeit. *Z. Zellforsch.,* 119:77–98.
47. Skoglund, C. R. (1942): The response to linearly increasing currents in mammalian motor and sensory nerves. *Acta Physiol. Scand.* [*Suppl. 12*], 4:1–75.
48. Swadlow, H. A., and Waxman, S. G. (1976): Variations in conduction velocity and excitability following single and multiple impulses of visual callosal axons. *Exp. Neurol.,* 53: 128–150.

49. Tasaki, I. (1953): *Nervous Transmission,* pp. 81–85. Charles C Thomas, Springfield, Ill.
50. Tasaki, I. (1959): Conduction of the nerve impulse. In: *Handbook of Physiology, Sect. 1: Neurophysiology,* pp. 75–121. American Physiological Society, Washington, D.C.
51. Tasaki, I., and Fujita, M. (1948): Action currents of single nerve fibers as modified by temperature changes. *J. Neurophysiol.,* 11: 311–315.
52. Vallbo, Å. (1964): Accommodation of single myelinated nerve fibres from Xenopus laevis related to type of end organ. *Acta Physiol. Scand.,* 61:413–428.
53. Vizoso, A. D., and Young, J. Z. (1948): Internode length and fibre diameter in developing and regenerating nerves. *J. Anat.,* 82: 110–134.
54. Waxman, S. G., and Bennett, M. V. L. (1972): Relative conduction velocities of small myelinated and non-myelinated fibres in the central nervous system. *Nature [New Biol.],* 238:217–219.
55. Waxman, S. G., and Swadlow, H. A. (1976): Ultrastructure of visual callosal axons in the rabbit. *Exp. Neurol.,* 53:115–127.

Physiology and Pathobiology of Axons, edited by
S. G. Waxman. Raven Press, New York © 1978.

On Sodium Conductance Gates in Nerve Membranes

John W. Moore

*Department of Physiology, Duke University Medical Center,
Durham, North Carolina 27710*

In their monumental and classic work of the 1950s, Hodgkin and Huxley (8) showed that the bases of excitation and recovery of the specific ionic conductances in axon membranes were extremely voltage-sensitive. They stated simply (8): "It seems difficult to escape the conclusion that the changes in ionic permeability depend on the movement of some component of the membrane which behaves as though it had a large charge or dipole moment." Because they were unable to observe such currents experimentally, Hodgkin and Huxley (8) concluded that the density of ionic channels in the membrane must be low. Later a careful attempt by Chandler and Meves (4) to detect these currents was unsuccessful and led them to the conclusion that the number of channels (in invertebrate giant axons) must be less than $100/\mu m^2$. This prediction of a small number of channels has been borne out by estimates of the sodium channel density in nonmyelinated fibers by tetrodotoxin binding (15,20). During the last few years improved techniques have provided experimental observations of currents which are thought to be associated with molecular rearrangements responsible for the opening and closing of the ionic channels in response to changes in the membrane field. These charge movements are now frequently referred to as asymmetrical currents or, more hopefully, "gating" currents. The putative gating currents have been observed now in several laboratories (2,3,10,11), not only in squid axons but also at frog nodes of Ranvier (18).

Chandler and Meves (4) attempted to measure gating currents in internally perfused axons by removing permeant ions from inside and outside. Although this virtually eliminated all ionic currents, they were not able to detect gating currents and, from the resolution of their method, reasoned that there could be no more than 100 channels/μm^2.

The discoveries that tetrodotoxin (TTX) selectively blocked the sodium conductance (17,22) in squid axons and that tetraethylammonium (TEA) ions selectively blocked the potassium channel (23) opened new possibilities to observe the small asymmetrical currents. Our group (14) used TTX on the exterior of the squid axon to eliminate the sodium conductance and perfused it with TEA to eliminate the potassium, leaving only capacitative and leakage currents. We looked for gating currents but saw none and reported that the transient currents were symmetrical although they decayed with multiple time constants. Perhaps one reason we failed to observe any asymmetry at that time was that our analog-to-digital converter had limited resolution (1/256) and band width.

Most investigators have used these same ion blocking agents, added the capacitive currents from pulses of opposite polarity, and employed averaging techniques to enhance any small net current signal. More recently electronic bridge circuits have been developed to subtract several linear capacitative and leakage components and allow the net or "gating" current to be viewed directly for a single pulse. The electronic bridge is also useful in showing the outward gating current preceding the normal inward sodium current (before the addition of TTX), as can be seen in Fig 1.

The asymmetrical currents measured to date have been associated with the rapid turn-on and turn-off process for the sodium conductance, g_{Na}. None have been found to be asso-

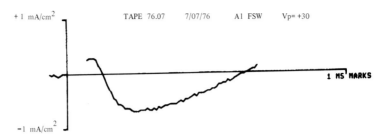

FIG. 1. Asymmetrical displacement current (upward) followed by inward sodium currents for a step depolarization of a squid axon membrane. An active electronic bridge has subtracted the leakage and four linear capacitative currents. The voltage pulse chosen was near the sodium equilibrium potential in order to reduce the sodium current peak to the same order of magnitude as that of the gating current. The latter part of the gating current is obscured by the early part of the sodium current.

ciated with the much slower processes of inactivation of the sodium conductance or activation of the potassium conductance.

Asymmetrical displacement or "gating" currents have also been reported for skeletal muscles. However, the major portion of these is thought to result from charge movement across the large membrane area associated with the transverse tubular system. In the context of this volume, we concern ourselves with only axon membranes.

SODIUM GATES "SHOULD"

We can extend Hodgkin and Huxley's anticipation of the gating charge movement and explicitly set forth general characteristics that gates must have. We can use these to eliminate from consideration some observations that are entirely out of keeping with these requirements for gates.

Asymmetrical Displacement Currents

Because the sodium conductance is turned on strongly with the polarization and shut-off under hyperpolarization, the charge movement should be larger in the depolarizing than in the hyperpolarizing region, or asymmetrical. Hodgkin and Huxley's expectation that the control mechanism is in the membrane and consists of rotation of dipoles or movement of charges through the membrane is equivalent to the expectation that the current be a displacement of charge from a nonlinear capacitor. Because there is a constraint on the distance a charge can move (or a dipole can

rotate) and still remain within the membrane in response to an applied electric field, the gating charge should saturate. This is consistent with the observed saturation of the ionic conductance mechanism. Gating currents must *precede* the turning on of the sodium conductance and therefore will be largely masked by the charging and discharging current of the linear component of membrane capacity. These expectations have been fulfilled by the observations of Bezanilla and Armstrong (3), Keynes and Rojas (11), and Meves (13).

Equality of Charge Movement

For an ideal dielectric, the displacement charge moved when the voltage is changed is identical to that moved on restoration of the original voltage. Axon membranes have a non-ideal dielectric (non-90° phase angle as described by Cole and Cole (5). The observed charge movements in the two directions may differ if measured during unequal times.

In 1974 the equality of the onset and reset charge movements was first used as evidence that the asymmetry currents were indeed gating currents (2,10). The next year Rojas (21) and Bezanilla and Armstrong (3) reported that this equality does not hold for longer and stronger pulses, where the reset charge movement may be as low as one-third of the onset.

Onset Time Course

One cannot state what the time course of the gates "should" be from first principles, because it is model-dependent. As an example, the time course expected from the Hodgkin-Huxley model is described later.

Inactivation

Again, no *a priori* prediction can be made, but expectations for the various models are different.

Channel Density

The gating charge movement should provide the basis of a channel density estimate in agreement with estimates from other independent measurements. The number of charges involved that move across the membrane at each channel can be estimated from the slope of the peak sodium conductance with voltage. Hodgkin and Huxley (8) pointed out that the extreme steepness of this relation, an *e*-fold change in conductance in 4 mV (rather than the usual 25 mV for a single charge) implies that six charges ($RT/F = 25$ mV $\simeq 6 \times 4$ mV) were involved per channel. The maximum reported (11) asymmetry charge moved is in the order of 34 nC/cm². This indicates

that the number of channels should be in the order of $530/\mu m^2$. This is in agreement with estimates of the channel density from TTX-binding experiments (12).

Distinguishing True Gating Currents from Other Asymmetrical Charge Movements

Many of the phospholipids that form the backbone of the membrane contain charge groups, and it is now generally accepted that there are many protein molecules plugged into biological membranes. Alterations in the electrical field across the membrane may give rise to displacement charge movement in both types of molecules, although just how much is uncertain. Such charge movement may be difficult to distinguish from that which actually controls the sodium channel. The only way to distinguish gating charge movements from the (perhaps large) background of unrelated displacement currents seems to be from their relationship with the sodium conductance system. For example, these ions, toxins, and drugs which effect the kinetics of the sodium conductance onset should also in some way effect movement of the gating charges. One must assume that the background asymmetrical dis-

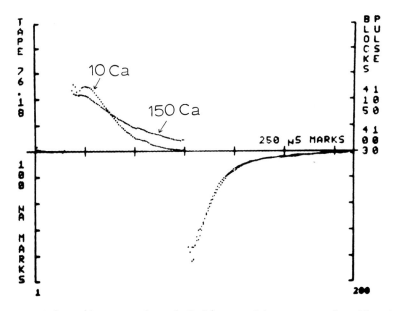

FIG. 2. Gating currents in squid axon membrane bathed in two calcium concentrations. Note that the onset currents associated with depolarization change in amplitude and shape, but the reset currents following repolarization overlay.

placement current from other molecules would not change in the presence of these agents.

A few experiments have been initiated to pursue this question and to determine what part, if any, of the observed asymmetrical charge movement is associated with the sodium channel. For example, calcium is known to have a marked effect on the kinetics of the onset of the sodium conductance and an even greater effect on the time constant of the sodium tail conductances (7). Recently we (16) studied the effect of external calcium ions on the asymmetry currents. When the external calcium concentration was increased (Fig. 2), there was a decrease in the peak amplitude of the onset asymmetry current and a marked increase in the longer of the two time constants describing its decay (see Fig. 4, below, which shows that the onset asymmetry current decays with two time constants). However, there was no significant change in the reset asymmetry current.

These observations are baffling. Although the change in the onset current is distinct enough to suggest that the charge movements do come from gates, the lack of change in the reset current with altered calcium level is not compatible with the marked change that occurs in the conductance time course.

MODEL DISCRIMINATION

Perhaps one of the most important contributions of the measurement of gating currents to our understanding of the opening and closing the ionic channels will be in finding the correct model, or mechanism. The sodium conductance system has been described in many models that are compatible with some of the variety of voltage clamp data in transient conductances. The measurement of ionic conductances restricts us to the events of the opening and closing of the conductance channel. From this limited point of view, it is almost impossible to distinguish between a variety of models or even to eliminate classes of models from consideration. The addition of the entirely independent measurement of the gating currents that precede the conductance changes gives another important set of constraints. The requirement that a putative model must fit both the ionic conductance and the

gating current data should help to eliminate most of them from consideration and help us focus on a narrow class of mechanisms.

Hodgkin-Huxley Model

The importance of gating current observations is demonstrated by examining current observations in the context of the Hodgkin-Huxley (HH) model, the classic and most popular for the squid axon membrane. In this model each sodium channel is governed by the position of three charged, identical but mutually independent particles (designated m), which can be imagined to flip from one side of the membrane to the other under the influence of the electrical field. If such a particle is on the side preferred for hyperpolarization, m has a value of zero, whereas a location at the other side of the membrane in response to depolarization gives m a value of unity. All three of the m particles must be on one side of the membrane for the sodium channel to be "open" and to conduct ions.[1] The probability that all three are on one side at any time is given by m^3. Thus the time course of the sodium conductance following a depolarization from rest follows the value of m^3, but the gating current is produced by the movement of these particles and is proportional to the time rate of change of m.

$$\frac{dm}{dt} = \alpha_m(m - m_\infty) - \beta_m m \qquad (1)$$

where the rate constants α_m and β_m have a strong dependence on the electrical field across the membrane. For a step depolarization, the magnitude of the rate constant α_m becomes very much larger than β_m, and the gating current predicted by this model shows a positive jump followed by an exponential decay to zero with a time constant equal to $1/(\alpha_m + \beta_m)$. In this model a step repolarization causes β_m to be much larger than α_m, and the gating cur-

---

[1] An inactivation particle (h) must also be on the correct side. However, the rate constants driving this particle are so much smaller (0.1) than those for the m particle that their rate of gating charge movement is so low as to be negligible in comparison. Because of this and because no putative "inactivation or h gating" currents have been reported, we neglect inactivation in this treatment.

rent jumps to a negative value and then decays exponentially to zero with the time constant given by the same expression. For these cases, the gating currents for this model approaches, respectively

$$m \simeq \alpha_m(m - m_\infty) \qquad (1a)$$

for depolarization and

$$m = -\beta_m m \qquad (1b)$$

for hyperpolarization.

Tsien and Noble (24) developed a very enlightening frame of reference from which to view the rate constants in the HH formulation. They point out that Hodgkin and Huxley used a constant field theory model for α_m and α_n but a single energy barrier model for the rate constants β_m and β_n, which change much more steeply with voltage. In the single energy barrier model, rate constants increased e-fold with each 25 mV change in potential for univalent charges. Compared to a single barrier model matched at midrange, rate constants governed by a constant field model[2] change more steeply for small rate constants, but above the midrange change less steeply and approach a maximum value. Keynes and Rojas (11) chose the simpler single energy barrier expression to describe both putative rate constants for the sodium channel and were able to show a moderately good correlation of the distribution of time constants of this model with that of their observations of "gating currents." They argued that this agreement indicates that they are related.

Figure 3 presents the forward and backward rate constants (on a logarithmic scale) for the m process of HH as a function of voltage. β_m is a straight line because of the choice of the single barrier model for this rate; its slope is 18 mV per e-fold. α_m deviates from a straight line with a slope of 25 mV. The time constant for the reaction is $1/(\alpha_m + \beta_m)$ and has a maximum at the voltage where the curves intersect (i.e., $\alpha_m = \beta_m$). The dashed lines give the Keynes and Rojas rate curves chosen to match their observations of gating currents.

[2] I am indebted to Dr. James Hall for pointing out that the single energy barrier model can give varying voltage sensitivity also by assuming that the distance between the energy well and top of the barrier varies with applied voltage.

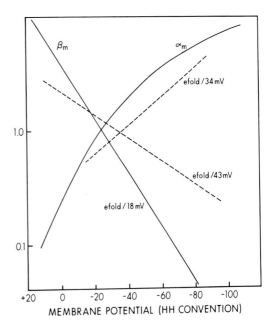

FIG. 3. Rate constants for the m process as a function of voltage. The solid lines are the HH values for α_m and β_m. The dashed lines are calculated from the values given by Keynes and Rojas (11), with the assignment of a resting potential of -65 mV for the HH equations.

Onset Time Course

If the gating process is a first-order reaction such as the m-reaction in the HH model, the onset gating current for a depolarization from strong holding potential should, after an initial jump, decay exponentially with a single time constant, as described in Eq. 1.

Initially it was observed that the decay of the onset gating currents could be fitted with single time constants (2,10,13). More recent measurements of asymmetry currents by Armstrong (1) show two time constants. The same phenomena occurred in our laboratory. That is, a single exponential fitted most of our early observations, but as the quality of our measurements and resolutions improved it became clear that more than one exponential decay process is involved in the onset current, as shown in Fig. 4. Such a multiple time constant decay is not compatible with the HH or any other first-order reaction process (but it could be compatible with two first-order processes).

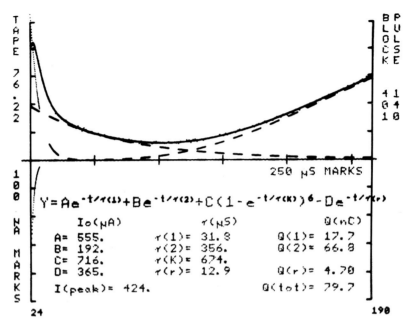

FIG. 4. Asymmetry current observed for a very strong depolarization (to +40 mV). The 200 data points are well overlaid by a solid curve (given by the expression for Y) fitted to them by a computer algorithm. The late rising phase is a residual potassium current because the 4-aminopyridine applied externally to the intact axon to block potassium conductance is not fully effective for positive internal potentials; it is fitted by a first-order lag raised to the sixth power. The remaining asymmetry current decays with two distinct time constants separated by an order of magnitude.

Inactivation

If the gating mechanism consists of two entirely independent processes such as postulated by Hodgkin and Huxley for m and h for the sodium channel, the onset gates, governed by Eq. 1, should be independent of the inactivation of the sodium conductance. It was reported that the gating currents do not inactivate (11,13), but others later reported that there is inactivation (3). We (Moore, Westerfield, and Jaslove, *unpublished*) observed that the onset asymmetry current partially inactivated with increasing duration of the depolarizing test pulse (Fig. 5).

Reset Time Constants

Because the sodium conductance in the Hodgkin and Huxley description is taken as m^3, repolarization when m is large causes the rate of change of the sodium conductance to be three times as fast as dm/dt. The value of

the ratio of these time constants provides a crucial test of the HH formulation.

It has been reported that the time constant of the rapid sodium decay or "tail" is approximately the same as that for the "tail gates" (3,10). In 1974 Meves (13) reported that the time constant of the tail gate increased 3-fold as the amplitude of the test pulse was increased. The next year, Rojas (21) reported that this time constant increased by 1.6-fold as the test pulse duration increased. In 1976 Keynes and Rojas (11) reported that the ratio of time constants of the tail gate to the sodium tail was 3 but decreased to 1.6 as they reduced the test pulse and holding potential. It is not very satisfactory to have the HH (or any other model invoked) to hold for only a restricted range of potentials.

It is unsettling when a pair of investigators change their conclusion from a ratio of 1 to a ratio of over 3. It is even more disconcerting to learn that the ratio changes as a function of the amplitude and duration of the test pulse

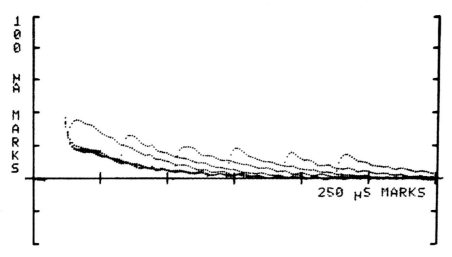

FIG. 5. Partial inactivation of onset asymmetry current for a depolarization of 80 mV when preceded by depolarization of 60 mV of increasing duration.

as well as the holding potential. There has been no experimental evidence to indicate that the tails of sodium conductance vary with either the amplitude or duration of the test pulse. As originally reported by Hodgkin and Huxley, they continue to appear to be almost dependent on the potential to which a return is made, with the exception that the decay is sometimes not described by a single exponential for all pulse widths, especially when the medium is low in calcium (7).

In order to obtain insight into this problem, preliminary studies have been carried out in which, following short test pulses, the potential was returned to different levels above or below resting. We (16) found that the ratio of the time constants of these two processes can vary over a considerable range (Fig. 6). For repolarization to very negative levels, the sodium conductance recovers faster than the "gating" current; but for repolarization to potential levels near rest, they have the same time constant. If the voltage is returned to a moderate negative value, the sodium conductance recovers more slowly than the "gating" current.

Series Resistance

The resistance in series with the membrane exerts a marked influence on the time course of current patterns observed in a voltage clamp (9,19). Therefore it is important to compensate for it as well as possible so that it does not affect the kinetics of the voltage clamp currents and thus the fit of any given model.

Keynes and Rojas (11) state that their earlier conclusion that the ratio of the conductance and gate off time constants was 1 was "evidently due to inadequate series resistance compensation." They also note that Bezanilla and Armstrong, who reported the same result in 1975, may have been "using less complete compensation than they supposed." Therefore it seems important to resolve this question with great care given to measurement and compensation of series resistance.

SUMMARY

The detection of gating currents is very difficult because they represent small differences in large surges of current. Their accurate measurement poses many more problems than the measurement of ordinary ionic currents, which occur later and are much larger in magnitude. Special methods and careful attention to detail is required.

Perhaps these problems account for much of the discrepancy in the observations re-

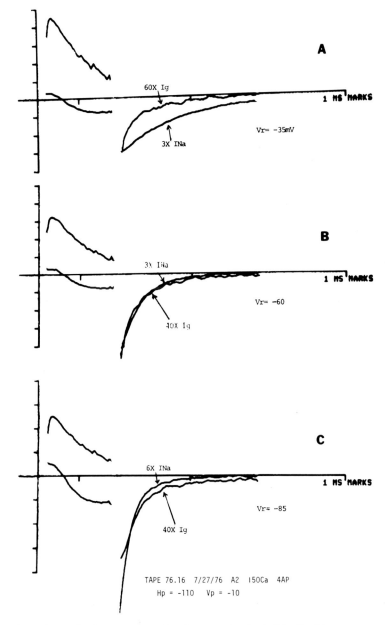

FIG. 6. Comparison of records of asymmetry and sodium currents (as in Fig. 1) with pure asymmetry currents at higher gain taken later after the axon was bathed in TTX. The membrane potential was held at -110 mV, depolarized to -10 mV for 0.5 msec and returned to the voltage levels indicated by V_r for each pair. For a return to -60 mV, the time constant of the sodium conductance turn-off equals that for the asymmetry current, but the ratio increases and decreases as the return voltage is returned to levels more or less negative than resting.

ported to date. Not only are there wide gulfs between the results of different investigators, but the same investigators report very different results at different times. There are several examples of changes in so-called gating currents when the sodium conductance shows no change, and there are the contrary observations where the "gates" do not change when there are marked changes in the conductance.

The curious differential effect of calcium on

the onset gates and the total lack of effect of calcium on the reset or "tail" gates is certainly another baffling observation and may need further investigation. The changes in the onset gates are distinct enough so that one can distinguish putative models on the basis of this. However, the lack of a calcium effect on the tail gates when it is known that the sodium tails are drastically affected may be a unique experiment with which to distinguish among models.

In conclusion, it is clear that we are in the early stages of investigation of the gating currents. Much more work needs to be done to resolve the discrepancies and differences in observations. Although the experiments are technically difficult, continuing gating current measurements seems to be fully worthwhile because of the unique opportunity to distinguish among various putative models.

REFERENCES

1. Armstrong, C. M. (1975): Currents associated with the ionic gating structures in nerve membrane. *Ann. NY Acad. Sci.*, 264:265–277.
2. Armstrong, C. M., and Bezanilla, F. (1974): Charge movement associated with opening and closing of the activation gates of the Na channels. *J. Gen. Physiol.*, 63:533–552.
3. Bezanilla, F., and Armstrong, C. M. (1975): Properties of the sodium channel gating current. *Symp. Quant. Biol.*, 40:297–304.
4. Chandler, W. K., and Meves, H. (1965): Voltage clamp experiments in internally perfused giant axons. *J. Physiol. (Lond)*, 180: 788–820.
5. Cole, K. S. and Cole, R. H. (1942): Dispersion and absorption in dielectrics. II. Direct current characteristics. *J. Chem. Phys.*, 10:98–105.
6. FitzHugh, R., and Cole, K. S. (1973): Voltage and current clamp transients with membrane dielectric loss. *Biophys. J.*, 13:1125–1140.
7. Frankenhaeuser, B., and Hodgkin, A. L. (1957): The action of calcium on the electrical properties of squid axons. *J. Physiol. (Lond)*, 137:217–244.
8. Hodgkin, A. L., and Huxley, A. F. (1952): A quantitative description of membrane current and its application to conduction and excitation in nerve. *J. Physiol. (Lond)*, 117: 500–544.
9. Hodgkin, A. L., Huxley, A. F., and Katz, B. (1952): Measurement of current-voltage relations in the membrane of the giant axon of Loligo. *J. Physiol. (Lond)*, 116:424–445.
10. Keynes, R. D., and Rojas, E. (1974): Kinetic and steady-state properties of charged system controlling sodium conductance in the squid giant axon. *J. Physiol. (Lond)*, 239:393–434.
11. Keynes, R. D., and Rojas, E. (1976): The temporal and steady-state relationships between activation of the sodium conductance and movement of the gating particles in the squid giant axon. *J. Physiol. (Lond)*, 255: 157–189.
12. Levinson, S. R., and Meves, H. (1975): The binding of tritiated tetrodotoxin to squid giant axons. *Philos. Trans. R. Soc. B.*, 270:349–352.
13. Meves, H. (1974): The effect of holding potential in the asymmetry currents in squid giant axon. *J. Physiol. (Lond)*, 243:847–867.
14. Moore, J. W., Narahashi, T., Poston, R., and Arispe, N. (1970): Leakage currents in squid axon. *Biophys. Soc. Abstr.* 10:180a.
15. Moore, J. W., Narahashi, T., and Shaw, T. I. (1967): An upper limit to the number of sodium channels in nerve membrane? *J. Physiol. (Lond)*, 188:99–105.
16. Moore, J. W., Westerfield, M., and Jaslove, S. (1977): Calcium affects kinetics of sodium onset gates, but not reset gates. *Biophys. J.*, 17:14a.
17. Narahashi, T., Moore, J. W., and Scott, W. R. (1964): Tetrodotoxin blockage of sodium conductance increase in lobster giant axons. *J. Gen. Physiol.*, 47:965–974.
18. Nonner, W., Rojas, E., and Stämpfli, R. (1975): Displacement currents in the node of Ranvier: Voltage and time dependence. *Pfluegers Arch.*, 354:1–18.
19. Ramón, F., Anderson, N., Joyner, R. W., and Moore, J. W. (1975): Axon voltage-clamp simulations. IV. A multicellular preparation. *Biophys. J.*, 15:55–69.
20. Ritchie, J. M., Rogart, R. B., and Strichartz, G. R. (1976): A new method for labelling saxitoxin and its binding to non-myelinated fibres of the rabbit vagus, lobster walking leg, and garfish olfactory nerves. *J. Physiol. (Lond)*, 261:477–494.
21. Rojas, E. (1975): Gating mechanism for the activation of the sodium conductance in nerve membranes. *Symp. Quant. Biol.*, 40:305–320.
22. Takata, M., Moore, J. W., Kao, C. Y., and Fuhrman, F. A. (1966): Blockage of sodium conductance increase in lobster giant axon by Tarichatoxin (tetrodotoxin). *J. Gen. Physiol.*, 49:977–988.
23. Tasaki, I., and Hagiwara, S. (1957): Demonstration of two stable potential states in the squid giant axon under tetraethylammonium chloride. *J. Gen. Physiol.*, 40:859–885.
24. Tsien, R. W., and Noble, D. (1969): A transition state theory approach to the kinetics of conductance changes in excitable membranes. *J. Memb. Biol.*, 1:248–273.

Physiology and Pathobiology of Axons, edited by
S. G. Waxman. Raven Press, New York © 1978.

Voltage Clamp Studies on the Node of Ranvier

Michael Cahalan

Department of Physiology, University of California, Irvine, California 92717

One of the outstanding feats in electrobiology has been the development of a method to control the potential and measure current across the membrane at a single node of Ranvier from a myelinated nerve fiber. The node itself, a 1-μm gap between tightly wrapped Schwann cells, can barely be seen under a high-power dissection microscope. The axon membrane at a node has a surface area of less than 50 μm^2, and the membrane currents are at the nanoampere level. Yet the node voltage clamp preparation is reasonably easy to learn, requires no microelectrodes, and lends itself to quantitative biophysical experiments. In this chapter the technique is briefly outlined, advantages and disadvantages of the preparation are considered, and properties of ionic channels at the node are reviewed.

SINGLE FIBER VOLTAGE CLAMP TECHNIQUE: TAKING ADVANTAGE OF MYELIN

During the late 1920s and early 1930s workers in Kato's laboratory in Japan discovered how to isolate single nerve fibers from the sciatic nerve bundle of a frog (61). Two needles are used to spread the fibers in a desheathed bundle laterally, leaving approximately 5% of the fibers in the middle between the needles, usually with a few individual fibers separated from the rest for a distance of several millimeters. The best looking single fiber can be isolated from the rest by simply cutting away all fibers except the one chosen. Then the isolated fiber is transferred under water to a nerve chamber for recording. The dissection techniques are described more fully by Stämpfli (84,86), and are illustrated in Fig. 1.

Myelin enables the action potential to be transmitted at high conduction velocity by small fibers with a great saving of metabolic energy compared with conduction by unmyelinated fibers. By limiting current flow across the axon membrane to the nodal region, conduction velocity is increased to the extent that a 15-μm myelinated frog fiber conducts faster than a squid giant axon with a diameter of 1 mm. In addition to the fact that thousands of the myelinated fibers could fit inside the giant axon, myelin results in a several-thousand-fold reduction in the energy expenditure per impulse for a unit length of fiber. The influx of sodium is limited to the nodes, and hence the sodium–potassium pump uses much less ATP to restore the ionic concentrations inside the fiber.

Nearly all techniques of recording membrane potentials and currents in myelinated nerve fibers have taken advantage of the insulating properties of myelin. The high resistance (300 k$\Omega \cdot$ cm^2) Schwann cell wrappings around the axon make it possible to record the membrane potential across the patch of nodal membrane through the axoplasmic access resistance without using microelectrodes. In essence, the internodal segment is used as a high-resistance pipette (10–20 MΩ) to record the membrane potential at the node. As Cole (22) expressed it, several investigators decided by the mid-1950s that "a node had been designed for voltage clamping."

The methods developed by Tasaki and Takeuchi (89,90), Huxley and Stämpfli (60), and Frankenhaeuser (38) to record the nodal membrane potential depend on reducing the flow of extracellular current next to the fiber. Figure 2 depicts the equivalent circuit of the nerve fiber in the recording chamber with

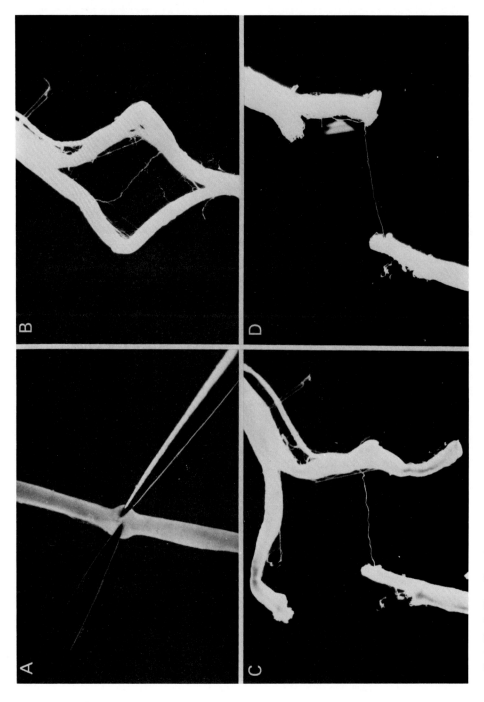

FIG. 1. Single fiber dissection. A desheathed frog sciatic nerve bundle is spread by two needles in **A** and **B**, revealing at least two single fibers. One is chosen, and the rest are removed (**C**), leaving the single fiber in **D** connecting the remaining nerve stumps.

Vaseline seals in place. Consider point D just inside the patch of membrane in pool A as being attached to the end pools C and E through the axoplasmic resistance (r_i). Typically, $r_i = 10$–20 mΩ when the fiber ends are cut in pools C and E. One possible way to record the membrane potential across the patch of membrane in pool A would be to make a very high resistance seal on top of the fiber from the A pool to the end pool (C) and record the potential difference between C and A. The problem with this method is that the membrane potential is attenuated by short circuit current from C to A outside the fiber underneath the seals. In practice, seals cannot be made with high enough resistance to prevent attenuation.

An alternative method is to record the current around the loop D→C→A→D, and then offset the current, generated by the membrane potential, with a variable potential. The applied potential must equal the membrane potential to satisfy the condition that no current flow in the loop. When the C pool is at ground, point D is also at ground, with no current flowing down the axoplasmic resistance. Then the full membrane potential appears as $-E_m$ in the A pool. This is the principle of the method used by Huxley and Stämpfli (60) to record the size of the resting and action potentials. The first feedback amplifier (A1),

introduced by Frankenhaeuser (38), varies the applied voltage automatically to keep the C pool at virtual ground. In contrast to most techniques of recording a membrane potential, the inside of the fiber is kept at ground while the extracellular solution in pool A is made to follow the time course of any change in membrane potential. In order to control the membrane potential, a second amplifier is added whose output injects enough current through the E pool to keep the membrane potential equal to the command voltage (28). In practice, this amplifier arrangement results in the ability to follow the time course of ionic current across the membrane following a step of potential with approximately 50 μsec time resolution.

The preparation is continuing to evolve as new ways are found to increase the speed of the voltage clamp. Nonner (75) improved the time resolution for current measurement to 10 μsec. Another important development has been applying the node clamp to single muscle fibers (41,53). Because the muscle fiber has much lower longitudinal access resistance, the speed of the muscle fiber clamp is improved compared to the myelinated nerve fiber. The technique has also been used to record miniature end-plate currents and acetylcholine-sensitive current fluctuations (J. H. Steinbach, *personal communication*). In general, the node

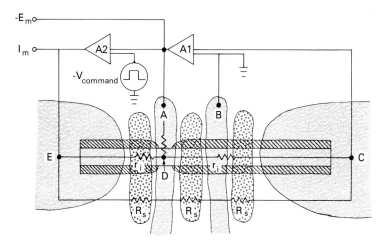

FIG. 2. A single fiber in the recording chamber. Vaseline seals separate four pools (E, A, B, and C). The nerve fiber width is magnified approximately 25 times relative to the chamber, and the nodal region in pool A is even more highly enlarged in this view. Amplifier A1 keeps point D inside the fiber near virtual ground. The A pool voltage follows changes in the membrane potential (E_m). Current (I_m) is injected by amplifier A2 through pool E to voltage clamp the nodal membrane to the command signal ($V_{command}$).

clamp should be applicable to most large cells with cylindrical geometry.

A favorable feature of the node preparation is the relative absence of diffusion barriers between the external solution and the membrane. The Schwann cell layer around a squid giant axon leads to accumulation of potassium ions following large outward potassium currents in the space (Frankenhaeuser–Hodgkin space) between the axon membrane and the Schwann cells (39). Potassium accumulation can result in distortion of the time course of potassium conductance, since the driving force for potassium ions is varying during a large outward current. Potassium accumulation in the perinodal space has been observed at the node of Ranvier for some species (8,32). However, in *Rana pipiens* from Vermont this barrier seems to be absent as no potassium accumulation is observed (8).

In a squid giant axon the Schwann cell layer around the axon also makes rapid solution changes at the axon membrane impossible. In contrast, external solution changes equilibrate rapidly at the surface of the nodal membrane. Following a sudden change in the external sodium concentration, the concentration at the membrane surface equilibrates within 100 msec (92). The relative absence of an external diffusion barrier makes the node preparation especially attractive for pharmacological experiments, because the rate of action of many agents on the ionic conductance mechanisms can be followed.

In a perfused squid axon, solution changes can be completed more rapidly inside the axon than outside. Substances can also be introduced to the inside of a Ranvier node by diffusion from the cut ends within 10–20 min, although the exchange is incomplete (67).

PROPERTIES OF IONIC CHANNELS AT THE NODE

The voltage clamp experiments by Hodgkin and Huxley (56–59) on squid giant axon provided a framework for understanding the action potential in terms of voltage-dependent changes in membrane permeability to sodium and potassium ions. In their elegant kinetic analysis, ionic current across the membranes is divided into three independent components: an early inward current carried by sodium responsible for the upstroke of the action potential, a delayed outward current carried by potassium ions responsible for repolarization, and a leakage current, which also helps to repolarize the axon and set the resting potential. The remainder of this chapter is devoted to describing ideas and speculation concerning the nature of the permeability mechanisms, focusing especially on evidence from the frog myelinated nerve fiber voltage clamp preparation.

It seems that evolution has been rather conservative with regard to the invention of excitability, for the most important finding of comparative axonology has been the overall

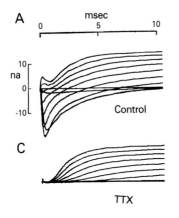
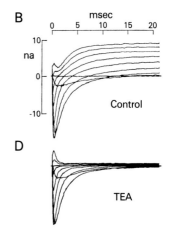

FIG. 3. Voltage clamped sodium and potassium currents. **A** and **B** show ionic currents for two time scales. **C** illustrates blockage of sodium currents by 300 nM TTX. In **D** the potassium currents have been blocked by 6 mM TEA, leaving just sodium currents that turn on and then inactivate. (From ref. 47.)

similarity of permeability mechanisms in a variety of vertebrate and invertebrate nerve fibers. From worms to squid to frogs to mammals, the same ionic current pattern is observed with voltage steps to varying levels, shown for the frog in Fig. 3A and B. The Hodgkin and Huxley analysis applies to the frog node with only minor modifications (27).

Hille (47) summarized the evidence that the early and late components of ionic current are carried by independent sodium and potassium channels, respectively. The discovery of selective blocking agents for different components of ionic current is part of the evidence supporting the idea that the kinetic separation of ionic currents into independent components in the Hodgkin and Huxley model has a molecular basis. As shown in Fig. 3C and D, tetrodotoxin selectively eliminates the early sodium current, and tetraethylammonium ions block the late outward potassium current. These agents are valuable tools in the study of ionic channels because they enable direct observation of the entire time course of either sodium or potassium current.

To perform their job of transmitting the impulse, ionic channels must be able to discriminate between different ionic species, and they must have the ability to open and close. The next two sections discuss the selectivity of sodium and potassium channels for different ions, as well as the gating mechanism that enables channels to open and close.

Selectivity

The node preparation has been important in the development of ideas about ion selectivity largely through the work of Hille, who set out to find a comprehensive list of permeant ions for both sodium and potassium channels. His work resulted in a set of phenomenological dimensions for the narrowest part of a conducting channel, the selectivity filter. In a sodium channel the following ions are measurably permeant, in decreasing order: sodium, hydroxylammonium, lithium, hydrazinium, thallium, ammonium, formamidinium, guanidinium, hydroxyguanidinium, potassium, and aminoguanidinium (48,49). From the size of the large, barely permeant ions, the minimum size of an open sodium channel in cross section is postulated to be 3×5 Å. Larger ions

such as methylated cations with diameters greater than 3.8 Å cannot go through. Potassium channels seem to be narrower than sodium channels, as only thallium, potassium, rubidium, and ammonium are measurably permeant (50). The dimensions of a potassium channel are thought to be 3×3 Å. There is no comprehensive physical theory explaining the relative permeability to different ions in either channel, although steric factors and electrostatic interactions between the ions and sites inside the channel are thought to interact in determining the sequence of selectivity (51).

Gating

The voltage clamp technique is an essential tool in studying the permeability properties of excitable membranes because the membrane potential is the controlling factor that determines the opening and closing rates of ionic channels. Figure 3D illustrates the transient nature of the sodium conductance; sodium current is activated with rapid kinetics and then inactivated with slower kinetics following a step depolarization. Sodium inactivation has the function of making the membrane easier to repolarize when potassium channels are activated during an action potential. In the HH model, activation and inactivation of sodium channels are represented by two independent gating parameters, m^3 and h, respectively, each of which is a function of membrane potential and time. These parameters are probability functions whose product m^3h equals the probability that a sodium channel is open. The opening and closing of a potassium channel is controlled by another gating parameter, n^4, with slower kinetics representing the slower activation of potassium current (Fig. 3C).

Since the Hodgkin and Huxley model was formulated, other very slow gating processes have been discovered in myelinated nerve fibers. Potassium channels inactivate slowly under a maintained depolarization with two time constants: 0.6 sec and 4–20 sec (81). In addition to h, sodium channels have at least two and perhaps three other inactivation processes for very long depolarizations with time constants of 150–300 msec (77), 4–7 sec, and 94–123 sec (35). Another type of very slow inactivation may represent the turnover of ionic channels in the membrane. During the course of an experiment the maximum sodium and potassium currents gradually decline, with a time constant of 1–3 hr depending on potential and temperature (36). Interestingly, thiamine and thiamine phosphates can prevent or reduce the slow rundown of the currents, suggesting an axoplasmic metabolic role in maintaining functioning ionic channels in the membrane.

The design requirements for a voltage-sensitive gating process suggested to Hodgkin and Huxley (59) the presence of charges or dipoles within the membrane whose position or orientation depends on the local electrical field. When the membrane is depolarized, the change in electrical field would result in a net movement of charge associated with the opening of the channel. More than 20 years after the prediction, sodium channel gating movement was detected in the squid axon (6,62) and frog node (76). Now that there is a direct measure (gating currents) of molecular events within the membrane linked to the gating process, new lines of experimentation have opened up, which are reviewed by Moore (*this volume*).

Several pharmacological agents have been found to interfere selectively with the inactivation (*h*) process of the sodium channel (see below under gating modifiers). One agent, *Centruroides sculpturatus* scorpion venom, alters the activation (*m*^{3}) process, leaving inactivation only slightly modified (17). It seems from this kind of pharmacological evidence that there are separate factors or processes underlying *m*^{3} and *h*. Evidence is now accumulating that these two processes (*m*^{3} and *h*) are coupled mechanistically. Perhaps the strongest evidence in favor of coupling between the activation and inactivation of the sodium channel is the inactivation of gating currents discovered by Armstrong and Bezanilla (6,7). The exact nature of coupling is now a topic of considerable controversy and excitement.

Surface Charges

For many years it has been known that raising the extracellular calcium concentration increases the threshold for a nerve action potential (16). Recently the effects of calcium ions on threshold have been given a complete explanation by several authors on the basis of fixed negative charges at the membrane near the sodium channels. In the preceding section a view of excitability was presented in which a change of the electrical field within the membrane causes the opening and closing of ionic channels. The charges or dipoles that produce gating currents "sense" the field by moving or orienting in it. In voltage clamp experiments a change in the divalent cation concentration resembles a change in membrane potential from the point of view of how many ionic channels are open. Specifically, for an *e*-fold increase in calcium concentration, the membrane must be depolarized by approximately 10 mV more to open a given fraction of sodium channels (46). In this sense, increasing the calcium concentration is like hyperpolarizing the membrane or increasing the electrical field across the membrane near the channels.

An explanation for the voltage shifting effect of calcium, originally advanced by A. F. Huxley (40) and since tested by several experimenters, postulates the existence of fixed negative charges at the outer surface of the membrane. The surface charges create a negative surface potential extending into the external solution for some 10–20 Å. Cations in solution, especially divalent cations, are attracted toward the surface charges, forming a layer of net positive charge next to the membrane, which "screens" the negative surface potential. If the divalent cation concentration is increased, the surface potential is more effectively screened, thereby altering the electrical field that controls the gating processes.

Voltage clamp experiments can provide an estimate for the surface charge density near sodium or potassium channels by using the gating process as a detector of the electrical field. Conductance–voltage curves for sodium and potassium channels are shifted along the membrane potential axis by different amounts for a given calcium concentration change (46, 95). Estimates for the density of surface charges vary to some degree, but it seems clear that the density is approximately three times higher near sodium channels than potassium channels, with approximately one negative charge per 100 Å^2 near sodium channels (55, 95) and one negative charge per 200 Å^2 (95), 300 Å^2 (17), or 600 Å^2 near potassium channels (68). Some theories (55) also allow for specific binding of calcium and other divalent ions to the surface charges. Sodium channel activation (m^3) is consistently shifted more by calcium than is inactivation (h) (40,46,94), which may indicate the existence of separate potential sensing mechanisms for m^3 and *h,* even though from other evidence it seems likely that the two processes are coupled.

Pharmacology

The node preparation is attractive for pharmacological studies. The relative absence of an external diffusion barrier facilitates kinetic studies to determine the rate of action of many compounds. One milliliter of solution is enough to exchange the solution bathing the node several times. Agents can also be applied internally by diffusion from the end pools. Voltage clamp experiments are needed to determine the mechanism of action of agents that alter the action potential. For example, long-duration action potentials can be produced in two fundamentally different ways: by blocking potassium current with TEA or by removing and slowing sodium inactivation with a number of agents. Some pharmacological agents are useful tools for further study of ionic channels by selective blockade of one current component, permitting direct observation of another. Other agents reveal properties of channels that give hints about their normal functioning. Roughly speaking, many pharmacologically active compounds can be classified as conductance blockers or gating modifiers.

Conductance Blocking Agents

Tetraethylammonium Ions

Comparing the block of potassium current by external or internal tetraethylammonium (TEA) reveals the asymmetry of a potassium channel. From the outside, TEA blocks potassium current within 100 msec of application (93) by simply scaling the size of the current without altering its kinetics (44). The dose dependence of block fits the simple model of one TEA molecule per receptor, with a dissociation constant (K_d) of 0.4 mM. The K_d is increased by raising the extracellular calcium

concentration (69), an effect which has been interpreted as evidence for accumulation of positive TEA ions at negative surface charges near the TEA receptor or blocking site. The measured increase in K_d of 1.6 to 1.7 on changing the calcium from 2 mM to 20 mM predicts a surface potential change of 11 mV to 13 mV, in good agreement with the surface potential change by calcium ions near the potassium channel gating mechanism (17).

Externally applied TEA is often useful in frog node voltage clamp experiments to reveal the entire time course of the sodium current (Fig. 3D). Squid axons are insensitive to externally applied TEA.

In contrast to external TEA, internal TEA ions and particularly more hydrophobic derivatives of TEA alter the kinetics of potassium current, apparently interacting only with open channels (9,67). A time-dependent block of potassium current resembling sodium inactivation is observed with a nine-carbon chain derivative of TEA (9). The block is strong for larger depolarizations. Furthermore, block by internal TEA is partially relieved by raising the extracellular potassium concentration. It seems that the receptor for internally applied TEA is within the channel where a blocking TEA ion can be knocked away by potassium ions entering the channel from the outside. Since TEA gains access to its blocking site after the channel is open, by implication the gates of the potassium channel are thought to be located near the axoplasmic side of the membrane. The results with internal TEA also suggest that the inner part of a potassium channel might be over 8 Å in diameter to accommodate the TEA ion (5).

Tetrodotoxin, Saxitoxin, and Ultraviolet Light

Tetrodotoxin (TTX) and saxitoxin (STX) each block sodium channels selectively in a nanomolar concentration range (45,80). It is remarkable that the complex structure of the TTX molecule has evolved twice in the animal kingdom—once in the puffer fish and again in certain salamanders of the western United States. STX, which bears some molecular resemblance to TTX, is produced by a marine dinoflagellate and is concentrated to toxic proportions by shellfish. Both compounds are ineffective from the inside of the membrane (67, 70), and it is hypothesized that the block of TTX and STX from the outside is due to interaction between the charged guanidinium group of the blocking molecule and the selectivity filter region of the sodium channel (52). The kinetics of binding and unbinding to the sodium channel are readily observed on a scale of several seconds following a rapid solution change (80,96), with STX having four times faster rates of block and washout than TTX. Like the block of potassium current by external TEA ions, TTX block of sodium channels is partially antagonized by raising the calcium concentration (54); divalent STX is even more strongly affected by calcium. A surface charge density near the TTX and STX binding site with one-half the magnitude of the charge density near the gating mechanism could explain the effects of calcium on TTX and STX block.

TTX and STX have been used to count the number of sodium channels in nerve membrane by measuring the amount of bound radioactivity after incubating a nerve with tritiated toxin (2,78). The density of toxin-binding sites and hence sodium channels in most nerve membranes is extremely low, with fewer than 50 sites/μm^2 for small unmyelinated nerves (23). On the other hand, as is discussed later, it appears that a frog node of Ranvier may have approximately 100 times as many sodium channels per square micrometer.

Sodium current is also selectively blocked by ultraviolet (UV) light, with a sharp peak of sensitivity at 280 nm (34). Sodium channel gating currents are reduced by UV light (37), whereas TTX has no effect on gating currents (74), indicating a different site of action for UV light compared with TTX.

Blockage by Ions

Hydrogen ions block sodium and potassium currents, and alter the voltage dependence for opening the channels (29,30,46,97). The shifts of the voltage dependence for opening sodium and potassium channels are explained by negative surface charges modified by hydrogen ions near the gating mechanism, whereas the block of ionic currents is thought to represent the titration of a site in the channel. Potassium channels have a titration curve with an apparent pK_a of approximately 4.5 (30,50), whereas sodium channels are approximately 10 times more sensitive to an increase in hydrogen ion concentration, having a pK_a of approximately 5.4. Of particular interest is the fact that the pK_a for the sodium channel site is potential-dependent, suggesting that block by a hydrogen ion occurs part way across the membrane (97).

Several other types of ion in addition to TEA and its derivatives can block potassium channels. Internal sodium, cesium, lithium, and methylammonium ions interfere with outward potassium current but not inward current through potassium channels (13,15,31,51). External cesium but not sodium interferes with inward potassium current (31). These kinds of ionic blockage are evidence for interactions between ions inside the potassium channel.

Permeant ions can also block the passage of ions through channels. The size of current through the sodium channel appears to saturate as the concentration of many ions, even sodium, is increased (51). Sodium channel selectivity ratios can be altered by the concentration of internal ions (19). New theories of how ions pass through ionic channels are needed to explain these recently discovered phenomena, which can be classified broadly as deviations from the independence principle formulated by Hodgkin and Huxley (56) to express the idea that the passage of an ion through a channel is not affected by the presence of other ions.

Local Anesthetics

The block of sodium current by local anesthetic molecules differs in several respects from the action of TTX or STX. First, anesthetic molecules are active when applied on the inside of the membrane (64,71,88). When applied externally, tertiary amine anesthetics can diffuse through the membrane to their site of action. Permanently charged quaternary derivatives of local anesthetics are active only from the inside (42,88). In addition, the amount of block depends on membrane potential and the previous pulse history of the axon membrane (26,88) for many tertiary anesthetic compounds and their quaternary derivatives. It appears that the site of anesthetic block becomes available to these more hydrophilic anesthetic species present in the axoplasm when the sodium channel is opened, just as TEA gains access to its blocking site inside a potassium channel when the channel opens. In fact, in squid axons treated with pronase to remove normal sodium inactivation, the entry rate of anesthetic molecules into the channel can be directly observed as a time-dependent block of the sodium current (1). The degree of block depends on how much the channel is used. For example, after a long rest period, if the axon is then given test clamp pulses at a fixed rate, the current decreases with each pulse until a steady level of inhibition is reached, which depends on the frequency of stimulation. Viewed in this way, it is easy to see why certain tertiary amine anesthetics have an antiarrhythmic type of action; the more the channel is used, the more it becomes blocked. This is why many anesthetic molecules limit the frequency of firing to low rates (26). An anesthetic molecule like benzocaine, which is permanently uncharged, lacks this sort of use dependence.

Gating Modifiers

The shape of an action potential depends critically on the sodium channel gating processes. Many toxins from the plant and animal kingdoms owe their pharmacological activity to modifications of the normal opening and closing of sodium channels. These agents often bring about hyperexcitability in the nervous system by producing long-duration action potentials or repetitive firing. Several may be useful in attempts to isolate and purify components of sodium channels.

Several agents have been found that selectively alter the inactivation process of sodium channels either by slowing the kinetics of inactivation or by completely removing inactivation. The best example of complete inactivation removal is the action of pronase on the inside of a squid axon (8). Pronase is a mixture of proteolytic enzyme from the bacterium *Streptomyces griseus,* and its specific action suggests that sodium inactivation depends on a protein accessible from the axoplasmic side of

the membrane. In the node of Ranvier, iodate ions have a similar action in selectively removing sodium inactivation from the inside (85). On the other side of the membrane, inactivation can be selectively slowed and partially removed by certain types of scorpion venom—*Leiurus* (65,66) and *Buthus* (72)—and by toxin isolated from the sea anemone (14). Both scorpion venom and anemone toxin are composed of polypeptide components of molecular weight 3,000–8,000. Interestingly, scorpion venom is inactive when applied internally (72). These agents bring about long-duration action potentials.

Venom from a different scorpion, *Centruroides sculpturatus,* produces repetitive firing through a selective alteration of the activation process of sodium channels (18). *Centruroides* venom shifts the voltage dependence for activation in a fraction of sodium channels by 50–60 mV in the hyperpolarizing direction. The fraction of altered channels is increased by depolarization. This is the only known case in which inactivation can be removed in channels that are already activated. The result is a steady inward sodium current near the normal resting potential.

Another class of sodium channel gating modifier includes batrachotoxin (63), aconitine (79), and grayanotoxin (82). Each of these agents shifts the voltage dependence and slows the kinetics for activating sodium current, and in addition completely removes inactivation in a fraction of the channels.

Finally, there is another group of agents including DDT and veratrine alkaloids that override the normal closing of sodium channels by the inactivation route during a maintained depolarization and by the normal rapid closing of the activation process at hyperpolarized potentials. With DDT the time course of closing the sodium channel is on the order of tens of milliseconds (45), whereas with veratridine, one of the veratrine alkaloids, the time course is more on the order of seconds (91).

Several of these agents can be put to use as pharmacological tools to depolarize and induce sodium fluxes in a variety of preparations (10,20,21,43,94). Because of their tight binding, scorpion venoms may be useful as affinity agents in attempts to isolate sodium channels. Finally, some of the gating modifiers have been useful in studying sodium conductance fluctuations, as described in the next section.

Conductance Fluctuations

The opening and closing of ionic channels is a probabilistic process in which the membrane potential sets the odds for how many channels are open. A close look at records of ionic current at the node of Ranvier with high enough gain reveals a certain graininess above the normal background noise that stands out when ionic currents are activated. By studying the characteristics of the fluctuating current record, it is possible to estimate the size of the unitary event underlying the fluctuations (i.e., the conductance of a single open channel) and to determine the kinetic properties for the spontaneous opening and closing of the channel.

Ideally, one would like to have sufficiently good resolution to observe directly the ionic current passing through a single channel. This was recently accomplished for the channel activated by acetylcholine in denervated muscle (73) by recording current from a 10-μm^2 patch of membrane through a pipette pressed against the membrane. Unfortunately, single-channel currents have not yet been observed for the potential-sensitive sodium and potassium channels, because the signal is too small and rapid to be detected above the background noise with present techniques. However, by activating a fraction of the available channels and measuring the variance about the mean of ionic current that develops as the number of open channels fluctuates around some mean value, the conductance of a single channel (γ) can be estimated from the formula

$$\gamma = \frac{\sigma^2}{\mu_g(1-p)}$$

where σ^2 is the variance, μ_g is the mean conductance, and p is the probability that a channel is open. In addition, the fluctuating current record can be subjected to Fourier analysis to evaluate the power of different frequency components that make up the record (87).

To study potassium current fluctuations, TTX is applied to block sodium currents, and the membrane is depolarized to activate a steady potassium current with fluctuations about a mean value. When the variance and mean current measurements are made before potassium inactivation has a chance to develop, the single-channel potassium conductance is estimated to be 4×10^{-12} mho, independent of the membrane potential (11). Sodium current fluctuations are more difficult to study because sodium inactivation prevents the development of a large steady sodium current. Dubois and Bergman (32) measured the amount of noninactivating sodium current to be approximately 2% in sensory fibers and much lower in motor fibers. There have been three approaches to this problem. First, the very small sodium currents that do not inactivate were analyzed either as voltage fluctuations (12) or as current fluctuations under a voltage clamp depolarization after the transient sodium currents reached a small but still measurable level (24). Second, steady-state sodium currents were induced by using pharmacological agents that alter the inactivation process (25) or by using *Centruroides* venom to alter sodium activation (3). Finally, the ensemble fluctuations were measured by studying the variance of transient sodium currents, not over time but between individual current records for a fixed depolarization (83). Each method yielded an estimate for the conductance of a single sodium channel of approximately $5-10 \times 10^{-12}$ mho. For comparison, the conductance of an acetylcholine-sensitive channel at the frog neuromuscular junction is approximately 25×10^{-12} mho (4). Fluctuation analysis should also prove useful as a test for kinetic models of the gating process.

These estimates for single-channel conductance enable calculation of the total number of sodium and potassium channels at a single frog node of Ranvier. Taking the maximum conductances for sodium and potassium as 0.75 and 0.13 μmho, respectively (27), reveals that there are approximately 100,000 sodium channels and 30,000 potassium channels at a single node. For a node with a surface area of 35 μm^2, there are approximately 3,000 sodium channels and 850 potassium channels per square micrometer. For a driving force of 100 mV, a sodium channel passes 10^{-12} amperes of ionic current, representing the movement of 3,000–6,000 sodium ions each millisecond.

CONCLUSION

The patch of axon membrane at a node of Ranvier is highly specialized for the transmission of the action potential, having approxi-

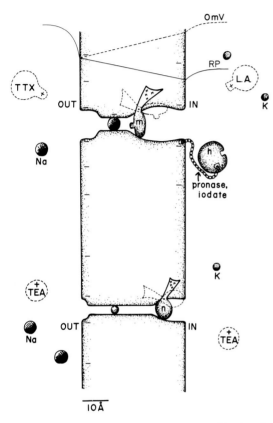

FIG. 4. Imaginary view of a sodium channel (*top*) and a potassium channel (*below*). Charges linked to the m and n gates move when the nerve is depolarized to the dotted line position, opening the channel. The potential profile from the outside to the inside is depicted above the channels for the normal resting potential (RP, *solid line*) and for a depolarization to 0 mV (*dotted line*). Negative surface charges modify the field within the membrane (slope of potential profile). The second gating factor (h) of the sodium channel in this figure is capable of interacting with the m gate by binding, one of several possible coupled gating schemes. The h factor is attacked by pronase or iodate. A sodium ion is shown inside the channel at a negatively charged site, the selectivity filter. TTX can block the channel from the outside, and local anesthetics (L.A.) can block from the inside. The potassium channel is a bit narrower and can be blocked by TEA from inside or outside.

mately 100 times the density of sodium channels as do the small unmyelinated fibers. Modern voltage clamp experiments seek to explore molecular properties of the ionic channels in order to gain clues concerning their structure and function. Channels are likely to be made of protein specialized for the detection of electrical fields and for discrimination between ions. Many of the conceptual features of channels in the membrane are depicted in Fig. 4. Through a combination of biochemical and electrophysiological experimentation, our picture will hopefully continue to become clearer.

ACKNOWLEDGMENT

This work was supported in part by NIH grant NS-12547-02 and by a fellowship from the Muscular Dystrophy Association. I am grateful to Joanne Weinstock for typing the manuscript and to Janet K. Cahalan for help with the illustrations.

REFERENCES

1. Almers, W., and Cahalan, M. D. (1977): Interaction between a local anesthetic, the sodium channel gates and tetrodotoxin. *Biophys. J.*, 17:205a.
2. Almers, W., and Levinson, S. R. (1975): Tetrodotoxin binding to normal and depolarized frog muscle and the conductance of a single sodium channel. *J. Physiol.*, 247:483–509.
3. Anderson, C. R., and Cahalan, M. (1974): Gating kinetics and conductance of single Na⁺ channels in excitable membrane: Studies of current fluctuations in voltage-clamped node of Ranvier. *Proc. Int. Un. Physiol. Sci.*, 11:8.
4. Anderson, C. R., and Stevens, C. F. (1973): Voltage clamp analysis of acetylcholine produced end-plate current fluctuations at frog neuromuscular junction. *J. Physiol. (Lond)*, 235:655–691.
5. Armstrong, C. M. (1975): Potassium pores of nerve and muscle membranes. In: *Membranes—A Series of Advances*, Vol. 3, edited by G. Eisenman. Marcel Dekker, New York.
6. Armstrong, C. M., and Bezanilla, F. (1974): Charge movement associated with the opening and closing of the activation gates of the Na channels. *J. Gen. Physiol.*, 63:533–552.
7. Armstrong, C. M., and Bezanilla, F. (1975): Currents associated with the ionic gating structures in nerve membrane. *Ann. NY Acad. Sci.*, 264:265–277.
8. Armstrong, C. M., Bezanilla, F., and Rojas, E.

(1973): Destruction of sodium inactivation in squid axons perfused with pronase. *J. Gen. Physiol.*, 62:375–391.

9. Armstrong, C. M., and Hille, B. (1972): The inner quaternary ammonium ion receptor in potassium channels of the node of Ranvier. *J. Gen. Physiol.*, 59:388–400.

10. Barnola, F. V., and Villegas, R. (1976): Sodium flux through the sodium channels of axon membrane fragments isolated from lobster nerves. *J. Gen. Physiol.*, 67:81–90.

11. Begenisich, T., and Stevens, C. F. (1975): How many conductance states do potassium channels have? *Biophys. J.*, 15:843–846.

12. Berg. R. J., van den DeGoede, J., and Verveen, A. A. (1975): Conductance fluctuations in Ranvier nodes. *Pfluegers Arch.*, 360:17–23.

13. Bergman, C. (1970): Increase of sodium concentration near the inner surface of the nodal membrane. *Pfluegers Arch.*, 317:287–302.

14. Bergman, C., Dubois, J. M., Rojas, E., and Rathmeyer, W. (1976): Decreased rate of sodium conductance inactivation in the node of Ranvier induced by a polypeptide toxin from sea anemone. *Biochim. Biophys. Acta*, 455:173–184.

15. Bezanilla, F., and Armstrong, C. M. (1972): Negative conductance caused by entry of sodium and cesium ions into the potassium channels of squid axons. *J. Gen. Physiol.*, 60:588–608.

16. Brink, F. (1954): The role of calcium ions in neural processes. *Pharmacol. Rev.*, 6:243–298.

17. Brismar, T. (1973): Effects of ionic concentration on permeability properties of nodal membrane in myelinated nerve fibers of Xenopus laevis. *Acta Physiol. Scand.*, 87:474–484.

18. Cahalan, M. D. (1975): Modification of sodium channel gating in frog myelinated nerve fibres by Centruroides sculpturatus scorpion venom. *J. Physiol. (Lond)*, 244:511–534.

19. Cahalan, M., and Begenisich, T. (1976): Sodium channel selectivity: Dependence on internal permeant ion concentration. *J. Gen. Physiol.*, 68:111–125.

20. Catterall, W. A. (1975): Cooperative activation of action potential Na ionophore by neurotoxins. *Proc. Natl. Acad. Sci. USA*, 72:1782–1786.

21. Catterall, W. (1976): Purification of a toxic protein from scorpion venom which activates the action potential ionophore. *J. Biol. Chem.*, 251:5528–5536.

22. Cole, K. S. (1968): *Membranes, Ions and Impulses.* University of California Press, Berkeley.

23. Colquhoun, D., Henderson, R., and Ritchie, J. M. (1972): The binding of labelled tetrodotoxin to non-myelinated nerve fibres. *J. Physiol. (Lond)*, 227:95–126.

24. Conti, F., Hille, B., Neumcke, B., Nonner, W., and Stämpfli, R. (1976): Measurement of the conductance of the sodium channel from current fluctuations at the node of Ranvier. *J. Physiol. (Lond)*, 262:699–728.

25. Conti, F., Hille, B., Neumcke, B., Nonner, W., and Stämpfli, R. (1976): Conductance of the sodium channel in myelinated nerve fibres with modified sodium inactivation. *J. Physiol. (Lond)*, 262:729–742.

26. Courtney, K. R. (1975): Mechanism of frequency-dependent inhibition of sodium currents in frog myelinated nerve by the lidocaine derivative GEA 968. *J. Pharmacol. Exp. Ther.*, 195:225–236.

27. Dodge, F. A. (1963): A study of ionic permeability changes underlying excitation in myelinated nerve fibres of the frog. Thesis, The Rockefeller University. University Microfilms, Ann Arbor, Michigan (No. 64–7333).

28. Dodge, F. A., and Frankenhaeuser, B. (1958): Membrane currents in isolated frog nerve fibre under voltage clamp conditions. *J. Physiol. (Lond)*, 143:76–90.

29. Drouin, H., and Neumcke, B. (1974): Specific and unspecific charges at the sodium channel of the nerve membrane. *Pfluegers Arch.*, 351:207–229.

30. Drouin, H., and The, R. (1969): The effect of reducing extracellular pH on the membrane currents of the Ranvier node. *Pfluegers Arch.*, 313:80–88.

31. Dubois, J. M., and Bergman, C. (1975): Cesium induced rectifications in frog myelinated nerve fibres. *Pfluegers Arch.*, 355:361–364.

32. Dubois, J. M., and Bergman, C. (1975): Late sodium current in the node of Ranvier. *Pfluegers Arch.*, 357:145–148.

33. Dubois, J. M., and Bergman, C. (1975): Potassium accumulation in the perinodal space of frog myelinated axons. *Pfluegers Arch.*, 358:111–124.

34. Fox, J. M. (1974): Selective blocking of the nodal sodium channels by ultraviolet radiation. *Pfluegers Arch.*, 351:287–301.

35. Fox, J. M. (1976): Ultra-slow inactivation of the ionic currents through the membrane of myelinated nerve. *Biochim. Biophys. Acta*, 426:232–244.

36. Fox, J. M., and Duppel, W. (1975): The action of thiamine and its di- and triphosphates on the slow exponential decline of the ionic currents in the node of Ranvier. *Brain Res.*, 89:287–302.

37. Fox, J. M., Neumcke, B., Nonner, W., and Stämpfli, R. (1976): Block of gating currents by ultraviolet radiation in the membrane of myelinated nerve. *Pfluegers Arch.*, 364:143–145.

38. Frankenhaeuser, B. (1957): A method for recording resting and action potentials in the isolated myelinated nerve fibre of the frog. *J. Physiol. (Lond)*, 135:550–559.

39. Frankenhaeuser, B., and Hodgkin, A. L. (1956): The after effects of impulses in the

giant nerve fibres of Loligo. *J. Physiol.* (*Lond*), 131:341–376.

40. Frankenhaeuser, B., and Hodgkin, A. L. (1957): The action of calcium on the electrical properties of squid axons. *J. Physiol.* (*Lond*), 137:218–244.

41. Frankenhaeuser, B., Lindley, B. D., and Smith, R. S. (1966): Potentiometric measurement of membrane action potentials in frog muscle fibres. *J. Physiol.* (*Lond*), 183:152.

42. Frazier, D. T., Narahashi, T., and Yamada, M. (1970): The site of action and active form of local anesthetics. II. Experiments with quaternary compounds. *J. Pharmacol. Exp. Ther.*, 171:45–51.

43. Henderson, R., and Strichartz, G. (1974): Ion fluxes through the sodium channels of garfish olfactory nerve membranes. *J. Physiol.* (*Lond.*) 238:329–342.

44. Hille, B. (1967): The selective inhibition of delayed potassium currents in nerve by tetraethylammonium ion. *J. Gen. Physiol.*, 50:1287–1302.

45. Hille, B. (1968): Pharmacological modification of the sodium channels of frog nerve. *J. Gen. Physiol.*, 51:199–219.

46. Hille, B. (1968): Charges and potentials at the nerve surface. Divalent ions and pH. *J. Gen. Physiol.*, 51:221–236.

47. Hille, B. (1970): Ionic channels in nerve membranes. *Prog. Biophys. Mol. Biol.*, 21:1–32.

48. Hille, B. (1971): The permeability of the sodium channel to organic cations in myelinated nerve. *J. Gen. Physiol.*, 58:599–619.

49. Hille, B. (1972): The permeability of the sodium channel to metal cations in myelinated nerve. *J. Gen. Physiol.*, 59:637–658.

50. Hille, B. (1973): Potassium channels in myelinated nerve: Selective permeability to small cations. *J. Gen. Physiol.*, 61:669–686.

51. Hille, B. (1975): Ionic selectivity of Na and K channels in nerve membranes. In: *Membranes—A Series of Advances,* Vol. 3, Chap. 4, edited by G. Eisenman. Marcel Dekker, New York.

52. Hille, B. (1975): The receptor for tetrodotoxin and saxitoxin: A structural hypothesis. *Biophys. J.*, 15:615–619.

53. Hille, B., and Campbell, D. (1976): An improved Vaseline gap voltage clamp for skeletal muscle fibers. *J. Gen. Physiol.*, 67:265–293.

54. Hille, B., Ritchie, J. M., and Strichartz, G. (1975): The effect of surface charge on the nerve membrane on the action of tetrodotoxin and saxitoxin in frog myelinated nerve. *J. Physiol.* (*Lond*), 250:34–35p.

55. Hille, B., Woodhull, A. M., and Shapiro, B. I. (1975): Negative surface charge near sodium channels of nerve: Divalent ions, monovalent ions, and pH. *Philos. Trans. R. Soc. Lond. B,* 270:301–318.

56. Hodgkin, A. L., and Huxley, A. F. (1952): Currents carried by sodium and potassium ions through the membrane of the giant axon of Loligo. *J. Physiol.* (*Lond*), 116:449–472.

57. Hodgkin, A. L., and Huxley, A. F. (1952): The components of membrane conductance in the giant axon of *Loligo. J. Physiol.* (*Lond*), 116:473–496.

58. Hodgkin, A. L., and Huxley, A. F. (1952): The dual effect of membrane potential on sodium conductance in the giant axon of Loligo. *J. Physiol.* (*Lond*), 116:496–506.

59. Hodgkin, A. L., and Huxley, H. F. (1952): A quantitative description of membrane current and its application to conduction and excitation in nerve. *J. Physiol.* (*Lond*), 117:500–544.

60. Huxley, A. F., and Stämpfli, R. (1951): Direct determination of membrane resting potential and action potential in single myelinated nerve fibers. *J. Physiol.* (*Lond*), 112:476–495.

61. Kato, G. (1934): *The Microphysiology of Nerve.* Maruzen, Tokyo.

62. Keynes, R. D., and Rojas, E. (1974): Kinetics and steady-state properties of the charged system controlling sodium conductance in the squid giant axon. *J. Physiol.* (*Lond*), 239:393–434.

63. Khodorov, B. I., Peganov, E. M., Revenko, S. V., and Shishkova, L. D. (1975): Sodium currents in voltage clamped nerve fiber of frog under the combined action of batrachotoxin and procaine. *Brain Res.*, 84:541–546.

64. Khodorov, B., Shishkova, L., Peganov, E., and Revenko, S. (1976): Inhibition of sodium currents in frog Ranvier node treated with local anesthetics: Role of slow sodium inactivation. *Biochim. Biophys. Acta,* 433:409–435.

65. Koppenhöfer, E., and Schmidt, H. (1968): Die wirkung von skorpiongilt auf die ionenströme des Ranvierschen schnürrings. I. Die Permeabilitäten P_{Na} und P_K. *Pfluegers Arch.*, 303:133–149.

66. Koppenhöfer, E., and Schmidt, H. (1968): Die wirkung von skorpiongift auf die ionenströme des Ranvierschen scnnürrings. II. Unvollstärdize Natriuminaktivierung. *Pfluegers Arch.*, 303:150–161.

67. Koppenhöfer, E., and Vogel, W. (1969): Effects of tetrodotoxin and tetraethylammonium chloride on the inside of the nodal membrane of Xenopus laevis. *Pfluegers Arch.*, 313:361–380.

68. Mozhayeva, G. N., and Naumov, A. P. (1970): Effect of surface charge on the steady-state potassium conductance of nodal membrane. *Nature* (*Lond*), 228:164.

69. Mozhayeva, G. N., and Naumov, A. P. (1972): Tetraethylammonium ion inhibition of potassium conductance of the nodal membrane. *Biochim. Biophys. Acta,* 290:248–255.

70. Narahashi, T. (1971): Neurophysiological basis for drug action. In: *Biopnysics and*

Physiology of Excitable Membranes, edited by W. J. Adelman, pp. 423–462. Van Nostrand Reinhold, New York.

71. Narahashi, T., Frazier, D. T., and Yamada, M. (1970): The site of action and active form of local anesthetics. I. Theory and pH experiments with tertiary compounds. *J. Pharmacol. Exp. Ther.,* 171:32–44.

72. Narahashi, T., Shapiro, B., Deguchi, T., Scuka, M., and Wang, C. M. (1972): Effects of scorpion venom on squid axon membranes. *Am. J. Physiol.,* 222:850–857.

73. Neher, E., and Sakmann, B. (1976): Single-channel currents recorded from membrane of denervated frog muscle fibres. *Nature (Lond),* 260:799–801.

74. Neumcke, B., Nonner, W., and Stämpfli, R. (1976): Asymmetrical displacement current and its relation with the activation of sodium current in the membrane of frog myelinated nerve. *Pfluegers Arch.,* 363:193–203.

75. Nonner, W. (1969): A new voltage clamp method for Ranvier nodes. *Pfluegers Arch.,* 309:176–192.

76. Nonner, W., Rojas, E., and Stämpfli, R. (1975): Displacement currents in the node of Ranvier: Voltage and time dependence. *Pfluegers Arch.,* 354:1–18.

77. Peganov, E. M., Khodorov, B. I., and Shishkova, L. D. (1973): Slow sodium inactivation related to external potassium in the membrane of Ranvier's node: The role of external K. *Bull. Exp. Biol. Med.,* 9:15–19 (in Russian).

78. Ritchie, J. M., Rogart, R. B., Strichartz, G. R. (1976): A new method for labelling saxitoxin and its binding to nonmyelinated fibres of the rabbit vagus, lobster walking leg, and garfish olfactory nerve. *J. Physiol.* 261:477–494.

79. Schmidt, H., and Schmitt, O. (1974): Effect of aconitine on the sodium permeability of the node of Ranvier. *Pfluegers Arch.,* 349:133–148.

80. Schwarz, J. R., Ulbricht, W., and Wagner, H. H. (1973): The rate of action of tetrodotoxin on myelinated nerve fibers of Xenopus laevis and Rana esculenta. *J. Physiol. (Lond),* 233:167–194.

81. Schwarz, J. R., and Vogel, W. (1971): Potassium inactivation in single myelinated nerve fibres of Xenopus laevis. *Pfluegers Arch.,* 330:61–73.

82. Seyama, I., and Narahashi, T. (1976): Sodium conductance kinetics of squid axon membranes poisoned by grayanotoxin. I. *Biophys. J.,* 16:87a.

83. Sigworth, F. (1977): Na-current fluctuations give estimates of single-channel conductance in frog nerve. *Biophys. J.,* 17:10a.

84. Stämpfli, R. (1969): Dissection of single nerve fibres and measurement of membrane potential changes of Ranvier nodes by means of the double air gap method. In: *Laboratory Techniques in Membrane Biophysics,* edited by H. Passow and R. Stämpfli. Springer, New York.

85. Stämpfli, R. (1974): Intraaxonal iodate inhibits sodium inactivation. *Experientia,* 30:505–508.

86. Stämpfli, R., and Hille, B. (1977): Electrophysiology of frog peripheral myelinated nerve. In: *Neurobiology of the Frog,* edited by R. Llinas and W. Precht. Springer, New York.

87. Stevens, C. F. (1972): Inferences about membrane properties from electrical noise measurements. *Biophys. J.,* 12:1028–1047.

88. Strichartz, G. R. (1973): The inhibition of sodium currents in myelinated nerve by quaternary derivatives of lidocaine. *J. Gen. Physiol.,* 62:37–57.

89. Tasaki, I., and Takeuchi, T. (1941): Der am Ranvierschen kroten entstehende aktiovsstrom und reine Bedetung für die erregungslirtung. *Pfluegers Arch.,* 244:696–711.

90. Tasaki, I., and Takeuchi, T. (1942): Weitere studien über den aktronsstrom der markhaltigen nervenfasern und über die elektrosaltatorische ubertragung des nervenimpulses. *Pfluegers Arch.,* 242:764–782.

91. Ulbricht, W. (1969): The effect of veratridine on excitable membranes of nerve and muscle. *Ergeb. Physiol. Biol. Chem. Exp. Pharmakol.,* 61:18–71.

92. Vierhaus, J., and Ulbricht, W. (1971): Effect of a sudden change in sodium concentration on repetitively evoked action potentials of single nodes of Ranvier. *Pfluegers Arch.,* 326:76–87.

93. Vierhaus, J., and Ulbricht, W. (1971): Rate of action of tetraethylammonium ions on the duration of action potentials in single Ranvier nodes. *Pfluegers Arch.,* 526:88–100.

94. Villegas, J., Sevcik, C., Barnola, F. V., and Villegas, R. (1976): Grayanotoxin, veratrine and tetrodotoxin sensitive sodium pathways in the Schwann cell membrane of squid nerve fibers. *J. Gen. Physiol.,* 67:369–380.

95. Vogel, W. (1974): Calcium and lanthanum effects at the nodal membrane. *Pfluegers Arch.,* 350:25–39.

96. Wagner, H. H. and Ulbricht, W. (1975): The rates of saxitoxin action and of saxitoxin tetrodotoxin interaction at the node of Ranvier. *Pfluegers Arch.,* 359:297–315.

97. Woodhull, A. M. (1973): Ionic blockage of sodium channels in nerve. *J. Gen. Physiol.,* 61:687–708.

Physiology and Pathobiology of Axons, edited by
S. G. Waxman. Raven Press, New York © 1978.

Variations in Axonal Morphology and Their Functional Significance

Stephen G. Waxman

*Department of Neurology, Harvard Medical School, Beth Israel Hospital, Boston, Massachusetts
02215; and Harvard–MIT Program in Health Sciences and Technology, Massachusetts Institute
of Technology, Cambridge, Massachusetts 02139*

The remarkable differentiation of the neuronal surface is probably most elaborately displayed by the dendritic and axonal portions of the neuron. Even a cursory examination indicates that axons exhibit a very high degree of structural differentiation. This morphological differentiation is evident not only when comparing one axon with another, but also when comparing different regions along the course of a single axon. The structural specialization of cells usually reflects functional differentiation. Thus in studying cells or cell systems with a high degree of morphological differentiation, one is led to inquire about structure–function relations. In this chapter, we consider the structural differentiation of axons. We further consider some structure–function relations, and the physiological implications of the observed variations in morphology. Because it is especially amenable to experimental morphophysiological analysis, we concentrate on the myelinated axon.

GEOMETRY OF THE MYELINATED AXON: RELATION OF INTERNODE DISTANCE TO FIBER DIAMETER

For most normal myelinated axons in the peripheral nervous system (22,53), and many myelinated axons in the central nervous system (23,33), the ratio of internode distance (L) to axon diameter (d) has a value of 100–200. Rushton (47) and Huxley and Stämpfli (25) suggested that this value of the ratio L/d is such as to maximize conduction velocity at any given diameter. At other sites in the central nervous system, however, the ratio L/d is considerably smaller. Fibers with closely spaced ($L/d < 20$) nodes of Ranvier have been described, for example, in teleost oculomotor (54) and electromotor (35,55) systems, mammalian oculomotor nucleus and mesencephalic reticular formation (61), cerebral cortex (12), and superior olivary nucleus (30). Moreover, it has been shown that the ratio L/d may change along the course of single fibers (55). Figure 1 shows a myelinated preterminal fiber from the pacemaker region of the electromotor nucleus of the gymnotid *Sternopygus.* Fiber diameter is approximately 3 μm. Four nodes of Ranvier are present, and the internode distances are all less than 10 μm.

L/d is also decreased in remyelinated fibers in the peripheral (49) and central (19) nervous systems. However, as pointed out by McDonald (32), in view of the occurrence of closely spaced nodes at some sites in the normal central nervous system, short internode distances do not represent unequivocal evidence of prior demyelination.

Figure 2 shows the computed relation between internodal distance and conduction velocity for a 10-μm fiber (11). As predicted by Huxley and Stämpfli (25) and Rushton (47) on the basis of analytic arguments, there is a broad maximum in conduction velocity centered around the value of L/d observed in normal peripheral fibers. As L/d decreases from its normal peripheral nerve value (100–200), conduction velocity decreases (Fig. 2). For short internode lengths, conduction velocity is strongly dependent on small relative

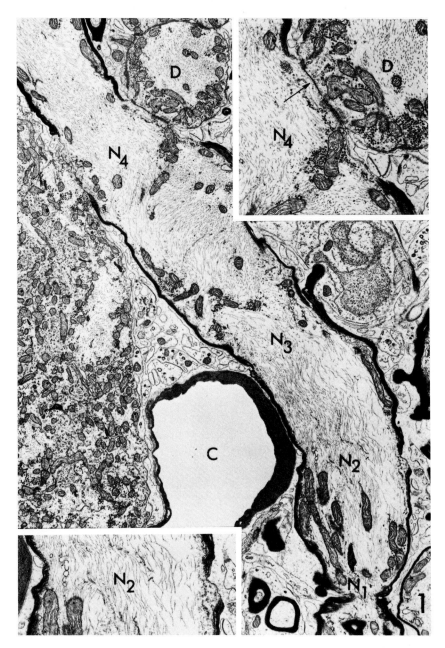

FIG. 1. Electron micrograph showing a myelinated preterminal fiber from the pacemaker electromotor nucleus of the gymnotid *Sternopygus*. Four nodes of Ranvier (N_1–N_4) are separated by internode distances of less than 10 μm. The surface area of node N_4 is larger than that of nodes N_1, N_2, and N_3. Nodes N_2 and N_4 are enlarged in the insets. At N_4 there is a close apposition (*arrow, upper inset*) with a dendrite (D). (C) Capillary. $\times 7,700$. **Inset:** $\times 13,400$.

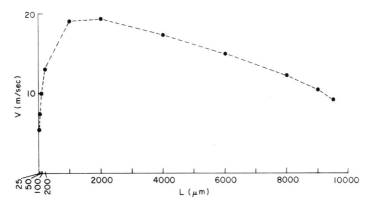

FIG. 2. Plot of impulse conduction velocity versus internodal distance (L) for a myelinated fiber with an axon diameter of 10 μm. The graph can be generalized to other axon diameters by scaling conduction velocity and internode length appropriately. (Modified from ref. 11.)

changes in *L*. Thus normal peripheral nerve fibers are expected to be relatively velocity-stabilized with respect to small changes in internode length. This prediction is consistent with the observation that, in remyelinated peripheral fibers with internode distances of 200–500 μm, conduction velocities are minimally reduced (49). On the other hand, pre-terminal fibers, in which the ratio L/d may be as small as 5–10 (54,55), should be highly sensitive to further changes in *L*. Meszler et al. (35), in fact, demonstrated values of the ratio L/d for axons in the *Electrophorus* electromotor system consistent with the delay line function of these axons. Since sensitivity to further changes in *L* increases as L/d becomes small (Fig. 2), local changes in internode length may provide a mechanism for presetting route-dependent travel times. In addition, as pointed out by Khodorov and Timin (27), decreases in internode distance may facilitate conduction into unmyelinated terminals.

GEOMETRY OF THE MYELINATED AXON: RELATION OF SHEATH THICKNESS TO FIBER DIAMETER

Dimensional arguments (47) suggest that conduction velocity should be maximal when the ratio *g* (axon diameter/total fiber diameter) $= 0.6$. Electron microscopic studies on peripheral nerve (17,50) indicate that for most fibers myelin thickness is nearly proportional to fiber diameter, and that the ratio *g* is usually close to 0.6 in the peripheral nervous system. Bishop et al. (6) studied the relation of sheath thickness to fiber diameter in dorsal column cuneate and gracile bundles, pyramidal tract, optic nerve and tract, and trigeminal and auditory nerves in eight mammalian species, and reported values of *g* to be 0.5–0.9 for the great majority of fibers. For myelinated fibers in the splenium of the rabbit corpus callosum (65), values of *g* range from 0.64 to 0.87 (mean 0.77, SD 0.05); a line fit to these points by the least-squares method has a slope of 0.074 and a *y*-intercept of 0.72 (Fig. 3). For small fibers in the lizard oculomotor nucleus, Waxman and Bennett (60) found values of *g* between 0.54 and 0.88 (mean 0.77); and in the cat oculomotor nucleus (58), values of *g* fall between 0.58 and 0.88 (mean 0.74). Thus values of *g* usually fall between 0.5 and 0.9 for most fibers in peripheral nerve and in white matter and gray matter of the central nervous system.

Variation of *g* within this range should have only small effects on conduction velocity. Rushton (47) predicted that conduction velocity would be maximal for a fiber of fixed diameter when $g = 0.6$, and calculated a variation in conduction velocity of less than 5% for values of *g* between 0.47 and 0.74. Computations by Smith and Koles (51) suggest that conduction speed is maximal for *g* between 0.6 and 0.7, with a variation in conduction velocity of less than 20% for values of *g* between 0.5 and 0.9, holding fiber diameter constant.

It should be kept in mind that several investigators (50,59) have called into question the practice of determining fiber diameter, or the relation of sheath thickness to fiber diameter, by light microscopy, since many fibers (especially in the central nervous system) fall close to the limit of resolution of the light microscope. When viewed by light microscopy, values of g for small fibers depart from the range 0.5–0.9 observed by electron microscopy and approach zero.

If conduction velocity for nonmyelinated fibers varies with diameter$^{1/2}$, and conduction velocity for myelinated fibers varies directly with diameter, it should be expected that the relationships between fiber diameter and conduction velocity should intersect at some point, below which myelinated fibers would be expected to conduct less rapidly than nonmyelinated fibers of the same diameter. Proportionality between conduction velocity and diameter for myelinated fibers depends on the assumptions that: (a) specific membrane properties are the same for all fibers; and (b) fibers exhibit "dimensional similarity" (47). The latter constraint, in simplified form, requires that the nodal area vary directly with fiber diameter and that the internodal length be proportional to the fiber diameter. Rushton (47) observed that, to a rough approximation, peripheral axons do exhibit dimensional similarity. He further noted that in the peripheral nervous system nearly all fibers larger than 1 μm are myelinated (15), and he presented a set of arguments leading to the conclusion that

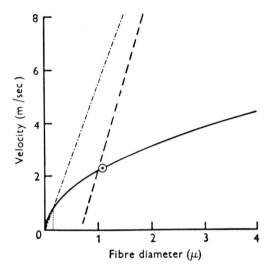

FIG. 4. Relations between conduction velocity and fiber diameter for small myelinated and nonmyelinated fibers. [Modified from Rushton's (47) Fig. 5 as indicated in the text.] The circled point represents Gasser's (18) measurements for the largest C-fibers. Rushton's relation (- - - -) intersects the parabolic relation for nonmyelinated fibers at approximately 1 μm. The revised linear relation (— · — · —) for myelinated fibers intersects the parabola at a point corresponding to a diameter of approximately 0.2 μm. This value, rather than the 1 μm intersection provided by Rushton's relation, is the critical diameter above which myelinated fibers should conduct more rapidly than nonmyelinated fibers of the same size. (From ref. 60.)

1 μm was a physiologically critical diameter below which "conduction is faster without myelination." This conclusion is based on the relations shown in Fig. 4, which is redrawn from Rushton's (47) Fig. 5. The diameter–conduction velocity relation for nonmyelinated fibers is a parabola perpendicular to the ordinate at the origin, drawn on the basis of the proportionality of conduction velocity to diameter$^{1/2}$, using Gasser's (18) measurements of diameter (1.1 μm) and velocity (2.3 meters/sec) for the largest unmyelinated fibers. The diameter–conduction velocity relation for myelinated fibers was derived from the relation

$$V \propto Dg\sqrt{-\log_e g}$$

where V = conduction velocity and D = total fiber diameter. Sanders' (48) measurements of the values of g were used to compute the left side of the equation, and the resulting curve

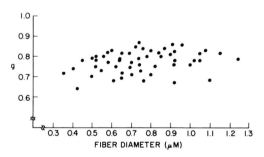

FIG. 3. Values of ratio g for fibers from rabbit visual corpus callosum. The g values range from 0.64 to 0.87 (mean 0.77) and do not show a strong dependence on diameter. (From ref. 65.)

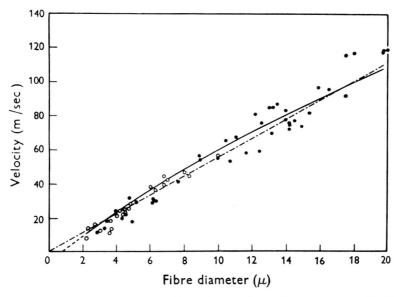

FIG. 5. Relations between conduction velocity and fiber diameter for myelinated axons, modified from Rushton (47). Open and closed circles represent Hursh's (24) observations on fibers from kittens and cats, respectively. Rushton's relation, computed using Sanders' measurements of the ratio *g*, is indicated by the solid curve with dashed extrapolation for small diameters. The linear relation, assuming constant *g*, is indicated by the broken line; its slope is 5.5 msec^{-1} μm^{-1}. (From ref. 60.)

was fit to Hursh's (24) data relating conduction velocity and fiber diameter, as shown in Fig. 5. The extrapolated region of the curve (dashed line) in Fig. 5 was plotted on an expanded scale (Fig. 4, dashed line) to give the relation between diameter and conduction velocity for myelinated fibers in Rushton's Fig. 5. The diameter–conduction velocity relation for myelinated fibers intersects the relation for nonmyelinated fibers at a point corresponding to a diameter of 1 μm, suggesting that with a diameter smaller than this myelinated fibers should conduct less rapidly than nonmyelinated fibers of the same size. Moreover, extrapolation of the relationship downward leads to intersection with the abscissa at 0.6 μm, suggesting that with a diameter smaller than this myelinated fibers should not conduct impulses at all.

Since myelinated fibers in the central nervous system may exhibit diameters as small as 0.2 μm (7,59), we re-examined the derivation of the relations shown in Fig. 4 (60). Sanders' data on the values of *g* were derived from light microscopic observations on rabbit peroneal nerve and suggest that the value of *g* decreases for small fibers, approaching a value of zero at

0.6 μm. This accounts for the predicted failure of conduction at 0.6 μm, since core resistance would be infinite for this value of *g*. Using the ultrastructural data (i.e., assuming that *g* = 0.6 for fibers of all diameters), a revised diameter–conduction velocity relation for myelinated fibers (broken line, Fig. 4) may be constructed. This revised relation intersects the origin and crosses the relation for nonmyelinated fibers at a point corresponding to a diameter of 0.2 μm, suggesting that 0.2 μm should be the critical diameter for myelination. In this regard, note that for a value of *g* = 0.6 fibers with the thinnest myelin sheaths (200 Å) would exhibit diameters of 0.1 μm.

There is some evidence that conduction velocity may not be strictly proportional to fiber diameter in myelinated axons. Paintal (37) observed that spike rise time and duration are inversely related to conduction velocity. Coppin and Jack (14) reported an inverse relation between internodal conduction time and internodal length. Furthermore, Boyd and Davey (10) found that, although the conduction velocity/fiber diameter ratio was 5.6 for α-motor axons, it was approximately 4.5 for γ-motor axons. These observations may be explained either by differences in the specific membrane properties of fibers of different diameter, or by a deviation from dimensional similarity. There is some evidence indicating that nodal surface area may not be proportional to fiber diameter, since the nodal diameter/internodal diameter ratio is greater for small than for large fibers (46). There have been no direct comparisons of specific membrane properties of large and small myelinated fibers.

DIFFERENTIATION OF THE AXONAL SURFACE

Let us now consider the structural differentiation of the surface of the myelinated axon. The structure of the myelin sheath, paranodal region, and the node of Ranvier were discussed in previous chapters. Transmission electron microscopy of thin-sectioned material indicates that the nodal axon membrane, which is directly accessible to the extracellular space, is characterized by an electron-dense undercoating that extends 100–200 Å subjacent to the axon surface at the node. A similar electron-dense undercoating is present at the axonal initial segment (38,42), and it was suggested on the basis of its distribution that it may represent a morphological specialization of the neuronal surface related to specific membrane properties (38).

Figure 6 shows a node of Ranvier fixed with a mixture of glutaraldehyde and paraformaldehyde in phosphate buffer, postfixed in osmium tetroxide in phosphate buffer, and stained with ferric ion and ferrocyanide (29). The bound ferric ion is distributed as a fine precipitate in the perinodal extracellular space. As described by Landon and Langley (29), the perinodal Schwann cell microvilli are seen in negative contrast. Under these conditions, little stain appears within the axon. Landon and Langley interpreted their findings on similarly stained nodes to indicate the presence of a cation-binding substance, which they considered to be composed predominantly of protein-linked mucopolysaccharide, in the perinodal extracellular region. They further suggested that the ion-binding properties of the extracellular matrix at the node might be significant in terms of maintaining the extra-

cellular environment at the node, and that electrophysiological properties would reflect the properties of the node in its entirety, including the perinodal matrix.

Although it is abundantly clear that direct accessibility of the axon membrane to the external milieu is limited to the nodes, and that the extracellular matrix at the node may be specialized, a question remains as to whether the nodal membrane is intrinsically different from the internodal axon membrane of the myelinated fiber. It is known that conduction block occurs at sites of demyelination along both peripheral (31) and central (34) axons. Does this observation allow us to make any inference about the properties of the internodal axon membrane? Conduction block at a demyelinated internode could reflect shunting of current through bared inexcitable internodal axon membrane. Alternatively, conduction block could occur at a demyelinated internode in the presence of electrically excitable internodal axon membrane if the current density in the demyelinated area were sufficiently small owing to the increased surface area of bared axon membrane in the demyelinated region. We simulated impulse conduction in demyelinated axons, under the assumption that the demyelinated internodal axon membrane is electrically excitable, with the same specific membrane properties as the nodal axon. Computational methods and parameters are described elsewhere (11). Figure 7 shows the simulated behavior of a fiber totally demyelinated at the seventh internode (i.e., the internode between nodes 7 and 8), in which the demyelinated internodal axon membrane has the same specific membrane properties as those of normal nodes. Despite the assumption of normal nodal membrane properties for the demyelinated axon membrane, propagation fails at the focally demyelinated region, presumably because of impedance mismatch. It thus becomes apparent that one cannot, from observations of conduction failure in demyelinated fibers, predict whether the internodal membrane is excitable or inexcitable.

We approached the question of possible differentiation of nodal and internodal regions of the axon membrane using ion-binding techniques. Our studies (44,63,64) of ferric ion–ferrocyanide binding in nerves fixed in Karnov-

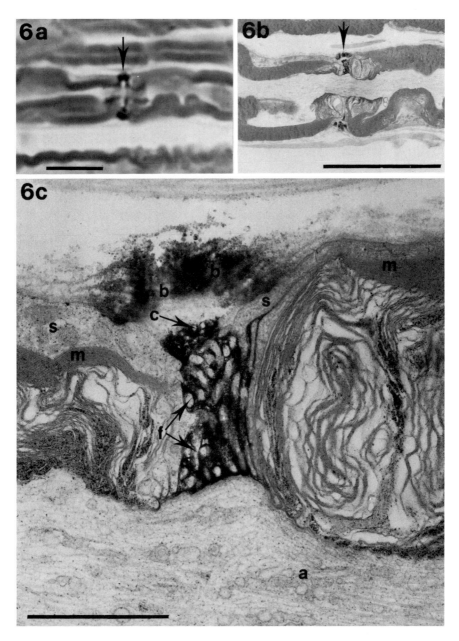

FIG. 6. Extracellular matrix at node of Ranvier in rat sciatic nerve, visualized by staining with ferric ion and ferrocyanide following fixation in phosphate-buffered aldehydes and osmium tetroxide. **A:** Light microscopy of a node (arrow) reveals a colorless, optically refractile deposit in inner portions of the gap, with a blue stain in outer regions. 3 μm section, yellow filter; scale = 10 μm. **B:** In survey electron micrograph of the same node (arrow) following resectioning, the nodal gap substance is seen as electron-dense, scale = 10 μm. **C:** At higher magnification, the electron-dense deposit is located in the extracellar gap substance and adjacent endoneurium, such that Schwann cell fingers (f) and collagen fibrils (c) are seen in negative contrast. That part of the stain which appears blue by light microscopy (b) is amorphous-to-crystalline, and appears to have migrated away from the nodal gap region. (a), axoplasm, (m) myelin, (s), Schwann cell cytoplasm. Scale = 1 μm. **A:** ×1,500. **B:** ×3,200. **C:** ×38,000.

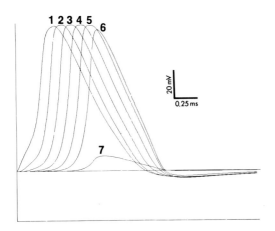

FIG. 7. Computed action potentials at nodes 1–7 for a 10-μm fiber totally demyelinated at internode 7–8, in which the demyelinated internodal axon membrane had the same specific membrane properties as the nodal membrane. Conduction failure occurs at node 7, presumably due to impedence mismatch at the demyelinated region. (From Brill et al., *unpublished results.*)

sky's (26) aldehyde fixative and postfixed in osmium tetroxide, both in cacodylate buffer, indicate that there are structural differences between the axon membrane at the nodes compared with the axon membrane beneath the myelin. Using this method, both peripheral (44,63) and central (64) nodes of Ranvier are intensely stained as viewed by light and electron microscopy. Initial segments are similarly stained (64). In ultrathin sections observed by electron microscopy, the stain is deposited as a layer of dense aggregates (200–1,000 Å thick) located immediately subjacent to the axon membrane at the node of Ranvier (Figs. 8 and 9). Unmyelinated C-fibers do not stain (Fig. 9, inset), even in regions directly exposed to the extracellular milieu (63). In all cases the dense aggregates are confined to the non-myelinated nodal axon membrane and do not appear subjacent to the paranodal myelin loops or the internodal axon membrane. Thus staining of the axon membrane is confined to the nodes of Ranvier. Axoplasmic filaments are often stained in the center of the axon, several micrometers from the axolemma (Figs. 8 and 9), indicating diffusion of stain through the fixed axoplasm. In some experiments nerves were severed after fixation and before exposure to staining solutions. Examination of

the cut ends of the axons revealed an absence of staining of the internodal axon membrane, in contrast to adjacent nodes of Ranvier, which were heavily stained. The last two observations demonstrate that specific staining of the nodal axon membrane with ferric ion and ferrocyanide is not due to accessibility to stain but rather to biochemical differentiation of the inner surface of the axon membrane at the nodes. We interpreted these observations as indicating a structural differentiation of the axon membrane between normal nodes and internodes (44). As described below, binding of ferric ion and ferrocyanide under these conditions, in one model system, appears to be related to specific membrane properties.

Ritchie and Rogart (45) recently estimated the density of sodium channels in mammalian myelinated fibers from measurements of the binding of [³H]saxitoxin to rabbit sciatic nerve. Binding to both intact and homogenized nerve was studied. Their results indicate a much higher density of sodium channels at the nodes ($> 10,000/\mu$m² nodal membrane) than in non-myelinated nerve or muscle, and a low density of sodium channels at the internodes ($< 25/\mu$m²). These values are consistent with the requirement that nodal current density must be considerably greater than at other excitable membranes.

The available experimental data thus indicate that the plasma membrane of the normal mammalian peripheral myelinated fiber is not a homogeneous structure. On the contrary, *nodal and internodal domains of the membrane of the normal myelinated fiber appear to exhibit distinct structural differences.* Whether this differentiation of the axon membrane represents an invariant property is, however, open to question since, under some conditions, abnormally myelinated fibers may conduct impulses in a continuous manner (see Rasminsky, *this volume*). It is, in fact, quite possible that the organization of the axolemma may change during development or in various pathological conditions (45,63).

REGIONAL DIFFERENTIATION OF ELECTROCYTE AXONS

The electrocyte axons of sternarchid fish provide a highly accessible system for studying

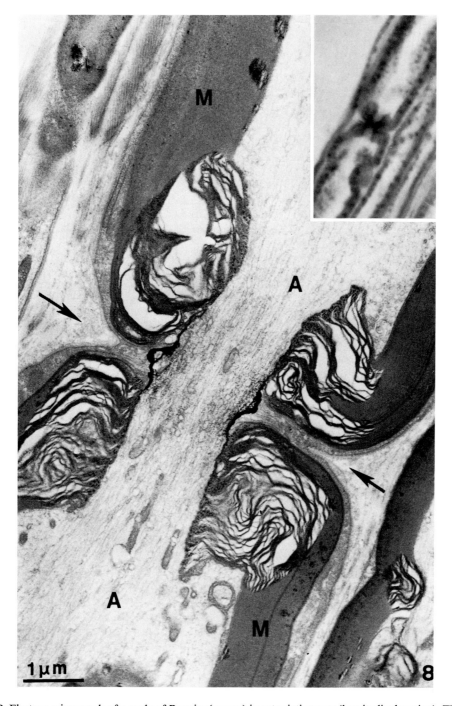

FIG. 8. Electron micrograph of a node of Ranvier (*arrows*) in rat sciatic nerve (longitudinal section). The thin section shown in this figure was cut from the 5-μm section shown in the inset. Ferric ion–ferrocyanide staining, as described in the text, results in a dense deposit of electron-opaque stain located immediately subjacent to the nodal axolemma. Other parts of the axon membrane are not stained. (A) Axoplasm. (M) Myelin. ×16,000. (From ref. 44.)

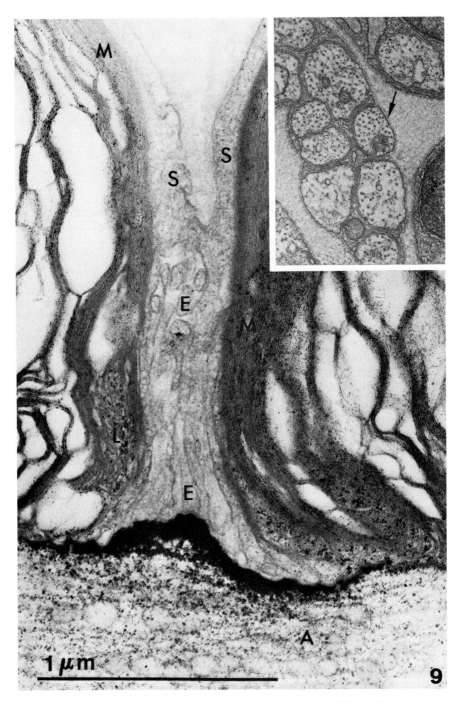

FIG. 9. Higher-magnification electron micrograph of the same node shown in Fig. 8. The densest aggregations of stain are located subjacent to the axon membrane. Lesser deposits of stain are seen in the axoplasm (A), compact myelin (M), and myelin terminal loops (L). Very little stain is present in the Schwann cell cytoplasm (S) or its finger-like extensions (E), or in the gap substance that lies between the fingers. ×66,000. **Inset:** C-Fibers stained under the same conditions. No precipitate is observed in these fibers, even where directly exposed to the extracellular milieu (*arrow*). ×26,000. (From ref. 44.)

differentiation of the axon. In the knifefish *Sternarchus albifrons,* the electric organs are neurogenic (i.e., derived from peripheral axons) in contrast to most other gymnotid electrocytes, which are derived from muscle (4,5). As would be expected from the neurogenic origin of these electrocytes, the electric organ discharge, which is of high frequency (700–1500 Hz), is not significantly affected by curare (4). The electrocyte axons originate in the spinal cord. The axons run from their origin in the spinal cord to the electric organ, where they initially run anteriorly for several spinal segments, then turn sharply to run posteriorly for several segments, and finally taper and end blindly in a connective tissue filament. Light microscopic studies show distinct differences in morphology at different regions along the axon (5,62). In the areas where the fibers enter the electric organ and where they turn around, they are approximately 20 μm in diameter. Anteriorly and posteriorly running regions of the axons dilate to a diameter of approximately 100 μm. In the areas where the fibers enter the electric organ and where they turn around, the nodes of Ranvier exhibit normal morphology, and the nonmyelinated gap in the nodes extends approximately 1 μm along the fiber axis. In proximal parts of the anteriorly and posteriorly running regions of the axons, the gaps in the nodes also appear small. In distal regions of the anteriorly and posteriorly running axonal regions, the nodes are much larger, extending for 50 μm or more along the axis of the fiber (Fig. 10).

Electron microscopy of the nodes of Ranvier in this system show that they fall into two classes (62). In regions where the fibers enter the electric organ and where they turn around, and in proximal parts of the anteriorly and posteriorly running regions of the axons, nodal ultrastructure (Fig. 11) is similar to that of typical peripheral nodes of Ranvier (16,46). The nonmyelinated gap in the myelin extends less than 1 μm along the fiber axis. An electron-dense cytoplasmic undercoating is present subjacent to the nodal axon membrane. As at other normal peripheral nodes, finger-like extensions of the paranodal Schwann cytoplasm often extend into the nodal region. The large nodes in distal parts of the anteriorly and

posteriorly running regions exhibit a different structure (Fig. 12). The nonmyelinated gap extends for as far as 50 μm or more along the axon. The axonal surface is elaborated to form a layer of polypoid processes, further increasing surface area. At these enlarged nodes, the cytoplasmic dense undercoating is not present.

A difference in the electrophysiological properties of the large and small nodes was elucidated by Bennett (4,5) in his studies on the cellular basis for the electric organ discharge. The discharge is generated by the synchronous activity of many electrocytes and is diphasic (initially head-positive). The electrophysiological studies showed that impulses in the electrocyte axons propagate to involve both the anteriorly and posteriorly running segments (Fig. 13A). Spikes are generated only by nodes with narrow gaps and normal morphology; the enlarged nodes in distal portions of the anteriorly and posteriorly running axonal regions do not exhibit spike electrogenesis. Initially, the nodes with normal morphology in the proximal part of the anteriorly running axonal region are active. Enlarged nodes in the distal part of the anteriorly running region are inexcitable and pass outward current. The external currents therefore run posteriorly, generating the head-positive phase of the organ discharge. Normal-appearing nodes in the region where the fiber turns around are subsequently excited. The large nodes in the distal part of the posteriorly running region are inactive, so that external currents flow in an anterior direction, generating the head-negative phase of organ discharge (4,5). The data further suggest that in these axons the enlarged nodes act as a series capacity (Fig. 13B), since there is no direct current (DC) component to the discharge, indicating that there is no net current flow averaged over a single discharge cycle. In cases where propagation into the posteriorly running segment is blocked by anoxia, there is no net current flow, demonstrating that the outputs of the anteriorly and posteriorly running segments exhibit no net current flow. Furthermore, Bennett (4,5) showed that in other sternarchids where the anteriorly running segment is reduced or absent, the head-positive phase is reduced or absent but the discharge still exhibits no DC component.

Figure 14 shows the staining properties of

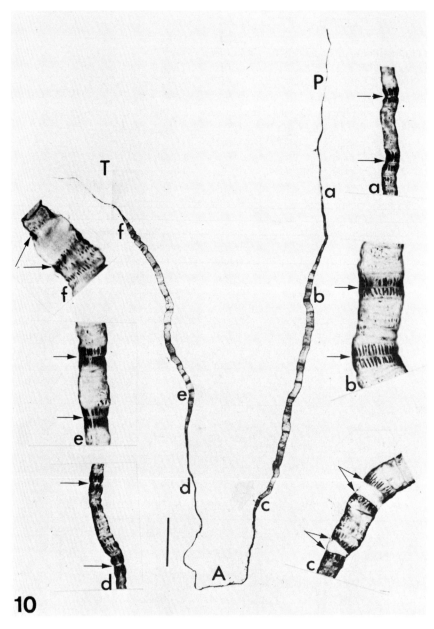

FIG. 10. Photomontage of a dissected single axon from the electric organ of *Sternarchus*. The proximal part of the fiber, near its entry into the organ, is marked P. The anteriorly running portion extends from P to A, where the fiber turns around. The posteriorly running portion extends from A to T, where the fiber terminates. Nodes from different parts of the fiber are enlarged in the insets. The nodal gaps in the myelin are indicated by arrows. In thin regions near the site of entry into the organ (a) and near the point at which the fiber turns around (d), the nodal gap is small. Nodes exhibit a similarly small gap in the proximal and central part of the anteriorly running segment (b) and in the proximal and central part of the posteriorly running segment (e). Distal nodes of the anteriorly running segment (c) and in the posteriorly running segment (f) are large. The fiber ends in a tapering collagenous filament (T). The vertical bar between A and d represents 1 mm for the fiber (150 μm in the insets). ×13. **Insets:** ×88.

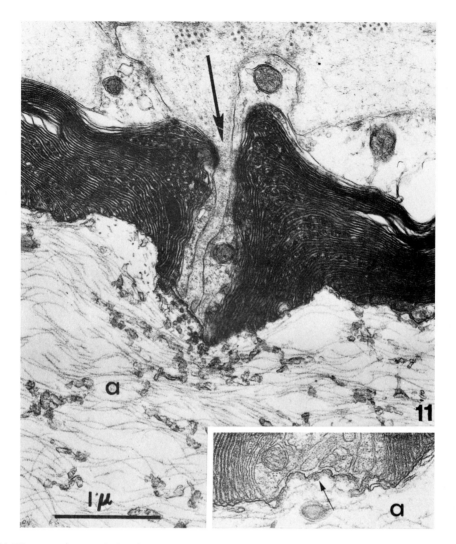

FIG. 11. Electron micrograph showing a node of Ranvier from an electrocyte axon in the efferent nerve to the *Sternarchus* electric organ. The axoplasm (a) contains neurofilaments, vesicles, and elements of a tubular reticulum. Associated with the axon surface at the node is a dense cytoplasmic layer approximately 200 Å thick. A distinct extracellular channel, less than 0.5 μm wide, is indicated by the arrow. ×27,000. **Inset:** The axon membrane at a narrow node from a larger electrocyte axon. Note the dense cytoplasmic undercoating associated with the axon membrane at the node (*arrow*). ×42,000. (From ref. 62.)

the *Sternarchus* electrocytes when exposed to ferric ion and ferrocyanide after fixation in cacodylate-buffered aldehydes and osmium tetroxide (44). Although the narrowest nodes are usually stained, the very wide (5–50 μm) nodes are not, either in tissue blocks in which nearby narrow nodes are stained or in teased fiber preparations in which adjacent narrow nodes of the same axon are stained. The results are consistent with a biochemical dif-

ferentiation of the axon surface, in this case in a neural system with active and inactive nodes of Ranvier.

Kristol et al. (28) examined the *Sternarchus* electrocytes using freeze-fracture techniques. Their results indicate a differentiation of E-face particle density at active and inactive nodes. A higher particle density was observed at the active nodes in contrast to the larger inactive nodes, whose particle density values were

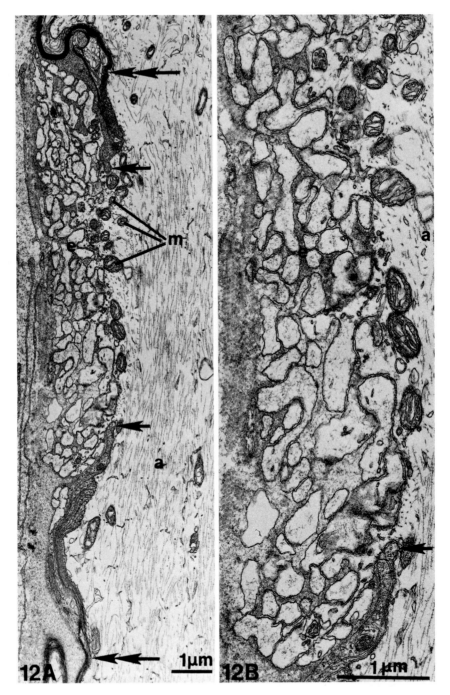

FIG. 12. A: An elaborated enlarged *Sternarchus* electrocyte axon node. The axis of the fiber runs from top to bottom. The paranodal region begins at the double-headed arrows. The axon surface is elaborated to form a layer of polypoid processes (e). The axon (a) contains numerous neurofilaments and mitochondria (m), which are especially common subjacent to the surface elaborations. Thin fibroblast processes surround the network of processes at the node. Bar = 1μm. ×11,400. **B:** Part of the axon surface from A at higher magnification. The irregular axonal processes contain electron-lucent cytoplasm with few organelles. There is no dense undercoating of the axon membranes in this region. Bar = 1 μm. ×25,000. (From ref. 62.)

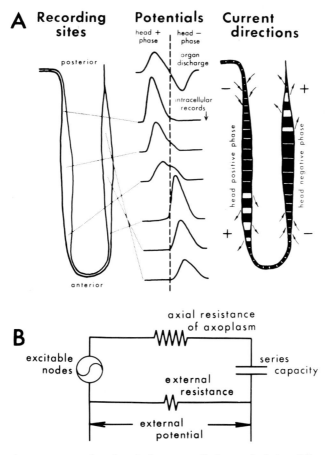

FIG. 13. *Sternarchus* electrocyte axon function during organ discharge. **A:** Intracellular potentials and directions of current flow during electrocyte activity generating the head-positive and head-negative phases of organ discharge. The central column represents organ discharge on the upper line and intracellular recordings on the lower lines at the sites indicated in the diagram of an electrocyte on the left. The responses from the regions of the large nodes are delayed and reduced in magnitude. The directions of current flow during the two phases are indicated on the right diagram. (Modified from Bennett, ref. 5.) **B:** Equivalent circuit of an electrocyte segment to illustrate the effect of a series capacity. (From ref. 62.)

nearly in the same range as those of the internodal axon.

The electrocyte axons in *Sternarchus* provide an example of two principles of axonal design. First, they demonstrate that axons need not be uniform structures with invariant properties along their entire course but, rather, may exhibit a high degree of regional specialization in terms of morphological and physiological properties. Second, they illustrate that axons need not function as simple conduits in which rapidity and reliability of impulse transmission are primary criteria of design. In this case the axons mediate a spatiotemporal transformation of spikes into diphasic external signals.

VARIATIONS IN THE STRUCTURE OF CENTRAL NODES OF RANVIER

Central myelinated fibers, and in particular those in the neuropil, differ from peripheral nerve fibers in that the nodes of Ranvier exhibit a high degree of structural differentiation. The nonmyelinated gap at nodes of Ranvier in the peripheral nervous system usually extends approximately 1 μm along the axis of the fiber (23,46). At central nodes of Ranvier, the

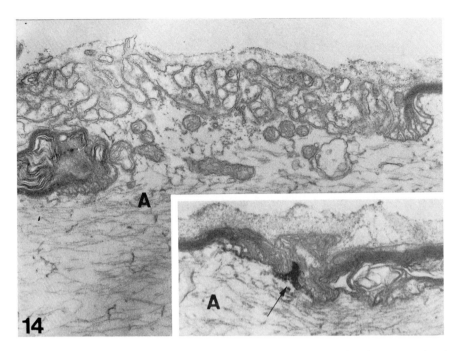

FIG. 14. Two nodes of Ranvier from a single axon dissected from *Sternarchus* electric organ and stained with ferric ion–ferrocyanide after fixation in cacodylate-buffered aldehydes and OsO_4 (44). A 4-μm wide node with elaborated surface shows no staining. A narrow node **(inset)** from the same fiber exhibits a dense aggregation of electron-opaque stain subjacent to the nodal axolemma. (A) Axon. $\times$18,000. **Inset:** $\times$25,000.

nodal gap can extend for less than 1 μm or can be considerably larger. Hess and Young (23) commented, on the basis of light microscopic studies, that a longer stretch of axon could be left bare at central nodes than in peripheral nerve. Ultrastructural studies confirmed the existence of nodes extending 10 μm or more in the central nervous system (20, 36,57). Moreover, as shown in Fig. 1, nodal size can vary along single fibers. Synapses may also arise at central nodes (9,39,54). These may be of either the chemical or electrotonic type. In at least one site, nodes of Ranvier comprise the postsynaptic element of chemical synapses (1), suggesting the possibility that synaptic conductance changes may modify nodal conduction properties.

Ultrastructural studies also suggest a possible differentiation of central axons in terms of the distribution of nodal membrane properties (56,57). At most peripheral and central nodes, a dense cytoplasmic undercoating approximately 200 Å thick (Fig. 11, inset) is present subjacent to the axon surface (16,41). As noted above, at the larger nodes along the electrocyte axons in the gymnotid *Sternarchus,* which are known to be inexcitable (4), the dense undercoating is absent (62). A dense cytoplasmic undercoating is present at most central nodes, where it forms a continuous layer beneath the unmyelinated nodal membrane. However, as shown in Fig. 15, the undercoating is absent or attenuated at some nodes at which synapses arise or at which unmyelinated collaterals emerge. Serial or appropriately oriented single sections of axon collaterals show that the dense undercoating in most cases extends for only several micrometers along the axon membrane into the collateral; more distant membrane is devoid of the dense cytoplasmic layer (56). The extent of the undercoating varies widely. The morphological data thus suggest a mosaic structure for the central axonal membrane, in which differences in the distribution of nodal membrane properties, in addition to the previously considered variations in internode distance and in nodal surface area and geometry, might contribute to differentiation of the surface of central myelinated axons.

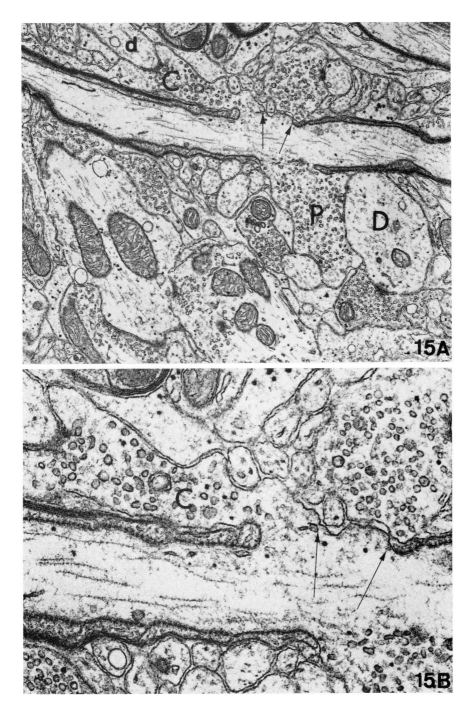

FIG. 15. A: Node of Ranvier from the oculomotor nucleus of the lizard *Anolis carolinensis*. A collateral (C) arises at the node and extends to the upper left of the figure, where it forms synaptic contact with adjacent dendritic profile (d). Process (P) forms a synaptic contact with dendrite (D). **B:** The origin of the collateral is shown at higher magnification. The cytoplasmic dense undercoating extends for only a short distance along the nodal membrane from which the collateral arises (between *arrows*). **A:** ×25,000. **B:** ×58,000.

IMPLICATIONS FOR AXONAL FUNCTION

We now briefly consider the physiological implications of structural differentiations of the axon surface. Figure 16 summarizes the various modes of axonal function. For most normal peripheral myelinated fibers (22,53) and for many normal central myelinated fibers (23,33), the internode length/fiber diameter ratio is close to the value that would maximize conduction velocity at any given diameter (25,47). Similarly, the myelin thickness/fiber diameter ratio is close to the value that would maximize conduction velocity (51). The safety factor is approximately 5–6 (52). For these fibers, maximization of conduction velocity and reliability of transmission appear to be primary design criteria, and the axons may be treated, as a first approximation, as *simple transmission lines.*

At other sites, axons appear to function as *delay lines.* Pumphrey and Young (43) showed, in studies on innervation of the mantle of the cephalopods *Sepia* and *Loligo,* that conduction velocities of the giant fibers innervating the mantle muscles increased with the 0.614 power of diameter. In *Sepia* the conduction distances to the various muscles are approximately equal, and the diameters of the nerves are similar. In *Loligo,* on the other hand, the muscles are located at varying distances from the command nucleus, and the axons exhibit a spectrum of sizes, with muscle closer to the stellate ganglion innervated by thinner axons of slower conduction velocity. Thus the axon conduction velocities are "matched" to conduction distance so as to mediate near-synchrony of contraction of muscles at different distances from the stellate relay ganglion. A similar principle applies to teleost electromotor systems in which electroplaque cells located at different distances from command or relay nuclei must fire synchronously so as to generate the electric organ signal. Bennett (3) suggested three compensatory mechanisms for presynaptic timing in electromotor systems: equalization of path length, compensatory differences in conduction velocity, and localized compensatory delays determined by variations in conduction properties of preterminal axon branches. Compensation for differences in conduction path length in the eel *Electrophorus* involves increased delay at spinal relays and increased delay from activity in the ventral roots to spike initiation in the electrocytes (5). Morphological studies indicate a reduction in the internode distance/fiber diameter ratio along some preterminal fibers (53). Studies on bulbospinal and electromotor axons also show differences in fiber diameter, and in the ratios of myelin thickness and internode length to fiber diameter, which could account for compensatory delays in conduction to rostral and caudal electrocytes (35). Thus the data indicate a second function for some axons, viz., the introduction of appropriate delays in signal travel times within the nervous system.

Finally, there is evidence that axons may function as complex *transformational elements.* Even in relatively uniform axonal trunks, conduction velocity and excitability may vary as a result of prior activity in that axon (Swadlow and Waxman, *this volume*). As discussed by Raymond and Lettvin (*this volume*), in the case of branching axons evidence points toward differential conduction of impulse trains into the secondary arbors, or *filtering.* As early as 1935, Barron and Matthews (2) recognized intermittent conduction in the recurrent branches of dorsal column fibers and suggested that this could provide "a mechanism of nerv-

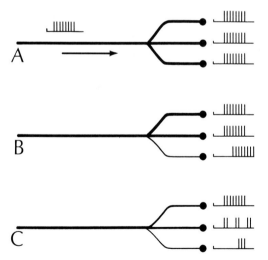

FIG. 16. Modes of axonal function. **A:** Simple transmission line model. **B:** Delay line (phase-shifting) model. **C:** Intermittent conduction (transformational element) model.

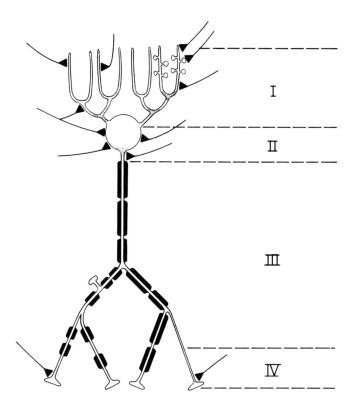

FIG. 17. Multiplex neuron model. Impulse initiation sites in the dendrites and cell body are indicated by shading. Transformation of neural information occurs sequentially, first in the dendritic zone (phase I), then by initiation of a series of impulses at the axon initial segment (phase II) and by transformations within the axonal tree (phase III), and finally by modulation of activity at axonal terminals by presynaptic inhibition (phase IV).

ous integration . . . which does not involve a synapse." Chung et al. (13) confirmed and extended these findings, and presented evidence that single fibers in the visual system could signal several stimulus parameters, with temporal impulse patterns being transformed into spatial patterns of activity within the axonal tree. Other examples of filtering at axonal branch points include those of Bittner (8), Parnas (40), and Grossman et al (21), who showed that differential channeling of spike trains may take place at points of axonal branching. It thus appears that the differentiation of axonal structure at branch points and in the preterminal region may be reflected by an equally complex set of functional differentiations, so that the axon may, in some cases, function as both a spatial and a temporal filter of neural information.

The integrative properties of axons have important implications for neuronal function (55). Interposed between perikaryon and terminal, the axon occupies a crucial site in the path traversed by neural information. Thus we may view neural messages as being sequentially transformed (Fig. 17), first in the dendrites (I) and at the perikaryon and initial segment trigger zone (II), then in the axon (III), and finally in the terminals (IV). The single neuron, according to this model, exhibits a complex logical infrastructure. Even minor changes in axonal function may alter this logical infrastructure and either adaptively or pathologically change the functional properties of the entire nerve cell.

ACKNOWLEDGMENTS

Work in the author's laboratory has been supported by grants NS-12307, RR-05479, GM-1674, and Research Career Development Award K04-NS-00010 from the National Institutes of Health, and by grant RG-1133A1 from the National Multiple Sclerosis Society.

REFERENCES

1. Andersen, P. (1975): Organization of hippocampal neurons and their interconnections. In: *The Hippocampus, Vol. I: Structure and Development,* edited by R. L. Isaacson and K. H. Pribram, pp. 155–175. Plenum Press, New York.

2. Barron, D. H., and Matthews, B. H. C. (1935): Intermittent conduction in the spinal cord. *J. Physiol. (Lond),* 85:73–103.

3. Bennett, M. V. L. (1968): Neural control of electric organs. In: *The Central Nervous System and Fish Behavior,* edited by D. Ingle, pp. 147–169. University of Chicago Press, Chicago.

4. Bennett, M. V. L. (1970): Comparative physiology: Electric organs. *Annu. Rev. Physiol.,* 32:471–528.

5. Bennett, M. V. L. (1971): Electric organs. In: *Fish Physiology,* Vol. 5, edited by W. S. Hoar and D. J. Randall, pp. 347–491. Academic Press, New York.

6. Bishop, G. H., Clare, M. H., and Landau, W. M. (1971): The relation of axon sheath thickness to fiber size in the central nervous system of vertebrates. *Int. J. Neurosci.,* 2:69–78.

7. Bishop, G. H., and Smith, J. M. (1964): The sizes of nerve fibers supplying cerebral cortex. *Exp. Neurol.,* 9:483–501.

8. Bittner, G. D. (1968): Differentiation of nerve terminals in the crayfish opener muscle and its functional significance. *J. Gen. Physiol.,* 51:731–758.

9. Bodian, D., and Taylor, N. (1963): Synapse arising at a node of Ranvier, and a note on fixation of the central nervous system. *Science,* 139:330–332.

10. Boyd, I. A., and Davey, M. R. (1968): *Composition of Peripheral Nerves.* Livingstone, Edinburgh.

11. Brill, M. H., Waxman, S. G., Moore, J. W., and Joyner, R. W. (1977): Conduction velocity in myelinated fibers: Computed dependence on internode distance. *J. Neurol. Neurosurg. Psychiatry,* 40:769–774.

12. Chang, H-T. (1952): Cortical and spinal neurons: Cortical neurons with particular reference to the apical dendrites. *Cold Spring Harbor Symp. Quant. Biol.,* 18:189–202.

13. Chung, S. H., Raymond, S. A., and Lettvin, J. Y. (1970): Multiple meaning in single visual units. *Brain Behav. Evol.,* 3:72–101.

14. Coppin, C. M. L., and Jack, J. J. B. (1972): Internodal length and conduction velocity of cat muscle afferent nerve fibres. *J. Physiol. (Lond),* 222:91P–93P.

15. Duncan, D. (1934): A relation between axon diameter and myelination as determined by measurement of myelinated spinal root fibers. *J. Comp. Neurol.,* 60:437–471.

16. Elfvin, L-G. (1961): The ultrastructure of the nodes of Ranvier in cat sympathetic nerve fibers. *J. Ultrastruct. Res.,* 5:374–387.

17. Friede, R. L., and Samorajski, T. (1967): Relation between the number of myelin lamellae and axon circumference in fibers of vagus and sciatic nerves of mice. *J. Comp. Neurol.,* 130:223–232.

18. Gasser, H. S. (1950): Unmedullated fibers originating in dorsal root ganglia. *J. Gen. Physiol.,* 33:651–690.

19. Gledhill, R. F., Harrison, B. M., and McDonald, W. I. (1973): Pattern of remyelination in the CNS. *Nature (Lond),* 244:443–444.

20. Gray, E. G. (1970): The fine structure of nerve. *Comp. Biochem. Physiol.,* 36:419–488.

21. Grossman, Y., Spira, M. E., and Parnas, I. (1973): Differential flow of information into branches of a single axon. *Brain Res.,* 64:379–386.

22. Gutrecht, J. A., and Dyck, P. J. (1970): Quantitative teased-fiber and histologic studies of human sural nerve during postnatal development. *J. Comp. Neurol.,* 138:117–130.

23. Hess, A., and Young, J. Z. (1952): The nodes of Ranvier. *Proc. R. Soc. B,* 140:301–319.

24. Hursh, J. B. (1939): Conduction velocity and diameter of nerve fibers. *Am. J. Physiol.,* 127:131–139.

25. Huxley, A. F., and Stämpfli, R. (1949): Evidence for saltatory conduction in peripheral myelinated nerve fibres. *J. Physiol. (Lond),* 108:315–339.

26. Karnovsky, M. J. (1965): A formaldehyde-glutaraldehyde fixative on high osmolality for use in electron microscopy. *J. Cell Biol.,* 27:137a–138a.

27. Khodorov, B. I., and Timin, E. N. (1975): Nerve impulse propagation along non-uniform fibers. *Prog. Biophys.,* 30:145–184.

28. Kristol, C., Akert, K., Sandri, C., Wyss, U., Bennett, M. V. L., and Moor, H. (1977): The Ranvier nodes in the neurogenic electric organ of the knife fish Sternarchus: A freeze-etching study on the distribution of membrane-associated particles. *Brain Res.,* 125:197–212.

29. Landon, D. N., and Langley, O. K. (1971): The local chemical environment of nodes of Ranvier: A study of cation binding. *J. Anat.,* 108:419–432.

30. Lindsey, B. G. (1975): Fine structure and distribution of axon terminals from the cochlear nucleus on neurons in the medial superior olivary nucleus of the cat. *J. Comp. Neurol.,* 160:81–104.

31. McDonald, W. I. (1963): The effects of experimental demyelination on conduction in peripheral nerve: a histological and electrophysiological study. II. Electrophysiological observations. *Brain,* 86:501–524.

32. McDonald, W. I. (1974): Pathophysiology in multiple sclerosis. *Brain,* 97:179–196.

33. McDonald, W. I., and Ohlrich, G. D. (1971): Quantitative anatomical measurements on single isolated fibres from the cat spinal cord. *J. Anat.,* 110:191–202.

34. McDonald, W. I., and Sears, T. A. (1970): The effects of experimental demyelination on conduction in the central nervous system. *Brain,* 93:583–598.

35. Meszler, R. M., Pappas, G. D., and Bennett, M. V. L. (1974): Morphology of the electromotor system in the spinal cord of the electric eel, Electrophorus electricus. *J. Neurocytol.,* 3:251–261.

36. Metuzals, J. (1965): Ultrastructure of the nodes of Ranvier and their surrounding structures in the central nervous system. *Z. Zellforsch.,* 65:719–759.

37. Paintal, A. S. (1967): A comparison of the nerve impulses of mammalian nonmedullated nerve fibres with those of the smallest diameter medullated fibres. *J. Physiol. (Lond),* 193:523–533.

38. Palay, S. L., Sotelo, C., Peters, A., and Orkand, P. M. (1968): The axon hillock and the initial segment. *J. Cell Biol.,* 38:193–201.

39. Pappas, G. D., and Waxman, S. G. (1972): Synaptic fine structure: morphological correlates of chemical and electrotonic transmission. In: *The Structure and Function of Synapses,* edited by G. D. Pappas and D. P. Purpura, pp. 1–44. Raven Press, New York.

40. Parnas, I. (1971): Differential block at high frequency of branches of a single axon innervating two muscles. *J. Neurophysiol.,* 35: 903–914.

41. Peters, A. (1966): The node of Ranvier in the central nervous system. *Q. J. Exp. Physiol.,* 51:229–236.

42. Peters, A., Proskauer, C. C., and Kaiserman-Abramof, I. R. (1968): The small pyramidal neuron of the rat cerebral cortex: The axon hillock and initial segment. *J. Cell Biol.,* 39: 604–619.

43. Pumphrey, R. J., and Young, J. Z. (1938): The rates of conduction of nerve fibres of various diameters in cephalopods. *J. Exp. Biol.,* 15:453–466.

44. Quick, D. C., and Waxman, S. G. (1977): Specific staining of the axon membrane at nodes of Ranvier with ferric ion and ferrocyanide. *J. Neurol. Sci.,* 31:1–11.

45. Ritchie, J. M., and Rogart, R. B. (1977): The density of sodium channels in mammalian myelinated nerve fibers and the nature of the axonal membrane under the myelin sheath. *Proc. Natl. Acad. Sci. USA,* 74:211–215.

46. Robertson, J. D. (1960): The molecular structure and contact relationships of cell membranes. *Prog. Biophys.,* 10:343–418.

47. Rushton, W. A. H. (1951): A theory of the effects of fibre size in medullated nerve. *J. Physiol. (Lond),* 115:101–122.

48. Sanders, F. K. (1948): The thickness of the myelin sheaths of normal and regenerating peripheral nerve fibres. *Proc. R. Soc. B,* 135: 323–357.

49. Sanders, F. K., and Whitteridge, D. (1946): Conduction velocity and myelin thickness in regenerating nerve fibres. *J. Physiol. (Lond),* 105:152–174.

50. Schnepp, P., and Schnepp, G. (1971): Faseranalytische Untersuchungen an peripheren Nerven bei Tieren verschiedener Grösse. II. Verhaltnis Axon durchmesser/Gesamtdurchmesser und Internodallänge. *Z. Zellforsch.,* 119:99–114.

51. Smith, R. S., and Koles, Z. J. (1970): Myelinated nerve fibers—computed effect of myelin thickness on conduction velocity. *Am. J. Physiol.,* 219:1256–1258.

52. Tasaki, I. (1959): Conduction of the nerve impulse. In: *Handbook of Physiology, Section I, Vol. I: Neurophysiology,* edited by J. Field, pp. 75–121. American Physiological Society, Washington, D.C.

53. Thomas, P. D., and Young, J. Z. (1949): Internode lengths in the nerves of fishes. *J. Anat.,* 83:336–350.

54. Waxman, S. G. (1970): Closely spaced nodes of Ranvier in the teleost brain. *Nature (Lond),* 227:283–284.

55. Waxman, S. G. (1972): Regional differentiation of the axon: A review with special reference to the concept of the multiplex neuron. *Brain Res.,* 47:269–288.

56. Waxman, S. G. (1974): Ultrastructural differentiation of the axon membrane at synaptic and non-synaptic central nodes of Ranvier. *Brain Res.,* 65:338–342.

57. Waxman, S. G. (1975): Integrative properties and design principles of axons. *Int. Rev. Neurobiol.,* 18:1–40.

58. Waxman, S. G. (1975): Electron-microscopic observations on preterminal fibers in the oculomotor nucleus of the cat. *J. Neurol. Sci.,* 26:395–400.

59. Waxman, S. G., and Bennett, M. V. L. (1970): An analysis of the pattern of myelination of some preterminal fibers in the teleost central nervous system. *J. Cell Biol.,* 47:222a.

60. Waxman, S. G., and Bennett, M. V. L. (1972): Relative conduction velocities of small myelinated and non-myelinated fibres in the central nervous system. *Nature [New Biol.],* 238:217–219.

61. Waxman, S. G., and Melker, R. J. (1971): Closely spaced nodes of Ranvier in the mammalian brain. *Brain Res.,* 32:445–448.

62. Waxman, S. G., Pappas, G. D., and Bennett, M. V. L. (1972): Morphological correlates of functional differentiation of nodes of Ranvier along single fibers in the neurogenic electric

organ of the knife fish Sternarchus. *J. Cell Biol.*, 53:210–224.

63. Waxman, S. G., and Quick, D. C. (1977): Cytochemical differentiation of the axon membrane in A- and C-fibers. *J. Neurol. Neurosurg. Psychiatry*, 40:379–386.

64. Waxman, S. G., and Quick, D. C. (1977): Intra-axonal ferric ion-ferrocyanide staining of nodes of Ranvier and initial segments in central myelinated fibers. *Brain Res. (in press)*.

65. Waxman, S. G., and Swadlow, H. A. (1976): Ultrastructure of visual callosal axons in the rabbit. *Exp. Neurol.*, 53:115–128.

Physiology and Pathobiology of Axons, edited by
S. G. Waxman. Raven Press, New York © 1978.

Activity-Dependent Variations in the Conduction Properties of Central Axons

Harvey A. Swadlow and Stephen G. Waxman

*Department of Neurology, Harvard Medical School, Beth Israel Hospital, Boston, Massachusetts
02215; Harvard–MIT Program in Health Sciences and Technology, Massachusetts Institute of
Technology, Cambridge, Massachusetts 02139*

This chapter deals with the aftereffects of impulse activity in central axons. Although it is generally accepted that conduction velocity and excitability are somewhat decreased during the relative refractory period, the conduction properties of axons are otherwise considered to be relatively invariant in the temporal domain. There have, however, been a number of demonstrations of increased conduction velocity and excitability following the relative refractory period of the axon. In the central nervous system, activity-dependent variations in conduction velocity and excitability have been studied in parallel fibers of cat cerebellum (9) and in visual callosal axons of the rabbit (22,24,25,30). Parallel fibers are nonmyelinated and demonstrate a "supernormal" period of increased conduction velocity and excitability which lasts more than 100 msec following prior activation. In the peripheral nervous system, variations in conduction properties have been shown to follow activation of nonmyelinated reptilian olfactory nerve axons (5) and axons in the sciatic nerve of the frog (7,15,16). Increases in excitability have also been shown to follow activation of axons in the human median (11) and ulnar (3) nerve. In this chapter we review our work on the conduction properties of visual callosal axons of the rabbit. In particular, we show that impulse activity is followed by a sequence of events: relative refractory period → supernormal period → subnormal period. Conduction velocity and excitability are decreased during the relative refractory period. An increase in conduction velocity and excitability

(*supernormal period*) occurs after the relative refractory period following a single impulse in both myelinated and nonmyelinated visual callosal axons. A subsequent decrease in conduction velocity and excitability lasting from several hundred milliseconds to over a minute (*subnormal period*) results from a greater number of prior impulses. Both increases and decreases in conduction velocity thereby occur, depending on the history of impulse activity along the axon.

ANATOMY OF THE VISUAL CALLOSAL SYSTEM

Before describing the conduction properties of visual callosal axons, we briefly present some anatomical considerations. The cell bodies of visual callosal axons are located in the lateral portion of visual area I and in visual area II of the cerebral cortex (23). Most cells of origin of callosal axons are pyramidal cells, which are located primarily in cortical layer II–III (26). The visual component of the corpus callosum (splenium) contains myelinated and nonmyelinated axons (31). Approximately 45% of callosal axons are nonmyelinated and have diameters of 0.08–0.60 μm (mean 0.20 μm). Nonmyelinated axons usually occur in clusters of at least three or four axons (Figs. 1 and 2). In some cases as many as 10–20 nonmyelinated axons are clustered together with no intervening glial process. Nonmyelinated axons are separated from other axons by an extracellular space at least 100 Å wide. Myelinated axons comprise approxi-

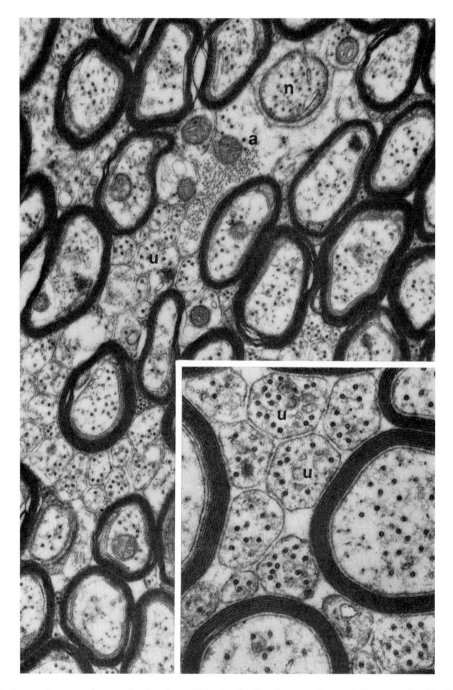

FIG. 1. Survey electron micrographs showing rabbit visual callosal axons. Some of the axons in this field are cut slightly obliquely. Nonmyelinated axons are grouped in clusters (u) between myelinated axons. (n) A cross section through a myelinated axon at a node of Ranvier. There is an electron-dense cytoplasmic undercoating subjacent to the axon membrane at the node. An astrocytic process (a) partially surrounds the nodal axons. **Inset:** A cluster of nonmyelinated axons (u) at higher magnification. An extracellular space at least 200 A wide separates adjacent nonmyelinated axons. ×33,000. **Inset:** ×52,000.

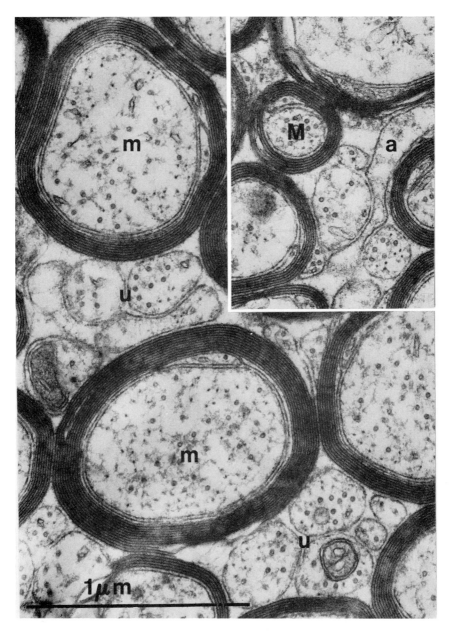

FIG. 2. Electron micrograph showing rabbit visual callosal axons in transverse section at higher magnification. Myelinated (m) and nonmyelinated (u) axons are present. The largest nonmyelinated fibers have a diameter of 0.6 μm. Myelinated fibers as small as 0.3 μm are present. **Inset:** A myelinated fiber with a diameter of 0.4 μm. (a) Astrocytic process. Bar = 1 μm. $\times$60,000.

mately 55% of the axons in the splenium and have diameters of 0.3 μm to approximately 2 μm (mean 0.74 μm). The myelin sheath has a spiral configuration with a periodicity of approximately 120 Å. The nonmyelinated gap at the node usually extends 0.75–1.25 μm and exhibits a typical electron-dense undercoating within the cytoplasm subjacent to the axon membrane (Fig. 3). Branching was not observed along the midline of callosal axons, nor

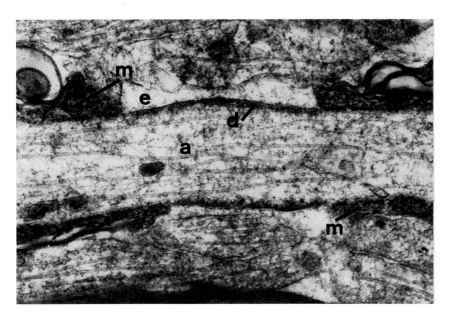

FIG. 3. Electron micrograph showing a longitudinal section through a node of Ranvier in the splenium of the rabbit corpus callosum. The nonmyelinated gap extends approximately 1.1 μm along the axis of the fiber. Note the dense cytoplasmic undercoating (d) subjacent to the axon membrane at the node. As at other central nodes, there is an extensive perinodal extracellular space (e). $\times$50,000. (a) Axon. (m) Terminating myelin.

has it been inferred from physiological studies using appropriate collision techniques (21).

The ultrastructural data on the visual callosal system provide a basis for choosing a criterion value for the identification of myelinated and nonmyelinated axons on the basis of measurements of conduction velocity. The largest nonmyelinated axons in peripheral nerve (1.1 μm) have a conduction velocity of 2.3 meters/sec (10). Since conduction velocity is proportional to diameter$^{0.5}$ (20), the expected conduction velocity for a peripheral nonmyelinated axon with a diameter equal to the largest nonmyelinated axon in the rabbit splenium (0.6 μm) would be 1.7 meters/sec. In view of the lack of definitive data on the relationship between diameter and conduction velocity for central fibers, we added a large margin for error and chose 3.4 meters/sec as a physiological criterion for the identification of myelinated fibers. A peripheral myelinated axon with a diameter equal to that of the smallest myelinated axon from the rabbit splenium would have a conduction velocity of 1.35–1.8 meters/sec, based on various estimates (6,14,28). We again added a large margin of error and chose 0.8 meter/sec as

the physiological criterion for the identification of nonmyelinated axons.

CONDUCTION PROPERTIES OF VISUAL CALLOSAL AXONS

We studied impulse conduction along visual callosal axons of the *unanesthetized, unparalyzed rabbit*. Our strategy was to study the conduction velocity and excitability of callosal axons by measuring latency and threshold to antidromic activation via stimulating electrodes located at one or several sites along the course of the callosal axon. Neurons which are antidromically activated by stimulation of the callosal axon are identified by the tests for collision of impulses and postcollision recovery (4,21). Examination of refractory periods and spike wave forms (4,18,19) to double volley stimulation provide further evidence of antidromic activation. When a unit is demonstrated to be antidromically activated by stimulation of the callosal axons, latency to a single pulse is determined at various intervals following either a single conditioning pulse or a train of conditioning pulses. Conditioning and test pulses in most cases are delivered via the same stimu-

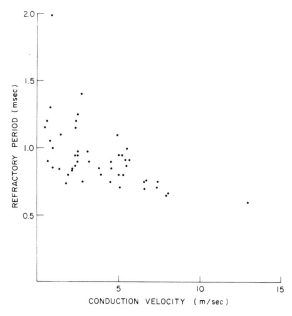

FIG. 4. Refractory periods and conduction velocities of rabbit visual callosal axons that were activated by double volley stimulation at decreasing intervolley intervals. Each volley was delivered at 2 times the control threshold.

lating electrode. Since variations in both threshold and latency to a test volley follow conditioning volleys, the stimulus threshold is determined at each conditioning stimulus–test stimulus interval, and the intensity of the test stimulus is adjusted to 1.2 times threshold value at that particular conditioning stimulus–test stimulus interval.

The estimated conduction velocity of 75 axons studied in a recent series (25) ranged from 0.3 to 12.9 meters/sec (median 2.8 meters/sec). These values are quite similar to those which would be expected on the basis of the diameter spectrum of visual callosal axons (31), assuming that the relationship between conduction velocity and axon diameter is similar to that for peripheral nerve (6,14,28). The *refractory period* was determined for most units and is shown in Fig. 4. Refractory periods range from 0.6 to 2.0 msec, with faster conducting axons generally having shorter refractory periods than slower axons.

Supernormal Phase

Following the relative refractory period, the great majority of visual callosal axons show a period of increased conduction velocity and excitability. This is demonstrated by measuring the latency and threshold to a test stimulus presented at various intervals following a conditioning stimulus. At conditioning stimulus–test stimulus intervals of less than 2 msec, the latency to the test stimulus is usually greater than control values. This is probably due to the relative refractory period of the axons. At intervals of 2–4 msec, antidromic latency is reduced and reaches a minimum latency at conditioning stimulus–test stimulus intervals of 3–17 msec. Thereafter, latency slowly increases and reattains control values at intervals of 18–169 msec. As shown below, the reduction in antidromic latency is due to an increase in axonal conduction velocity.

Figure 5A_1–C_1 shows the antidromic latency to a test stimulus as a function of conditioning stimulus–test stimulus interval for three units with control axon conduction velocities of 0.3, 1.3, and 4.1 meters/sec, respectively. In each case the test stimulus is presented at 1.2 times threshold at each conditioning stimulus–test stimulus interval, whereas the conditioning stimulus is presented at 1.5 times threshold. Closed circles represent the latency at each conditioning stimulus–test stimulus interval. Figure 5A₁ shows the slowest callosal axon that we studied, with a control antidromic latency of 37.5 msec (conduction velocity = 0.3 meter/sec). Latency decreased to approximately 34.7 msec at conditioning stimulus–test stimulus intervals of 10 and 17 msec. Latency slowly increased to reattain the control value at an interval of approximately 170 msec. Figure 5B₁ and C₁ shows decreases in latency for two faster conducting units. Although the proportional magnitude of the maximal decrease in latency was similar for the three units (7.5–11% of control values), the duration of the decrease in latency was greater for the slower conducting axons. In Fig. 5A₂–C₂, variations in threshold are plotted

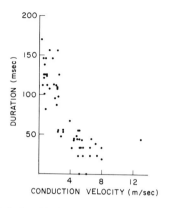

FIG. 6. Relationship between conduction velocity and the duration of the decrease in latency for callosal axons. Each point represents a single unit.

for the same three units presented in Figs. 5A₁–C₁, respectively. The variations in threshold for these and for other cells follow roughly the same time course, or a slightly longer time course than the variations in latency.

Figure 6 presents the relationship between the duration of the increase in conduction velocity (manifested by a decrease in latency) and the control conduction velocity of the axon. It is clear that there is an approximate inverse relationship between the control conduction velocity and the duration of the increase in conduction velocity. The sample contains many myelinated axons (conduction velocities > 3.4 meters/sec) and some nonmyelinated axons (conduction velocities < 0.8 meters/sec). The duration of the increase in conduction velocity, however, appears to vary continuously with conduction velocity, and there is no discrete change that might indicate a qualitative difference between myelinated and nonmyelinated axons. As shown in Fig. 4, the refractory period also appears to vary continuously with the conduction velocity of the axon. These findings on central axons are similar to those of Paintal (17; see also Paintal, *this volume*), who observed that although rise time, fall time, and spike duration of peripheral myelinated and nonmyelinated axons vary systematically with conduction velocity there is no obvious qualitative difference between the two types of fiber.

Figure 7 presents the relationship between the conduction velocity of the axon and the absolute and proportional magnitude of the

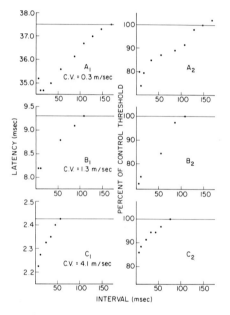

FIG. 5. A₁–C₁: The latency to antidromic activation to a test stimulus as a function of conditioning stimulus–test stimulus interval for three rabbit visual callosal neurons with axon conduction velocities of 0.3, 1.3, and 4.1 meters/sec. Points show the antidromic latency at each conditioning stimulus–test stimulus interval. Pairs of stimuli were delivered at a rate of 1/3.3 sec. Each conditioning stimulus is presented at 1.5 times threshold intensity, and the test stimulus is presented at 1.2 times the threshold at each conditioning stimulus–test stimulus interval. A₂–C₂: Variations in threshold to antidromic test volley following a single antidromic conditioning volley for the same three units presented in Fig. 5 A₁–C₁. The changes in threshold follow a similar time course to the changes in latency.

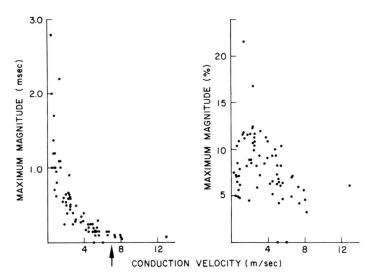

FIG. 7. Relationship between conduction velocity and magnitude of the decrease in latency. **Left**: The maximum absolute magnitude of the decrease in latency. **Right**: The relative magnitude (percent decrease) of the decrease in latency.

decrease in latency. The proportional magnitude of the maximal latency decreases ranged from 3% to 22% of control latency and was not clearly related to the conduction velocity of the axon. As would be expected, the absolute magnitude is much less for fast-conducting than for more slowly conducting axons. It is interesting that neurons with an axon conduction velocity of greater than 7.0 meters/sec had a maximum decrease in latency of 0.1 msec or less (arrow), a figure often cited as a criterion for the maximum latency variability, or "jitter," that is acceptable for an antidromically activated unit. All but four units with conduction velocities of 6.0 msec or less had a latency decrease of 0.1 msec or more. Had collision and other tests for the identification of antidromically activated units not been employed, many of these units would probably have been inappropriately classified as synaptically activated. Neither the magnitude nor the duration of the decrease in latency was consistently augmented by an increase in the number of conditioning volleys. An increase in the number of conditioning volleys resulted in either no change in the magnitude or a decrease in the magnitude of the decrease in latency, whereas the effect on the duration of the decrease in latency was variable.

Control experiments indicate that the reduction in latency resulted from the prior impulse in the axon under study, rather than from some nonspecific effect of the prior electrical stimulation or from activity in neighboring axons. One such experiment is shown in Fig. 8. In Fig. 8A an antidromic spike is elicited 4.9 msec after electrical stimulation of the corpus callosum near the midline (arrow).

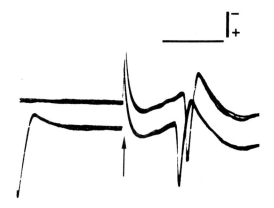

FIG. 8. Oscilloscope tracing demonstrating decreased antidromic latency after a spontaneous spike. **Upper trace**: Antidromic activation of a callosal neuron to a test stimulus (*arrow*) presented at 1.2 times threshold intensity. **Lower trace**: The test stimulus is preceded by a spontaneous spike which triggers the oscilloscope. Note the reduction in latency to the test stimulus. Calibration bar = 5 msec.

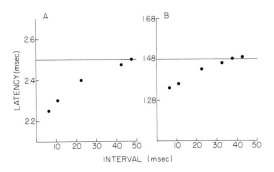

FIG. 9. Demonstration that the magnitude of the decrease in latency is proportional to conduction path length, and that changes in conduction velocity occur along the axonal trunk *within* the corpus callosum. **A:** Both conditioning and test stimuli are delivered through a stimulating electrode located approximately 2 mm to the right of midline. **B:** Both stimuli are delivered via a stimulating electrode located approximately 2 mm to the left of the midline. Points represent the latency to the test stimuli. The conditioning stimulus was delivered at 1.5 times threshold, and the test stimulus was delivered at 1.2 times threshold at each conditioning stimulus–test stimulus interval. The horizontal line represents antidromic control latency at 1.2 times threshold.

In Fig. 8B the antidromic volley is preceded by a spontaneous spike, which triggers the oscilloscope. Antidromic latency was reduced to approximately 4.4 msec. Additional control experiments have shown that: (a) although the latency does not decrease in response to a test stimulus that follows a subthreshold conditioning stimulus, decreases in latency of a similar magnitude and time course occur to a test stimulus that follows a conditioning stimulus presented at either 1.1 or 1.5 times threshold; and (b) when the intensity of a conditioning stimulus is just at threshold, the latency decreases in response to the test stimulus only when the initial conditioning stimulus results in a spike (25).

Control experiments also show that the activity-dependent variations in conduction velocity occur along the main axonal trunk. In these experiments two pairs of stimulating electrodes activate the axon at different distances from the cell body. In Fig. 9A, for example, latency to antidromic activation to a test stimulus is presented as a function of conditioning stimulus–test stimulus interval for a unit in which stimulation was presented via electrodes 2 mm to the right of the midline

(contralateral to the recording microelectrode). In Fig. 9B the same neuron is activated by stimulation 2 mm to the left of the midline. Although the duration of the latency decreases are approximately equal, the magnitude of the latency decreases following stimulation at the two sites are approximately proportional to the control latency at each stimulation site. The demonstration of proportional changes in latency following stimulation on both sides of the corpus callosum indicates that the latency decrease occurs along the main axonal trunk and is not dependent on changes which occur only in the nonmyelinated terminals and/or nonmyelinated segments near the cell body.

We also observed activity-dependent variations in conduction velocity and excitability in each of a small number of somatosensory callosal axons and in most of the corticotectal axons studied. For the somatosensory callosal axons, the variations in conduction properties were very similar to those found in visual callosal axons. Four of six corticotectal axons showed a decrease in antidromic latency, whereas all six showed a decrease in threshold following the relative refractory period. For the corticotectal axons, the magnitude and duration of the supernormal phase were less than for callosal axons.

Subnormal Phase

After a single antidromic conditioning volley, a slight increase in latency to a test stimulus sometimes follows the initial decrease in latency. This increase in latency is augmented in magnitude and duration by an increase in the number of conditioning pulses. Even those axons that exhibited no increase in latency to a test stimulus following a single conditioning volley showed a clear increase in latency after a conditioning stimulus consisting of a train of pulses (24,25). Thus after a train of prior impulses, a subnormal period of decreased conduction velocity (as manifested by an increase in latency) follows the supernormal period. This is illustrated in Fig. 10, which shows the response to a test stimulus of a unit that received a conditioning stimulus consisting of 1, 20, or 54 pulses (333 pulses/sec). In this, as in all other similarly tested axons, the magnitude of the increase in latency was related to the

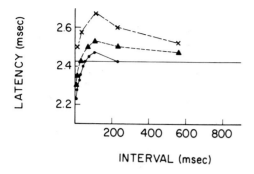

FIG. 10. Time course of the increase in latency for one unit when the conditioning stimulus consisted of a single pulse (● — ●), 20 pulses (△ — △), or 54 pulses (x — — x) delivered at 330 pulses/sec.

number of conditioning pulses. For some units the duration of the increase in latency that followed a conditioning stimulus consisting of 20 pulses was as long as 1.5 sec. Two lines of evidence (25) indicate that the increases in latency are a result of previous spike activity along the axon under study: (a) Increases in latency do not occur following a conditioning train that is just subthreshold; and (b) increases in latency occur during and following periods of heightened "spontaneous" or orthodromically driven activity.

Most units which show an increase in latency following a train of conditioning pulses also show a concomitant increase in threshold. Changes in threshold, however, do not parallel increases in latency as closely as they do decreases in latency, and some units show clear latency increases with no concomitant increases in threshold.

Subnormality is demonstrable for more than a minute following tetanic stimulation of some axons. Figure 11 illustrates an experiment in which we attempted to determine the temporal limitations of the increase in latency following tetanic stimulation. A unit with a control conduction velocity of 5.3 meters/sec is shown. Closed circles to the left of the solid bar represent antidromic latency during a period in which baseline latency was determined. Antidromic volleys were presented at 1 pulse/3.3 sec. The width of the solid bar represents the duration of a period of tetanic stimulation (33 pulses/sec). Latency was not measured during this period of stimulation. Closed circles to the right of the bar represent antidromic latency at various intervals following the tetanic stimulation. During this period a single test pulse was presented every 3.3 sec. All stimuli in the experiment were presented at 1.5 times the control threshold. Following a 40-sec train (Fig. 11a), the latency increased from just over 2.4 msec to approximately 2.65 msec, and returned to baseline latency within approximately 60 sec. The latency of this unit increased to over 2.7 msec following a 60-sec train and did not return to control levels for more than 90 sec (Fig. 11b).

CONCLUSIONS AND IMPLICATIONS

The studies summarized above show that the conduction properties of myelinated and

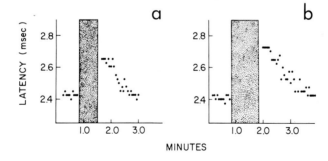

FIG. 11. Demonstration of a long-lasting increase in antidromic latency for a single unit with a conduction velocity of 5.3 meters/sec. Points to the left of the bar represent a period during which baseline latency was obtained. Antidromic volleys were presented at 1 pulse/3.3 sec. The width of the bar represents the duration of a period of tetanic stimulation (33 pulses/sec). Latency was not measured during this period of tetanic stimulation. Points to the right of the bar represent antidromic latency at various intervals following the tetanic stimulation. During this period a single test pulse was presented every 3.3 sec. All stimuli were presented at 1.5 times the control threshold. **a:** 40-sec conditioning train. **b:** 60-sec conditioning train.

nonmyelinated callosal axons are not invariant; on the contrary, they vary dynamically with the history of impulse conduction along the axon. Increases and decreases in conduction velocity and excitability occur, depending on the number and temporal distribution of prior impulses and the conduction velocity of the axon. At those sites in the central nervous system where such aftereffects of impulse activity do occur, they may be significant with respect to the temporal and spatial coding of neural information. Activity-dependent variations in threshold could modulate the spatial distribution of impulses along the terminal arbors that are invaded via branch points of low safety factor. This idea was explored by Chung et al. (8) and is more fully discussed in the chapter by Raymond and Lettvin in this volume. Transmitter dynamics might also be expected to vary with variations in terminal excitability (13,27). Moreover, since axons taper in the preterminal region, the magnitudes and durations of the aftereffects (Figs. 6 and 7) might be expected to be greater in the preterminal region than along the main axonal trunk.

Activity-dependent variations in conduction velocity may also influence the temporal summation of neural information. For some callosal axons we observed a range of activity-dependent increases and decreases in antidromic latency of as much as 3 msec. Although some postsynaptic neurons may be relatively insensitive to the fine temporal patterning of incoming impulses, other neurons are sensitive to small differences in the timing of presynaptic spikes. Some neurons in the Mauthner spinal motor system, for example, are sensitive to differences as small as 150 μsec in the timing of the incoming impulses (32). In the accessory superior olivary nucleus of the cat, some neurons are sensitive to interaural intervals of less than 100 μsec (12). For axons that are part of a system in which preservation of fine temporal relationships are important, the interval between spike initiation near the cell body and the time of arrival of the impulse at the axon terminal might be expected to be nearly constant. Conduction of impulses along most visual callosal axons could meet this requirement only if no prior impulse had occurred for at least several hundred milliseconds. It

should be noted in this regard that the great majority of visual callosal neurons in the rabbit exhibit spontaneous firing rates of less than 1 spike/sec (21).

In addition to the above considerations, our observations on variations in conduction velocity have important methodological significance with respect to the identification of antidromically and synaptically activated neurons. Since conduction velocity varies with the history of impulse activity along the axon, a constant latency does not constitute a necessary condition for the identification of antidromically activated neurons. Conversely, a variable latency does not constitute a sufficient condition for the identification of synaptically activated neurons. The careful use of impulse collision tests, examination of refractory periods and waveform changes following the second of two closely spaced volleys, and systematic exploration of latency and threshold variability provide, in our view, the most appropriate criteria for differentiating antidromic from synaptic activation.

Activity-dependent variations in conduction properties are not limited to the visual callosal system of the rabbit. Similar aftereffects have been documented in axons in other regions of the central nervous system (somatosensory callosal and corticotectal axons of the rabbit, parallel fibers of the cat) and peripheral nervous system (sciatic nerve of frog, radial and ulnar nerve of humans). We recently examined the conduction properties of callosal axons of the macaque monkey; for the (41) axons thus far studied, we found activity-dependent variations in conduction velocity and excitability which are very similar in both time course and proportional magnitude to those found in callosal axons of the rabbit. Furthermore, the morphology of visual callosal axons (31) is very similar to that of axons in many regions of the central nervous system. A sequential set of events (action potential → relative refractory period → supernormal period → subnormal period) may therefore represent a rather general feature of axonal physiology. With respect to these changes, the question arises as to why the supernormal and subnormal phases of impulse conduction along central axons have not been more widely observed. It should be emphasized in this regard that the corpus callosum is a fine-fibered system, with more than 85% of visual callosal axons of the rabbit having conduction velocities of less than 6 meters/sec. Most of the axonal systems that have been studied by physiological means are composed of larger axons. As shown in Figs. 6 and 7, the duration and absolute magnitude of the period of supernormal impulse conduction is minimal in the faster-conducting callosal axons. The magnitude of the maximal decrease in latency of any visual callosal axon with a conduction velocity of greater than 6.0 meters/ sec was only 150 μsec. For corticotectal axons, the maximal decrease in latency was 125 μsec. We would probably not have noted such decreases in latency had we not been alerted by observations of larger latency changes in more slowly conducting axons. That such latency variations do occur in neuronal systems other than those referred to above is suggested by occasional references to "jitter" in the latency of antidromically activated units (e.g., ref. 1).

The above considerations may have some relevance to the evolutionary constraints that have determined the diameters of axons within a given system. In the rabbit splenium, for example, the diameter of the largest axon is approximately 20 times that of the smallest, and the volume is thus greater by a factor of 400. Increases in axonal diameter are achieved at a biological cost of a decreased number of independent axonal channels. On the other hand, increases in axon diameter result in a number of changes in conduction properties. The most obvious of these is an increase in the velocity of conduction. This may be of functional value, not only in terms of decreasing the absolute conduction time but also in terms of mediating synchrony (2,29; see also Waxman, *this volume*). Secondly, as demonstrated by Paintal (17) in peripheral nerve and as shown above for central axons, the refractory period is briefer for more rapidly conducting axons; thus the maximum possible impulse frequency is greater for larger-diameter axons. Finally, the finding that the magnitude and duration of activity-dependent variations in conduction velocity are smaller for fast-conducting than for slowly conducting axons suggests that large axons may provide the most

appropriate channels when it is important to preserve the temporal interval between spike initiation near the soma and the arrival of the impulse at the axon terminals.

ACKNOWLEDGMENTS

Work reported in this chapter was supported in part by grant NS-21307 from the National Institute of Neurological and Communicative Disorders and Stroke and by grant RG 1133-A-1 from the National Multiple Sclerosis Society. Dr. Waxman is the recipient of Research Career Development Award K04-NS-00010 from the National Institutes of Health.

REFERENCES

1. Atkinson, D. H., Sequin, J. J., and Wiesendanger, M. (1974): Organization of corticofugal neurons in somatosensory area II of the cat. *J. Physiol. (Lond)*, 236:663–679.
2. Bennett, M. V. L. (1968): Neural control of electric organs. In: *The Central Nervous System and Fish Behavior,* edited by D. Ingle, pp. 147–169. University of Chicago Press, Chicago.
3. Bergmans, J. (1973): Physiological observations on single human nerve fibres. In: *New Developments in Electromyography and Clinical Neurophysiology,* Vol. 2, edited by J. E. Desmedt, pp. 89–127. Karger, Basel.
4. Bishop, P. O., Burke, W., and Davis, R. (1962): Single-unit recording from antidromically activated optic radiation neurons. *J. Physiol. (Lond)*, 162:432–450.
5. Bliss, T. V. P., and Rosenberg, M. E. (1974): Supernormal conduction velocity in the olfactory nerve of the tortoise. *J. Physiol. (Lond)*, 239:60–61P.
6. Boyd, I. A., and Davey, M. R. (1968): *Composition of Peripheral Nerves.* Livingstone, Edinburgh.
7. Bullock, T. H. (1951): Facilitation of conduction rate in nerve fibers. *J. Physiol. (Lond)*, 114:89–97.
8. Chung, S., Raymond, S. A., and Lettvin, J. (1970): Multiple meaning in single visual units. *Brain Behav. Evol.,* 3:72–101.
9. Gardner-Medwin, A. R. (1972): An extreme supernormal period in cerebellar parallel fibers. *J. Physiol. (Lond)*, 22:357–371.
10. Gasser, H. S. (1950): Unmedullated fibers originating in dorsal root ganglia. *J. Gen. Physiol.,* 33:651–690.
11. Gilliatt, R. W., and Willison, R. G. (1963): The refractory and supernormal periods of the human median nerve. *J. Neurol. Neurosurg. Psychiatry,* 26:136–143.

12. Hall, J. L. (1965): Binaural interaction in the accessory superior-olivary nucleus of the cat. *J. Acoust. Soc. Am.,* 37:814–823.

13. Hubbard, J. I., and Willis, W. D. (1962): Hyperpolarization of mammalian motor nerve terminals. *J. Physiol. (Lond),* 163:115–137.

14. Hursh, J. B. (1939): Conduction velocity and diameter of nerve fibers. *Am. J. Physiol.,* 127:131–139.

15. Lass, Y., and Abeles, M. (1975): Transmission of information by the axon. I. Noise and memory in the myelinated nerve fiber of the frog. *Biol. Cyb.,* 19:61–67.

16. Newman, E. A., and Raymond, S. A. (1971): Activity dependent shifts in excitability of frog peripheral nerve axons. *Q. Prog. Rep. MIT Res. Lab. Electronics,* 102:165–187.

17. Paintal, A. S. (1967): A comparison of the nerve impulses of mammalian nonmedullated nerve fibres with those of the smallest diameter medullated fibres. *J. Physiol. (Lond),* 193:523–533.

18. Phillips, C. G. (1959): Actions of antidromic pyramidal volleys on single Betz cells in the cat. *Q. J. Exp. Physiol.,* 44:1–25.

19. Phillips, C. G., Powell, T. P. S., and Shepherd, G. M. (1963): Responses of mitral cells to stimulation of the lateral olfactory tract in the rabbit. *J. Physiol. (Lond),* 168:65–88.

20. Rushton, W. A. H. (1951): A theory of the effects of fibre size in medullated nerve. *J. Physiol. (Lond),* 115:101–122.

21. Swadlow, H. A. (1974): Properties of antidromically activated callosal neurons and neurons responsive to callosal input in rabbit binocular cortex. *Exp. Neurol.,* 43:424–444.

22. Swadlow, H. A. (1974): Systematic variations in the conduction velocity of slowly conducting axons in the rabbit corpus callosum. *Exp. Neurol.,* 43:445–451.

23. Swadlow, H. A. (1977): The relationship of the corpus callosum to visual areas I and II of the rabbit. *Exp. Neurol.* 57:516–531.

24. Swadlow, H. A., and Waxman, S. G. (1975): Observations on impulse conduction along central axons. *Proc. Natl. Acad. Sci. USA,* 72:5156–5159.

25. Swadlow, H. A., and Waxman, S. G. (1976): Variations in conduction velocity and excitability following single and multiple impulses of visual callosal axons in the rabbit. *Exp. Neurol.,* 53:128–150.

26. Swadlow, H. A., Waxman, S. G., and Hartweig, E. (1977): The cells of origin of the visual component of the corpus callosum of the rabbit. In preparation.

27. Takeuchi, A., and Takeuchi, N. K. (1959): Active phase of frog's end-plate potential. *J. Neurophysiol.,* 22:395–411.

28. Waxman, S. G., and Bennett, M. V. L. (1972): Relative conduction velocities of small myelinated and non-myelinated fibres in the central nervous system. *Nature [New Biol.],* 238:217–219.

29. Waxman, S. G., and Melker, R. J. (1971): Closely spaced nodes of Ranvier in the mammalian brain. *Brain Res.,* 32:445–448.

30. Waxman, S. G., and Swadlow, H. A. (1976): Morphology and physiology of visual callosal axons: Evidence for a supernormal period in central myelinated axons. *Brain Res.,* 113:179–187.

31. Waxman, S. G., and Swadlow, H. A. (1976): Ultrastructure of visual callosal axons in the rabbit. *Exp. Neurol.,* 53:115–127.

32. Yasargil, G. M., and Diamond, J. (1968): Startle-response in teleost fish: An elementary circuit for neural discrimination. *Nature (Lond),* 230:241–243.

Physiology and Pathobiology of Axons, edited by
S. G. Waxman. Raven Press, New York © 1978.

Aftereffects of Activity in Peripheral Axons as a Clue to Nervous Coding

S. A. Raymond and J. Y. Lettvin

Research Laboratory of Electronics and Department of Electrical Engineering, Massachusetts Institute of Technology, Cambridge, Massachusetts 02139

Almost every axon ultimately arborizes into a teledendron of thin, bare twigs that by virtue of their differences in anatomy from the stouter, often myelinated trunk can be expected to pose more stringent limitations on conduction of impulses. In 1935 Barron and Matthews (4) reported the discovery of periodic conduction blocks occurring in the extensive arbors of primary afferent fibers in cats. In the same system, conduction block between the main fibers and their descending collaterals was identified in 1955 (40) and shown to be contingent on previous activity. A few years later, Krnjević and Miledi (43) reported intermittent conduction in peripheral nerve. Conduction block in the ectodromic primary afferent fibers of Barron and Matthews was again studied during the late 1960s (59,66), and it was noted that the activity of a fiber influenced its pattern of impulse conduction. So did activity in its neighbors. Notions that branch points in axonal arbors were generally regions of lowered conduction safety and that switching of impulses occurred throughout the teledendron were proposed, emphasizing that since the state of the switch was determined contingently, a good deal of information handling must occur prior to synapse (17,59).

At this juncture there were two questions of central importance to further understanding. The first was essentially structural. What were the structural and anatomical features of axons and their branches such that regions of low conduction safety would develop? The second was essentially physiological. How did activity, intrinsic and extrinsic, so change the state of the membrane at a branch that impulse conduction would be altered and switching occur?

To pursue the second issue appeared to be a difficult problem, at least in mammalian spinal cord, because simultaneous interacting influences prevented unambiguous isolation of any one factor. The density of neuropil is so great in dorsal horn that currents between adjacent fibers and cells influence both conduction and threshold (6,21,37,40,59). Furthermore, strong synaptic inputs are claimed to act on these fibers (24).

In order to study the aftereffects of impulses on axon membrane, we therefore turned away from mammalian central nervous system (CNS) to work on peripheral nerve of frogs. Here the axons travel in longitudinal parallel strands surrounded by connective tissue sheaths. The interweaving of the axons is spatially less complex, and fiber geometry is better delineated. The nerve trunk can be excised from the animal and bathed in a defined medium. No synapses ending on the axon now exist, and as we mention below the effects of extracellular currents can be controlled. Observations emerging from this system may be interpreted as direct effects of impulse activity on axon membrane. The intent of the experiments was to discover the general pattern of aftereffects of activity in axon membrane and thus to clarify the interpretations of activity-dependent phenomena observed in cells and axons enmeshed in neuropil.

EXPERIMENTAL APPROACHES

Figure 1 shows the basic features of our peripheral nerve experiments. A monopolar

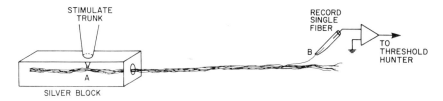

FIG. 1. Representation of experiment. The stimulating chamber was machined from a block of silver, with its interior bore plated with Ag/AgCl to serve as diffuse electrode for the monopolar stimulus. System ground is an Ag/AgCl plate in the recording bath also filled with recirculating Ringer's solution.

current pulse provides stimulation to the entire nerve at point A. Impulses occurring in response to this stimulus propagate from the stimulating chamber and are recorded using a flexible plastic suction electrode at B. The nerve is teased apart until a single unit can be picked up with forceps and electrode. CO_2 in O_2 and breathing air are bubbled through a Boyle Conway Ringer's solution (14), holding it at a steady pH near 7.2. The medium is pumped and recirculated so as to flow continuously along the nerve.

We adopted the threshold of the nerve fibers as a measure of the aftereffects of impulse activity in the nerve. Threshold was chosen for two reasons. First, the level of threshold is a function of many interdependent parameters (membrane voltage, conductances and other cable parameters, E_{Na}, E_K, noise, pump metabolism, temperature, etc.). Activity-dependent changes of any of the parameters can therefore be expected to appear in records of threshold. The second reason is that the threshold of an axon segment is directly related to its ability to invade, a feature that is important in interpreting the implications of the results for impulse conduction in axonal arbors.

A device called a threshold hunter was developed (63) to generate plots of threshold as a function of activity and time (threshold curves). It is an adaptation of the "method of constant response" (7) wherein the duration of the stimulus is adjusted automatically until the axon is firing in response to 50% of the stimulus presentations. This is accomplished by incrementing the stimulus duration by an amount $\Delta\tau$ (usually 1.5 μsec) after each failure and decrementing the duration by the same $\Delta\tau$ after every success. The record of stimulus size versus time shows the tracking of the threshold curve. To measure threshold changes

after "activity," supramaximal conditioning stimuli are repeated at long intervals (usually 2–5 sec), and the hunting stimulus is presented at slowly increasing delays following the conditioning spike(s). Records of the hunting stimulus as a function of delay interval from a repeated pattern of conditioning impulses give the early portion of the threshold curve after that pattern of activity. Since the threshold changes slowly in later portions of the curve, it can be directly hunted versus time without repeating conditioning events.

The following sections present the threshold curves phase by phase. All time delays and conduction velocities, unless otherwise mentioned, apply to frog sciatic nerve. Threshold curves in mammalian nerve fibers are essentially similar, but the phases are sped up (32, 49).

REFRACTORY PERIOD

The absolute refractory period begins with the onset of an impulse and lasts until it first becomes possible to stimulate another conducted impulse in the same nerve. Since Adrian (1), many laboratories have studied the refractoriness of nerve membrane (32,48,56), and they introduced some variety into its definition and measurement. An absolute refractory period defined by initiation of a nontraveling impulse can be measured (26,57), but the value obtained depends critically on the particular conditions of stimulation (57; Paintal, *this volume*). For the experiments presented here we measured the absolute refractory period from the beginning of the conditioning stimulus to the beginning of the earliest successful test stimulus as diagrammed in Fig. 2. Thus we require not only initiation but conduction of the impulse to define the onset of

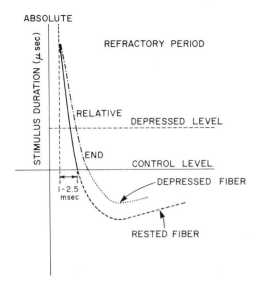

FIG. 2. Definition of absolute and relative refractory periods. Vertical axis marks onset of first stimulus. Times denote delay to onset of first hunting stimuli to fire conducted impulses. Note that threshold of depressed fibers cannot reach control level as quickly as it does for rested fibers. It may cross the depressed level of threshold within the interval corresponding to the refractory period measured in the rested fiber.

the relative refractory period. The threshold hunter produces a longest test stimulus of approximately 304 μsec, three times resting threshold duration. Stimulus current was fixed at the level giving resting threshold durations of approximately 100 μsec. Under these conditions we measured absolute refractory periods lasting 1.5–2 msec following single impulses in axons with conduction velocity of 15–20 meters/sec (15°–20°C). For mammalian A fibers, Paintal (57) reports that slowly conducting fibers have longer absolute refractory periods than ones with high conduction velocity. The slope of this relation becomes steep at low conduction velocities. We noticed little variation in absolute refractory periods of different fibers, but since we tested mainly large fibers, our results are not inconsistent with Paintal's.

The earliest successful test stimulus marks the beginning of the relatively refractory period. Since impulses can be recorded during this interval, the threshold hunter could be used to track the steep monotonic decline of threshold as it descended through the control level. In Fig. 2 the control level precedes the discontinuity occasioned by the absolute refractory period. Control levels were drawn from threshold hunter records of hunting stimuli presented every 2 sec while no conditioning stimuli were given. This is our operational approximation of the ideal *resting* threshold measured without any activity at all. This definition of resting and control (experimental) threshold applies to all other experiments reported here. A sample of 22 axons held at 17° ± 1°C, with conduction velocities between 8 and 30 meters/sec, were measured. The relative refractory period began within 2 msec and lasted until 3–4.5 msec after the conditioning pulse, at which interval the threshold crossed the control level. Thus the vaunted relative refractory period (9,25) occupies only approximately 1–2.5 msec of the interval after a spike and is the shortest phase in the threshold curve.

Activity alters the duration of the refractory period. Long conditioning bursts or increased steady activity increase the relative refractory period by 1–2 msec at most. The prolongation stems from the activity-produced depression (described below) that hinders the return of threshold to control level. As diagrammed by the dashed lines of Fig. 2, crossing of the raised level of threshold associated with depression often happens after an interval approximately equal to that of the relative refractory period measured in the same nerve at rest. Average activity rates of 20/sec produce such high depression that the threshold never drops to the control level following an impulse, and the relative refractory period as defined here does not exist. Even with such strong depressions, however, a refractory period defined by the return of threshold to the depressed level is essentially the same as the refractory period defined by return to resting threshold (64). A consequence of these observations is that whether an activity-dependent shift in the ending of the relative refractory period is reported under conditions of high activity depends essentially on definition. Furthermore, even if processes producing refractoriness are not much affected by activity, interactions with other mechanisms producing later phases alter the duration of the refractory period.

Figure 3 summarizes the principal features of the remaining phases and their relation to

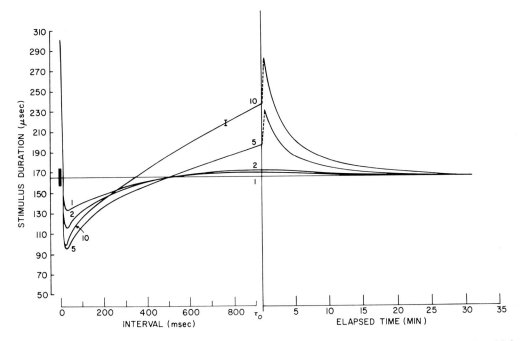

FIG. 3. Threshold curves following bursts of impulses. The figure was traced directly from a colored multiple graph generated by the threshold hunter and x–y plotter. Additional results from later plots were used to sketch out the last 20 min of the two longest recovery periods. To the left of τ_0 the x-axis gives the interval between the last conditioning stimulus at 0 and the hunting stimulus. At τ_0 conditioning stimuli were turned off and threshold during recovery was hunted every 2 sec for approximately 20 min. The dark bar (*at left*) shows the duration change required to vary probability of response from nearly 0 to nearly 1. The range mark on the curve associated with bursts of 10 impulses shows the extent of variation in the duration of the threshold hunter with respect to the smooth traced line. Approximately 400 tests for threshold were made to compile each trace during the 900 msec interval after conditioning pulses. Bursts were repeated every 2 sec; pH 7.45, temperature 17°C, conduction velocity of axon used was 16 meters/sec.

activity. The threshold of a frog sciatic nerve fiber is plotted as a function of delay from the last impulse of conditioning trains. Conditioning trains were repeated every 2 sec, and one test with the hunter stimulus was made each cycle. The plot was formed from hundreds of such tests, each one at a successively longer delay from $t = 0$ than the one preceding it. Figure 3 is a tracing of the plot.

SUPEREXCITABLE PHASE

As seen in Fig. 3, a phase of enhanced excitability and low threshold, called either the supernormal or superexcitable period, begins as the descending threshold crosses the control threshold after the refractory period. Superexcitability is maximal between 7 and 20 msec and ends after a slow return to control threshold level that lasts approximately 1 sec.[1] It has been observed often in nerve and muscle fibers (e.g., refs. 15,33,47,48,50,53,84). It is not an artifact of injury or poor condition, a possibility raised by Adrian (1) and by Graham and Lorente de Nó (35), but is present in fresh nerve and, as shown by Swadlow (75), is seen in CNS axons and cells recorded from awake animals. It is absent or attenuated in depolarized and unhealthy fibers, as we note below.

If the repetition rate is changed to 1 cycle every 1.5 sec (or if 2 conditioning impulses 10 msec apart are used, every 2 sec), a very slight overshoot in the return can be discerned. In

---

[1] The reader is referred to the chapter by Swadlow and Waxman in this volume for a description of the super- and subnormal phases in mammalian CNS fibers.

Fig. 3 some overshoot occurred with 1 conditioning spike every 2 sec. The overshoot is the first sign of yet another phase called depression. Depression becomes more obvious with higher average rates of activity, as does superexcitability. Note that the conditioning trains of 2, 5, and 10 impulses generate a pronounced increase in maximum superexcitability. There is an accumulation of the superexcitability from each spike. This accumulation can be clarified by a two-spike experiment as follows. The threshold curves following each of two spikes are sampled as the interval between the pair is reduced in stages from 500 to 10 msec. Only at the briefer intervals is the maximum superexcitability after the second spike substantialy greater than it is after a single spike (64). The closer the paired pulses are, the more of an additive effect is produced. So far we have studied pairs at least 5 msec apart. Results confirm that one aspect of the accumulation of superexcitability depends on the interval between preceding spikes.

The extent of the increase in superexcitability depends also on the number of conditioning pulses given. Earlier work by Gasser and his colleagues concentrated mainly on the afterpotentials. The negative afterpotential was strongly associated with superexcitability of whole nerve, and it was shown to increase after brief tetani (31). Zucker (84) reports that superexcitability of motor nerve terminals in crayfish is greater after tetani of 6 spikes than after 1 spike. We found that giving more than 6–8 impulses produces only marginal increases, if any, in the superexcitability of single fibers. In some axons 4 impulses suffice to achieve a maximum additive effect; for others a slight increment in superexcitability can be achieved by the 10th spike. Nevertheless, the accumulation invariably saturates after only a handful of conditioning spikes. In Fig. 3 note that the peak superexcitability for a 10-spike conditioning train was actually a little less than for a train of 5. Before saturation each additional impulse in the burst contributes additional superexcitability, and the magnitude of superexcitability is correlated with the number of spikes in the conditioning train.

The return from the superexcitable peak has similar dynamics whether the peak is small (after 1 spike) or large (after 8). The time to return to baseline is a bit prolonged after a large peak (by as much as 40% in smaller axons). This feature does not show in Fig. 3, since it is revealed only in experiments that repeat the larger conditioning train so seldom that significant depression fails to develop. After the larger maximal superexcitabilities in Fig. 3, the returns are steeper than for the smaller ones. Repetitive presentation of conditioning trains of 5 and 10 pulses every 2 sec implies average activity on the order of 2.5 and 5 spikes/sec. This is sufficient to produce quite notable depression, even for large fibers of sciatic nerve. As can be seen in Fig. 3, depression offsets superexcitability. Strong depression attenuates the superexcitable maximum. The larger depression associated with repeated bursts of 10 impulses accounts for the slight diminution of maximal superexcitability observed.

A superexcitable "fraction" continues to influence the threshold even after it has climbed past control level into the depressed phase. This influence can be revealed usually for more than a second after the last impulse. The method, which was used for Fig. 3, is to turn off the conditioning pulses, thus eliminating renewal of superexcitability. In Fig. 3 the section showing threshold curves during refractory and superexcitable phases is followed by a section that gives threshold as a function of time following the extinction of conditioning activity. In this portion it is clear that, without the aftereffects of a preceding burst (875 msec earlier), the threshold rises quickly and substantially before beginning to recover. The peak of this rise occurs within 3–4 sec of the last impulse. Even with manual overrides, the threshold hunter requires approximately 10 sec to converge on the new level. However, recovery of depression takes so long that threshold remains near the peak during this time.

DEPRESSION

Buildup

The threshold level during depression rises as activity rates increase. In Fig. 3 the dependence of depression on activity is shown in the differences between depressions after bursts of 1, 2, 5, and 10 impulses. The average rate of activity even for 10-impulse bursts is only 5 impulses/sec, indicating that quite modest rates (in comparison to the maximum impulse frequency such fibers can carry) produce substantial depression. In order to note depressions after mild activity, it is essential that baseline thresholds be obtained from a well-rested nerve. If the temperature falls below 15°C, rates as low as 1 impulse every 6 sec raise some depression (11).

Experiments using intermittent tetanic bursts to condition the axon, and hunting the threshold at a fixed interval (e.g., 2 sec) after each burst, show the development of depression after the commencement of a constant average activity. The first trace of Fig. 5 (below) is drawn directly from such an experiment. The threshold can be seen to begin climbing away from the control level as soon as the intermittent tetanus begins. Threshold climbs slowly over the course of the next 10 min to an equilibrium value that depends on average activity (53,67). By measuring the initial slope of the rise in threshold at the onset of intermittent conditioning, we observed that the rate of buildup is proportional to average activity. Each pulse appears to add a constant increment to the upward threshold displacement. The value of this constant and hence the buildup rate at a given impulse frequency differs substantially among axons. Buildup is slower and the approach to equilibrium takes longer in large axons. First-order models based on the notion of constant threshold increment per pulse generate activity-dependent depressions that grow and equilibrate with the same dependence on impulse frequency shown by experimental preparations (60,67).

Recovery

An equilibrium arises because the rate of recovery depends on the severity of depression and buildup does not. Recovery becomes faster as threshold grows more depressed, whereas the rate at which depression is generated is a fixed constant proportion of the activity rate. A membrane beginning to fire at a given average impulse frequency immediately generates depression at a rate depending only on that frequency. The threshold rapidly begins to climb, since recovery rate at low levels of depression is lower than buildup rate. Threshold slows its climb at higher levels of depression as recovery rate progressively increases. Eventually each firing frequency engenders its own equilibrium level of depression. The rate of buildup and the equilibrium level also depend on temperature; depression is substantially augmented by cooling (12).

Although rate of recovery increases with depression, it is not strictly proportional to depression level. At very strong depressions, recovery times appear to be longer than one would expect if recovery rate depended only on the instantaneous level of threshold, as in a first-order process. For example, we superimpose two recovery traces from the same fiber, one of which followed a mild depression and the other a strong one. We arrange it so that the peak depression following the mild depression intersects the descending recovery curve recorded after the strong one. Further recovery in the two records thus ensues from the same threshold level. Instead of overlapping, the remainders of the recovery curves proceed at quite different rates. The curve associated with the strong depression takes as much as five times longer than the mild one's curve to reach control level. We are still investigating this issue, but our present results strongly indicate that different histories of impulse activity in a fiber are reflected not only in the level of depression but also in the slope of the recovery curve at each threshold level.

Taken together, the preceding observations allow prediction of threshold curves during and following any arbitrary activity in a fiber. Thus the curves imply the particular activity patterns that generate them, and we can state generally that membranes "remember" their previous patterns of firing in their threshold curves (47,53).

If physiological rates of firing during the daily life of a frog exceed 1 or 2 impulses/sec, our results indicate that even large axons are normally depressed. Wild axons more active than this can be expected to be strongly depressed. Further, since smaller axons are most easily depressed, the distributing end of a large parent axon may show substantial depression in its branches at activities having only slight influence on resting threshold of the trunk. As seen in Fig. 3, depression has the effect of increasing the magnitude of the threshold transients following an impulse. It also prolongs the total duration of aftereffects. After the last conditioning impulse at the highest activity rate in Fig. 3, threshold had still not completely recovered 30 min later.

ROLE OF ELECTRODE CHANGES, ACTIVITY IN OTHER FIBERS, AND EXTRACELLULAR CURRENTS

We interpreted the above observations as direct aftereffects of impulses conducted by an axon on its threshold. It is important to substantiate this statement, since the conditions of the experiment allow for another interpretation. The aftereffects could instead arise from pulse-dependent changes in the stimulator, in the electrode, and in the coupling of the currents from the electrode to the axon being studied. It is also possible that activity in neighboring fibers acts to retard or augment the effect of a stimulus on the recorded fiber. To determine if such effects were present we ex-

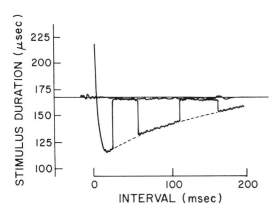

FIG. 4. Superexcitability after subthreshold stimuli. The solid horizontal line shows resting threshold. At a time corresponding to 0, a conditioning stimulus was presented every 2 sec. Hunting stimuli were given at progressively longer intervals from the conditioning stimulus. The conditioning stimulus was made barely subthreshold during two periods corresponding to the intervals 22–58 msec and 110–160 msec. At other times the conditioning stimulus strength was varied from three times to just above the threshold. Without a conditioning nerve spike, the conditioning stimulus itself produced no discernible effects. (Modified from ref. 53.)

amined the consequences of changing the magnitude of the conditioning current pulses on the threshold curves. If the strength of the conditioning pulses were to change the threshold measured, we could then look to an effect of adjacent activity or electrode degradation to explain it. However, we observe that changes of conditioning stimulus only result in a variation of the threshold curve if they alter whether or not a conditioning spike is generated in the recorded fiber. Even very small changes of stimulus ($\sim 1\%$) can account for 100% of the threshold curve changes providing only that one level produces conditioning spikes and the other does not. Figure 4 was drawn from one such experiment performed during the superexcitable phase. Experiments done during the depression phase have analogous results (63). What matters is whether a conditioning impulse is present in the recorded fiber. Thus the aftereffects are those of the nerve spike and not of the stimulus. Large increases or decreases in stimulus that do not change whether a conditioning impulse occurs in the recorded fiber produce substantial increases and decreases in the number of surrounding axons that are firing and in the current density through the electrode. They have no discernible effect on threshold curves measured by the hunter circuit. Similar results have been observed in mammalian preparations (30,76).

MECHANISM

What processes underlie the threshold curves? The refractory period always follows an impulse. No drugs or procedures have been found to eliminate it or reverse it. We have not studied it ourselves, except for noting its slight prolongation by activity rates generating depression. Hodgkin and Huxley accounted for refractoriness as a period of high sodium inactivation and high potassium conductance, rendering the axon leaky to current and less prone to reinforce a depolarization (39). It seems to be a function of the same processes and structures that give rise to the impulse itself.

One possible explanation for the superexcitable phase is that superexcitability originates in a depolarization that shifts the membrane potential closer to a "threshold voltage." The shift would be Nernstian, stemming mainly from the local decrease in equilibrium potential for potassium following an impulse. Higher internal sodium concentration may also be a factor by altering the resting relation between depolarization and sodium activation. A second explanation can be developed around the fact that there is no "threshold voltage," only a system of processes that interact (65). If the membrane were to be slightly hyperpolarized, inactivation would be reduced, membrane conductance would be low, and an increased excitability could occur independent of the increment of external potassium concentration. Mechanisms resulting in threshold and how they are modified by the state of the membrane are discussed by Bennett et al. (8) and Fitzhugh (27). There are several recent studies on K^+ depolarization and excitability changes in CNS (19,44–46,54).

Our observations indicate that the processes producing superexcitability generate a slight reversed effect when the membrane is depolarized (Fig. 5). This suggests that such processes act to depolarize the membrane during superexcitability. Furthermore, the accumulation effect of several closely timed pulses emerges as an expected consequence of a hypothesis based on an external pool of potassium that becomes more concentrated with each pulse. Except for Zucker's experiments showing attenuation of superexcitability by raised external K^+ in crayfish (84), we know of no work devoted to measuring the effects of changed external potassium on superexcitability in nerve fibers. Spear and Moore (73), working with excised Purkinje fibers from dog heart, report that raising external potassium from 2.7 to 5 mM "eliminated" the superexcitable phase. At 5 mM concentrations of external potassium, however, fibers were more excitable at rest than they had been at maximum superexcitable levels measured in the 2.7 mM $[K_o^+]$. Higher concentrations of potassium (7 mM) diminished resting excitability with respect to that measured in 2.7 mM Tyrode's solution, and superexcitability remained absent (73). These observations are consistent with the first type of explanation for superexcitability that stresses the role of transient increments of external potassium. Zucker accounts for supernormality of crayfish terminals in this way (84). According to this view, concentration increases after impulses provoke depolarizations that act to make the nerve more excitable unless the membrane has become depolarized through deterioration, through poisoning as in Fig. 5, or by experimental manipulation of the external potassium concentration. One expects that such depolarized membranes will, if anything, only become

$\longrightarrow$

FIG. 5. Effect of ouabain on depression and superexcitability. 1: Establishment of equilibrium depression. Depression was produced by bursts of 10 spikes each with interspike intervals of 30 msec and burst intervals 4 sec. The y-axis shows threshold in terms of hunting stimulus duration. The hunting stimulus was given 1.5 sec after the end of each burst. All records in the figure are direct tracings of the x–y plotter graphs from one experiment. This first trace shows one cycle of buildup and recovery from a relatively mild depression. Note that buildup during the next tetanus results in equilibrium at the same level. 2: Superexcitability in depressed nerve before ouabain. Successive records are continuous, and the elapsed time scale shows time in hours from the beginning of the experiment. In this record an additional conditioning impulse was given at 1.5 sec, and the threshold was hunted through the refractory period (high threshold transient) and throughout the 1.5-sec interval following the impulse. The level of depression after 11 spikes was slightly greater than for 10. Some superexcitable effect shows well beyond 1 sec after the conditioning pulse. 3: Addition of ouabain during equilibrium depression, and spot tests of the level of maximum superexcitability. A threshold drop follows application of ouabain into the Ringer's solution. This forms the "descending limb" of the "ouabain trough." In several places the record was interrupted to test maximum superexcitability. The labels show the interval between these tests and the conditioning impulse. At the bottom of the trough, a full superexcitability plot as in 2 was run, as seen in 4, then the trough continues in 3. 4: Superexcitability after ouabain. The refractory period shows as a spike in the threshold plot, but otherwise the trace is flat. Even dense hunting near the former peak results only in a slight, brief drop in threshold, if any. Essentially the superexcitable transient is eliminated. 5: Secondary rise in threshold. A progressively steeper rise in threshold on the other side of the trough finally exceeds the maximum stimulus duration. After saturation, two attempts with anodal stimuli, the first at 0.5 mA (five times control threshold current) and the second at 5.0 mA, were temporarily able to generate impulses. A test for superexcitability at 16 msec shows a transient elevation of threshold from the rising baseline.

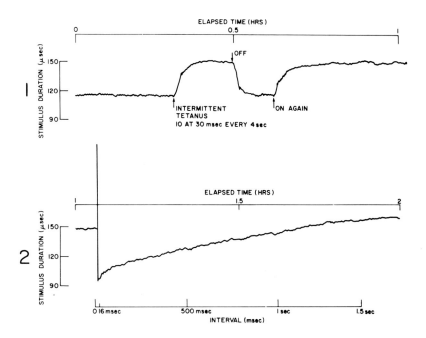

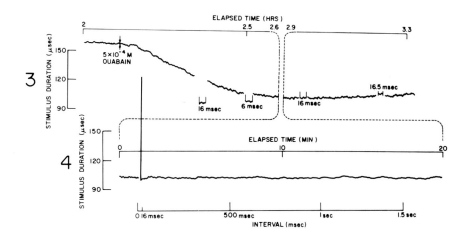

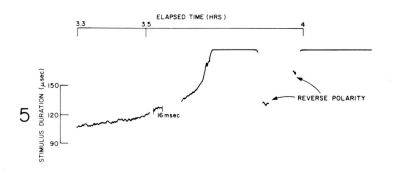

further inactivated by the transient additional depolarization following impulses. A number of other hypotheses can be invented for super-excitability as well as the two sketched above, but since the problem is tractable experimentally, we expect the domain of possible mechanisms to narrow during the next few years.

Depression accompanied by hyperpolarizing voltage shifts measured by Connelly and others (18,48,74), seems to result from a metabolic ion pump that depends on internal sodium concentrations (62). Temperature changes affect depression in complicated ways, probably owing to changes in the time course and magnitude of the conditioning impulses as well as alterations of membrane metabolism (10). Such experiments therefore reveal little that is unequivocal about the operation of the pump.

Figure 5 shows the effect of ouabain on a nerve fiber depressed by repeated tetanic bursts of impulses. Ouabain not only eliminates equilibrium depression, it also renders the membrane more excitable than it is at the resting or control level. In fact, threshold approaches are seen at the maximum of the superexcitable phase, as shown by comparing 2 and 4 of Fig. 5. Furthermore, after the threshold has reached the bottom of the ouabain trough, tracking it during the interval that corresponds normally to maximum superexcitability (6–20 msec) reveals that the threshold becomes slightly *higher*. Near the end of the trough, as the threshold begins to rise again, this reversal of the superexcitable phase is more distinct (3 of Fig. 5). Earlier in the trough the entire superexcitable interval is essentially flat. The threshold is slightly higher than the preouabain level (2 of Fig. 5), and this is reflected in the upward migration of short interval threshold levels during descent and the first 10–20 min of the trough. At the rising end of the trough the reversal of superexcitability at short intervals persists, but there is essentially no difference between the threshold at an interval of 2 sec and the threshold during most of the superexcitable phase. This contrasts sharply with measurements during the descending limb of the trough, showing short intervals strongly superexcitable and long ones depressed. The membrane is thus in different states during descent and rise. Impulse activity during the

trough hastens the second rise, suggesting that the membrane is depolarizing during the trough. This is supported by the brief success of anodal stimuli after maximal cathodal stimuli begin to fail at the end of the second rise (5 of Fig. 5).

Ouabain shuts off metabolic extrusion of Na^+ (42). One interpretation of the results obtained from experiments like that in Fig. 5 is that the sodium pump produces a hyperpolarization that increases in proportion to intracellular Na^+ levels (18). These in turn rise with activity rate as each impulse contributes an increment to the internal sodium debt. The exact quantity in each increment is a function of the activity pattern (64) and of temperature (11) but can be approximated by a constant (67). The larger the hyperpolarizing current is, the harder it will be to fire the cell, and higher threshold levels will be measured.

The ouabain results hold some further meaning for the superexcitable phase. If superexcitability is associated with the change in E_{K^+}, to which the axon responds at least transiently as a K^+ electrode, that change should lead to a larger, if shorter, superexcitable phase in depressed axons since hyperpolarizations associated with depression augment sensitivity of the membrane voltage to external potassium (5,28). In Fig. 3 the starting threshold just before each burst of 5 or 10 impulses is near peak depression and is hence much farther from the superexcitable peak. The resulting changes in superexcitability are very large. This augmentation is consistently observed in other experiments (53,63). One anticipates a limit on the increase in extracellular K^+ that could be maintained by impulse activity, given bulk flow, diffusion, and glial or neuronal uptake (44). As mentioned above, the saturation of superexcitability as conditioning trains become longer than 6–8 impulses could have its origin in such a saturation of extracellular K^+.

The reversal of threshold during the superexcitable phase observed after ouabain may be a form of cathodal block (sodium inactivation) resulting from depolarization of a nerve that has already been brought near its maximum excitability by poisoning the pump. It is consistent with this notion that the reversal becomes larger as the membrane depolarizes further near the far end of the ouabain trough.

Even in rested nerve the effect of ouabain is to lower the threshold until it is close to super-excitable level, although the trough lasts much longer at low activity rates (62).

Why is recovery slowed after strong depressions? An attractive hypothesis is that Na^+ debt becomes so great at strong depressions that sodium diffuses at high concentration into the internodes, prolonging the time during which amounts of sodium adequate to support substantial hyperpolarization can be delivered to the pump situated near the membrane at the nodes. An alternative is that high activity leads to consumption of residual ATP stores, so that availability of ATP becomes the limiting factor on pump rate, not internal Na^+. Metabolism would slowly build up ATP, accounting for the slow recovery. Both processes probably occur, but it is not yet known which is dominant.

UBIQUITY OF THRESHOLD OSCILLATIONS

The preceding brief sketches of cellular mechanisms behind the threshold curves enforce the perspective that the curves are rooted in the structure and metabolism of axon membrane. Since these features belong generally to nerve (and muscle) membrane, we may expect cells and fibers everywhere to show an activity dependence with the same general features born from the same mechanisms.

The frog nerve threshold curves are slower than those obtained from mammals, but the picture of a damped after-oscillation with three phases is consistent (32,48), although Gasser and Grundfest observed "distinctly unphysiological distortions" at high activity rates consisting of an extra damped cycle of super-excitability, depression, and recovery. The threshold curves in both frogs and mammals are rather large, and they last much longer than the impulse. The effects that such prolonged activity-dependent aftereffects might have on conduction velocity or on probability of conduction past a region of low conduction safety depend on the condition of the membrane. For instance, in cat dorsal horn there was evidence for two kinds of conduction block, each at a different region of the primary afferent fiber (59). In this and similar cases threshold oscillations after an impulse would

be expected to have opposing phase relations for effects on conduction in the two regions. That is, in a region of cathodal block, the processes associated with the superexcitable phase ought to render the region less passable, whereas the same influence might facilitate conduction at a region of anodal or hyper-polarization block. Two recent experimental studies assigning opposite roles to the same phase of the threshold curve are particularly interesting in this light (20,72).

LATENCY CHANGES

The same processes that interact to produce the threshold curves may be monitored with other measures. Conduction velocity change following activity has also been noted consistently (1,16,34,47,58). Supernormal conduction velocities were studied during the superexcitable interval in callosal axons of rabbits (75,76) and in parallel fibers of cat cerebellum (30). The later studies emphasize that the latency changes depended on activity in the particular fibers tested. We were interested to determine the degree of correlation between threshold changes and latency changes in peripheral nerve. They are tightly associated, as can be seen in Fig. 6, which shows latency changes and threshold changes measured simultaneously during a variety of conditioning impulse patterns and experimental conditions. These results are compatible with the notion that the same activity-dependent processes are manifest in both measures. In the excised frog nerve, the steadiness of stimulating conditions makes threshold a more sensitive and stable measure. For the rabbit callosum, stable thresholds are harder to obtain and activity dependence can apparently be investigated unambiguously with latency measures alone (75).

INTERMITTENT CONDUCTION

Many experimental observations of impulse conduction in cells and axons can be interpreted in terms of activity-dependent threshold curves. An excellent case in point is intermittent conduction. Periodic alternation between conduction and block was first noticed and

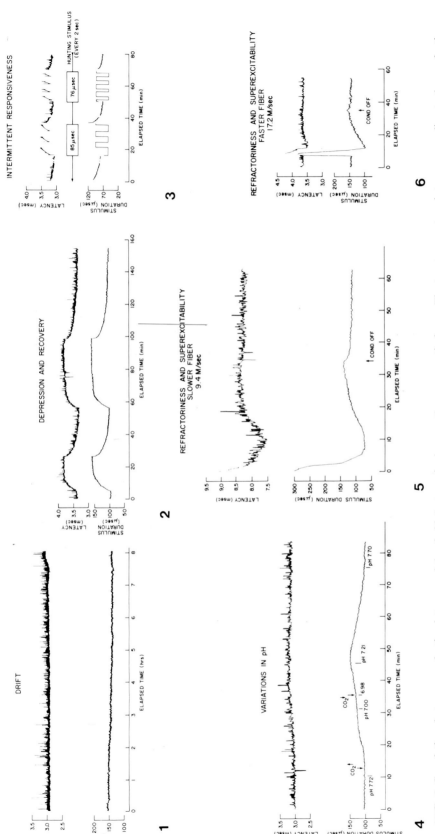

FIG. 6. Correlations between conduction latency and threshold. Latency is given on the upper vertical axes. The trace connects points corresponding to the conduction latency of each response to the hunting stimulus. Long gaps of no response show as blank interruptions of the trace. Threshold is plotted as a function of time on the lower trace. All records are direct tracings from a two-pen chart recorder. **1:** Threshold drifted slowly shorter as threshold descended. Conduction velocity 19.1 meters/sec; temperature 20.5°C; pH 7.34. **2:** Threshold was hunted every 2 sec for 8 hr. Latency drifted slowly shorter as threshold descended. Conduction velocity 19.1 meters/sec; temperature 20.5°C; pH 7.34. **2:** Periods of repeated bursts of 10 impulses every 2 sec generated buildup and recovery of depression associated with lengthening and shortening of conduction latency. Conduction velocity 13.7 meters/sec. **3:** Intermittent responsiveness. The record begins by showing recovery of both latency and threshold after a period of conduction. Hunting stimuli were given every 2 sec except during two blocks of repeated stimulation at 100-msec intervals at the fixed durations indicated in the blocks. During the blocks, periods of conduction are marked by the threshold trace being low, and periods of block are indicated when the trace is high. The first impulse of a period of conduction has a relatively long conduction latency; later impulses travel faster since they are affected by superexcitability. Then conduction latency rises. Just before failure, the record of latency becomes noisy, as it is for near-threshold stimuli. Note that cycle time is less for the 76-μsec conditioning stimulus (closest to threshold) than it is for the longer stimulus (85 μsec). Conduction velocity 18.7 meters/sec; 0.40 mA. **4:** Numbers denoting the pH measured are placed opposite the threshold trace. Latency changes are associated with the threshold shifts brought about by varying the pCO_2 in the gas bubbled through the Ringer's. $CO_2 \uparrow$ means raised pCO_2 was begun at the moment indicated by $\downarrow$ (18.3°C; conduction velocity 23.3 meters/sec). **5:** The x-axis is elapsed time, not interval, accounting for the apparent prolongation of the superexcitable phase. Sampling of threshold must be dense where the slope is steep. Conduction velocity 9.4 meters/sec. **6:** Consistent with other traces, the refractory period is associated with slower conduction velocity. Changes in

named by Barron and Matthews in 1935 (4). The work was questioned by Toennies (77, 78), who thought the impulses could be dorsal root reflexes, and later by Habgood, working with Matthews (38). In 1967 we studied intermittent conduction in cat dorsal root and confirmed the findings of Barron and Matthews regarding periodic variation of impulse conduction in single axons of dorsal horn (66). The periodicity depended at least in part on the activity of the fiber, tending to alternate at more regular and slower intervals as impulse frequency increased. Besides cat spinal cord,

where intermittent conduction was observed again in 1973 (51), other systems show the same phenomenon of long periods of conduction alternating with periods of block, particularly at high activity rates. Intermittent conduction has been seen in rats (3,43), frog spinal cord or roots (29), crayfish and lobster (2,36), and leech giant sensory neurons (81, 82). The first explanation in terms of activity-dependent changes in threshold at the region of low conduction safety was made in 1970 (53). The threshold curves were numerically modeled using exponential functions, and a

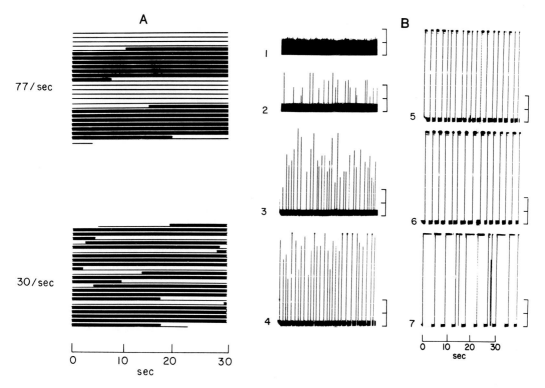

FIG. 7. Relation between impulse frequency and period of intermittent responsiveness. **A:** Records are results from experiments done on frog sciatic axons using near-threshold stimulus trains. Each sweep is 30 sec, and successive sweeps are stacked like lines of type in a book. Two long periods of conduction and three long periods of nonresponse occur during stimulation at 77/sec. At this rate successive stimuli are 13 msec apart, occurring near the maximum of superexcitability. There are six periods of conduction during the slightly shorter record made at 30 impulses/sec. Magnitude and duration of stimulus were held constant during both records. **B:** Seven records show changes in the pattern of intermittent conduction as the impulse frequency was increased for an ectodromic 1A muscle spindle afferent from a cat. Traces are composed of vertical ramps that return to zero after each conducted spike. Gaps of a few blocked impulses show up as vertical lines with length proportional to the gap duration. In record 1 the thick trace of successive ∼75-msec ramps shows that at approximately 14 impulses/sec there are no blocks. As impulse frequency progressively increased from 1 to 7, periods of conduction block appear. Brief, irregularly timed blocks occur at lower frequencies. At higher frequencies (records 4–7), the block durations are long enough to exceed maximum ramp duration (400 msec). At these frequencies (750/sec), periods of block become longer and the alternation with periods of conduction becomes more regular. Vertical time markers show height of a 100-msec ramp.

simulation was run of intermittent conduction on a visual computer graphics display (61,67, 69). This fuller account of the relation between threshold curves and intermittent conduction permitted the scripting and production of a film made from the display and presenting a detailed description of the origins of the periodicity (68).

We report here results of additional experimental studies on threshold and periodicity of intermittent conduction. Our experiments on intermittent conduction in sciatic nerve axons at artificial regions of low conduction safety were made using a point of near-threshold electrical stimulation. Conduction blocks engendered by pressure, cold, and drugs are not

stable, although they show intermittent conduction.

Figure 7 shows a very long intermittent periodicity obtained at high rates of stimulation at constant magnitude near threshold. Once conduction begins, it persists for a number of minutes. The first few blocked impulses are the harbingers of a long period of uninterrupted failed stimuli. The second record was taken of the same fiber at the same stimulus intensity and shows the effect of slowing the rate of stimulation—a decrease in period length for both phases. This same rate–periodicity correlation is shown for an intermittently conducting cat dorsal root fiber in the adjacent records.

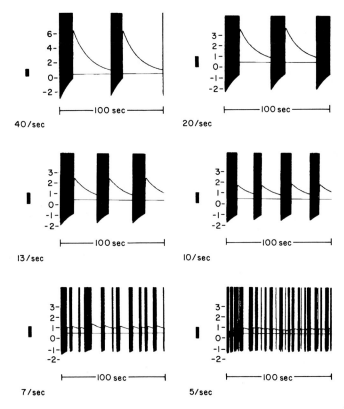

FIG. 8. Relation between stimulation rate and periodicity of threshold functions. Each record is a hard copy print from a PDP-9 programmed to give stimuli at resting threshold intensity and at the designated repetition rates to a system of exponential functions used as a numerical model of threshold curves of frog axons. Refractory and superexcitable thresholds after impulses produce the black bands. These become wider with each successful response, showing the duration of the on period. The diminishing of the maximum superexcitability during conduction shows in the cusps at the bottom of each band. Off periods are identified by the depression and recovery of threshold. Black bars to the left of each record mark the variation in stimulus duration needed to span the probabilistic region of response (65). Vertical axes are calibrated in multiples of this amount. Note the scale change at 40/sec required so that the large depression would not be off scale. (Adapted from ref. 69.)

Figure 8 shows the periodic behavior of threshold functions designed to generate threshold curves of the sort measured in frog sciatic nerve (68). Each record shows the threshold as it changes during continuous stimulation at the rate shown in the margin. During periods of conduction, depression accumulates until the threshold is too high for a successful stimulus. After the failure, the threshold climbs further and no stimulus is successful. Recovery ensues and eventually a single firing puts the next stimulus in the superexcitable phase, ensuring a new period of conduction. At low rates, neither superexcitability nor depression is very great, and the periodicity is noisy and sporadic. At higher frequencies the stimuli are closer to peak superexcitability, and more dramatic depressions develop. These two facts are accompanied by the following changes in threshold. The nearness of stimuli to peak superexcitability means that more depression must develop before becoming sufficient to offset the superexcitable aftereffects and lead to a failed spike. Thus the periods of conduction will be longer. Further, the high depressions take longer to recover, and hence the off portion of the cycle of intermittent conduction is also longer (70).

PHYSIOLOGICAL ROLE OF ACTIVITY-DEPENDENT THRESHOLD SHIFTS

Consider the results showing that threshold changes are sufficiently large to modulate conduction at regions of low conduction safety in a variety of preparations. Also recollect that the changes may persist for more than an hour, and that they bear a lawful relation to activity.

A third essential point to be discussed is that axons vary in safety factor along their length, particularly in the terminal arbors. The number of experimental studies of regions of low conduction safety seems to be steadily increasing, and the findings in a variety of systems are consistent. Regions of low conduction safety have been observed in studies of activity-dependent conduction block or delay that do not mention intermittent block (22,23,

41,52,55,72,79). Such regions do not appear to us to be preventable accidents; instead, they seem to be required for the successful operation of some systems. Surely a system less prone to failure or to interaction could have evolved than today's nervous system with its thousands of bare fine branches only 200 Å away from high-voltage fields of neighbors, each of which is fed impulses by parent fibers capable of conducting at 10 times the frequencies the daughter segments can sustain! In one example of a region of low conduction safety, the nodes of Ranvier elongate to form current sinks that generate the electric discharges of the fish *Sternarchus* by shaping the currents of the dying electromotor spikes (80; Waxman, *this volume*). In crayfish (13) and lobster (36) investigators have demonstrated that the distribution of impulses among branches of motor nerve axons changes with frequency. Although Grossman et al. wrote intriguingly of differential *information* flow, the meaning or behavioral significance, if any, of the differential blocking they observed remains difficult to prove (55). Arrangement of node position, the crucial determinant at the region of low conduction safety of the frog dorsal root ganglion (41), and variation of Na^+ channel density (71,83) are other principal ways to produce regions of slow conduction safety.

Taken together, the observations reported so far in this chapter suggest that the role of threshold shifts is to govern dynamically the connectivity of the nervous system, which in turn depends on impulse activity. More specifically, the history of impulses traveling through axonal arbors is reflected in threshold changes. These threshold changes condition the decisions of succeeding impulses as to which branches to invade. Information encoded in temporal patterns can be filtered by axon trees in this way, and study has begun of the information-handling properties of the class of time-pattern filters to which such trees belong (17,61). However, many questions remain regarding both mechanism and theory of operation.

In the next section we treat some of these questions, showing that threshold changes not only act in the differential distribution of nerve impulse trains, but they must also figure in the encoding and compilation of such trains at the initial segment.

ROLE OF THE AXON IN CODING AND DECODING

The preceding section leads directly to notions about coding. To assess those notions, we must first agree on the relevant physiological facts. When these are stated baldly, the argument that leads to the notion of coding is seen not merely as possible but necessary.

Any theory of nervous action must begin with an account of the neuron as an element. Enough is now known to set up such an account provisionally, but the kind of element that takes form is not familiar in terms of current notions of processing. This finding, however, had been expected by von Neumann, who remarked of theories about brain that "logic [may] have to undergo a pseudomorphosis to neurology to a much greater extent than the reverse."

For the argument presented here, we consider only the membrane of the neuron: the vast intracellular machinery, the genetics, metabolism, internal transport, and special biochemistry we believe to provide the forming and supporting actions that make the membrane what it is. We deal with the membrane only in terms of its electrical properties.

Ions are the charge carriers across membrane. They are imagined to pass through minute pores of channels that are species-specific. Thus mainly Na^+ passes through Na^+ pores, K^+ through K^+ pores, etc. Each Na^+ pore is like every other Na^+ pore, and the same holds for the other species-specific pore types. Each pore can be treated as a small fixed conductance over physiological ranges of voltage.

Through a patch of membrane, any specific ion conductance is given by the density of available pores for that ion. The maximum of such density is signified by a barred conductance per area, for example, $\bar{g}_{Na}$. However, under most conditions the actual density is much less, so the $g_{Na} = X\bar{g}_{Na}$, where $0 \leqslant X \leqslant 1$ and $g_K = Y\bar{g}_K$ where $0 \leqslant Y \leqslant 1$. X and Y are determined in different parts of the membrane by different factors. In keeping with Hodgkin and Huxley's formulation for axon, we use

only Na^+ and K^+ ions, comprising all other ionic species under L. As will be evident, the argument handling these two cations can be extended for more than two but does not change in character.

The only other feature that needs mention is I_p, an ionic pump, that maintains the concentration ratios across the membrane by using metabolism to move Na^+ (or Na^+ and K^+) against their concentration gradients across the membrane. The current is a function of the internal activity of Na^+ and the external activity of K^+.

A single patch of membrane in this simplified scheme then has the circuit equivalent shown in Fig. 9. V_{Na}, V_K, and V_L are assumed to be much the same everywhere along the nerve membrane. Two patches may differ intrinsically in terms of $\bar{g}_{Na}$, $\bar{g}_K$, and g_L. They differ extrinsically in terms of X and Y. For example, $X = m^3h$ and $Y = n^4$ in the Hodgkin–Huxley equations, where m, n, and h are functions of V_m and time. In subsynaptic regions, X is a function of excitatory transmitter concentration and time, and Y is a function of inhibitory transmitter and time.

It is obvious that g_{Na} and g_K are not two-terminal elements but three-terminal elements; they are governable conductances in much the same way as is any junction transistor that is run below collector saturation voltage or any field effect transistor (FET) below drain saturation voltage. In an analogous way, the governing lead may be made voltage-sensitive, pressure-sensitive, light-sensitive, and the like. Such three-terminal devices are simple amplifiers if, as in this case, there is a power gain between input and output.

A single membrane patch is then potentially

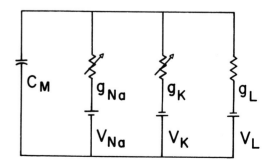

FIG. 9. Single patch of membrane.

capable of performing any operation that can be had from using, at most, two discrete amplifiers; e.g., it can build (a) a blocking oscillator, as is the case for axonal membrane; (b) a bistable flip-flop, as occurs in certain invertebrate neurons; or (c) a simple amplifier that transduces concentration of substances as occurs in subsynaptic patches. One can imagine many such engines. However, these active circuits divide into two types—regenerative devices such as produce pulses or are bistable, and simple amplifiers.

Any neuron can now be divided into two regions—the receiver and the distributor. This division cannot always be set anatomically (e.g., as for amacrine cells), but otherwise it is fairly obvious for most neurons. The receiver is that region over which most patches are simple amplifiers, and both X and Y are governed by influences external to the membrane. The distributor is that region over which most patches are regenerative devices, and both X and Y are governed by functions of the membrane voltage. The latter is usually called "electrically excitable membrane" and the former "electrically inexcitable membrane." The term "electrically inexcitable" is a little misleading for it covers two conditions: (a) where neither X nor Y can be changed; and (b) when X or Y can be changed but are not regeneratively coupled to each other.

The distributor is clearly the axon and teledendron. The receiver is the cell body and dendrites of a central neuron or a sensillum, e.g., a pressure receptor or a stretch receptor. Conceive an imaginary neuron, much stripped down, so that it consists of a single long tubular dendrite connected to a single long tubular axon. The physical image in Fig. 10 then corresponds to the circuit analog shown.

On the left is the dendrite on which synapses end in great profusion so that a dendritic segment between the dotted lines is a mosaic of subsynaptic patches. At the right is the axon, also shown as segmented. The unit patch of axon is P_A, the unit patch of dendrite is P_D; and the dendrite and axon are connected by a transitional region. The description of P_A is the Hodgkin–Huxley formulation or any of its variants which are species-dependent. The description of P_D is simple but needs explanation.

Each synapse on the dendrite is either *excitatory* or *inhibitory*. On receiving an impulse, an excitatory synapse transiently exerts an influence, and the X of the corresponding subsynaptic patch transiently measures how much of that influence the patch gets. Similarly, an inhibitory synapse transiently exerts another influence, and the Y of the corresponding subsynaptic patch transiently measures how much of that influence it gets. Let all of the excitatory responses be more or less similar to each other in terms of effect on X, and all inhibitory responses be similar to each other with respect to effects on Y. Then we can define a g_E as the unit change in an excitatory patch and g_I as the unit change in an inhibitory patch. In a dendritic segment the excitement of all excitatory patches can be expressed as a limit Na^+ conductance ($\bar{G}_E$) and excitement of all inhibitory patches as a limit K^+ conductance ($\bar{G}_I$). Whereupon, in a dendrite segment, X_D is the fraction of all E patches excited and Y_D the fraction of all I patches excited.

In the circuit diagram, G_D and G_A are each the sum of external and internal conductances between adjacent segments of dendrite and axon, respectively.

Given that the resting membrane of the dendrite has the same V_M as that of resting axon, changing X_D has a somewhat different effect from changing Y_D. An increase in Y_D alone acts mainly as a shunt with a small attendant current flowing outward through that segment and inward everywhere else. The current is small because V_M is close to V_K. An increase in X_D alone also gives a decreased impedance,

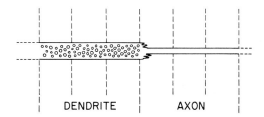

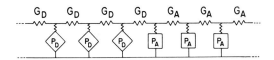

FIG. 10. Simplified scheme of junction between receiver (dendrite) and distributor (axon).

but the change is attended by a proportionately much larger current flowing inward through that segment and outward everywhere else. The current is large because V_M is fairly removed from V_{Na}.

However, we cannot deal with isolated segments and steady-state E and I but with segments strung together to make a transmission line and with transient E and I events. Handling such a line analytically is not a pleasant job if segments differ in X_D and Y_D as well as $\overline{G}_E$ and $\overline{G}_I$. Thus to calculate the current flow through the initial segment of axon and to calculate the dendritic impedance loading that segment is not at all appealing.

At this point, the physiologist as quondam physicist is assailed by a great temptation. Because there are so very many synapses on the dendrite, is it not easiest to assume that the relative densities of E and I change uniformly everywhere? That assumption of homogeneity makes tractable, if only barely, the problem of calculating the current through the initial segment of axon and its time course as well as the impedance seen from the initial segment and its time course. The temptation must be resisted.

The assumption of homogeneity flies in the face of anatomy, for it is generally true that synapses of different provenance are distributed differently over the dendrite so that inputs from one set of fibers may barely overlap those from another set (e.g., consider the apical dendrites of the large pyramidal cells in cortex or the dendritic arborizations of retinal ganglion cells in the inner plexiform layer). The different inputs, furthermore, need not be correlated in activity. Thus the assumption of homogeneity, although giving solutions, applies to no practical case of an extended dendrite.

The axon terminates this varying and nonuniform transmission line with a regenerative active element that itself is mutable by its own history, as the first part of this chapter shows. Axon membrane is described electrically by Hodgkin and Huxley's model, wherein $X = m^3h$ and $Y = n^4$. The three functions of V_M (m, n, and h) are dimensionless and vary between 0 and 1. Both m and n vary directly with V_M, and h varies inversely with V_M. All three are sigmoid and go from 0.1 to 0.9 in a few centivolts. The function $1 - h$ is twice as

steep as m and reaches its 0.5 value several centivolts below the 0.5 value of m^3. The time it takes for each of the three functions to adopt its new value on incremental change of V_M is also a function of V_M, but this settling time is much shorter for m than for n or h.

In this scheme $m^3h(\bar{g}_{Na})$ is a transient negative conductance, for if V_M is driven incrementally toward V_{Na} m increases, bootstrapping the change, whereas h (decreasing, but more slowly in time) damps out the effect. Thus $m^3h(\bar{g}_{Na})$ is a frequency-dependent negative conductance, with h providing the low-frequency cutoff. (That is why Cole's impedance-versus-frequency plots show an inductive loop at the high-frequency end, for that is what a $-g/C$ looks like.)

The terminating of the receiver by the regenerative axon then specifies a resonant system whose periods depend not only on m, n, and h and their time behavior but on the receiver acting as tank circuit for the axon. The interval between pulses reflects not only the current passing across the axon membrane but also the states of the receiver. Yet for all the precision with which we may know the parts and how they are connected, an exact account of the receiver as seen from its port to the axon is neither useful nor needed. Furthermore, given the first half of this chapter, which shows how mutable the axon is, computing the current–voltage–time relations in such a coupled system becomes an expensive folly. At this point it is better to conceive of crude guiding notions rather than interminable computations.

There is no familiar model for the device that is shown. The dendrite itself, as seen from the axon, behaves as a variable voltage generator with a variable internal impedance. All dendritic states that have the same Thevenin equivalence are indistinguishable for the axon, isomeric. Yet, because the axonal spike is followed by a long recovery cycle that changes the threshold and shaping factors for the next spike, two long, identical running histories of current across the axon membrane will not specify the same sequence of spike intervals unless the concurrent running histories of the impedance are the same in the Thevenin equivalent of the dendrite. Even if the history of both current and impedance is nicely periodic, the same periodicity need not show in the axonal time series of pulses, but rather some subharmonic regularity. That is all that is sufficient to show that running histories of pulse interval encode running histories of dendritic states, not in any precise, analytical way but certainly with more discrimination than present opinion admits. To put it briefly, because any pulse interval in the axon reflects the history of what leads to it as well as the present state, the history of states must be distributed over the history of pulse intervals and is vaguely encoded therein.

However, the dendrite shown, for all the care we have taken to lay it out, is an improperly stripped-down version of a real dendrite. The receiver does not consist exclusively of subsynaptic patches but has a complement of axon-like membrane as well. We know this by two observations. First, dendrites can show oscillations at a fair distance from the axon, and, under pathological conditions (e.g., poor impalement by a microelectrode) these oscillations can become pronounced and spike-like, signifying local damage. Second, a spike initiated in the axon can spread decrementally up into the dendrites as if there were some local regeneration but not enough to sustain a propagating spike. The presence of such intrinsically regenerative components in the membrane of the receiver makes the picture more complex and interesting. Now the spectrum for axonal pulse intervals may show contingent "forbidden" regions (as actually occur in our studies of retinal ganglion cells in the frog) and a variety of other such effects of nonlinear coupling in the dendrite. In turn, these effects, rather than increasing the messiness, can be used to sharpen the coding and its style as if the axon can more distinctly resolve the history of dendritic states because those states themselves have also become more history-dependent.

Note that it is not necessary to import the latter, more realistic model of the dendrite to treat the axonal time series of pulses as a meaningful, if not easily analyzed, code. The weakest possible assumptions about the dendrite as embodied in the first description, are enough. For both models it is the case that, if the multicausality behind the time series of axonal pulses is lawful, the time series itself is a lawful representation of those causes. In this

view, the time series is complex; it cannot be noisy, whatever its spectrum.

Yet if the running message of a neuron is distributed over the running sequence of pulse intervals, any reading system will need a memory. The subsynaptic patches of the next neurons respond only with unit transients that last a few milliseconds, and there is in them no memory beyond the short time course of such transients to distinguish one message from another. This is, of course, the problem that was treated in earlier works from this laboratory (17,59,61). For what was shown there is proof of an element which, taken iteratively, parses time series or, rather, distinguishes phrases of pulse intervals in a reliable way. In effect, the teledendron is a shaped filter in the time domain. Let us review how that comes to be.

A bifurcation of an axon is often a region of lowered safety factor. This lowering may be due in part to geometrical reasons (e.g., the sudden increase of membrane loading at a bifurcation) and in part to changes in the density of Na^+ pores. Whatever the cause, a bifurcation often acts as a two-bit switch, wherein one branch or the other (or both or neither) can be invaded by an oncoming impulse. The switch state is a function of time since the last invasion; i.e., there is a postspike exaltation and depression for each branch quite as for the parent fiber. The time sequence of threshold for a branch after firing is a function, in part, of its diameter. Branchings are seldom symmetrical. Furthermore, in a teledendron the branching-out forms a tapered tree.

In such a system, a first impulse invading the teledendron occupies some subtree. The next impulse that comes along invades another subtree, and that subtree is contingent in form on the first subtree invaded and the time between first and second pulses. The third impulse invades a subtree contingent on the subtree to the second impulse and time from the second impulse, and also on the subtree to the first impulse and time from the first. The result is that the subset of terminals of a teledendron occupied by a pulse reflects the sequence of pulse intervals leading to that pulse. This kind of system can be modeled on a computer. It is interesting to note that over a wide range, whatever rules one uses for the bifurcations, a tree inevitably "parses" time series in the sense of providing different pattern sequences of terminal invasions for different time series of input pulses.

Although this system sounds almost tractable, unfortunately it is not. Experiments on animals and computer models show that contingency at a bifurcation also depends on external influences. So, for example, the passage of current from neighboring trees through a bifurcation changes, as it should, the switching bias. Thus the figure of excited terminals from one teledendron in a neuropil reflects not only the history of its own invasion but the history and present state of neighbors, so that the message is altered by context. In this case we can only revert to the argument that regularities in action and interaction result in stylistic and contingent representations, but heaven alone knows how they are to be read by an external observer.

Suppose in our model neuron the receiver were very small, perhaps no more than the sensitive surface of a pressure, tension, or taste transducer, and only variable in the excitatory channel. The state of the receiver can then be represented by an elementary circuit— a voltage source with a variable internal impedance. The influence it would have on the initial segment would be direct and tightly coupled. The axon's response would then be expected to be a regular oscillation (perhaps intermittent) whose frequency is governed by the receiver and precisely expresses the state of the receiver. As the receiver grows in length and complexity and the number of influences playing on it increases, as the influences (inhibitory and excitatory) become ordered along the dendrite and some local regeneration occurs, pulse interval becomes less and less regular. One is not surprised to get a multicausal chatter that vaguely expresses, in the morphically based style of the neuron, the passing state of the receiver.

From an informational point of view, the best that a neuron can do is report the state of its own receiver; and the more states it can discriminate in its report, the better. However, since the nerve spike is essentially all-or-none, the only usable parameter for the report is time between spikes. Thus the longer

time it takes to report a state, the less temporal resolution is had of states; whereas the shorter the time for a message, the fewer states can be expressed. Furthermore, there is no way of expressing different states except by different time patterns. These constraints, together with the general rules for making codes, impel us to believe that in a short run any neuron with large receiver will look "noisy," but in a long run will show statistical regularities in densities and sequences of intervals that constitute a style by means of which one can read the passing state of the receiver (17).

These time series of pulse intervals are, in a manner of speaking, phrased in terms of markers which are the running account of longest pulse intervals, and the duration of the markers as well as the fine structure of activity between those markers carry the discrimination of states (17). Such phrased sequences of pulse intervals, whether regular or complex, can then be "parsed" by the teledendron, which acts as an interval-dependent switching system in the simplest case (e.g., the fiber to the opening muscle of the crayfish claw) or as a message classifier and distributor in more complex cases.

The self-same axonal mechanism encodes at one end the passing state of the receiver into a time series and at the other end converts the running history of the time series into a running sequence of different spatial distributions of active endings. Conceive all the terminals attributable to a single fiber to be laid out on a surface, and every time a terminal is invaded it gives a visible sign. Then, by this argued action of the teledendron, each impulse brings into view a subset or display, which, like an ideogram, expresses by its form (distribution) the recent history of pulse intervals in the context of the interval just terminated by the illuminating pulse.

This image of the neuron is not speculative. It emerges by necessity from the nature of axonal membrane, subsynaptic patches, and bifurcations. However, by this system the time series of pulse intervals takes on the character of a natural language in that the message carried is multicausal. From such a view, neurons are distinctly not logical elements, at least by the current notions of what is logic.

ACKNOWLEDGMENTS

This research was supported in part by the National Institutes of Health (research grant 3 R01 EY01149) and in part by the Bell Telephone Laboratories, Inc.

REFERENCES

1. Adrian, E. D. (1921): The recovery process of excitable tissues. Part II. *J. Physiol. (Lond)*, 55:193–225.
2. Bammann, S., Franck, J., and Raymond, S. A. (1974): Nerve spike conduction block in crayfish motor-neuron axon branches. *Res. Lab. Electronics (MIT) Q. Prog. Rep.*, 112: 132.
3. Barron, D. H. (1940): Central course of 're-current' sensory discharges. *J. Neurophysiol.*, 3:403–406.
4. Barron, D. H., and Matthews, B. H. C. (1935): Intermittent conduction in the spinal cord. *J. Physiol. (Lond)*, 85:73–103.
5. Baylor, D. A., and Nicholls, J. G. (1969): After effects of nerve impulses on signalling in the central nervous system of the leech. *J. Physiol. (Lond)*, 203:571–589.
6. Beall, J. E., Applebaum, A. E., Foreman, R. D., and Willis, W. D. (1977): Spinal cord potentials evoked by cutaneous afferents in the monkey. *J. Neurophysiol.*, 40:199–211.
7. Bekesy, G. von (1947): A new audiometer. *Acta Otolaryngol. (Stockh.)*, 35:411–422.
8. Bennett, M. V. L., Hille, B., and Obara, S. (1970): Voltage threshold in excitable cells depends on stimulus form. *J. Neurophysiol.*, 33:585–594.
9. Berkenblit, M. B. (1971): The periodic blocking of impulses in excitable tissues. In: *Models of the Structural-Functional Organization of Certain Biological Systems,* edited by I. M. Gelfand with V. S. Gurfinkel, S. V. Fornin, and M. L. Trettin. Translated by R. Beard. Maple Press, M.I.T., Cambridge.
10. Binder, M. (1975): Effects of temperature on nervous threshold. MS thesis, M.I.T.
11. Binder, M. H., and Raymond, S. A. (1975): Some effects of temperature changes on the threshold of frog sciatic nerve fibers. *Rep. Res. Lab. Electronics MIT*, 116:281–287.
12. Binder, M. Y., and Raymond, S. A. (1975): Effect of temperature upon threshold changes following impulses in frog nerve fibers. *Neurosci. Abstr.*, p. 604.
13. Bittner, G. D. (1968): Differentiation of nerve terminals in crayfish opener muscle and its functional significance. *J. Gen. Physiol.*, 51:731–758.
14. Boyle, P. J., and Conway, E. J. (1941): Potassium accumulation in muscle and associated changes. *J. Physiol. (Lond)*, 100:1–63.
15. Buchthal, F., and Engbaek, L. (1963): Refractory period and conduction velocity of the striated muscle fiber. *Acta Physiol. Scand.*, 59:199–220.
16. Bullock, T. H. (1951): Facilitation of conduction rate in nerve fibres. *J. Physiol. (Lond)*, 114:89–97.
17. Chung, S. H., Raymond, S. A., and Lettvin, J. Y. (1970): Multiple meaning in single visual units. *Brain Behav. Evol.*, 3:72–101.
18. Connelly, C. M. (1959): Recovery processes and metabolism of nerve. In: *Biophysical Science,* edited by J. L. Oncley. Wiley, New York.
19. Cordingley, G., and Somjen, G. (1976): Clearance of locally accumulated extracellular potassium in the spinal cord of cats. *Neurosci. Abstr.*
20. Dudek, F. E., and Blankenship, J. E. (1976): Neuroendocrine (bag) cells of Aplysia: Spike blockade and a mechanism for potentiation. *Science*, 192:1009–1010.
21. Dun, F. T. (1951): Studies on the conduction of sensory impulses through the dorsal root ganglion in the frog. *J. Cell Comp. Physiol.*, 38:131–133.
22. Dun, F. T. (1954): Blockage of impulses in the dorsal root ganglion by curare. *J. Cell Comp. Physiol.*, 44:322–324.
23. Dun, F. T. (1955): The delay and blockage of sensory impulses in the dorsal root ganglion. *J. Physiol. (Lond)*, 127:252–264.
24. Eccles, J. C. (1964): *The Physiology of Synapses,* pp. 220–232. Springer-Verlag, New York.
25. Erlanger, J., and Gasser, H. S. (1937): *Electrical Signs of Nervous Activity.* University of Pennsylvania Press, Philadelphia.
26. Evans, C. L. (1956): *Principles of Human Physiology,* 12th ed., p. 184. Churchill, London.
27. Fitzhugh, R. (1966): Theoretical effect of temperature on threshold in the Hodgkin Huxley nerve model. *J. Gen. Physiol.*, 49: 989–1005.
28. Frankenhauser, B., and Hodgkin, A. L. (1956): The after-effects of impulses in the giant nerve fibres of Loligo. *J. Physiol. (Lond)*, 131:341–376.
29. Fuortes, M. G. F. (1950): Action of strychnine on the "intermittent conduction" of impulses along dorsal columns of the spinal cord of frogs. *J. Physiol. (Lond)*, 112:42P.
30. Gardner-Medwin, A. R. (1972): An extreme supernormal period in cerebellar parallel fibres. *J. Physiol. (Lond)*, 222:357–371.
31. Gasser, H. S. (1937): The excitability cycle. In: *Electrical Signs of Nervous Activity,* edited by J. Erlanger and H. S. Gasser. University of Pennsylvania Press, Philadelphia.
32. Gasser, H. S., and Grundfest, H. (1936): Action and excitability in mammalian A fibers. *Am. J. Physiol.*, 117:113–133.

33. Gilliatt, R. W., and Willison, R. G. (1963): The refractory and supernormal periods of the human median nerve. *J. Neurol. Neurosurg. Psychiatry*, 26:136–143.

34. Graham, H. T. (1934): Supernormality, a modification of the recovery process in nerve. *Am. J. Physiol.*, 110:225–242.

35. Graham, H. T., and Lorente de Nó, R. (1938): Recovery of blood-perfused mammalian nerves. *Am. J. Physiol.*, 123:326–340.

36. Grossman, Y., Spira, M. E., and Parnas, I. (1973): Differential flow of information into branches of a single axon. *Brain Res.*, 64:379–386.

37. Grundfest, H., and Magnes, J. (1951): Excitability changes in dorsal roots produced by electrotonic effects from adjacent efferent activity. *Am. J. Physiol.*, 164:502–508.

38. Habgood, J. S. (1953): Antidromic impulses in the dorsal roots. *J. Physiol. (Lond)*, 121:264–274.

39. Hodgkin, A. L., and Huxley, A. F. (1952): A quantitative description of membrane current and its application to conduction and excitation in nerve. *J. Physiol. (Lond)*, 117:500–544.

40. Howland, B., Lettvin, J. Y., McCulloch, W. S., Pitts, W. H., and Wall, P. D. (1955): Reflex inhibition by dorsal root interaction. *J. Neurophysiol.*, 17:1–17.

41. Ito, M., and Takahashi, I. (1960): Impulse conduction through spinal ganglion. In: *Electrical Activity of Single Cells*, edited by Y. Katsuki. Ikagu Shoin, Tokyo.

42. Kerkut, G. A., and York, B. (1971): *The Electrogenic Sodium Pump*. Scientechnica, Bristol.

43. Krnjević, K., and Miledi, R. (1959): Presynaptic failure of neuromuscular propagation in rats. *J. Physiol. (Lond)*, 149:1–22.

44. Krnjević, K., and Morris, M. E. (1974): Extracellular accumulation of K^+ evoked by activity of primary afferent fibers in the cuneate nucleus and dorsal horn of cats. *Can. J. Physiol. Pharmacol.*, 52:852–871.

45. Krnjević, K., and Morris, M. E. (1975): Correlation between extracellular focal potentials and K^+ potentials evoked by primary afferent activity. *Can. J. Physiol. Pharmacol.*, 53:912–922.

46. Krnjević, K., and Morris, M. E. (1975): Factors determining the decay of K^+ potentials and focal potentials in the central nervous system. *Can. J. Physiol. Pharmacol.*, 53:923–934.

47. Lass, Y., and Abeles, N. (1975): Transmission of information by the axon. 1. Noise and memory in the myelinated nerve fiber of the frog. *Biol. Cybernet.*, 19:61–67.

48. Lorente de Nó, R. (1947): *A Study of Nerve Physiology*, Vols. I and II. Studies from the Rockefeller Institute, Vols. 131 and 132. Rockefeller Institute, New York.

49. Lorente de Nó, R., and Graham, H. T. (1936): Recovery of mammalian nerve fibres in vivo. *Proc. Soc. Exp. Biol. Med.*, 33:512–514.

50. Lucas, K. (1917): *The Conduction of the Nervous Impulse*. Longmans Green, London.

51. Matheson, G. K., and Wurster, R. D. (1973): Analysis of spike activity of the dorsal root reflex. *Neurosci. Abstr.*, p. 103.

52. Morris, M. E. (1971): The action of carbon dioxide on synaptic transmission in the cuneate nucleus. *J. Physiol. (Lond)*, 218:671–689.

53. Newman, E. A., and Raymond, S. A. (1971): Activity dependent shifts in excitability of frog peripheral nerve axons. *Q. Prog. Rep. Res. Lab. Electronics MIT*, 102:165–189.

54. Oswald, R. E., and Freeman, J. A. (1976): Extracellular potassium changes associated with the control of retinotectal synaptic transmission in Bufo marinus. *Neurosci. Abstr.*, p. 995.

55. Paintal, A. S. (1973): Conduction in mammalian nerve fibres. In: *New Developments in Electromyography and Clinical Neurophysiology*, Vol. 2, edited by J. E. Desmedt, pp. 19–41. Karger, Basel.

56. Parnas, I. (1972): Differential block at high frequency of branches of a single axon innervating two muscles. *J. Neurophysiol.*, 35:903–914.

57. Pecher, C. (1939): La fluctuation d'excitabilité de la fibre nerveuse. *Arch. Int. Physiol.*, 49:129–152.

58. Poussart, D. J-M. (1965): Measurements of latency distributions in peripheral nerve fibers. M.S. thesis, MIT.

59. Raymond, S. A. (1969): Physioiogical influences on axonal conduction and distribution of nerve impulses. Ph.D. thesis, MIT.

60. Raymond, S. A. (1974): Description and characterization of threshold changes in frog peripheral nerve axons. *Q. Prog. Rep. Res. Lab. Electronics MIT*, 112:130.

61. Raymond, S. A. (1974): Distribution of nerve impulses among branches of axonal trees. *Q. Prog. Rep. Res. Lab. Electronics MIT*, 112:130.

62. Raymond, S. A. (1976): The effect of ion pump poisons on threshold curves of frog sciatic nerve. *Neurosci. Abstr.*, p. 417.

63. Raymond, S. A. (1977): Fluctuation of threshold in frog sciatic axons during subliminal stimulation and firing in adjacent fibres. Submitted.

64. Raymond, S. A. (1977): Effects of nerve impulses on threshold of frog sciatic nerve fibres. Submitted.

65. Raymond, S. A., Binder, M. J., Odette, L. L., and Lettvin, J. Y. (1975): Membrane processes. *Prog. Rep. Res. Lab. Electronics MIT*, 115:317–318.

66. Raymond, S. A., and Lettvin, J. Y. (1969): Influences on axonal conduction. *Q. Prog. Rep. Res. Lab. Electronics MIT*, 92:431–435.

67. Raymond, S. A., and Pangaro, P. (1974): Development of a model frog nerve showing threshold oscillations. *Q. Prog. Rep. Res. Lab. Electronics MIT,* 112:129–130.

68. Raymond, S. A., and Pangaro, P. (1975): *Nerve Threshold and Intermittent Conduction.* Color film, 17 min. Research Lab. Electronics, Copyright MIT. Distributed by MetaMetrics, Carlisle, Mass.

69. Raymond, S. A., and Pangaro, P. (1975): Explanation of intermittent conduction based on activity dependent changes in nerve threshold. *Q. Prog. Rep. Res. Lab. Electronics MIT,* 116:273–281.

70. Raymond, S. A., and Pangaro, P. (1977): Intermittent conduction arising from activity induced changes in nerve threshold. Submitted.

71. Ritchie, J. M., and Rogart, R. B. (1977): The density of sodium channels in mammalian myelinated fibers and the nature of the axonal membrane under the myelin sheath. *Proc. Natl. Acad. Sci.,* 74:211–215.

72. Smith, D. O., and Hatt, H. (1976): Axon conduction block in a region of dense connective tissue in crayfish. *J. Neurophysiol.,* 39:794–801.

73. Spear, J. F., and Moore, E. N. (1974): Supernormal excitability and conduction in the His-Purkinje system of the dog. *Circ. Res.,* 35:782–792.

74. Straub, R. W. (1961): On the mechanism of post-tetanic hyperpolarization in myelinated nerve fibres from the frog. *J. Physiol. (Lond),* 159:19–20P.

75. Swadlow, H. A. (1974): Systematic variations in the conduction velocity of slowly conducting axons in the rabbit corpus callosum. *Exp. Neurol.,* 43:445–451.

76. Swadlow, H. A., and Waxman, S. G. (1976): Variations in conduction velocity and excitability following single and multiple impulses of visual callosal axons in the rabbit. *Exp. Neurol.,* 53:128–150.

77. Toennies, J. F. (1938): Reflex discharge from the spinal cord over the dorsal roots. *J. Neurophysiol.,* 1:378–390.

78. Toennies, J. F. (1939): Conditioning of afferent impulses by reflex discharges over the dorsal roots. *J. Neurophysiol.,* 2:515–525.

79. Van Essen, D. C. (1973): The contribution of membrane hyperpolarization to adaptation and conduction block in sensory neurons of the leech. *J. Physiol. (Lond),* 230:509–549.

80. Waxman, S. G., Pappas, G. D., and Bennett, M. V. L. (1972): Morphological correlates of functional differentiation of nodes of Ranvier along single fibers in neurogenic electric organ of the knife fish, Sternarchus. *J. Cell Biol.,* 53:210–224.

81. Yau, K-W. (1975): Conduction block at branch points of sensory neurons in leech CNS. *Neurosci. Abstr.,* p. 583.

82. Yau, K-W. (1976): Receptive fields, geometry and conduction block of sensory neurones in the central nervous system of the leech. *J. Physiol. (Lond),* 263:513–538.

83. Zeevi, Y. (1972): Structural functional relationships in single neurons: Scanning electron microscopy and theoretical studies. Ph.D. thesis, University of California, Berkeley.

84. Zucker, R. S. (1974): Excitability changes in crayfish motor nerve terminals. *J. Physiol. (Lond),* 241:111–126.

Physiology and Pathobiology of Axons, edited by
S. G. Waxman. Raven Press, New York © 1978.

Models of Conduction in Nonuniform Axons

Steven S. Goldstein

*Zimmerman Medical Clinic, and Department of Neurology, University of Texas, Medical School
at Houston, Houston, Texas 77054*

Most previous theoretical or computational treatments of action potential propagation have assumed uniform electrical and geometric properties along the length of the nerve membrane. Any irregularity in the velocity or shape of the action potential has been dismissed as an "end effect." These analyses have yielded much insight into the mechanisms of propagation and suggest a constant action potential shape and velocity. This velocity is predicted to vary with the square root (13) of axonal diameter (in nonmyelinated nerve) or linearly (9,15) with axonal diameter (in myelinated nerve).

More recently, experimenters have noted several results that are not in agreement with this theory. In areas of axonal branching, axonal propagation has been noted to proceed in one branch and not to the other (12,31; Raymond and Lettvin, *this volume*). Impulse conduction has also been noted to vary with the previous history of impulse conduction along the fiber (29; Swadlow and Waxman, *this volume*). Changes in the shape of the action potential have also been noted (3,7,10,11,21). Fiber diameter has not always been a reliable predictor of velocity (24).

Because of these observations, it would be useful to explore theoretically and computationally the effect of branching and other nonuniform geometries in the propagation of the action potential. Thus one could try to separate the effects of changes in electrical–chemical properties of the nerve from the effect of geometry. Such computations have been performed by several groups (4,8,17,18,22) and have shown that, depending on the type and the degree of geometric change, the action potential can slow down, speed up, or remain unchanged as it approaches a region of geometric change; also, it can fail to propagate or can continue with or without delay. Under certain conditions it can propagate both forward and backward from this region.

These predictions have been obtained by numerical solution of the Hodgkin–Huxley model (17) or of a simpler, yet related model —the VEJ model—devised by Rall. See Goldstein and Rall (8) for further details. The effects of geometry are reflected in the boundary conditions. What follows is an analysis of the expected changes in action potential propagation for the geometries shown in longitudinal section in Fig. 1. Correlation with experiment and experimental models is then attempted.

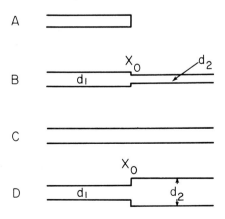

FIG. 1. Summary of the geometric regions considered, shown in longitudinal section.

THEORETICAL AND COMPUTATIONAL RESULTS

Case of Membrane Cylinder with Sealed End

A sealed end implies that no current can leak across the "seal" closing the cylinder (Fig. 1A). Mathematically, this implies that the voltage gradient at this point is zero. Katz and Miledi (16) noted that exactly the same condition occurs at the point of action potential collision. Figure 2 depicts a computed action potential as it travels from left to right toward the sealed end (or toward the point of collision with a second action potential, not shown, traveling in the opposite direction). The curves in the figure show the action potential at six equally spaced points along the cylinder. From left to right, these curves show a decreasing temporal displacement; i.e, it arrives at each successive point faster. In addition, the shape changes as the action potential approaches the sealed end; the peak voltage increases, and the half-width narrows.

An understanding of these changes may be obtained by reviewing the computations. One notes that far from the boundary or point of collision, the leading core current[1] flows downstream for a considerable distance and crosses the nerve membrane at relatively low current density. The sealed end blocks core current from traveling downstream further. Thus the core current builds up in the vicinity of the block and is forced to cross the nerve membrane at a relatively high current density. This causes a more rapid membrane depolarization than "normal" and a more rapid attainment of threshold, implying an increased velocity.[2] Also, the increase in local current augments the amplitude of the peak.

Step Reduction in Diameter

A cross section of this geometry is shown in Fig. 1B. Figure 3 shows the changes in the shape and velocity of the action potential near X_0, the point of a step reduction in diameter, as computed using the VEJ model. The dashed curves show a reference action potential in a uniform cylinder of the initial diameter. The action potential (solid curves) speeds up, increases in peak voltage, and becomes narrower as it approaches X_0. These changes are similar to those of the sealed end but lesser in degree. After passing X_0, it slows to the slower velocity corresponding to the smaller diameter as expected (13). Similar changes in velocity have also been calculated from a square wave potential (23) and using the Hodgkin–Huxley equations (17).

Figure 4 shows the same action potential in the distance domain. Instead of recording the action potential at a given location as voltage versus time, we are enabled by our simulation to take a "snapshot" of the action potential. Each curve of Fig. 4 is a recording of voltage versus distance at a given instant of time.

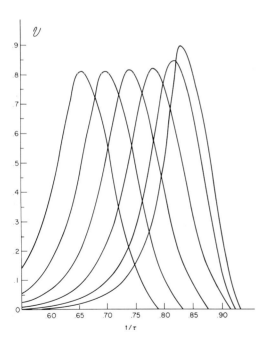

FIG. 2. Computed action potential approaching a sealed end. Each shape represents the action potential, "recorded" in time, at six equally spaced locations along the cylinder.

---

[1] Core current is that current which flows longitudinally along the axon (or core conductor) and is generated by the longitudinal voltage gradient along the nerve membrane.

[2] One must be careful when discussing "velocity" of a wave whose shape is changing (8). In this chapter we are referring to the velocity of the voltage peak as it moves from one point to another. Note that the peak voltage itself may change in amplitude from point to point.

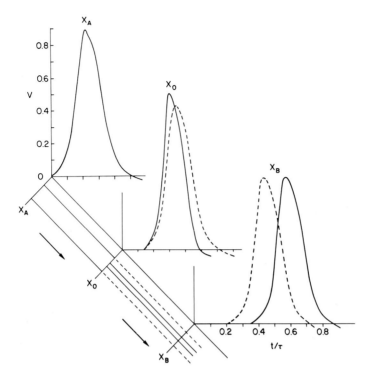

FIG. 3. Computed action potential for a step reduction (at X_0) of cylindrical diameter. Propagation is in the direction of the arrows. The shape is "recorded" in time at X_A, X_0, and X_B. The closed curves show the action potential as it would appear had no step reduction in diameter occurred. τ is a constant (membrane time constant) which need not concern us here.

Action potential propagation is from left to right. Note the rather remarkable changes in shape near X_0. In addition to velocity and peak voltage changes, slopes and half-width change rather dramatically. The discontinuity of slope occurs because of the sudden change in core resistance and the physical constraint that both current and voltage must be continuous. The progressively narrower half-width can be seen to occur because of the relatively slow movement of the rising phase of the action potential as it enters the region of smaller diameter.

One concludes that the action potential never fails (for geometric reasons) to enter a region of smaller diameter. Also, one suspects from these data that a subthreshold wave mov-

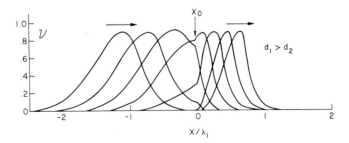

FIG. 4. Computed action potential for a step reduction (at X_0) of cylindrical diameter. A longitudinal section of the geometric region is shown in Figs. 1B and 3. Propagation is from left to right as shown by the arrows. Each shape is a "snapshot" (a plot of voltage versus distance) of the action potential at equal time intervals. λ_1 is a constant (length constant) which does not concern us here.

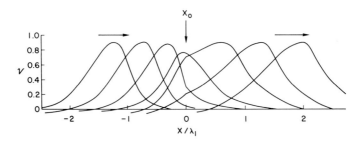

FIG. 5. Computed action potential for a step increase (at X_0) of cylindrical diameter. A longitudinal section of the geometric region is shown in Fig. 1D. Propagation is from left to right as shown by the arrows. Each shape is a "snapshot" (a plot of voltage versus distance) of the action potential at equal time intervals. λ_1 is a constant (length constant) which does not concern us here.

ing passively toward X_0 might reach threshold near X_0.

Step Increase of Diameter

In this situation (Fig. 1D) simulations show that the velocity of the action potential slows as one approaches the point of diameter change (8,17,23,33). However, qualitative differences occur depending on the amount of step increase.

For very large increases in diameter, propagation failed. In fact, failure of propagation occurs before the point of step increase and will fail at greater distances from X_0 for greater increases in diameter. The actual point of failure depends on the degree of the membrane excitability as well as the definition of failure.[3] Even though "failure" occurs, a subthreshold wave of decreasing amplitude spreads farther. This does not spread "electrotonically" because potentials near threshold do evoke some excitatory conductance change and a corresponding increment in transmembrane voltage. Since this increment is not self-sustaining, its spread may be referred to as decremental conduction.

For smaller increases in diameter, failure

---

[3] Failure of the action potential usually means failure to reach "threshold" at any particular location. In a propagating action potential, it is difficult to define threshold voltage because both excitatory and inhibitory conductance changes are taking place in time. Thus a given voltage may be above "threshold" if depolarization occurs rapidly but below threshold if depolarization occurs slowly. Various conventions may be used to define failure.

does not occur but conduction velocity initially slows and more complicated changes in shape are seen. Figure 5 illustrates these changes with a step increase in diameter at X_0. Each curve shown is the action potential voltage distribution (in distance) at equal time intervals. Propagation is from left to right. The velocity decrease as one approaches X_0 is illustrated by the decreasing displacement of the peak. The fall in peak voltage is shown slightly in the third and maximally in the fourth wave from the right. Most remarkable, however, is the change in shape illustrated by the fifth curve from the right. The almost flat top implies that the entire region immediately distal to X_0 reached threshold almost simultaneously. This may be viewed as a consequence of the slowing of velocity just proximal to X_0. During this slowing, there is a greater time for subthreshold electronic spread distal to X_0. The resulting distribution of subthreshold voltage becomes more uniform than usual, and threshold would be reached more synchronously as well. This implies a large increase in velocity as the wave passes X_0, followed by slowing to the constant velocity appropriate to the diameter of the larger cylinder.

An intermediate behavior was noted when the step increase in diameter was not quite great enough to cause failure. This is illustrated in Fig. 6. Here the action potential slows as it approaches X_0; the peak height falls as the peak passes X_0, and it is approximately threshold. After a delay, the potential reaches threshold and is able to continue forward propagation; however, it is also able to propagate in the reverse direction. In this example, the delay

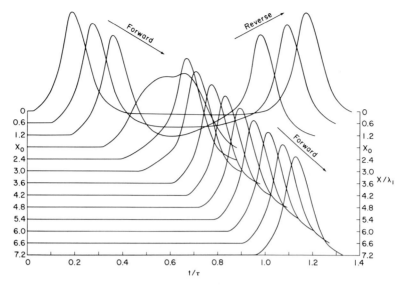

FIG. 6. Forward and reverse propagation of a computed action potential in a region of step increase. The potentials are "recorded" in time at successive locations indicated on the vertical scale, with X_0 being the point of step increase. λ_1 and τ are constants which do not concern us here.

is sufficiently long to exceed the refractory period for the membrane of the smaller cylinder. Thus, the action potential is able to propagate in both directions. If the delay is slightly less, the reverse wave occurs during the refractory period of the smaller cylinder, and one expects the wave to decay decrementally as it propagates in reverse (17,33), i.e., reverse decremental condition.

Models of Axon–Soma Region

The soma and axon hillock region is one location which might correspond to the diameter changes we have been discussing. Experimentally, there have been recordings of both orthodromic and antidromic potentials from the soma and the axon hillock region in several classes of neurons (1,3,5,7,10,11,30). Recently there was an experimental model of the soma using the giant squid axon (27). The authors reasoned that by lowering the internal (core) resistance of the axon they would cause the same effects on action potential propagation as with a sudden increase in diameter. This was accomplished by inserting an electrically floating wire along the axis of a squid giant axon for a short distance. They were then able to record the action potential at

multiple locations as it propagated "antidromically" toward the wire. As shown in Fig. 7, they were able to record a double-humped action potential at the wire tip. This is similar to the double-humped potential calculated from the VEJ model shown in Fig. 6, except that Fig. 7B shows an example of reverse decremental conduction rather than reverse propagation. These authors note that the "hump" on the action potential shifted from the falling to the rising phase of the action potential as it entered the axial wire region. The shapes noted in Fig. 7 are quite similar to the antidromic potentials recorded experimentally at the soma and axon hillock by Coombs et al. (3) (Fig. 8) and Fuortes et al. (7).

Although alternative explanations are possible, the computer simulations and the experiments with the giant squid axon provided a geometric explanation for these shape changes. They suggest that the sudden change in diameter over a short distance in the axon soma region can explain these changes in shape. Shape changes that are qualitatively different from the squid model were reported by Granit et al. (11). They noted that when cat and rat motoneurons were stimulated antidromically a "delayed depolarization" was recorded in the soma in place of the hyperpolarized portion of

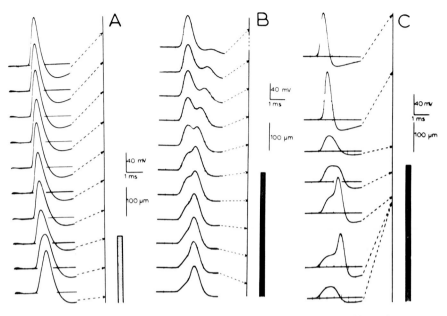

FIG. 7. Action potentials recorded experimentally in a squid axon with floating wire inserted part way as shown. **A:** There is relatively little change in the potential. **B:** An example of reverse decremental conduction. **C:** Failure of active propagation. (From ref. 27.)

the action potential. In the terms of the squid model of the soma, this meant that the "hump" would be on the falling phase after entering the axial wire region, a result that was not found. Nelson and Burke (21) confirmed this "delayed depolarization" but found some cells where it was not present and also noted that the amplitude of this hump was not constant but varied in a sequence of antidromic potentials. The authors suspected that the humps are due to an interaction with dendrites.

Further evidence of a dendritic role in the postspike hump was noted in an invertebrate preparation. Using the lobster stretch receptor neuron, Gramp (10) recorded activity in the dendritic region extracellularly. After an antidromic action potential, dendritic depolarization was still present at a time when the initial segment had regained its excitability. This depolarization was then able to re-excite the cell. Post spike "humps" were also recorded in the soma. Intracellular recordings by Calvin and Hartline (1) confirm the postspike hump. They noted this hump to be present at the soma during orthodromic action potentials.

How can we explain the postspike hump? Why is it found on orthodromic potentials?

Why is the hump not present in some cells, and why is the amplitude not constant with successive potentials? Although we did not model the axon, soma, and dendrites together, the simulations performed so far provide a possible explanation to these questions. Here, we assume the dendrites to be equivalent to a cylinder of larger diameter than the soma. [See Rall (25,26) for an explanation of how dendrites can be considered an equivalent cylinder.] Thus, an action potential invading the soma could be delayed as it approached the dendrites, and a retrograde wave would travel from the soma–dendritic junction toward the axon hillock. This wave would be recorded as a postspike hump. The decrease in diameter as the retrograde wave travels toward the axon, the initial delay at the soma–dendritic junction, as well as the postulated increase in membrane excitability of the initial segment (3,5,7) would tend to cause re-excitation of the cell.

In the case of orthodromic potentials, one would expect to record the postspike hump in the soma if the initial action potential originated at the initial segment and traveled retrograde through the soma. It would then encounter the dendrites and cause a postspike hump

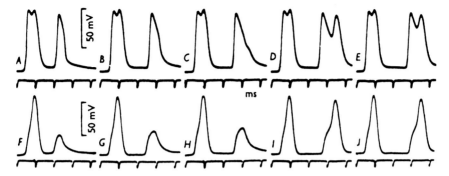

FIG. 8. Experimentally recorded action potentials at the soma and axon of cat motoneurons. (From ref. 3.)

in the same manner as the antidromic potential.

If this geometric explanation of the postspike hump were correct, we would expect to find it only in the fraction of cells where the dendrites did represent the equivalent of a sudden expansion in diameter and where the amount of expansion corresponded to the kinetic properties of the membrane to produce the appropriate delay. Also, we would expect such a model to be quite sensitive to any additional membrane depolarization present in the soma–dendritic region. Any depolarization would clearly shorten the time to reach threshold in the dendrites, and the retrograde wave, if any developed at all, would be of smaller amplitude. Thus synaptic activity or prior antidromic activity would be expected to influence the postspike hump adversely.[4] All these characteristics of our model "postspike hump" agree with the experimental findings of Nelson and Burke (21).

Rhythmical Activity

In studying action potential propagation, it has become clear that action potentials are not transmitted accurately on a one-to-one basis from soma to terminal branches of the axon. In invertebrate neurons "double spikes" are sometimes seen in the axon when recording a

single spike in the soma (1). These recordings are consistent with the idea that the first spike originating in the trigger zone is "reflected" backward as it enters the soma. The development of the double spike was not seen consistently but depended on a previous history of repetitive firing. This is consistent with the idea that small changes in membrane excitability are important in this phenomenon.

With repetitive firing through a point of sudden expansion, a retrograde action potential would collide with the next potential in sequence, causing it to be canceled. Thus, after the point of expansion, the frequency would be halved. In expansions with retrograde decremental conduction, lesser degrees of block would be expected. This has been shown in theoretical computations by Khodorov (17) and experimentally by Spira et al. (28). In theoretical computations, Parnas et al. (22) showed that the experimental data of Spira et al. (28) can be fitted by a region of gradually increasing diameter, with the assumption that potassium accumulates extracellularly.

Reflections at Other Sites

A reflected wave has been found experimentally in damaged nerve (14). The proposed mechanism for the reflection is similar to that of the reflection at a sudden increase in cylindrical diameter. The core current presumably has a low resistance path across the damaged membrane. Thus the leading core current of the action potential preferentially flows downstream and across the damaged membrane rather than across adjacent, more-proximal undamaged membrane. A slower velocity results

[4] On the other hand, in neurons where the increase in dendritic equivalent diameter was so great as to cause failure of propagation into the dendrites, additional dendritic depolarization might result in a postspike hump or an invading action potential.

in this undamaged membrane, since it takes progressively longer to reach threshold as the potential approaches the area of damage. When this slowing takes place, it is possible for a retrograde potential to arise. The authors question whether this mechanism is important in the pathophysiology of tic douloureux (2).

In myelinated nerve, a similar slowing of velocity has been predicted at areas of demyelination (18). Velocity decreases as the myelin thickness becomes less. Changes in shape noted were similar to those of Fig. 6, but their curves (not shown) depicted only decremental reverse conduction.

The idea that slowed conduction in a depressed area might yield a reflected wave has also been thought to be important in cardiac conduction. Wit et al. (32) found experimentally in excised cardiac Purkinje fibers that a local depression of the fiber can result in forward and reversed (re-entrant) conduction. They postulate that this may be important in the production of ventricular extrasystoles.

The F wave as recorded electromyographically in man (19) is thought by many to be the "reflection" of the antidromic action potential after it invades the cell soma. It is thought to have the following characteristics. A "delay" of 1 msec is usually assumed to occur (20). The amplitude of the muscle response is much lower than the original orthodromic (M) response. The response is variable and depends on the time of previous stimulation. These facts are consistent with the idea that "reflection" occurs only in that fraction of neurons with the appropriate diameter increase at the soma for the kinetic properties of the membrane. Thus the action potential is reflected only in a small fraction of axons and yields a lower-amplitude response in the muscle. The sensitivity to previous antidromic activity could be expected because residual depolarization would upset the delicate balance that results in reverse propagation.

As stated above, the models are not proof that the physiological mechanisms proposed here are correct, but they are consistent with the experimental evidence. One does not have to invoke changes in membrane excitability, ion changes, or multiple synapses to explain the experimental observations.

Branching

The behavior of the action potential as it approaches a branch point is variable and is dependent on the diameters of the branches. The dependence can be expressed in terms of the geometric ratio

$$\text{G.R.} = \sum_i d_j^{3/2}/d_a^{3/2},$$

where d_a is the diameter of the axon along which the action potential approaches the branch point, and d_j is the diameter of the jth branch. Thus to obtain G.R., we sum the 3/2s power of the diameters of the branches and divide by the 3/2s power of the approaching axon. Note that G.R. is not solely dependent on geometry but on which branch the action potential approaches the branch point.

It can be shown that when G.R. = 1 there is absolutely no change in action potential propagation and that shape and velocity remain constant until the branch point is reached. The velocity in the individual unmyelinated branches immediately assumes a value proportional to the square root of the branch diameter. The action potential shape (as recorded in time from a single point) remains unchanged. This was demonstrated formally by FitzHugh (6) using dimensional analysis and verified by computation. For further discussion of the geometric ratio see Goldstein and Rall (8). For a theoretical discussion of the basis by which cylindrical branches may be considered as an equivalent cylinder, see Rall (25.26).

When G.R. is less than 1, the action potential undergoes changes similar to those that occur with a step decrease in diameter (Fig. 1B). When G.R. is greater than 1, changes that occur are similar to a step increase in diameter (Fig. 1D). However, the situation becomes more complicated when two action potentials approach the branch point from two different branches. If they reach the branch point simultaneously, the core currents are additive and any delay of propagation is lessened. If they do not occur simultaneously, the potential reaching the branch point first could propagate into the other branches and cause a collision with the second potential. If the first potential is unable to propagate past the branch point, subthreshold current would spread into the other branches passively. This would depolarize the membrane and result in an increasing velocity of the second potential (23). The possibility for retrograde conduction in the first branch is enhanced when the waves do not reach the branch point simultaneously. However, none of the theoretical models can explain preferential conduction of an action potential into a large branch while failing in a small branch, or vice versa. This result suggests that those preferential effects found experimentally (for discussion and review see Raymond and Lettvin, *this volume*) are due to changes in the membrane properties, changes in intracellular resistivity, or to preferential changes in local ion accumulation.

REFERENCES

1. Calvin, W. H., and Hartline, D. K. (1976): Retrograde invasion of lobster stretch receptor somata in control of firing rate and extraspike patterning. *J. Neurophysiol.*, 39:106–118.
2. Calvin, W. H., Loeser, J. D., and Howe, S. F. (1977): A neurophysiological theory for the pain mechanism of tic douloureux. *Pain*, 3: 147–154.
3. Coombs, J. S., Curtis, D. R., and Eccles, J. C. (1957): The interpretation of spike potentials in motoneurons. *J. Physiol. (Lond)*, 139:198–231.
4. Dodge, F. A., Jr., and Cooley, J. W. (1973): Action potential of the motoneuron. *IBM J. Res. Dev.*, 17:219–229.
5. Edwards, C., and Ottoson, D. (1958): The site of impulse initiation in a nerve cell of a crustacean stretch receptor. *J. Physiol. (Lond)*, 143:138–148.
6. FitzHugh, R. (1973): Dimensional analysis of nerve models. *J. Theor. Biol.*, 40:517–541.
7. Fuortes, M. F. G., Frank, K., and Becker, M. D. (1957): Steps in the production of motoneuron spikes. *J. Gen. Physiol.*, 40:735–752.
8. Goldstein, S. S., and Rall, W. (1974): Changes of action potential shape and velocity for changing core conductor geometry. *Biophys. J.*, 14:731–757.
9. Goldman, L., and Albus, J. S. (1968): Computation of impulse conduction in myelinated fibers: Theoretical basis of the velocity diameter relation. *Biophys. J.*, 8:596–607.
10. Gramp, W. (1966): Impulse activity in different parts of the slowly adapting stretch receptor of the lobster. *Acta Physiol. Scand.* [*Suppl. 262*], 66:3–36.
11. Granit, R., Kernell, D., and Smith, R. S. (1963): Delayed depolarization and the repetitive response to intracellular stimulation of mammalian motoneurons. *J. Physiol. (Lond)*, 168:890–910.
12. Grossman, Y., Spira, M., E. and Parnas, I. (1973): Differential flow of information into branches of a single axon. *Brain Res.*, 64: 379–386.
13. Hodgkin, A. L. (1954): A note on conduction velocity. *J. Physiol. (Lond)*, 125:221–224.
14. Howe, J. F., Calvin, W. M., and Loeser, J. D. (1976): Impulse reflection from dorsal root ganglia and from focal nerve injuries. *Brain Res.*, 116:139–144.
15. Hursh, J. B. (1939): Conduction velocity and diameter of nerve fibers. *Am. J. Physiol.*, 127: 131–51.
16. Katz, B., and Miledi, R. (1965): Propagation of electric activity in motor nerve terminals. *Proc. R. Soc. Lond. B*, 161:453–582.
17. Khodorov, B. I., and Timin, E. N. (1975): Nerve impulse propagation along nonuniform fibres. *Prog. Biophys. Mol. Biol.*, 30:145–184.
18. Koles, Z. J., and Rasminsky, M. (1972): A computer simulation of conduction in demyelinated nerve fibres. *J. Physiol. (Lond)*, 227:351–364.
19. Magladery, J. W., and McDougal, D. B., Jr. (1950): Electrophysiological studies of nerve and reflex activity in normal man. I. Identification of certain reflexes in the electromyogram and the conduction velocity in peripheral nerve fibers. *Johns Hopkins Hosp. Bull.*, 86:265–290.
20. Miglietta, O. E. (1973): The F-response after transverse myelotomy. In: *New Developments in Electromyography and Clinical Neurophysiology*, edited by J. E. Desmet. Karger, Basel.
21. Nelson, R. P., and Burke, R. E. (1967): Delayed depolarization in spinal motoneurons. *Exp. Neurol.*, 17:16–26.
22. Parnas, I., Hochstein, S., and Parnas, H. (1976): Theoretical analysis of parameters leading to frequency modulation along an inhomogenous axon. *J. Neurophysiol.*, 39:909–923.
23. Pastushenko, V. F., Markin, V. S., and Chizmadzhev, Yu. A. (1969): Propagation of excitation in a model of an inhomogenous nerve fibre. I–IV. *Biophysika*, 14:316–323, 517–520, 883–890, 1130–1138.
24. Pinsker, H., Feinstein, R., Sawada, M., and Coggeshall, R. (1976): Anatomical basis for an apparent paradox concerning conduction velocities of two identified axons in Aplysia. *J. Neurobiol.*, 7:241–253.
25. Rall, W. (1959): Branching dendritic trees and mononeuron membrane resistivity. *Exp. Neurol.*, 1:491–527.
26. Rall, W. (1962): Theory of physiological

properties of dendrites. *Ann. NY Acad. Sci.,* 96:1071–1092.

27. Ramon, F., Moore, J. W., Joyner, R. W., and Westerfield, M. (1976): Squid giant axons: A model of the neuron soma? *Biophys. J.* 16:953–963.

28. Spira, M. E., Yarom, Y., and Parnas, I. (1976): Modulation of spike frequency by regions of special axonal geometry and by synaptic inputs. *J. Neurophysiol.,* 39:882–899.

29. Swadlow, H. A., and Waxman, S. G. (1975): Observations on impulse conduction along central axons. *Proc. Natl. Acad. Sci. USA,* 72:5156–5159.

30. Tauc, L., and Hughes, G. M. (1963): Modes of initiation and propagation of spikes in the branching axons of molluscan central neurons. *J. Gen. Physiol.,* 46:533–549.

31. Waxman, S. G. (1972): Regional differentiation of the axon: A review with special reference to the concept of the multiplex neuron. *Brain Res.,* 47:269–88.

32. Wit, A. L., Hoffman, B. F., and Cranefield, P. D. (1972): Slow conduction and re-entry in the ventricular conduction system. I. Return extrasystoles in canine Purkinje fibers. *Circ. Res.,* 30:1–10.

33. Zeevi, Y. Y. (1972): Ph.D. thesis, University of California, Berkeley.

Physiology and Pathobiology of Axons, edited by
S. G. Waxman. Raven Press, New York © 1978.

Optical Probes of Axonal Membrane

Ichiji Tasaki and Gen Matsumoto*

Laboratory of Neurobiology, National Institute of Mental Health, Bethesda, Maryland 20014

The application of optical techniques to the study of excitable membranes at the millisecond time scale was initiated approximately 10 years ago (5,32). By measuring birefringence, light scattering, and extrinsic fluorescence in crab and squid nerve fibers, it was found possible to record *optical signals* of a rapid, reversible nature which could be attributed to transient changes in the state of membrane macromolecules or in the dye–membrane interaction during nerve excitation. This discovery opened up an entirely new approach in the study of the physicochemical basis of action potential production.

The major problem encountered in an attempt to record optical signals is how to handle a relatively high level of random noise superposed on these signals. The origin of this random noise is quite distinct from that encountered in recording small potential variations with a high-resistance electrode. In the latter case, the noise is generated by the thermal agitation of the charged particles within the resistor and is proportional to the square root of the resistance. In recording optical signals, the noise level is determined almost exclusively by the number of photons arriving at the photodetector and is proportional to the square root of the light intensity. Under ordinary experimental conditions, the amplitude of an optical signal increases directly with the light intensity reaching the photodetector; hence the signal-to-noise ratio increases with the square root of the light intensity. At a given intensity of illumination, the signal amplitude varies widely depending on the nature of the signal as well as on the experimental condition under which the measurements are made.

In the early studies with optical probes, the major effort was directed toward finding the experimental conditions favorable for recording large optical signals. Soon it was found possible to observe optical signals directly on the screen of an oscilloscope under favorable conditions (e.g., ref. 26). However, because of the relatively high noise levels encountered under ordinary experimental conditions, the use of a signal averager was found to be almost indispensable in recording optical signals.

The choice of 1-anilinonaphthalene-8-sulfonate (1,8-ANS) and 2-*p*-toluidinylnaphthalene-6-sulfonate (2,6-TNS) for studies of extrinsic fluorescence of nerve fibers was suggested initially by the investigators who employed these dyes to examine the conformational states of various biomacromolecules *in vitro* (1,13). The objective of all the experiments carried out in this laboratory with these and other probes was to elucidate the physicochemical basis of production of optical signals. In recent years the objective of the studies by Cohen and his collaborators with fluorescent dyes was directed toward monitoring excitation of nerve cells by purely optical means, i.e., without using recording electrodes (19). A comprehensive review of this approach can be found elsewhere (18).

In this chapter we discuss studies with optical probes, how these optical methods can be applied to the physicochemical study of the nerve membrane, and what information has been derived from such studies. The optical methods reviewed in this article include the use of dye molecules attached to nerve fibers

* Present address: Electrotechnical Laboratory, Optoelectronics Section, Tanashi, Tokyo 188, Japan.

either noncovalently or covalently, and the application of calcium-sensitive dyes. This article does not cover optical signals observed without using probe molecules (e.g., light scattering and birefringence signals), although there was significant advancement in the field of birefringent studies in recent years (35,36). Readers interested in other reviews dealing with the results obtained with optical techniques are referred to articles by Cohen (4), Conti (6), and Tasaki and Warashina (29).

FLUORESCENCE STUDIES

Optical Setup and Experimental Procedure

An experimental setup used to record a fluorescence signal is shown in Fig. 1A. This setup consists of a device to optically excite the fluorescent probe in a nerve (bottom) and an arrangement to detect the emitted fluorescent light from the nerve (top). The light source was either a 100-watt quartz–iodine lamp or a 200-watt xenon–mercury or xenon lamp operated with a stabilized power supply. Cylindrical quartz lenses were used to focus the incident light on a 10-mm long portion of the nerve. The light from the source was converted into quasimonochromatic lightwave by inserting an interference filter between the lenses and the nerve. [As a rule, a polarizer (Polaroid, KN or HN series) was placed between the filter and the nerve.] The light emitted by the stained nerve was collected with a lens (not shown in the figure) placed on the top of the nerve chamber. The portion of the incident light scattered by the nerve was effectively eliminated by the use of a secondary filter,

either a cutoff filter or an interference filter. To measure the degree of polarization of the emitted light, a Polaroid sheet inserted between the secondary filter and the photomultiplier was used.

The intensity of the xenon or xenon–mercury lamp usually shows a fluctuation of the order of 1% at the range of frequencies required to analyze fluorescent signals. Since the observed changes in the fluorescent intensity are far smaller than 1%, it is necessary to suppress the response of the detector system to this fluctuation. This can be achieved by reflecting a small portion of the incident light onto a reference photomultiplier. The phase of the output of the reference photomultiplier is inverted, and this inverted output is added to the output of the fluorescence-detecting photomultiplier. When an incandescent lamp (e.g., a quartz–iodine lamp) is used as a light source, there is little or no fluctuation in the light intensity. However, when strong ultraviolet (UV) light is required to excite the dye molecules optically, it is difficult to use an incandescent lamp. The techniques used to eliminate mechanical and electrical (60 and 120 Hz) disturbances in detection of fluorescent responses are discussed elsewhere (27).

Physicochemical Factors Contributing to Production of Fluorescent Signals

The results of a systematic study of the fluorescence signals (or responses) from eight positional isomers of aminonaphthalene sulfonate (AmNS) in squid axons and crab nerves is summarized in Fig. 2A. The results are expressed as the relative sizes of these

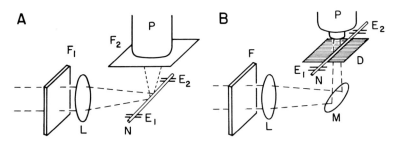

FIG. 1. Experimental setups used to record fluorescence signals (**A**) and absorption signals (**B**) from nerve fibers labeled with various optical probes. (F_1 and F) Interference filters. (L) Lens. (M) Mirror. (N) Squid giant axon or crab nerve. (E_1 and E_2) Stimulating and recording electrodes. (F_2) Cutoff filter. (D) Black Lucite plates. (p) Photodector, either photomultiplier or photodiode.

A

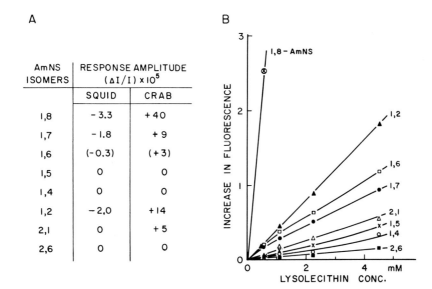

AmNS ISOMERS	RESPONSE AMPLITUDE $(\Delta I / I) \times 10^5$	
	SQUID	CRAB
1,8	− 3.3	+ 40
1,7	− 1.8	+ 9
1,6	(− 0.3)	(+ 3)
1,5	0	0
1,4	0	0
1,2	− 2.0	+ 14
2,1	0	+ 5
2,6	0	0

FIG. 2. A: Amplitude of fluorescence signals obtained from squid axons and crab nerves stained with various positional isomers of AmNS. **B:** Increase in fluorescence intensity (ordinate) plotted against the concentration of lysolecithin added to aqueous solutions of various AmNS isomers. (From ref. 29.)

fluorescence signals in terms of the ratio $\Delta I / I$, where ΔI denotes the change in the intensity of fluorescent light associated with nerve excitation and I the intensity of the fluorescent light emitted by the stained nerve at rest. Positive numerals in the table indicate that the observed signals represent a transient increase in the fluorescence intensity; the negative sign signifies the appearance of a transient decrease in the fluorescent light intensity during nerve excitation. Relatively large fluorescence signals were observed with 1-aminonaphthalene-8-sulfonate (1,8-AmNS) injected into the interior of squid giant axons. With many other AmNS isomers injected into squid axons, a change in fluorescence associated with nerve excitation was hardly detectable. When these AmNS isomers were applied *extracellularly* to crab claw nerves, it was found that the sign of the signal is opposite to that seen in *intracellularly* stained squid axons. In addition to 1,8-AmNS, 1,2-AmNS also produced sizable signals. The relative sizes of the signals seen in crab nerves were qualitatively the same as those from externally stained squid axon.

Physicochemical factors responsible for the difference among AmNS isomers in the nerves are now considered. First, the effect of solvent polarity on fluorescence emission of AmNS is

examined. The polarity dependence of the quantum yield of several AmNS isomers was examined previously by Turner and Brand (33). The major portion of their findings were confirmed in this laboratory. Furthermore, the properties of two isomers (1,2- and 2,1-AmNS), which were not examined previously, were clarified. According to these results, the fluorescence emission from 1,8-AmNS is highly sensitive to the solvent polarity, whereas the emission of 2,6-AmNS and 1,6-AmNS are practically unaffected by this factor. Such isomers as 1,7-AmNS, 1,5-AmNS, 1,2-AmNS, and 2,1-AmNS are moderately sensitive to the solvent polarity. These facts indicate that the sensitivity to solvent polarity is an important factor in production of fluorescence signals with these AmNS isomers.

It is evident that dye molecules must be bound to the nerve membrane in order to contribute to the generation of fluorescence signals. Therefore interaction of dye molecules with various biomacromolecules was examined as the second important physicochemical factor. This was done by measuring changes in fluorescence intensity brought about by addition of lysolecithin or bovine serum albumin to aqueous solutions of AmNS dyes. The integrated intensity of the fluorescence emission from each of the AmNS isomers in water is denoted by Φ_W; the corresponding value observed after addition of lysolecithin is represented by Φ_L. The increment ($\Delta\Phi$) is then defined by the following equation:

$$\Delta\Phi = \frac{\Phi_L - \Phi_W}{\Phi_W}$$

The values of increment are plotted in Fig. 2B against the concentration of lysolecithin used. It is seen that the effect on 1,8-AmNS fluorescence is very large. With isomers 1,2-, 1,6-, 1,7-, and 2,1-AmNS, a sizable increase in fluorescence is observed. With 1,5-, 1,4-, and 2,6-AmNS, very little or no detectable increase is seen. The order of these isomers arranged according to the magnitude of $\Delta\Phi$ is practically the same as that arranged in accordance with the size of the fluorescence signals. A qualitatively similar result was obtained when bovine serum albumin was used to increase the fluorescence emission of the aqueous solution of AmNS.

The increase in fluorescence intensity observed with these dyes *in vitro* is considered to be brought about by a decrease in the polarity of the microenvironment of the dye molecules resulting from binding of AmNS molecules to the added macromolecules. The fact that addition of the macromolecules does not enhance the fluorescence emitted by 1,5-AmNS must be attributed to a relatively weak tendency of this compound to bind to the macromolecules. This appears to explain why 1,5-AmNS, which has a reasonably high polarity sensitivity, fails to produce a fluorescence signal when applied to nerve fibers.

It was pointed out above that the sign of the optical signals observed with these dyes internally is opposite to that seen when the dyes are applied extracellularly. This fact can be understood on the following basis: The dye molecules used in these experiments are negatively charged at physiological pH. Reflecting the existence of negative fixed charges in the nerve membrane (24), negatively charged dye molecules do not pass through the membrane readily. Consequently, the binding sites of internally applied dye molecules are distinct from the sites for these dyes on the external surface of the nerve membrane. The effect of an action

potential on the dye binding is quite different on two sides of the nerve membrane.

Spectral Analyses of Fluorescence Signals

It is known that 1,8-ANS and 2,6-TNS are favorable membrane probes. The fluorescence emission of these compounds is highly polarity-sensitive. When dissolved in water, these compounds are practically nonfluorescent; they fluoresce intensely when dissolved in organic solvents (13,38). Light absorption by these compounds is rather insensitive to changes in solvent polarity. The observed change in the intensity of fluorescent light is brought about by changes in quantum yield. An increase in quantum yield caused by a fall in the solvent polarity is accompanied by a blue shift in the wavelength of emission maximum. The use of ANS and TNS in the investigation of the states of various macromolecules is based on these properties of the dyes (e.g., ref. 23).

Using squid giant axons intracellularly stained with 2,6-TNS and 2,6-ANS, the spectrum of the portion of the fluorescent light contributing to the optical signal was determined (25,31). The dye molecules in the axon were excited by polarized quasimonochromatic lightwave (365 nm) with its electric vector directed parallel to the longitudinal axis of the axon. In Fig. 3 the intensity (I) of fluorescent light emitted by the stained axon in its resting state was plotted against the center wavelength of the interference filter placed between the axon and the photomultiplier. The spectrum of the component of the fluorescent light that changes at the peak of the action potential (ΔI) was determined by the following procedure: Fluorescence signals were recorded at 440 nm and another wavelength alternately under constant illuminating and recording conditions, and the signal amplitudes at these two wavelengths were compared. By repeating this procedure of measuring the ratio of the signal amplitudes at two wavelengths, the entire spectrum of ΔI was determined.

The ΔI spectra of these probes inside a squid giant axon are strikingly different from the emission spectrum in the resting state of the axon (I). The ΔI spectra are sharp and narrow, having a maximum at approximately 420

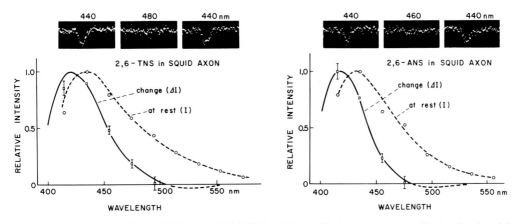

FIG. 3. Emission spectra of 2,6-TNS (*left*) and 2,6-ANS (*right*) in squid giant axons at rest (*broken lines*) and the spectra of the portion of the fluorescent light that changes during nerve excitation (*continuous lines*). The wavelengths of maximum transmission of the secondary filters used is indicated above each record on the top. (From ref. 37.)

nm and terminating abruptly at about 485 nm. It was impossible to find such a sharp and narrow spectrum from the spectra of this dye bound to common biomacromolecules, whereas the spectrum at rest is not very different from the spectra of this dye *in vitro*.

This sharp and narrow spectrum (ΔI) could be reconstructed by taking the difference between two spectra. When the emission spectrum of 2,6-TNS in 80% ethanol is subtracted from that in 100% ethanol, the resultant spectrum agrees very well with the observed ΔI spectrum. This agreement between these two spectra is significant because the wavelength of maximum emission and the band width of the spectrum are determined almost entirely by the solvent polarity (33). Therefore it appears reasonable to suggest that the transient decrease in fluorescence intensity from squid axons internally stained with 2,6-TNS (and also with 2,6-ANS) is brought about by an abrupt increase in the polarity of the environment of the bound probe molecules.

Fluorescence Polarization Studies

The polarization of the fluorescent light was examined to obtain information as to the orientation of probe molecules at or near the nerve membrane. In these observations, a polarizer and an analyzer were inserted in the light path. A squid giant axon internally

stained with 2,6-TNS was illuminated by a polarized light of 365 nm with its electric vector parallel to the long axis of the axon. With the polarizing axis of the analyzer oriented parallel to the axon, a distinct negative fluorescence signal was observed (Fig. 4, left); but when the analyzer was rotated through 90° under the same experimental conditions, only a record of random noise was obtained (right).

The degree of polarization (P), is calculated formally by the formula

$$P = \frac{\Delta I_{\parallel} - \Delta I_{\perp}}{\Delta I_{\parallel} + \Delta I_{\perp}}$$

where $\Delta I_{\parallel}$ and $\Delta I_{\perp}$ represent the fluorescence signal amplitudes observed with the analyzer axis parallel and perpendicular to the direction of the electric vector of the incident light, respectively. The value of P for this 2,6-TNS signal was larger than 0.7.

Similar polarization measurements were carried out using squid axons internally stained with 2,6-ANS and 1,8-ANS. With 2,6-ANS in the axon interior, no distinct signal was obtained under the "parallel (polarizer)–perpendicular (analyzer)" condition. In contrast, clear signals were obtained with 1,8-ANS under both the "parallel–parallel" and "parallel–perpendicular" conditions. A formal calculation of P for 1,8-ANS observed with the electric vector of the incident light parallel to the long axis of the axon yielded a value of approximately

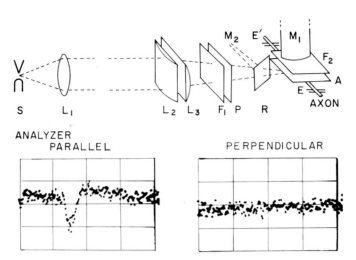

FIG. 4. **Top:** Experimental setup used to determine the polarization of fluorescence signals. (S) Light source (xenon or xenon–mercury lamp). (L_1–L_3) Lenses. (F_1) Interference filter. (P) Polarizer. (R) Quartz cover glass for reflecting a portion of the incident light. (E and E') Recording and stimulating electrodes. (A) Analyzer. (F_2) Secondary filter. (M_1 and M_2) Photomultipliers. **Bottom:** Fluorescence signals obtained from a squid giant axon stained internally with 2-p-toluidinyl-6-sulfonate (2,6-TNS). The incident light beam was polarized in the direction parallel to the axon. The orientations of the analyzer are indicated. (From ref. 31.)

0.35. The corresponding value for 2,6-ANS was found to be larger than 0.74. These results clearly indicated that there is a significant difference in polarization behavior between 1,8-ANS and 2,6-ANS.

With a view toward elucidating the molecular basis of the difference between 1,8-ANS and 2,6-ANS (or TNS), the following observations were made. These dye molecules were embedded in a sheet of polyvinyl alcohol (PVA) and then were stretched by the method described by Nishijima et al. (16) and Mc-Graw (14). A high degree of alignment of the probe molecules were obtained with 2,6-TNS (28). A theoretical analysis of the polarized fluorescent light from 2,6-TNS in a stretched PVA sheet indicated that the absorption and emission oscillators of this molecule are aligned roughly with the direction of stretching of the PVA sheet. The molecular orientation axis, which tends to coincide with the direction of stretching of the PVA sheet, is considered to be close to the straight line connecting the two side groups of 2,6-TNS. Similar results were obtained from 2,6-ANS in a stretched PVA sheet. In sharp contrast to these 2,6-derivatives, the polarization of fluorescent light of 1,8-ANS in a stretched PVA sheet was imperfect.

The high degree of alignment of either 2,6-TNS or 2,6-ANS may be considered evidence for the existence of a highly ordered macromolecular structure at or near the membrane. We suggest that the assembly of thread-like elements near the axolemma described by Metuzals and Izzard (15) is the structure that brings about a high degree of alignment of these molecules which participate in the production of the fluorescence signals. Quite recently this ordered submembranous structure was examined by the method of scanning microscopy (Metuzals and Tasaki, *in preparation*).

LIGHT ABSORPTION STUDIES

Optical Setup and Experimental Procedure

The experimental setup used to detect changes in light absorption by the dye molecules during nerve excitation is illustrated in Fig. 1B. A light beam from a 100-watt quartz–iodine lamp is focused on the stained part of the nerve by means of a lens. The white light from the source is converted into a polarized quasimonochromatic beam of light by the use of a polarizer and an interference filter. The direct beam of light (uninterrupted by the nerve) is prevented from reaching the photo-

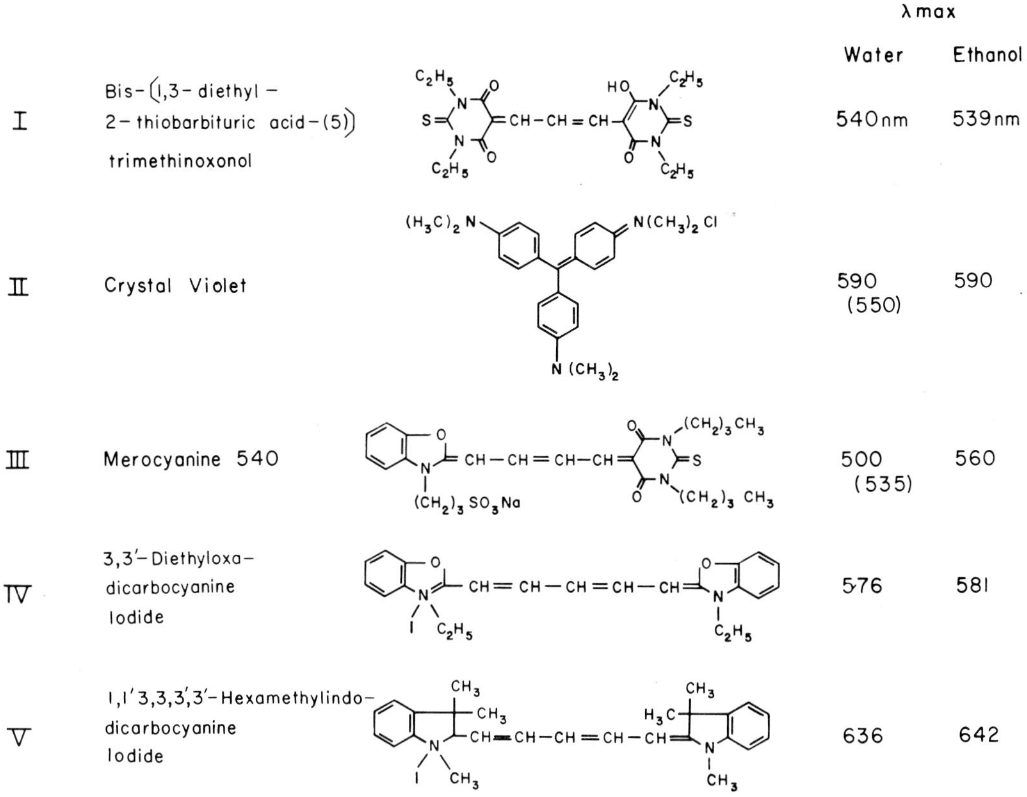

			λ max	
			Water	Ethanol
I	Bis-(1,3-diethyl-2-thiobarbituric acid-(5)) trimethinoxonol	C_2H_5 ... (structure)	540 nm	539 nm
II	Crystal Violet	(structure)	590 (550)	590
III	Merocyanine 540	(structure)	500 (535)	560
IV	3,3'-Diethyloxadicarbocyanine Iodide	(structure)	576	581
V	1,1'3,3,3',3'-Hexamethylindodicarbocyanine Iodide	(structure)	636	642

FIG. 5. Dyes used to label the nerve membrane for detection of absorption signals.

detector by a thin plate of black Lucite placed on each side of the nerve. The output of the photodetector, usually a photodiode, is led to a signal averager. In the optical setup used by Ross et al. (17), an additional interference filter (which has the same center wavelength as that of the primary filter) is inserted between the nerve and the photodetector. This secondary filter is required when the stained nerve emits intense fluorescent light.

The dyes used in the absorption experiments discussed in this article are listed in Fig. 5. The structural formulas, as well as the wavelength of maximum absorption of the main bands (λ_{max}) in water and ethanol, are also given.

Absorption Changes Associated with Nerve Excitation

With a variety of dyes, the intensity of light transmitted through the stained part of a nerve was found to change when an action potential was generated by the nerve. Optical signals generated by such absorbance changes usually have a duration comparable to that of the action potential. However, with certain dyes and/or under certain conditions, the absorption signals outlast the action potential by a great margin. Two examples of computer records of such absorbance signals are shown in Fig. 6. The records on the left were taken from a squid giant axon internally stained with crystal violet (dye II in Fig. 5). The optical signal on the top represents a transient decrease in the intensity of the transmitted light (i.e., an increase in absorption). The light wave used for measurements was polarized in the parallel direction in this case. The sign of the signal was reversed when perpendicularly polarized light was used. The bottom trace in Fig. 6 shows the intracellularly recorded action potential (slightly prolonged by intracellular application of tetraethylammonium).

CRYSTAL VIOLET
600 nm

OXONOL
550 nm

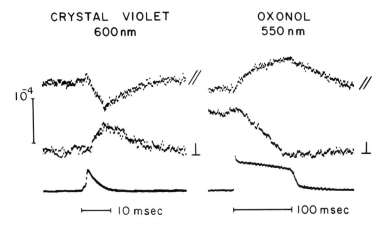

FIG. 6. Computer records of absorption signals (*upper traces*) taken from squid giant axons stained with crystal violet and with oxonol. The light beam used for measurements was polarized in a direction either parallel (*top*) or perpendicular (*middle*) to the axon and was permitted to pass only through the edge of the axon. The wavelengths of the light used are given. The bar indicates the magnitude of the deflection by a 0.01% change in the background light intensity. An upward deflection of the optical trace represents an increase in light intensity. The action potentials (recorded intracellularly) are shown at the bottom.

It is seen that the duration of the rising phase of the optical signal is very close to the action potential duration.

The records in the right-hand column of Fig. 6 show an absorption signal taken from a squid axon stained externally with oxonol (dye I in Fig. 5). With this dye, the decay of the optical signal following the end of the action potential is very slow.

Figure 7 shows that in a crab nerve stained with oxonol there is "summation" of the optical signals when the repetitive electric shocks are applied to the nerve. The binding sites for the dye molecules which generated long-lasting signals are distinct from the sites for the molecules giving rise to brief signals. With the

electric vector of the light wave directed parallel to the long axis of the nerve, the long-lasting absorption signal is negative, whereas the fast signal is positive and small (Fig. 7C). With the light polarized in the perpendicular direction, both the long-lasting and brief absorption signals are negative (Fig. 7A and B). Note that the action potentials never summate. The records presented in this figure look very similar to those published by Watanabe et al. (37).

Spectra of Absorption Signals

The spectrum of an absorption signal can be determined by the following procedure: At every wavelength of the lightwave used for

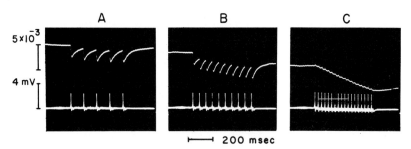

FIG. 7. Oscillograph records showing summation of optical signals produced by repetitive stimulation. A crab claw nerve stained with dye I (oxonol) was used. These single sweep records taken directly from the screen of an oscilloscope (without using a signal averager). Stimulating pulses were 0.2 msec in duration and twice the threshold in strength. The light used for measurements was 550 nm in wavelength and was polarized either perpendicular (**A** and **B**) or parallel (**C**) to the nerve.

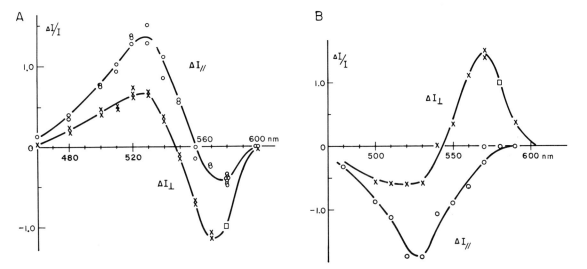

FIG. 8. A: Spectrum of absorption signals obtained from a crab nerve stained externally with M-540. **B:** Spectrum obtained from a squid giant axon stained internally with M-540. The polarizations of the light beam used for measurements are indicated. Unity on the ordinate indicates a change of 3×10^{-4} times the transmitted light intensity for **A** and 1×10^{-5} for **B**. (From ref. 29.)

measurements, the light intensity is adjusted so that the direct-current (DC) output of the photodetector remains constant irrespective of the wave length. The amplitudes of the signals produced by nerve stimulation plotted against the wavelength is the $\Delta I/I$ spectrum of the dye. This procedure automatically eliminates the effects of the wavelength dependence of the intensity of the incident light as well as that of the photodetector.

When the spectra of merocyanine-540 (M-540) were constructed, it was found that the polarization of the light wave seriously influences the spectra obtained (Fig. 8). The spectra obtained was diphasic; i.e., the sign of the signal was reversed at certain wavelengths. The wavelength at which the sign of the optical signal was reversed depended strongly on the polarization of the light used for measurements. Furthermore, when the same dye was introduced into the interior of the squid giant nerve fiber, the entire spectra were almost completely reversed. The dye used in this experiment is negatively charged. With a negatively charged dye, it is quite common that the sign of the signal with the molecules inside the nerve is opposite to that obtained by external application of the same dye.

A Physicochemical Interpretation of Absorption Signal Spectra

When the nerve membrane is thrown into the electrophysiologically excited state, there is a large change in the physicochemical properties of the dye-binding sites in and near the nerve membrane. The absorbance of dye molecules observed at a wavelength is affected by: (a) a change in the absorption spectrum associated with a transition of the dye-binding site from state 1 (at rest) to state 2 (reached at the peak of the action potential); and (b) a change in the angular distribution of the absorption oscillators of the dye molecules. The diphasicity of the signal spectrum is attributed to a change in the dye absorption spectrum. A difference in the orientation of the dye molecules in the two states of the dye-binding sites leads to a dichroism (i.e., polarization dependence) of the signal spectrum.

Based on these considerations, general mathematical expressions were derived describing relative change in the light intensities, $\Delta I_{\parallel}/I_{\parallel}$ and $\Delta I_{\perp}/I_{\perp}$, as functions of wavelength. They are

$$-\Delta I_{\parallel}/I_{\parallel} = [A_{\parallel}\epsilon_1(\lambda) - B_{\parallel}\epsilon_2(\lambda)]\,\Delta N$$

for light beams polarized in the parallel direction, and an analogous equation for the case of perpendicular polarization. Here the absorbance of the dye molecules in the two states of the membrane are denoted by $\epsilon_1(\lambda)$ and $\epsilon_2(\lambda)$. $A_\parallel$ and $B_\parallel$ above are the factors representing angular distribution of dye molecules for state 1 and state 2, respectively, of the nerve membrane and are independent of wavelength. The term ΔN denotes the total number of dye molecules contributing to the signals (34).

By comparing the observed spectra with the mathematical expressions stated above, it was possible to estimate quantitatively the statistical angular distribution of the dye molecules in the two states. In many dyes examined, the long axes of the dye molecules showed a strong tendency to be oriented perpendicularly to the membrane surface during nerve excitation. In some dyes (e.g., di- and tricarbocyanine in squid axons), there was no change in the angular distribution during nerve excitation (29).

Relationship Between the Membrane Potential and Absorption Signals

For each chemical species of dye molecule, there are in general more than one type of dye-binding sites in and near the nerve membrane. The response time and the rate of relaxation should be different at different sites. Therefore the time course of the signal is expected to vary significantly depending on the wavelength and the polarization of the light wave used for measuring the optical signals.

The records shown in Fig. 9 were obtained from a squid giant axon stained intracellularly with dicarbocyanine (dye V in Fig. 5). Using a pair of platinized–platinized electrodes inserted intracellularly along the long axis of the axon, the membrane potential was varied by the voltage-clamp technique. The light beam passing through the middle part of the axon was blocked by a narrow, rectangular piece of black tape, and the photodetector monitored only the polarized beam of light passing through the edge of the axon. In response to a rectangular hyperpolarizing voltage pulse applied across the axon membrane, the time course of the signal produced varied considerably depending on the polarization and wavelength of the light beam.

In general, the optical signals produced by rectangular voltage pulses do not have a rectangular time course. It seems possible to represent an optical signal observed under these conditions as a sum of an exponentially

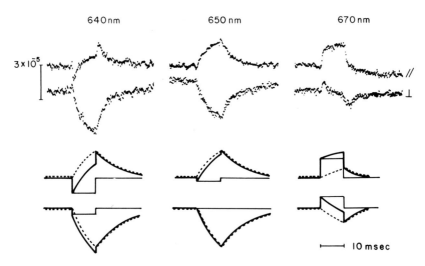

FIG. 9. Absorption signals obtained from the edge of a squid giant axon stained internally with dye V (Fig. 5). Rectangular hyperpolarizing voltage pulses 100 mV in amplitude were used to produce these absorption signals. The wavelengths and directions of polarization of the light beam used are indicated. The diagrams (*bottom*) indicate that these optical signals (*thick lines*) can be decomposed into two components, one with a rectangular time course (*thin lines*) and the other (*broken lines*) with a relaxation time of the order of 10 msec. (From Warashina, *unpublished.*)

changing term and a rectangular term (see the diagrams in the lower part of the figures). It was found that there are at least three distinct time constants of exponential change: 0.1 msec or shorter, 6–10 msec, and 50 msec or longer. The signal with the shortest time constant has an apparently rectangular time course. These different time constants represent different rates of rotation of dye molecules (34). It is reasonable to assume that these different rates indicate the existence of at least three distinct dye-binding sites involved in rotational movement of dye molecules. The amplitude of the signal with a 10-msec time constant is known to be markedly reduced when the Ca ions in the bathing sea water are replaced with Mg ions.

RESONANCE TRANSFER OF ENERGY BETWEEN DYE MOLECULES

Resonance energy transfer (3,9,10,22) takes place between two species of dye molecules separated by a very short distance. In this case the light energy absorbed by one species of molecules (the donor) is transferred to the other species (the acceptor) without involving emission and reabsorption of light. This type of energy transfer takes place only when there is a considerable overlap between the emission spectrum of the donor and the absorption spectrum of the acceptor.

In a recent study of this phenomenon (30), *p*-C1-anilinonaphthalene-sulfonate (*p*-C1-ANS) was chosen as the donor and M-540

as the acceptor. When applied externally to a crab nerve, *p*-C1-ANS produces negative fluorescence signals (i.e., transient decrease in fluorescent light during nerve excitation). M-540 gives rise to positive fluorescence signals when used extracellularly (7). There is a considerable overlap between the emission spectrum of *p*-C1-ANS and the fluorescence excitation spectrum of M-540. From the extent of this overlap, it is estimated that resonance energy transfer takes place with a high efficiency when the separation between *p*-C1-ANS and M-540 molecules is less than approximately 53 Å.

Figure 10 shows that the fluorescence of M-540 in a crab nerve can be excited by energy transfer from *p*-C1-ANS and that the intensity of this fluorescence emission is altered transiently when the nerve develops an action potential. The first record in the figure was taken after the nerve was stained with M-540 (without *p*-C1-ANS). The fluorescence emission excited at 550 nm was enhanced transiently by nerve stimulation. Since M-540 does not absorb 365-nm light wave significantly, no fluorescence signal was observed when the nerve prestained with M-540 was illuminated with this ultraviolet lightwave (see the second record). When *p*-C1-ANS was added to the surrounding medium, it became possible to detect a small change in the intensity of the fluorescent light generated by M-540 (see the third record). As staining of the nerve with *p*-C1-ANS progresses, the amplitude of the fluorescence signal increased (the fourth rec-

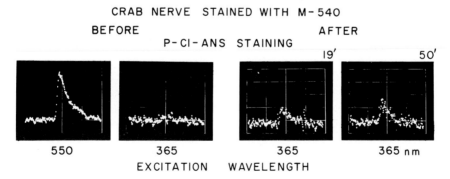

CRAB NERVE STAINED WITH M-540

BEFORE   AFTER

P-Cl-ANS STAINING

19′   50′

550   365   365   365 nm

EXCITATION   WAVELENGTH

FIG. 10. Demonstration of fluorescence signals mediated by resonance transfer of energy from *p*-Cl-ANS to M-540 in a crab nerve. The wavelengths of the light beam used for optical excitation of the dye molecules are indicated. The upward deflection of the computer trace indicates an increase in the intensity of the fluorescent light emitted by M-540. See text for further details. (From ref. 25.)

ord). The observed fluorescence signal cannot be attributed to *p*-C1-ANS molecules alone because the signal produced by *p*-C1-ANS in the absence of M-540 is negative. Furthermore, there was, in the experimental setup used, a secondary absorption filter between the nerve and the photodetector (for preventing the *p*-C1-ANS fluorescent light from reaching the photodetector). For these and other reasons, it was concluded that the two last records in Fig. 10 represent signals mediated by resonance energy transfer from *p*-C1-ANS to M-540 in a crab nerve.

CALCIUM-SENSITIVE PROBES

The tetracycline dyes, particularly chlorotetracycline, have been employed as probes of membrane-associated calcium during the excitation of nerve (12). Squid giant axons stained internally and lobster nerves stained externally show a small increase in fluorescent light during the action potential. Increasing the calcium concentration in the medium bathing a lobster nerve leads to a larger optical signal. Squid axons have been studied under conditions of voltage clamp and of generating hyperpolarizing responses. Chlorotetracycline injected into a squid giant axon appears to be monitoring calcium concentration near the inner surface of the nerve membrane.

Aequorin, a protein extracted from the jellyfish *Aequorea forskalea* (20,21), has been used as a Ca-sensitive probe in a large variety of excitable tissues. When bound to Ca ions, this protein becomes strongly luminescent (light emission occurring in the visible blue range). Baker et al. (2) injected aequorin into squid giant axons, and by using short trains of repetitive voltage-clamp pulses of different duration they obtained a distinct sign of Ca entry. They analyzed the time course of Ca influx during excitation by this method. Soon after this, Hallet and Carbone (11) detected changes in aequorin luminescence following an action potential in squid axons. The luminescent response produced by an action potential has a slow rising phase (approximately 0.1 sec in duration); the response lasts more than 1 sec. The time course of this response is governed by the rate of chemical reaction between calcium and aequorin; it does not

faithfully reflect the rise and fall of the calcium ion concentration in the axon.

Arnsenazo III (2,2'-[1,8-dihydroxy-3,6-bisulfo - 2,7 - naphthalene - *bis*(azo)] - dibenzene - arsenic acid) is a Ca-binding dye. When it encounters ionized Ca, its optical absorbance changes. Dipolo et al. (8) injected a 10 mM solution of this dye into a squid giant axon without any appreciable change in the action potential. They measured the Ca complex formation of such a dye by multichannel spectrophotometry. The concentration of ionized Ca was determined to be in the range 20–50 nM.

CONCLUSION

The method of detecting fluorescence and absorption signals with the aid of optical probes was developed with a view toward elucidating the mechanism of nerve excitation at the molecular level. With certain probes nerve excitation brings about a distinct shift of fluorescence emission and/or absorption spectrum of the probe molecules. Undoubtedly, this spectral shift is an indication of a sudden change in the properties of the milieu surrounding the probe molecules. We also showed that fluorescence signals obtained with certain probes are highly polarized, indicating the existence of a highly ordered macromolecular structure in and near the axonal membrane. Further, we presented the finding that the angular distribution of the probe molecules in or near the axonal membrane drastically changes during nerve excitation. This finding is interpreted as an indication of a rotational motion of the portion of the macromolecules to which the probe molecules are attached. From these and other findings, we arrive at the conclusion that membrane macromolecules undergo a drastic change when a large potential variation appears across the nerve membrane.

At present, our knowledge as to the mode of binding of probe molecules to proteins and lipids in and near the axolemma is limited. Our recent biochemical and electron microscopic studies showed that the highly ordered protein layer on the inner surface of the axolemma is essential to the maintenance of excitability. Electron microscopic studies of the freeze-fractured surface of the squid giant axon indicate the existence of intramembrane particles, which appear to play a crucial role in the process of nerve excitation.

Based on this picture of the axonal membrane, it seems possible to advance a reasonable interpretation of the relationship between the experimental results obtained with electrophysiological and optical methods. The main difficulty encountered in such an interpretation arises from the complexity, particularly the heterogeneity, of the axonal membrane at the molecular level. Furthermore, optical probes "report" to us only the state of the microenvironment around the probe-binding sites, and the information obtainable with an electrophysiological technique is limited to certain aspects of averaged electrochemical properties of the membrane. In order to overcome this difficulty, we are now carrying out comprehensive studies of the axonal membrane combining biochemical, morphological, electrophysiological, and optical techniques. We hope that these studies will promote a better understanding of the behavior of optical probe molecules within the axonal membrane.

REFERENCES

1. Aronson, J., Deter, A., and Morales, M. (1967): Myofibrillar shortening observed with a fluorescent "vital stain." *Fed. Proc.,* 26:553.
2. Baker, P. F., Hodgkin, A. L., and Ridgway, E. G. (1971): Depolarization and calcium entry in squid giant axons. *J. Physiol. (Lond),* 218:709–755.
3. Brand, L., and Witholt, B. (1967): Fluorescence measurements. *Methods Enzymol.,* 11:776–856.
4. Cohen, L. B. (1973): Changes in neuron structure during action potential propagation and synaptic transmission. *Physiol. Rev.,* 53:373–418.
5. Cohen, L. B., Keynes, R. D., and Hille, B. (1968): Light scattering and birefringence changes during nerve activity. *Nature (Lond),* 218:438–441.
6. Conti, F. (1975): Fluorescence probes in nerve membranes. *Annu. Rev. Biophys. Bioeng.,* 4:287–310.
7. Davila, H. V., Salzberg, B. M., Cohen, L. B., and Waggoner, A. S. (1973): A large change in axon fluorescence that provides a promising method for measuring membrane potential. *Nature [New Biol.],* 241:159–160.
8. Dipolo, R., Requena, J., Brinley, F. J., Jr.,

Mullins, L. J., Scarpa, A., and Tiffert, T. (1976): Ionized calcium concentrations in squid axons. *J. Gen. Physiol.,* 67:433–467.
9. Förster, Th. (1959): Transfer mechanisms of electronic excitation. *Discuss. Faraday Soc.,* 27:7–17.
10. Förster, Th. (1948): Zwischenmolekulare Energiewanderung und Fluorescenze. *Ann. Physik.,* 2:55–75.
11. Hallett, M., and Carbone, E. (1972): Studies of calcium influx into squid giant axons with aequorin. *J. Cell. Physiol.,* 80:219–226.
12. Hallett, M., Schneider, A. L., and Carbone, E. (1972): Tetracycline fluorescence as calcium-probe for nerve membrane with some model studies using erythrocyte ghosts. *J. Membr. Biol.,* 10:31–44.
13. McClure, W. O., and Edelman, G. M. (1966): Fluorescence probes for conformational studies of proteins. I. Mechanisms of fluorescence of 2-p-toluidinylnaphthalene-6-sulfonate, a hydrophobic probe. *Biochemistry,* 5:1909–1918.
14. McGraw, G. E. (1970): Study of molecular orientation in polymers by fluorescence polarization. In: *Structure and Properties of Polymer Films,* edited by R. W. Lenz and R. S. Stein, pp. 97–111. Plenum, New York.
15. Metuzals, J., and Izzard, C. S. (1969): Spatial pattern of threadlike elements in the axoplasm of the giant nerve fiber of the squid (Loligo pealii) as disclosed by differential interference microscopy and by electron microscopy. *J. Cell Biol.,* 43:456–479.
16. Nishijima, Y., Onogi, Y., and Asai, T. (1966): Fluorescence method for studying molecular orientation in polymer solids. *Polymer Sci.,* C15:237–250.
17. Ross, W., Salzberg, B. M., Cohen, L. B., and Davila, H. V. (1974): A large change in dye absorption during the action potential. *Biophys. J.,* 14:983–986.
18. Salzberg, B. M., and Cohen, L. B. (1977): Optical measurements of membrane potential. *Rev. Physiol. Biochem. Pharmacol. (in press).*
19. Salzberg, B. M., Davila, H. V., and Cohen, L. B. (1973): Optical recording of impulses in individual neurons of an invertebrate central nervous system. *Nature (Lond),* 246:508–509.
20. Shimomura, O., Johnson, F. H., and Saiga, Y. (1962): Extraction, purification and properties of aequorin, a bioluminescent protein from the lumimous hydromedusan Aequorea. *J. Cell. Comp. Physiol.,* 59:223–239.
21. Shimomura, O., and Johnson, F. H. (1969): Properties of the bioluminescent protein aequorin. *Biochemistry,* 8:3991–3997.
22. Stryer, L. (1960): Energy transfer in proteins and polypeptides. *Radiat. Res. (Suppl.),* 2:432–451.
23. Stryer, L. (1968): Fluorescence spectroscopy of proteins. *Science,* 162:526–533.

24. Tasaki, I. (1968): *Nerve Excitation.* Charles C Thomas, Springfield, Ill.
25. Tasaki, I., Carbone, E., Sisco, K., and Singer, I. (1973): Spectral analyses of extrinsic fluorescence of the nerve membrane labeled with aminonaphthalene derivatives. *Biochim. Biophys. Acta,* 323:220–233.
26. Tasaki, I., Carnay, L., Sandlin, R., and Watanabe, A. (1969): Fluorescence changes during conduction in nerves stained with acridine orange. *Science,* 163:683–685.
27. Tasaki, I., and Sisco, K. (1975): Electrophysiological and optional methods for studying the excitability of the nerve membrane. In: *Methods in Membrane Biology,* Vol. 5, edited by E. D. Korn, pp. 163–194. Plenum Press, New York.
28. Tasaki, I., Sisco, K., and Warashina, A. (1974): Alignment of anilinonaphthalenesulfonate and related fluorescent probe molecules in squid axon membrane and in synthetic polymers. *Biophys. Chem.,* 2:316–326.
29. Tasaki, I., and Warashina, A. (1976): Dyemembrane interaction and its changes during nerve excitation. *Photochem. Photobiol.,* 24: 191–207.
30. Tasaki, I., Warashina, A., and Pant, H. (1976): Studies of light emission, absorption and energy transfer in nerve membranes labelled with fluorescent probes. *Biophys. Chem.* 4:1–13.
31. Tasaki, I., Watanabe, A., and Hallett, M. (1971): Properties of squid axon membrane

as revealed by a hydrophobic probe, 2-p-toluidinylnaphthalene-6-sulfonate. *Proc. Natl. Acad. Sci. USA,* 68:938–941.
32. Tasaki, I., Watanbe, A., Sandlin, R., and Carnay, L. (1968): Changes in fluorescence, turbidity and birefringence associated with nerve excitation. *Proc. Natl. Acad. Sci. USA,* 61:883–888.
33. Turner, D. C., and Brand, L. (1968): Quantitative estimation of protein binding site polarity: Fluorescence of N-arylaminonaphthalene-sulfonates. *Biochemistry,* 7:3381–3390.
34. Warashina, A., and Tasaki, I. (1975): Evidence for rotation of dye molecules in membrane macromolecules associated with nerve excitation. *Proc. Jpn. Acad.,* 51:610–615.
35. Watanabe, A., and Terakawa, S. (1976): Alteration of birefringence signals from squid giant axons by intracellular perfusion with pronase solution. *Biochim. Biophys. Acta,* 436:833–842.
36. Watanabe, A., and Terakawa, S. (1976): A long-lasting birefringence change recorded from a tetanically stimulated squid giant axon. *J. Neurobiol.,* 7:271–286.
37. Watanabe, A., Terakawa, S., and Nagano, M. (1973): Axoplasmic origin of birefringence change associated with excitation of a crab nerve. *Proc. Jpn. Acad.,* 49:470–475.
38. Weber, G., and Laurence, J. R. (1954): Fluorescent indicators of adsorption in aqueous solution and on the solid phase. *Biochem. J.,* 56:xxxi.

Physiology and Pathobiology of Axons, edited by
S. G. Waxman. Raven Press, New York © 1978.

Axoplasmic Transport in Normal and Pathological Systems

S. Ochs and R. M. Worth

*Departments of Physiology and Neurosurgery, Indiana University School of Medicine,
Indianapolis, Indiana 46202*

Axoplasmic transport, the movement of perikaryally synthesized material into axons and dendrites, is the means by which the neurites are supplied with proteins and other constituents necessary for maintenance of their structural and functional integrity. This mechanism also carries neurotransmitters and some of their synthetic and degradative enzymes to the nerve terminals. Additionally, there is evidence of transsynaptic passage of trophic materials from the nerve endings of sensory and motor fibers to influence muscle and other cells. Since axoplasmic transport supports such basic neuronal functions, it is not surprising that changes in transport could lead to nerve or muscle pathology. In the first part of this chapter we briefly characterize the properties of axoplasmic transport, including recent information on the ionic requirement of the process. In the second part, some of those pathological entities where a defect in transport has been implicated are discussed.

CHARACTERISTICS OF AXOPLASMIC TRANSPORT

The pattern of outflow is shown by injecting a small volume of ^{3}H-leucine into a dorsal root ganglion or the anterior horn of the spinal cord where the precursor can be taken up by neuronal cell bodies and incorporated into proteins and polypeptides (Fig. 1). Following injections into the cat lumbar 7 (L7) dorsal root ganglion, the subsequent transport of labeled components into the sciatic nerve allows the pattern of downflow to be determined when sufficient time is allowed. As can be seen in the example given in Fig. 1, outflow is shown

by assaying the activity in 5-mm segments of the root, ganglion, and nerve. A high level of radioactivity remains in the ganglion, falling distally in the nerve to a plateau and then rising to a crest before rapidly dropping to baseline activity. Transport velocity is measured by taking the distance from the front of the crest back to the peak of activity at the injection site in the ganglion. The front of labeled material moves linearly down the nerve at a rate of 410 mm/day, as shown in Fig. 2, where a series of five nerves were taken at successively longer times following injection.

By extrapolating back to zero time, the activity is seen to move out into the axons with little noticeable lag after injection of the precursor. This finding indicates that the incorporation of ^{3}H-leucine into proteins and polypeptides is rapid, and that labeled components are quickly moved out into the fibers. The rapidity of incorporation was indicated by the effects of the protein synthesis-blocking agents cycloheximide or puromycin. If either of these agents were injected before ^{3}H-leucine, a block of synthesis and outflow of labeled material was seen as expected. If the inhibitor was injected only 10–15 min after the precursor, however, it was ineffective (103). This indicates that polypeptide synthesis is completed within this period of time.

A similar downflow pattern and rate of transport is seen in the motor fibers of the sciatic nerve when the ventral horn is injected (Fig. 1). The overall size of the nerve does not make any difference in the pattern or rate of axoplasmic transport, as was shown for a number of mammalian species ranging from the rat to the goat (88). The rate of transport

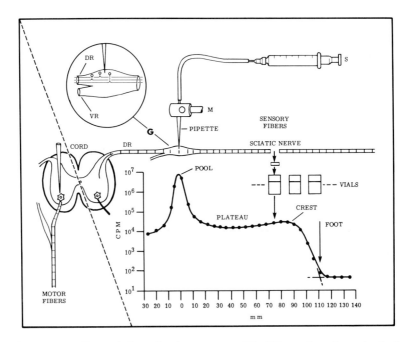

FIG. 1. Injection and sampling technique showing transport. The L7 ganglion shown in the insert contains T-shaped neurons with one branch ascending in the dorsal root, the other descending in the sciatic nerve. A pipette containing ³H-leucine is passed into the ganglion; after its injection and the incorporation of precursor, the downflow of labeled components in the fibers is sampled at various times by sacrificing the animal and sectioning the nerve. Each segment is placed in a vial, solubilized, scintillation fluid added, and the activity counted. The outflow pattern is displayed on the ordinate log scale; the abscissa is in millimeters, taking the distance from the center of the ganglion as zero. A high level of activity is seen remaining in the ganglion region; more distally, a plateau rises to a crest before abruptly falling at the front of the crest to baseline levels. The left-hand side of the cord shows for motoneurons an injection of the precursor into the L7 cell body region followed by removal of ventral root and sciatic nerve at a later time for a similar treatment and display of outflow.

also does not depend on the diameters of the individual nerve fibers. This was determined by taking small segments of nerve at the front of the crest and examining cross sections after radioautography. Nerve fibers of all diameters were seen to contain grains of activity, indicating that they all had the same rate of transport (88). Similar experiments using electron microscopic autoradiography demonstrated grains at the same position in nonmyelinated fibers, indicating that the same fast transport rate is present in these axons (98; and cf. ref. 16).

A similar rate appears to be present in the nerves of nonmammalian species. Using the garfish olfactory nerve, Gross and Beidler (44) found a similar outflow pattern in these non-myelinated fibers. When the authors corrected the results found in this poikilotherm to a temperature of 38°C using the Q_{10} they de-

termined for this nerve, they found a transport rate of 405 mm/day (43). Frog nerves *in vitro* also showed a transport rate of 400 mm/ day when the rate was similarly estimated at 37°C (29).

Another method for determining the transport of labeled components or materials present in the fibers is to assess their accumulation above ligations, crushes, or transections of nerves. Acetylcholinesterase (AChE) was found to accumulate just above nerve transections by Lubinská (77). After making two transections, the enzyme was seen accumulated in the isolated nerve segment, above the distal interruption and below the upper one as well. A redistribution of the enzyme within the segment was thereby demonstrated. In later work Lubinská and Niemierko (79) found a fast rate for AChE transport. In similar studies using double ligations (109), we found the rate

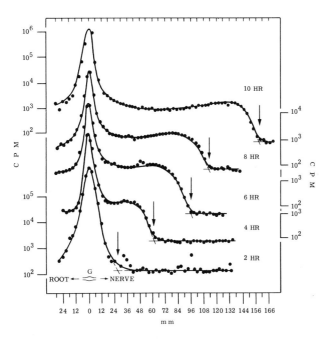

FIG. 2. Distribution of radioactivity. Activity present in the dorsal root ganglia and sciatic nerves of five cats taken 2–10 hr after injection of ³H-leucine into the L7 ganglia (G) is shown. The activity present in 5-mm segments of roots, ganglia, and nerves is given on the ordinate in logarithmic divisions. The ordinate scale for the nerve taken 2 hr after injection is shown at the bottom left. At the top left a scale is given for the nerve taken 10 hr after injection. Only partial scales are shown at the right for the nerves taken 4, 6, and 8 hr after injection. Abscissa is in millimeters, taking the distance from the center ganglion as zero.

for AChE to be 431 mm/day (109), practically the same as the 410 mm/day value determined for labeled proteins.

Dahlström (22) and her colleagues used a ligation technique to show a fast axoplasmic transport of norepinephrine (NE). Typically this neurotransmitter is present in adrenergic nerves in the form of dense-core membrane-bound granules measuring some 500 Å in diameter. These granules also contain the synthesizing enzyme dopamine-β-hydroxylase (DBH). Brimijoin and Helland (12,13) used a cold-block technique to assess the rate of movement of the granules revealed by DBH assay. Nerves were placed in a special chamber so that one part of the nerve was kept at a few degrees above 0°C, i.e., well below the temperature of 11°C at which transport completely stops (100). The remainder of the nerve was kept at 38°C, and in that portion of the nerve a continued transport causes the accumulation of granules to occur just above the cold-blocked region. After several hours the cooled region of the nerve was brought

back to a temperature of 38°C and the dammed-up DBH then moved as a wave into the previously cooled region. From the displacement of the wave with time, a rate of 360 mm/day was assessed for NE transport. The discrepancy between this rate and the value of 410 mm/day reported for labeled proteins may be due to changes in transport induced by the cold block of the nerve (100).

Grafstein (39) studied transport by the accumulation of isotope-labeled components at nerve terminals. In that system, one goldfish eye is injected with ³H-leucine for uptake by the ganglion cells of the retina, and the synthesized proteins and polypeptides are then transported to the contralateral optic nerve endings in the tectum. A similar technique was used to study accumulation in the tectum of birds (40) and in the lateral geniculate body of rodents (50). In these species nearly all the optic fibers from each eye cross to terminate in the tectum or lateral geniculate of the opposite side. There is considerable leakage of precursor from the injected eye into the circulation from which it can cross the blood–brain barrier, gaining entry to the tectum or lateral geniculate and becoming locally synthesized into proteins. To correct for such local incorporation, the activity present in the tectum or geniculate on the ipsilateral side is subtracted from the activity of the contralateral side. The difference gives the amount of transported activity. The precursor ³H-proline is better than ³H-leucine in this system because it does not as readily pass the blood–brain barrier (85).

PROTEIN AND OTHER MATERIALS TRANSPORTED

A wide range of labeled proteins and polypeptides were found to be transported in the nerve (115), as shown by differential centrifugation of nerves taken at various times after injecting ³H-leucine into the L7 ganglion or ventral horn region. After 3–5 hr, a period consistent with fast axoplasmic transport, the small particulate fraction was labeled to the greatest extent, with a somewhat smaller degree of labeling present in the high-speed supernatant. This fraction was shown by gel filtration to contain labeled soluble proteins of molecular weight (MW) greater than 450,000, proteins in the 50,000–200,000 MW range, and polypeptides below 10,000 MW. Additionally, some free labeled leucine was also transported. The latter amounted to approximately 30% of the total polypeptide fraction or 15% of the total fast-transported activity present in the soluble fraction (58,115). At times greater than 6 hr and up to several weeks, a period consistent with slow transport, higher MW soluble proteins showed progressively increased labeling (115). A shift in the isoelectric potential of the soluble proteins was also seen at the later times (60,67).

Using ³H-glucosamine or ³H-fucose as the precursor, a fast downflow of labeled glycoproteins and glycolipids was found (62). The glycoproteins may pass into the synaptic cleft to play a role in synaptic function. A fast downflow of mucopolysaccharide proteins (31), phospholipids (1), and ³H-cholesterol (113) has also been found. These components appear destined to supply axonal membrane or membrane-bound organelles within the fiber.

Large particulates that appear to be moving at fast rates can be seen using darkfield or Nomarski optics microscopy (68). A movement of mitochondria transported in both directions at times attains rates approaching the rate of fast-transported labeled proteins, with, however, a slow net translocation in the proximodistal direction (6,61,66).

After injecting the brain of mice with ³H-leucine and isolating the synaptosomes by differential centrifugation, labeled soluble proteins gradually accumulate over a period of days (4). However, some labeled activity accumulates rapidly, as expected from a fast transport (24). A transsynaptic passage of material also occurred (41,129).

RETROGRADE TRANSPORT

As noted above, Lubinská and her colleagues had shown an anterograde and a retrograde movement of AChE in isolated nerve segments. In our studies using double ligation, the rate of retrograde transport of AChE was 220 mm/day, approximately half that of the forward rate (109). Retrograde transport has also been shown for a number of other materials, including the marker horseradish peroxidase (HRP). This protein is taken up by nerve terminals and is carried to the cell bodies at a rate estimated to be > 84 mm/day (74). The technique is now extensively used to trace various pathways in the central nervous system (CNS) (3,19,73). Tetanus toxin and certain viruses also show a retrograde movement in nerve fibers (see below). Retrograde transport into dendrites was seen after injecting ³H-glycine into single motoneuron cell bodies and following the spread of labeled incorporated activity by radioautography (80).

Retrograde transport in the axons appears to be related to the regulation of protein synthesis in the cell bodies. The chromatolysis of nerve cell bodies seen several days after a nerve transection later followed by large increases in their levels of nucleic acids and proteins (11, 32,127) may be explained by the loss of a "signal" substance normally transported up the fibers acting as a negative feedback control over the level of protein synthesis (96).

Kristensson and Olsson (72) demonstrated in rats that the rate of retrograde transport of HRP correlates with the time of appearance of chromatolysis following nerve transections made at various distances in the nerve from the cell bodies.

ENERGETICS OF TRANSPORT

Fast axoplasmic transport was shown to be closely dependent on oxidative phosphorylation (89). Fast axoplasmic transport *in vitro* was blocked within 15 min after oxygen in the atmosphere was replaced by N_2 or when nerves were exposed to cyanide (CN), azide, or dinitrophenol (DNP). In this time the total $\sim$P (the combined level of ATP and creatine phosphate) measured in the nerve falls from a control level of 1.2–1.4 μM/g to approximately half this value (114).

When glycolysis was blocked by iodoacetic acid, transport ceased after 1.5–2.0 hr (114), correlated with a fall in $\sim$P to half-control levels. Similarly, when the citric acid cycle was blocked with fluoracetate (89), transport stopped within 1 hr and again $\sim$P fell to half of control levels at that time. Such evidence indicates that ATP is required to maintain axoplasmic transport.

The ATP appears to be present in a pool common to both the transport mechanism and the sodium pump, as indicated by the fact that both transport and action potentials fail at the same time after initiating a block of oxidative phosphorylation by anoxia (91).

When a local anoxia was produced by covering a small length of nerve with petrolatum jelly and Parafilm strips so that O_2 could not diffuse into that region, transport into the anoxic area was blocked, as shown by the damming of labeled activity above that site. This result indicates that a local supply of ATP is required for transport along the entire length of the nerve fibers (86).

Anoxic blocks lasting 1–1.5 hr are readily reversible. After long durations of anoxia, more time is required for recovery of fast axoplasmic transport. Long-lasting anoxias were produced *in vivo* by hind limb compression in cats using sphygmomanometer cuffs with pressures raised above 300 mm Hg to block circulation. Recovery of transport took several days after as much as 6 hr of anoxia (75). Irreversible block and Wallerian degeneration was seen after 7 hr (75).

MECHANISM OF TRANSPORT—THE TRANSPORT FILAMENT MODEL AND THE UNITARY HYPOTHESIS

The wide range of materials including particles, soluble proteins, smaller polypeptides, and free leucine carried at the same fast rate suggests a common carrier (91). The hypothesis proposed to account for transport is based on the sliding-filament theory of muscle (55). "Transport filaments" binding the various materials are moved along the microtubules by cross-bridges utilizing ATP as the source of energy (Fig. 3). A relatively high level of Mg^{2+}-Ca^{2+}-activated ATPase (MgCa-ATPase) with actomyosin-like properties found in peripheral nerve (65) could utilize ATP, supplying the energy required. The ATPase does not appear to be bound to the transport filament itself as indicated by its very slow accumulation above nerve ligations (65).

Slow and fast transport have been reported, with the implication that they are subserved by two mechanisms. Although fast transport is readily characterized, it is difficult to do so for the slow system. After injection of ^{32}P or ^{3}H-leucine, slow transport appears as a slope of declining activity, extending out from the perikaryon into the fiber and decreasing over a period of days eventually to flatten out (90,95). After several weeks, the slope may even reverse (82,123). By taking into consideration its known characteristics, it appears possible to account for slow transport by the transport filament model on a "unitary" hypothesis (92). These characteristics include: (a) the compartmentation of labeled components in the cell bodies with a later egress of materials into the axons for transport; (b) differences in the transport filament binding affinities of various materials with a consequent "fall-off" and deposition of components in the fibers; and (c) the subsequent redistribution of these materials in anterograde and retrograde directions. These factors, all demonstrated in cat sciatic nerves (95), can account for the

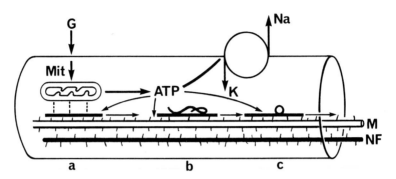

FIG. 3. Transport filament hypothesis. Glucose (G) enters the fiber, and after glycolysis oxidative phosphorylation in the mitochondrion (Mit) gives rise to ATP. The $\sim$P of ATP supplies energy to the sodium pump, controlling the level of Na^+ and K^+ in the fiber and also to the cross-bridges activating the transport filaments. These are shown as black bars to which the various components transported are bound and so carried down the fiber by cross-bridge activity. The components transported include the mitochondria (a) attaching temporarily (*dashed lines*) to the transport filament, this giving rise to either fast-forward or retrograde movement (although with a slow net forward movement); soluble protein (b) shown as a folded or globular configuration; and polypeptides and small particulates (c). Simpler molecules are also bound to the transport filaments. Thus a wide range of components are transported at the same fast rate. The cross-bridges between the transport filament and the microtubules presumably act in a fashion similar to the sliding filament theory of muscle, and the MgCa-ATPase found in nerve utilizes ATP as the source of energy. (M), microtubules. (NF), neurofilaments

pattern of outflow seen at later times, characterized as "slow" transport.

Some recent studies have shown what appear to be slow waves moving out at a rate of approximately 1–3 mm/day (17,54). In long-term studies of outflow in cat and rat sensory nerve fibers, such regular slow waves were not seen (122). Instead, those results and most likely the other studies appear to be best accounted for by the unitary theory.

ROLE OF CALCIUM

We might expect on the basis of the transport filament theory that Ca is required to maintain axoplasmic transport. However, in prior *in vitro* experiments carried out with isotonic sucrose replacing Ringer solution, transport in the nerve was maintained (28,48,87). The explanation is that the perineurium effectively maintains the usual ionic composition of the extracellular fluid, including Ca (20,33,34, 47). A desheathed peroneal nerve preparation was developed, and Ca (in a concentration of 3–5 mM) was shown to be required to maintain transport (97). Magnesium cannot substitute for Ca. Additionally, high Ca concentrations (above 25 mM) cause reduced transport, and block can actually occur within 2 hrs with Ca concentrations of 95 mM.

The level of ionized Ca present within myelinated nerve fibers is not yet known. In the giant axon it is estimated to be kept at a low level, approximately 10^{-7} M (2), by means of special regulating mechanisms, including compartmentation of Ca in the mitochondrion and possibly in the endoplasmic reticulum. Additionally, a carrier mechanism in the membrane acts to exchange Ca with entering Na (7,51, 84). The fact that little difference in the time required for transport block to occur in Ca-free media with and without Na present suggests that a mechanism for Ca efflux other than a Ca–Na shuttle is present (7).

In addition, another system which may regulate Ca was recently uncovered. ^{45}Ca is taken up by cell bodies and fast-transported in frog (48) and mammalian nerves (57). The Ca was found to be carried down in the fibers bound in part to a protein with a MW of

15,000 (56) and in part to a 1,100 MW polypeptide. These Ca-binding components may regulate Ca levels in the axon or perhaps be part of the transport mechanism itself.

MICROTUBULES AND MITOTIC BLOCKING AGENTS

In the transport filament model, the microtubules are considered to be the fixed elements along which the filaments are moved. The microtubules are seen in electron micrographs as hollow-walled structures approximately 250 A in diameter (119,130). The walls are composed of tubulin, a globular protein dimer of 110,000 MW, in turn composed of α- and β-monomers of 55,000 MW (119,130). Along the length of the microtubules spur-like projections or cross-arms are seen that could have ATPase activity. A protein with ATPase activity co-migrates with tubulin, indicating a possible association (111,112).

Colchicine injected into the nerve trunk blocks fast axoplasmic transport of NE (21) and AChE (70). A proposed action of colchicine and other mitotic blocking agents such as the *Vinca* alkaloids is that they bind to the free tubulin in equilibrium with the microtubules, thus causing the microtubules to become disassembled. This concept was first suggested by disruption of the spindles of mitotically dividing cells by these agents. However, colchicine and *Vinca* alkaloids can block axoplasmic transport without obvious loss of microtubular structure (35,49,63). A similar picture appears in studies (64) using halothane or the local anesthetic lidocaine (16). At low concentrations these agents block nerve impulse excitation without affecting axoplasmic transport. At higher concentrations, axoplasmic transport is blocked in addition, and at still higher concentrations disassembly of microtubules is seen (52). Additionally, colchicine may act preferentially on the endoplasmic reticulum, causing its disruption (51) and presumably also altering its Ca-storing ability.

Fink et al. (36) and Byers (15) recently suggested that microtubules may not be involved in transport at all. Desheathed vagal nerves treated with colchicine showed a continuation of transport despite a reduced number of microtubules. A likely explanation is

that the bulk of the radioactivity is carried in the larger myelinated axons, the microtubules of which are less affected by colchicine than those of the nonmyelinated fibers.

Properties of microtubules have been elucidated from studies of purified tubulin *in vitro*. At low temperatures they can disassemble into their tubulin subunits and then reassemble when the temperature is brought up to 37°C in the presence of small amounts of Mg^{2+} and GTP (37). The microtubules in frog nerves were reported to disappear at low temperatures (27), but mammalian nerve fibers are apparently not as obviously affected by cold (99). However, fast axoplasmic transport *in vitro* in mammalian nerve is blocked at temperatures below 11°C (100). Such "cold blocks" are reversed by returning the nerves to a temperature of 38°C with a lag time of approximately 0.5 hr. This time correlates with that required for microtubular reassembly. Another possibility considered to account for cold block was a greatly increased axoplasmic viscosity at low temperatures. Using the spin-label tempone for electron spin resonance measurements, nerve axoplasm was found to have a relatively low viscosity, approximately five times that of water (46,47; cf. ref. 128). A gradual increase in viscosity was seen at lower temperatures. This is due to water alone, and it was insufficient in degree to account for the cold-block phenomenon (46).

INTERRELATION OF MEMBRANE AND TRANSPORT MECHANISMS

Fast axoplasmic transport continued unchanged when tetrodotoxin (TTX) or procaine was present to block membrane excitability (94). However, some anesthetic agents may, in high concentrations, enter the fibers and block axoplasmic transport (16) by acting on some part of the transport mechanism.

The effect of electrical stimulation on transport was recently re-evaluated, and high stimulation rates of 350 pps were shown to slow the rate of axoplasmic transport approximately 15% (131). To evaluate the possibility that the effect may be due to increased entry of Na into the fibers, batrachotoxin (BTX) was used to hold Na channels open. Fast axoplasmic transport was found to be blocked by BTX at remarkably low concentrations of less than 0.2 μM (101). However, the effect is not likely due to an increased entry of Na because a similar block of transport with BTX was seen in desheathed peroneal nerves in a Na-free media (132). The action of BTX appears to be on the transport mechanism itself, the microtubules remaining intact (93).

PATHOLOGY RELATED TO AXOPLASMIC TRANSPORT

Axoplasmic transport may be involved in the production of nervous system pathology in two ways: Pathogenic agents may gain access to the nervous system by means of axoplasmic transport. Alternatively, a disease process may alter the kind or amount of material carried by axoplasmic transport required for neural maintenance.

Among agents proposed to move in a retrograde direction into the cell bodies are the viruses of poliomyelitis and herpes simplex. Goodpasture (38) earlier inferred that peripheral nerves may serve as portals of entry for the herpesvirus into the CNS. Recently Kristensson (71) found virus particles in Schwann cells and neuron cell bodies of the sensory or motor systems following viral innoculation in the skin or of the muscular distributions of the appropriate nerves, respectively. Barringer and Griffith (5) identified viral particles in the ganglion cells after corneal innoculations in the rabbit, and an intra-axonal location of viral particles in mice inoculated with herpes simplex virus was demonstrated by Hill et al. (53).

Tetanus toxin has also been considered to be transported in nerve fibers. Price et al. (106) injected ¹²⁵I-labeled toxin intramuscularly and demonstrated an accumulation of radioactivity within the fibers below a nerve crush in autoradiographs. The rate of retrograde transport of the toxin was calculated to be in excess of 75 mm/day. The tetanus toxin is transported specifically in the axons of α-motor neurons to the exclusion of the γ-fibers (42).

As discussed by Dyck (25), a distinction must be made between neuropathies giving rise to a picture of Wallerian degeneration, a primary segmental demyelination, or axonal atrophy with a secondary myelin degeneration. Wallerian degeneration has been variously

said to spread proximodistally in fibers from the point of transection or to occur synchronously all along the amputated parts of nerve. The consensus favors a synchronous appearance. Considering the fast rate of axoplasmic transport, transported materials rapidly traverse the length of the entire distal amputated segment of nerve in a few hours. This, and the redistribution of materials (90), acts to mask an early proximodistal gradient of degeneration recently found by Lubinská (78).

In those disease entities which exhibit axonal degeneration, the distal axon fails without obvious evidence of perikaryal involvement, and demyelination then follows secondarily. This must be distinguished from segmental demyelination due to a primary disorder of the myelin sheath. A number of neuropathies resulting from industrial toxins produce such a "dying-back" phenomenon. Among agents implicated are acrylamide, methyl-n-butyl ketone (MBK), and n-hexane. The characteristic ultrastructural changes can be produced experimentally and are also seen in "giant axonal neuropathy," a congenital hypertrophic type of neuropathy. Spencer and Schaumburg (120; see also *this volume*) suggested the name "central–peripheral distal axonopathy" to designate these disorders. They are characterized clinically by motor and/or sensory disturbances beginning in the distal extremities and progressing centrally accompanied by distal axonal degeneration and secondary demyelination (121). Three possible etiological mechanisms are: (a) a general metabolic defect of the perikaryon leading to a deficiency in the amount or alteration in the type of material transported; (b) a primary defect in the transport mechanism; and (c) a direct toxin action on the distal part of the axon. Pleasure et al. (105) reported a defect in axoplasmic transport in cats exposed to acrylamide, although they were unable to demonstrate any changes in triorthocresylphosphate (TOCP)-intoxicated animals. Their method did not allow transport rates greater than 100 mm/day to be determined; fast transport was therefore not assessed. Mendell et al. (81) found the usual axoplasmic transport rate of 412 mm/day in their control rat motor nerves with a progressive diminution of rate paralleling the behavioral severity of MBK neuropathy. Proliferating neurofilaments seen in the fibers were suggested to be responsible for the defect in axoplasmic transport.

Two patients with the distal peripheral neuropathy of Charcot–Marie–Tooth disease and one case of hypertrophic neuropathy of the Dejerine–Scottas type were demonstrated to have a decreased accumulation of DBH in human nerve biopsy studies made using a double-ligature technique (14). These results also tend to support the contention of Oppenheimer (104) that Friedreich's ataxia is related to the "loss of vitality of a long axon."

Conditions which impair metabolism and the supply of ATP would be expected to affect transport. Thiamine and pyridoxine act as enzyme cofactors and deficiencies of these vitamins lead to the axonal degenerations (107). Alcoholic polyneuropathy, essentially identical to the syndrome of beriberi caused by thiamine deficiency, appears to have a similar etiology (126). Schmidt et al. (117) reported decreases in the accumulation of AChE and choline acetylase in experimental diabetes, with no such changes apparent in insulin-treated animals.

Moorhead et al. (83), in a case of primary hyperoxaluria, revealed the presence of oxalate crystals within axons. This could perhaps cause a block of transport by binding Ca (see above). Interference with metabolism and ATP generation have also been reported as pathogenetic factors in the neuropathies associated with porphyria (18,110) and uremia (26). A number of pharmacological agents have been reported to produce peripheral neuropathies of the degenerative axonal type: diphenylhydantoin (30,76), isoniazid (116), dapsone (45), and hexachlorophene (125). The *Vinca* alkaloids must be included here because their chronic use at high levels as antitumor agents in clinical practice often produces a neuropathy (109,118). The identification of derivatives showing good antitumor activity and a reduction of the neuropathy would be of great value. The neurotoxicity of different *Vinca* derivatives can be evaluated by the time of block of axoplasmic transport *in vitro* (102).

Much attention has been paid to animal models of muscular dystrophy. The rate of transport has been variously reported to be much increased (69) or unchanged (9) in dystrophic mice. Similarly, the presence (8,

133) or absence (108) of a rate change has been noted in a dystrophic-like condition produced by pargyline. No alteration in anterograde transport was found in dystrophic chickens (123), and little difference in the retrograde accumulation of HRP has been seen in these dystrophic animals (23). Although the rate of transport may be unaffected in the disease, some components were reported to show an increase (124), whereas the transport of choline acetyltransferase activity was found to be reduced in dystrophic mice (59).

It is hoped that further study of axoplasmic transport and its alteration in various neuropathies, either of unknown causes or following exposure to various known toxic agents, will lead to a better understanding of this fundamental neuronal function and promote more effective therapy of these disabling disorders.

REFERENCES

1. Abe, T., Haga, T., and Kurokawa, M. (1973): Rapid transport of phosphatidylcholine occurring simultaneously with protein transport in the frog sciatic nerve. *Biochem. J.,* 136:731–740.
2. Baker, P. F. (1976): Regulation of intracellular Ca and Mg in squid axons. *Fed. Proc.,* 35:2589–2595.
3. Barber, P. C., and Field, P. M. (1975): Autoradiographic demonstration of afferent connections of the accessory olfactory bulb in the mouse. *Brain Res.,* 85:201–203.
4. Barondes, S. H. (1964): Delayed appearances of labeled protein in isolated nerve endings and axoplasmic flow. *Science,* 146: 779–781.
5. Baringer, J. R., and Griffith, J. F. (1970): Experimental herpes simplex encephalitis: Early neuropathological changes. *J. Neuropathol. Exp. Neurol.,* 29:89–104.
6. Barondes, S. H. (1966): On the site of synthesis of the mitochondrial protein of nerve endings. *J. Neurochem.,* 13:721–727.
7. Blaustein, M. P. (1976): The in and outs of calcium transport in squid axons: Internal and external ion activation of calcium efflux. *Fed. Proc.,* 35:2574–2578.
8. Boegman, R. J., Wood, P. L., and Pinaud, L. (1975): Increased axoplasmic flow associated with pargyline under conditions which induce a myopathy. *Nature (Lond),* 253:51–52.
9. Bradley, W. G., and Jaros, E. (1973): Axoplasmic flow in axonal neuropathies. II. Axoplasmic flow in mice with motor neuron

disease and muscular dystrophy. *Brain,* 96: 247–258.

10. Bradley, W. G., Lassman, L. P., Pearce, G. W., and Walton, J. N. (1970): The neuromyopathy of vincristine in man: Clinical electrophysiological and pathological studies. *J. Neurol. Sci.,* 10:107–131.

11. Brattgård, S-O., Edström, J-E., and Hydén, H. (1958): The productive capacity of the neuron in retrograde reaction. *Exp. Cell Res. (Suppl.),* 5:185–200.

12. Brimijoin, S. (1975): Stop-flow: A new technique for measuring axonal transport, and its application to the transport of dopamine-beta-hydroxylase. *J. Neurobiol.,* 6:379–394.

13. Brimijoin, S., and Helland, L. (1976): Rapid retrograde transport of dopamine-beta-hydroxylase as examined by the stop-flow technique. *Brain Res.,* 102:217–228.

14. Brimijoin, S., Capek, P., and Dyck, P. J. (1973): Axonal transport of dopamine-β-hydroxylase by human nerves in vitro. *Science,* 180:1295–1297.

15. Byers, M. R. (1974): Structural correlates of rapid axonal transport: Evidence that microtubules may not be directly involved. *Brain Res.,* 75:97–113.

16. Byers, M. R., Hendrickson, A. E., Fink, B. R., Kennedy, R. D., and Middaugh, M. E. (1973): Effects of lidocaine on axonal morphology, microtubules, and rapid transport in rabbit vagus nerve in vitro. *J. Neurobiol.,* 4:125–143.

17. Cancalon, P., and Beidler, L. M. (1975): Distribution along the axon and into various subcellular fractions of molecules labeled with ^{3}H-leucine and rapidly transported in the garfish olfactory nerve. *Brain Res.,* 89: 225–244.

18. Cavanaugh, J. B., and Mellick, R. S. (1965): On the nature of the peripheral nerve lesions associated with acute intermittent porphyria. *J. Neurol. Neurosurg. Psychiatry,* 28:320–327.

19. Cowan, W. M., Gottlieb, D. I., Hendrickson, A. E., Price, J. L., and Woolsey, T. A. (1972): The autoradiographic demonstration of axonal connections in the central nervous system. *Brain Res.,* 37:21–51.

20. Crescitelli, F. (1951): Nerve sheath as a barrier to the action of certain substances. *Am. J. Physiol.,* 166:229–240.

21. Dahlström, A. (1968): Effect of colchicine on transport of amine storage granules in sympathetic nerves of rat. *Eur. J. Pharmacol.,* 5:111–113.

22. Dahlström, A. (1971): Axoplasmic transport with particular respect to adrenergic neurons. *Philos. Trans. R. Soc. B.,* 261:325–358.

23. DeSantis, M., Hoekman, T., and Limwongse, V. (1977): Retrograde transport of per-

oxidase in motor neurons innervating slow and fast muscles: Absence of a difference between normal and dystrophic chickens. *Brain Res.,* 119:454–458.

24. Droz, B., and Barondes, S. H. (1969): Nerve endings—rapid appearance of labelled protein shown by electron microscope radioautography. *Science,* 165:1131–1133.

25. Dyck, P. J. (1975): Pathological alterations of the peripheral nervous system of man. In: *Peripheral Neuropathy,* Vol. 1, edited by P. J. Dyck, P. K. Thomas, and E. H. Lambert, pp. 296–336. Saunders, Philadelphia.

26. Dyck, P. J., Johnson, W. J., Lambert, E. H., and O'Brien, P. C. (1971): Segmental demyelination secondary to axonal degeneration in uremic neuropathy. *Mayo Clin. Proc.,* 46:400–431.

27. Echandia, R. E. L., and Piezzi, R. S. (1968): Microtubules in the nerve fibers of the toad Bufo arenarium Hensel: Effect of low temperature on the sciatic nerve. *J. Cell Biol.,* 39:491–497.

28. Edström, A. (1974): Effects of Ca^{2+} and Mg^{2+} on rapid axonal transport of proteins in vitro in frog sciatic nerves. *J. Cell Biol.,* 61:812–818.

29. Edström, A., and Hanson, M. (1973): Temperature effects on fast axonal transport of proteins in vitro in frog sciatic nerves. *Brain Res.,* 58:345–354.

30. Eisen, A. A., Woods, J. F., and Sherwin, A. L. (1974): Peripheral nerve function in long-term therapy with diphenylhydantoin: A clinical and electrophysiologic correlation. *Neurology (Minneap),* 24:411–417.

31. Elam, J. S., and Agranoff, B. W. (1971): Transport of proteins and sulfated mucopolysaccharides in the goldfish visual system. *J. Neurobiol.,* 2:379–390.

32. Engh, C. A., and Schofield, B. H. (1972): A review of the central response to peripheral nerve injury and its significance in nerve regeneration. *J. Neurosurg.,* 37:195–203.

33. Feng, T. P., and Gerard, R. W. (1930): Mechanism of nerve asphyxiation: With a note on the nerve sheath as a diffusion barrier. *Proc. Soc. Exp. Biol. Med.,* 27:1073–1076.

34. Feng, T. P., and Liu, Y. M. (1950): Further observations on the nerve sheath as a diffusion barrier. *Chin. J. Physiol.,* 17:207–218.

35. Fernandez, H. L., Huneeus, F. C., and Davison, P. F. (1970): Studies on the mechanism of axoplasmic transport in the crayfish cord. *J. Neurobiol.,* 1:395–409.

36. Fink, B. R., Byers, M. R., and Middaugh, M. E. (1973): Dynamics of colchicine effects on rapid axonal transport and axonal morphology. *Brain Res.,* 56:299–311.

37. Gaskin, F., Cantor, C. R., and Shelanski, M. L. (1975): Biochemical studies on the

in vitro assembly and disassembly of microtubules. *Ann. NY Acad. Sci.*, 253:133–146.

38. Goodpasture, E. W. (1929): Herpetic infection, with especial reference to involvement of the nervous system. *Medicine (Bolt)*, 3:223–243.

39. Grafstein, B. (1967): Transport of protein by goldfish optic nerve fibers. *Science*, 157: 196–198.

40. Grafstein, B. (1969): Axonal transport: Communication between soma and synapse. *Adv. Biochem. Psychopharmacol.*, 1:11–25.

41. Grafstein, B., and Laureno, R. (1973): Transport of radioactivity from eye to visual cortex in the mouse. *Exp. Neurol.*, 39:44–57.

42. Green, J., Erdmann, G., and Wellhöner, H. H. (1977): Is there retrograde axonal transport of tetanus toxin in both α and γ fibers? *Nature (Lond)*, 265:370.

43. Gross, G. W. (1973): The effect of temperature on the rapid axoplasmic transport in C-fibers. *Brain Res.*, 56:359–363.

44. Gross, G. W., and Beidler, L. M. (1973): Fast axonal transport in the C-fibers of the garfish olfactory nerve. *J. Neurobiol.*, 4:413–428.

45. Gutman, L., Martin, J. D., and Welton, W. (1976): Dapsone motor neuropathy—an axonal disease. *Neurology, (Minneap)*, 26:514–516.

46. Haak, R. A., Kleinhans, F. W., and Ochs, S. (1976): The viscosity of mammalian nerve axoplasm measured by electron spin resonance. *J. Physiol. (Lond)*, 263:115–137.

47. Haak, R. A., Kleinhans, F. W., Newhall, W. J., and Ochs, S. (1977): A step increase in nerve microviscosity at the temperature causing cold block of fast axoplasmic transport. *Biophys. J.*, 17:275a.

48. Hammerschlag, R., Dravid, A. R., and Chiu, A. Y. (1975): Mechanism of axonal transport—a proposed role for calcium ions. *Science*, 188:273–275.

49. Hansson, H-A., and Sjöstrand, J. (1971): Ultrastructural effects of colchicine on the hypoglossal and dorsal vagal neurons of the rabbit. *Brain Res.*, 35:379–396.

50. Hendrickson, A. E. (1972): Electron microscopic distribution of axoplasmic transport. *J. Comp. Neurol.*, 144:381–398.

51. Hindelang-Gertner, C., Stoeckel, M-E., Porte, A., and Stutinsky, F. (1976): Colchicine effects on neurosecretory neurons and other hypothalamic and hypophysial cells, with special reference to changes in the cytoplasmic membranes. *Cell Tissue Res.*, 170:17–41.

52. Hinkley, R. E., and Samson, F. E. (1972): Anesthetic induced transformation of axonal microtubules. *J. Cell Biol.*, 53:258–263.

53. Hill, T. J., Field, H. J., and Roome, A. P. C. (1972): Intra-axonal location of herpes simplex virus particles. *J. Gen. Virol.*, 15:253–255.

54. Hoffman, P. N., and Lasek, R. J. (1975): The slow component of axonal transport. Identification of major structural polypeptides of the axon and their generality among mammalian neurons. *J. Cell Biol.*, 66:351–366.

55. Huxley, A. F. (1957): Muscle structure and theories of contraction. *Prog. Biophys.*, 7:255–318.

56. Iqbal, Z., and Ochs, S. (1975): Fast axoplasmic transport of calcium binding components in mammalian nerve. *Abstr. Soc. Neurosci.*, 1:802.

57. Iqbal, Z., and Ochs, S. (1976): Calcium binding protein in brain synaptosomes. *Abstr. Soc. Neurosci.*, 2:47 (part 1).

58. Iqbal, Z., and Ochs, S. (1977): Unpublished observations.

59. Jablecki, C., and Brimijoin, S. (1974): Reduced axoplasmic transport of choline acetyltransferase activity in dystrophic mice. *Nature (Lond)*, 250:151–154.

60. James, K. A. C., and Austin, L. (1970): The binding in vitro of colchicine to axoplasmic protein from chicken sciatic nerve. *Biochem. J.*, 117:773–777.

61. Jeffrey, P. L., James, K. A. C., Kidman, A. D., Richards, A. M., and Austin, L. (1972): The flow of mitochondria in chicken sciatic nerve. *J. Neurobiol.*, 3:197–208.

62. Karlsson, J.-O., and Sjöstrand, J. (1971): Rapid intracellular transport of fucose-containing glycoproteins in retinal ganglion cells. *J. Neurochem.*, 18:2209–2216.

63. Karlsson, J.-O., Hansson, H. A., and Sjöstrand, J. (1971): Effect of colchicine on axonal transport and morphology of retinal ganglion cells. *Z. Zellforsch.*, 115:265–283.

64. Kennedy, R. D., Fink, B. R., and Byers, M. R. (1972): The effect of halothane on rapid axonal transport in the rabbit vagus. *Anesthesiology*, 36:433–443.

65. Khan, M. A., and Ochs, S. (1974): Magnesium or calcium activated ATPase in mammalian nerve. *Brain Res.*, 81:413–426.

66. Khan, M. A., and Ochs, S. (1975): Slow axoplasmic transport of mitochondria (MAO) and lactic dehydrogenase in mammalian nerve fibers. *Brain Res.*, 96:267–277.

67. Kidwai, A. M., and Ochs, S. (1969): Components of fast and slow phases of axoplasmic flow. *J. Neurochem.*, 16:1105–1112.

68. Kirkpatrick, J. B., Bray, J. J., and Palmer, S. M. (1972): Visualization of axoplasmic flow in vitro by Nomarski microscopy: Comparison to rapid flow of radioactive proteins. *Brain Res.*, 43:1–10.

69. Komiya, Y., and Austin, L. (1974): Axoplasmic flow of protein in the sciatic nerve of normal and dystrophic mice. *Exp. Neurol.*, 43:1–12.

70. Kreutzberg, G. W. (1969): Neuronal dynamics and axonal flow. IV. Blockage of intra-axonal enzyme transport by colchicine. *Proc. Natl. Acad. Sci. USA*, 62:722–728.

71. Kristensson, K. (1970): Morphological studies of the neural spread of herpes simplex virus to the central nervous system. *Acta Neuropathol. (Berl).*, 16:54–63.

72. Kristensson, K., and Olsson, Y. (1975): Retrograde transport of horseradish peroxidase in transected axons. II. Relations between rate of transfer from the site of injury to the perikaryon and onset of chromatolysis. *J. Neurocytol.*, 4:653–661.

73. Lasek, R. J., Joseph, B. S., and Whitlock, D. G. (1968): Evaluation of a radioautographic neuroanatomical tracing method. *Brain Res.*, 8:319–336.

74. LaVail, J. H., and LaVail, M. M. (1974): Intra-axonal transport of horseradish peroxidase following intravitreal injections in chicks. *Soc. Neurosci. Abstr.*, 4:299.

75. Leone, J., and Ochs, S. (1973): Reversibility of fast axoplasmic transport following differing durations of anoxic block in vitro and in vivo. *Abstr. Soc. Neurosci.*, 3:147.

76. Lovelace, R. E., and Horwitz, S. J. (1968): Peripheral neuropathy in long-term diphenylhydantoin therapy. *Arch. Neurol.*, 18:69–77.

77. Lubińská, L. (1964): Axophasmic streaming in regenerating and in normal nerve fibers. *Prog. Brain Res.*, 13:1–66.

78. Lubińská, L. (1977): Early course of Wallerian degeneration in myelinated fibres of the rat phrenic nerve. *Brain Res.* 130:47–63.

79. Lubińská, L., and Niemierko, S. (1971): Velocity and intensity of bidirectional migration of acetylcholinesterase in transected nerves. *Brain Res.*, 27:329–342.

80. Lux, H. D., Schubert, P., Kreutzberg, G. W., and Globus, A. (1970): Excitation and axonal flow: Autoradiographic study on motoneurons intracellularly injected with a ^{3}H-amino acid. *Exp. Brain Res.*, 10:197–204.

81. Mendell, J. R., Saida, K., Weiss, H. S., and Savage, R. (1976): Methyl-n-butyl ketone-induced changes in fast axoplasmic transport. *Neurology (Minneap)*, 26:349.

82. Miani, N. (1963): Analysis of the somato-axonal movement of phospholipids in the vagus and hypoglossal nerves. *J. Neurochem.*, 10:859–874.

83. Moorhead, P. J., Cooper, D. J., and Timperley, W. R. (1975): Progressive peripheral neuropathy in patients with primary hyperoxaluria. *Br. Med. J.*, 2:312–313.

84. Mullins, L. J. (1976): Steady-state calcium fluxes: Membrane versus mitochondrial control of ionized calcium in axoplasm. *Fed. Proc.*, 35:2583–2588.

85. Neale, J. H., Neale, E. A., and Agranoff, B. W. (1972): Radioautography of the optic tectum of the goldfish after intraocular injection of ^{3}H-proline. *Science*, 176:407–410.

86. Ochs, S. (1971): Local supply of energy to the fast axoplasmic transport mechanism. *Proc. Natl. Acad. Sci. USA*, 68:1279–1282.

87. Ochs, S. (1972): Membrane properties (excitability and osmoticity) and fast axoplasmic transport in vitro. *Soc. Neurosci. Abstr.*, 2:255.

88. Ochs, S. (1972): Rate of fast axoplasmic transport in mammalian nerve fibers. *J. Physiol. (Lond)*, 227:627–645.

89. Ochs, S. (1974): Energy metabolism and supply of nerve by axoplasmic transport. *Fed. Proc.*, 33:1049–1058.

90. Ochs, S. (1974): Retention and redistribution of fast and slow axoplasmic transported proteins in mammalian nerve. In: *Third International Congress on Muscle Diseases*, Vol. 334, edited by W. G. Bradley, D. Gardner-Medwin, and J. N. Walton, p. 26. Excerpta Medica, Amsterdam.

91. Ochs, S. (1974): Systems of material transport in nerve fibers (axoplasmic transport) related to nerve function and trophic control. *Ann. NY Acad. Sci.*, 228:202–223.

92. Ochs, S. (1975): A unitary concept of axoplasmic transport based on the transport filament hypothesis. In: *Third International Congress on Muscle Diseases*, Vol. 360, edited by W. G. Bradley, D. Gardner-Medwin, and J. N. Walton, pp. 189–194. Excerpta Medica, Amsterdam.

93. Ochs, S. (1975): Axoplasmic transport. In: *The Basic Neurosciences, Vol. 1: The Nervous System*, edited by D. B. Tower, pp. 137–146. Raven Press, New York.

94. Ochs, S. (1975): Mechanism of axoplasmic transport and its block by pharmacological agents. *Proceedings: 6th International Congress on Pharmacology, Vol. 2: Neurotransmission*, pp. 161–174. Finnish Pharm. Society, Helsinki.

95. Ochs, S. (1975): Retention and redistribution of proteins in mammalian nerve fibers by axoplasmic transport. *J. Physiol. (Lond)*, 253:459–475.

96. Ochs, S. (1976): Axoplasmic transport. In: *Basic Neurochemistry*, 2nd ed., edited by G. J. Siegel, R. W. Albers, R. Katzman, and B. W. Agranoff, pp. 429–444. Little Brown, Boston.

97. Ochs, S., Worth, R., and Chan, S. Y. (1977): Dependence of axoplasmic transport on calcium shown in the desheathed peroneal nerve. *Soc. Neurosci. Abst.*, 111:31.

98. Ochs, S., and Jersild, R. A. (1974): Fast axoplasmic transport in nonmyelinated mammalian nerve fibers shown by electron microscopic radioautography. *J. Neurobiol.*, 5:373–377.

99. Ochs, S., and Jersild, R. A. (1977): Unpublished studies.

100. Ochs, S., and Smith, C. (1975): Low temperature slowing and coldblock of fast axo-

plasmic transport in mammalian nerves in vitro. *J. Neurobiol.*, 6:85–102.

101. Ochs, S., and Worth, R. (1975): Batrachotoxin block of fast axoplasmic transport in mammalian nerve fibers. *Science*, 187:1087–1089.

102. Ochs, S., and Worth, R. (1975): Comparison of the block of fast axoplasmic transport in mammalian nerve by vincristine, vinblastine and desacetyl vinblastine amide sulfate (DVA). *Am. Assoc. Cancer Res. Abstr.*, 16:70.

103. Ochs, S., Sabri, M. I., and Ranish, N. (1970): Somal site of synthesis of fast transported materials in mammalian nerve fibers. *J. Neurobiol.*, 1:329–344.

104. Oppenheimer, D. R. (1976): Diseases of the basal ganglia, cerebellum and motor neurons. In: *Greenfield's Neuropathology*, edited by W. Blackwood and J. A. N. Corsellis. Edward Arnold, London, pp. 608–651.

105. Pleasure, D. E., Mishler, K. C., and Engel, W. K. (1969): Axonal transport of protein in experimental neuropathies. *Science*, 166:524–525.

106. Price, D. L., Griffin, J., Young, A., Peck, K., and Stocks, A. (1975): Tetanus toxin: Direct evidence for retrograde intraaxonal transport. *Science*, 188:945–947.

107. Prineas, J. (1970): Peripheral nerve changes in thiamine-deficient rats: An electron microscopic study. *Arch. Neurol.*, 23:541–548.

108. Ranish, N., and Dettbarn, W-D. (1977): The effect of pargyline and serotonin on fast axoplasmic transport in sciatic nerve. *Fed. Proc.*, 36:560.

109. Ranish, N., and Ochs, S. (1972): Fast axoplasmic transport of acetylcholinesterase in mammalian nerve fibers. *J. Neurochem.*, 19:2641–2649.

110. Ridley, S. (1969): The neuropathy of acute intermittent phophyria. *Q. J. Med.*, 38:307–333.

111. Rosenbaum, J. L., and Sloboda, R. (1977): Microtubule-associated-proteins (MAPs) and the assembly and function of microtubules. *Trans. Am. Soc. Neurochem.*, 8:114.

112. Rosenbaum, J. L., Binder, L. I., Granett, S., Dentler, W. L., Snell, W., Slobodo, R., and Haimo, L. (1975): Directionality and rate of assembly of chick brain tubulin onto pieces of neurotubules, flagellar axonemes, and basal bodies. *Ann. NY Acad. Sci.*, 253:147–177.

113. Rostas, J. A. P., McGregor, A., Jeffrey, P. L., and Austin, L. (1975): Transport of cholesterol in the chick optic system. *J. Neurochem.*, 24:295–302.

114. Sabri, M. I., and Ochs, S. (1972): Relation of ATP and creatine phosphate to fast axoplasmic transport in mammalian nerve. *J. Neurochem.*, 19:2821–2828.

115. Sabri, M. I., and Ochs, S. (1973): Characterization of fast and slow transported proteins in dorsal root and sciatic nerve of cat. *J. Neurobiol.*, 4:145–165.

116. Schlaepfer, W. W., and Hager, H. (1964): Ultrastructural studies of INH-induced neuropathy in rats. I. Early axonal changes. *Am. J. Pathol.*, 45:209–219.

117. Schmidt, R. E., Matschinsky, F. M., Godfrey, D. A., Williams, A. D., and McDougal, D. B., Jr. (1975): Fast and slow axoplasmic flow in sciatic nerve of diabetic rats. *Diabetes*, 24:1081–1085.

118. Shelanski, M. L., and Wiśniewski, H. (1969): Neurofibrillary degeneration: Induced by vincristine therapy. *Arch. Neurol.*, 20:199–206.

119. Soifer, D. (1975): The biology of cytoplasmic microtubules. *Ann. NY Acad. Sci.*, 253:1–848.

120. Spencer, P. S., and Schaumburg, H. H. (1976): Central and peripheral distal axonopathy—the pathology dying back neuropathies. In: *Progress in Neuropathology*, Vol. 3, edited by H. M. Zimmerman. Grune & Stratton, New York, pp. 253–295.

121. Spencer, P. S., and Schaumburg, H. (1977): *This volume.*

122. Stromska, D., and Ochs, S. (1977): Slow outflow patterns of labeled proteins in cat and rat sensory nerves. *Fed. Proc.*, 36:485.

123. Stromska, D., and Ochs, S. (1977): Unpublished observations.

124. Tang, R. Y., Komiya, Y., and Austin, L. (1974): Axoplasmic flow of phospholipids and cholesterol in the sciatic nerve of normal and dystrophic mice. *Exp. Neurol.*, 43:13–20.

125. Towfighi, J., Gonatas, N. K., and McCree, L. (1974): Hexachlorophene-induced changes in central and peripheral myelinated axons of developing and adult rats. *Lab. Invest.*, 31:712–721.

126. Victor, M. (1975): Polyneuropathy due to nutritional deficiency and alcoholism. In: *Peripheral Neuropathy*, edited by P. J. Dyck, P. K. Thomas, and E. H. Lambert, pp. 1030–1066. Saunders, Philadelphia.

127. Watson, W. E. (1965): An autoradiographic study of the incorporation of nucleic-acid precursors by neurones and glia during nerve regeneration. *J. Physiol. (Lond)*, 180:741–753.

128. Weiss, P. A. (1972): Neuronal dynamics and axonal flow. V. The semisolid state of the moving axonal column. *Proc. Natl. Acad. Sci. USA*, 69:620–623.

129. Wiesel, T. N., Hubel, D. H., and Lam, D. M. K. (1974): Autoradiographic demonstration of occular-dominance columns in the monkey striate cortex by means of transneuronal transport. *Brain Res.*, 79:273–279.

130. Wilson, L. (1974): Pharmacological and biochemical properties of microtubule proteins. *Fed. Proc.*, 33:151.

131. Worth, R. M., and Ochs, S. (1976): The effect of repetitive electrical stimulation on axoplasmic transport. *Soc. Neurosci. Abstr.*, 2:50 (part 1).

132. Worth, R. M., and Ochs, S. (1977): Unpublished observations.

133. Yu, M. K., Wright, T. L., Dettbarn, W-D., and Olson, W. H. (1974): Pargyline induced myopathies with histochemical characteristics of Duchenne muscular dystrophy. *Neurology*, 24:237–244.

Physiology and Pathobiology of Axons, edited by
S. G. Waxman. Raven Press, New York © 1978.

Pathobiology of Neurotoxic Axonal Degeneration

Peter S. Spencer and Herbert H. Schaumburg

Departments of Neuroscience and Pathology (Neuropathology), Saul R. Korey Department of Neurology, and Rose F. Kennedy Center for Research in Human Development and Mental Retardation, Albert Einstein College of Medicine, Bronx, New York 10461

The diseased axon offers the neurobiologist a unique opportunity to examine certain aspects of axonal biology that are inapparent or suppressed in the normal axon. An example of this principle is the discovery of a mechanism for the sequestration and removal of effete and abnormal organelles from the axon, a phenomenon barely recognizable in the normal state but a prominent feature of the diseased axon (42). Studies of the diseased nerve fiber have also provided an opportunity to dissect many other aspects of axonal biology, among them the symbiotic relationship shared by the axon and its ensheathing cells. The elucidation of these concepts has emanated in large part from experimental studies in which neurotoxic chemicals such as *n*-hexane and acrylamide have been employed to produce axonal degeneration (4,28,29). Not to be confused with other agents which share the same eponym, these neurotoxic chemicals display a common property of delayed neurological expression which depends on the slow or more rapid development of axonal disease and breakdown.

Two distinct and contrasting types of neurotoxin-induced axonal degeneration are considered in this chapter (Table 1). The first and most useful experimental model to study axonal pathobiology is the dying-back type of degeneration. This name was coined to describe a specific type of axonal disease in which foci of degenerative change move in space with time—the first signs of disease appearing in the distal axon and, later, in more proximal regions as the nerve fiber "dies back" toward the neuronal cell body. These *distal axonopathies* are especially useful for the study

of axonal pathobiology because of the slow pace of the degenerative process, the ability to manipulate velocity and degree of axonal damage, and the possibility for recovery of axonal integrity by reconstitution (central nervous system; CNS) or regeneration (peripheral nervous system; PNS) following the cessation of intoxication (26,36,38). Such recovery from the disease process is feasible because the proximal spread of axonal degeneration usually fails to reach the neuron cell body.

A second type of neurotoxin-induced axonal degeneration, that which accompanies a primary attack on the neuron cell body, is also briefly considered here because it represents the antithesis of the dying-back phenomenon. The disease process (neuronopathy) is expressed initially within the neuronal cell body and subsequently within the axon. In contrast to the slow, distal, and retrograde degeneration characteristic of the dying-back process, the entire axon appears to undergo a rapid breakdown in neuronopathies. Whether breakdown occurs simultaneously along the axon or the axon "dies forward" from the diseased neuronal cyton in this type of degeneration is unanswered at the present time.

ENVIRONMENTAL NEUROTOXINS

Distal Axonopathy

Several chemically unrelated neurotoxic substances are able to produce distal axonopathy in the CNS and PNS. The list includes such common industrial chemicals as the plastic monomer acrylamide (Sumner, *this volume*); the solvents *n*-hexane, methyl-*n*-butyl ketone,

TABLE 1. *Contrasting features of murine hexacarbon distal axonopathy and doxorubicin neuronopathy*

Parameter	Hexacarbon distal axonopathy	Doxorubicin neuronopathy
Toxin target	Axon	Neuron cell body
Axonal degeneration	Incomplete, giant axonal, distal, retrograde	Complete, probably simultaneous
	PNS:	PNS:
	Somatic, afferent and efferent; hindlimb, then forelimb nerves	Somatic, afferent; autonomic, afferent and efferent; hindlimb and forelimb nerves
	CNS:	
	Dorsal columns (gracile, then cuneate); spinocerebellar (dorsal); corticospinal; vestibulospinal; lateral geniculate and optic tract; fornix-mammillary tract	CNS:
		Dorsal columns (gracile and cuneate)
Neuronal degeneration	Late, transsynaptic only (gracile nucleus)	Primary (sensory and autonomic ganglia)
Behavior	Symmetrical limb weakness	Symmetrical limb incoordination
	Hindlimb before, and to greater degree than forelimb	Hindlimb and forelimb
Ataxia	Minor (cerebellar and sensory)	Pronounced (sensory)
Weakness	Insidious onset and slowly progressive to quadriparesis	Absent
Recovery	PNS: good	Unknown, probably poor
	CNS: poor	

and carbon disulfide; pesticides such as certain cresyl phosphates; and a number of therapeutic drugs such as vincristine (4,36,43). Typically, these neurotoxins damage the nervous system by repeated, low-level systemic exposure, but a few, such as tri-*o*-cresyl phosphate, may exhibit this delayed neurotoxic effect after a single, systemic administration.

The hexacarbon compounds (*n*-hexane, methyl *n*-butyl ketone, 2,5-hexanedione, and 2,5-hexanediol) have become among the most widely used neurotoxins in experimental neurobiology and form the principal subject of this chapter. These compounds form a metabolically interrelated class of neurotoxins that all produce the same type of central–peripheral distal axonopathy (36,39) (Fig. 1). Interest in these aliphatic hexacarbon compounds as

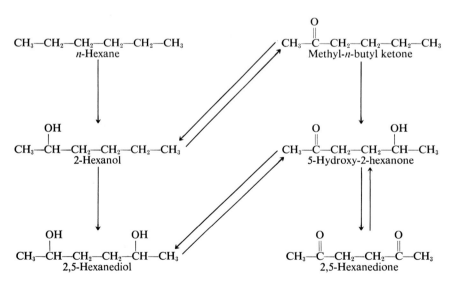

FIG. 1. Metabolism of methyl-*n*-butyl ketone and *n*-hexane in guinea pig serum. (Modified from ref. 9.)

experimental probes to study axonal patho-biology arose from reports of factory workers who developed symmetrical, distal polyneurop-athy following exposure to solvents contain-ing either *n*-hexane or methyl-*n*-butyl ketone (MBK) (1,13,46). Similar diseases developed in individuals who regularly inhaled glue va-pors containing *n*-hexane for their euphoric properties (17,45). The initial symptoms of disease consisted of intermittent tingling and numbness in the hands and feet. Motor signs included weakness in the feet or hands with the development of a slapping gait or an inability to grasp heavy objects. Lower limbs were always involved to a greater degree than upper limbs. In severe cases weakness ex-tended to the upper part of the leg, although sensory loss rarely ascended above the knee. Symmetrical limb weakness also developed in experimental animals chronically exposed to *n*-hexane, methyl *n*-butyl ketone, or their me-tabolites 2,5-hexanedione and 2,5-hexanediol (17,35,41). Intoxicated rats first developed a waddling gait in which the feet were everted and placed flat on the ground. A pronounced hindlimb weakness developed with further in-toxication, and later the forelimbs became weakened. This clinical picture, seen in pa-tients and intoxicated animals, suggested that the hexacarbons produced a distal (dying-back) axonopathy, a suspicion later confirmed by morphological study of the CNS and PNS of experimentally intoxicated animals, and of nerve biopsies obtained from patients with hexacarbon neuropathy (1,13,17).

Neuronopathy

In contrast to the large number of neuro-toxins which precipitate distal axonopathy, relatively few produce a neuronopathy. The best known examples are the mercurial com-pounds, which produce a rapid degeneration of dorsal root neurons and their central and peripheral axons (14,15). A similar, remark-ably selective pattern of neuropathology was recently recognized in animals intoxicated with the drug doxorubicin (Adriamycin) (5,6). Doxorubicin is an anthracycline anti-biotic which has emerged in recent years as an important antineoplastic agent because of the beneficial effects achieved in the treatment of a wide variety of malignant tumors. The cytotoxic effect of doxorubicin and related compounds (e.g., daunorubicin) is believed to result from their ability to bind with DNA by intercalation between the base pairs of the double helical structure (8,21). The selec-tive damage to the chromosomal DNA is ex-pressed at the cellular level by a striking loss of mitotic activity in a dividing cell popula-tion and, it appears, by cellular degeneration in a neuronal population.

Drug trials in rats first revealed the neuro-toxic property of doxorubicin (20). Animals treated with a single intravenous injection (10 mg/kg) developed a progressive limb incoor-dination which usually begins during the sec-ond week. An early sign of sensory damage in this disease is the adoption of asymmetrically folded hindlimbs when the animals' hind-quarters are raised by the tail, the normal re-sponse being that of limb extension. The limb clumsiness progresses with time, and by the third week profound ataxia is prominent al-though muscle strength appears to be retained. Doxorubicin intoxication produces a selective degeneration of dorsal root ganglia neurons, their centrally directed axons in dorsal roots and dorsal columns, and their distally directed axons within peripheral nerves (Fig. 2) (5,6). Pathological changes appear within the sensory neuron before alterations are detected in cen-tral or peripheral nerve fibers. Neuronal pa-thology is visible from 4 days after a single intravenous dose of doxorubicin (10 mg/kg). Toluidine blue staining reveals focal clear-ing of the nuclei of neurons located in tri-geminal and spinal ganglia. Nucleoplasm be-comes coarsely granular by day 9 and finely granular by day 12. Nuclear displacement and other features indicative of chromatolysis are also seen at this time. The larger neurons seem to be especially susceptible to doxorubi-cin and may undergo perikaryal vacuolation followed by total degeneration. These neurons are replaced by satellite cells in a pattern re-sembling nodes of Nageotte. These neuronal changes develop *pari passu* with central and peripheral nerve fiber degeneration. In the spinal cord, fiber breakdown occurs through-out the length of the cuneate and gracile tracts. Dorsal roots display marked fiber degeneration whereas ventral roots remain normal. In the

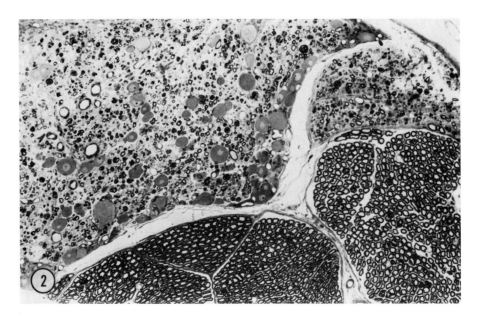

FIG. 2. Doxorubicin neuronopathy. Damaged lumbar spinal ganglion (*upper left*) and intact ventral root (*lower right*) from a rat 35 days after single i.v. injection of 10 mg/kg doxorubicin. This figure and Figs. 3–8 are light micrographs of 1-μm epoxy cross sections stained with toluidine blue. ×145. (From ref. 6.)

hindlimb the sural nerve displays a remarkable loss of fibers, a feature which is also pronounced in the peroneal and tibial nerves, except in the predominantly motor branches to the calf muscles which remain relatively well preserved.

The selective damage to sensory neurons with doxorubicin is probably related to its inability to cross the blood–brain (7,24) and nerve barriers, except at those sites where the barrier is normally incomplete, e.g., sensory ganglia. A similar explanation has been offered to explain the peripheral effects of mercury intoxication (15). Once doxorubicin enters the extracellular compartment of the ganglion, it presumably has access first to Schwann and satellite cells and then to neurons, but only the latter seem to degenerate. It seems likely that doxorubicin produces its primary lesion within the nuclear apparatus of the sensory neuron, the nerve fiber breakdown occurring as a secondary phenomenon. The selective degeneration of neurons might be related to an inability to regenerate damaged DNA in contrast to the other cells within the affected ganglia. Whatever the explanation, doxorubicin represents an important addition to the armamentarium of the neurobiologist

because it provides a tool to produce selective and rapid damage to sensory neurons. Because of its likely site of toxic action, the drug may prove useful in studies dissecting the production, packaging, and export of neuronal supplies to the axon.

EXPERIMENTAL DISTAL (DYING-BACK) AXONOPATHY

The experimental distal axonopathies produced by neurotoxic chemicals represent a group of diseases related by their broadly similar pattern of pathology (distal axonal degeneration of long CNS and PNS tracts) and clinical expression (weight loss and neuropathy). Within the group, it is useful to distinguish nuances in the pattern and distribution of neurological disease produced by the individual neurotoxins. For example, there are variations between the distribution of PNS axonal damage in the hindlimb of rats and cats intoxicated with acrylamide and that seen with the neurotoxic hexacarbons (39). Plantar sensory nerves in the rat are much more vulnerable to acrylamide than to hexacarbons. This is consistent with the observation that certain sensory terminals in the hindfeet of the cat (e.g., the pacinian corpuscle) commence degeneration before adjacent motor terminals. By contrast, pacinian corpuscles in the hindfeet of cats intoxicated with hexacarbon compounds show a remarkable resistance to damage and degenerate long after hindlimb weakness is profound (37). There are also reported variations in the morphological pattern of nerve fiber breakdown in response to different neurotoxins. For example, the hexacarbon compounds induce massive 10 nm neurofilament accumulations which lead to the production of spectacular, multifocal axonal swellings as a prelude to fiber destruction (38). Carbon disulfide and acrylamide may induce similar axonal swellings (34,43), although with acrylamide these are prominent only during very slow intoxication and may be absent if intoxication and fiber breakdown are rapid. The intensity and rapidity of intoxication therefore appear not only to determine the rate of fiber degeneration but also to affect the appearance of the diseased axon. Indeed it is possible that many of the neurotoxins produce a uniform, sequential evolution of axonal degeneration, the prominence of the individual steps in the sequence of change being related directly to the speed of breakdown.

Pattern and Distribution of Axonal Degeneration

The morphological hallmarks of experimental distal axonopathy are distal, temporally ascending degeneration of long nerve fiber tracts located in the CNS and PNS (3,22,23, 36). In the spinal cord, degenerative changes are first detected in the rostral limit of long ascending tracts (e.g., gracile and dorsal spinocerebellar) and in the caudal region of long descending tracts (e.g., corticospinal). Concurrently, in the peripheral nervous system the elongated nerve fibers supplying the hindlimb also begin to undergo distal axonal degeneration. The disease process always affects nerve tracts with bilateral symmetry and, as it progresses degenerative change moves retrograde along the affected pathways. The net effect of this pattern of change is a gradation of nerve damage, increasing in severity from proximal to distal regions. As the disease develops, progressively shorter nerve tracts commence distal and ascending degeneration. This phenomenon is well illustrated by the behavior at the cervico-medullary junction of the distal regions of the gracile and cuneate tracts, which contain, respectively, the *long* and *shorter* central axonal projections of sensory neurons located in the lumbar and cervical ganglia. Unlike the picture with doxorubicin, the distal extremities of vulnerable fibers located in the gracile tract commence ascending degeneration long before similar changes are seen in equivalent regions of the cuneate tract (Table 1). Thus when fibers in the cuneate tract display axonal swelling, neighboring fibers in the gracile tract show advanced fiber breakdown. The optic tract provides an example of an even shorter nerve fiber pathway that commences distal (lateral geniculate, superior colliculus) axonal degeneration very late in the disease process (27). The visual system damage seen in hexacarbon neuropathy probably accounts for the visual impairment in humans exposed to *n*-hexane (46). With pronounced neuropathy, distal axonal swellings may be found in several other, relatively short nerve fiber tracts located in the feline CNS (e.g., fornix–mammillary pathway) and in the PNS (e.g., forelimb nerves). The former may be associated with recent memory loss in man (45) and the latter responsible for the addition of forelimb weakness on the existing hindlimb paraparesis.

Fiber Vulnerability

It is apparent from the foregoing discussion that every nerve fiber pathway is potentially vulnerable in distal axonopathies, the degree of susceptibility being related directly to axonal *length*. One corollary of this hypothesis is that the anatomy of the experimental animal, the key factor determining axonal length, would affect the onset and distribution of the disease process. For example, an animal with arms and legs of similar length (e.g., orang-utan) might contemporaneously develop distal axonopathy in all four limbs. An animal with short legs and a long body (e.g., ferret, dachshund) might develop tractal degeneration in the spinal cord, medulla and cerebellum before distal axonopathy in the PNS. These considerations may also be relevant to the naturally occurring recurrent laryngeal nerve palsy in the horse, the nerve running twice the length of the elongated neck before arriving at its position of innervation (10).

Athough the length of the axon is a key factor in determining nerve fiber susceptibility, it is apparent from studies of the distribution of change in the PNS that the *diameter* of the axon also plays an important role. Susceptibility seems to be related directly to axonal diameter (and therefore to total axonal volume) since in distal axonopathies there is a relatively greater loss of large-diameter myelinated fibers than those of small caliber. Axons of unmyelinated fibers are the least susceptible. A striking example of the role of axon caliber is provided by the tibial nerve, which contains a special population of very large diameter myelinated fibers in the branches supplying the calf musculature. In murine and feline hexacarbon neuropathies, these nerve fibers undergo distal axonal degeneration long before similar events commence in the much longer but thinner sensory and motor fibers supplying the hindfeet. Since the degenerative process moves proximally with time, two independent ascending waves of giant axonal swelling appear in the tibial nerve. Because the ascending wave in the calf muscle branches precedes that in the plantar branches, scattered giant axonal swelling in the sciatic nerve precedes its appearance in the posterior tibial nerve below the calf branches (39). By examining only these two sites, one group was incorrectly led to the conclusion that damage is greater proximally than distally and therefore that nerve fibers were not engaged in the dying-back process (25).

The relative importance of axonal diameter versus axonal length might be tested in those somatic, efferent, myelinated fibers which normally display small-diameter, preterminal branches emanating from a larger-diameter parent axon. This problem has been examined (in collaboration with E. R. Peterson) in an organotypic tissue culture model of the PNS which displays distal axonopathy following chronic exposure to soluble neurotoxic hexacarbons. By observing the evolution of giant axonal swelling in the living nerve fibers for periods up to 1 year, it was possible to demonstrate that swellings first developed on the proximal side of the last node of Ranvier of the broad parent fiber and, subsequently, on the proximal sides of progressively more proximal paranodes. Giant axonal swelling was also seen in the thinner, preterminal branches of the parent fiber, but only *after* changes were pronounced in the parent fiber. A parallel evolution of multifocal paranodal changes occurring *in vivo* would account for the observation that giant axonal swelling is frequently visible in the tibial nerve branches to the calf muscles before swellings develop at the corresponding motor nerve terminals.

Evolution of Nerve Fiber Degeneration

On the basis of data obtained from the three-dimensional observation of single living fibers *in vitro* and of fixed, teased fibers *in*

→

FIGS. 3–8. Hexacarbon distal axonopathy. Stages of myelinated nerve fiber degeneration in longitudinal sections. (From ref. 38.)

FIG. 3: Paranodal giant axonal swelling(s) associated with an abnormally thin myelin sheath. 2,5-Hexanedione. ×1,485.

FIG. 4. Paranodal giant axonal swelling(s) displaying paranodal myelin retraction and differential density of the axoplasm. Methyl-*n*-butyl ketone. ×1,500.

FIG. 5. A corrugated myelinated fiber displaying intussusception and fracturing of the paranodal myelin sheath. MBK. ×1,760.

FIG. 6. Demyelination (d) and early remyelination (r). 2,5-Hexanedione. ×1,500.

FIG. 7. Fiber with a phagocytic cell (*arrow*) sited between the axon and the myelin sheath. Early remyelination (r). 2,5-Hexanedione. ×1,510.

FIG. 8. Phagocytic cell (*arrow*) associated with bubbling of the myelin sheath in a late phase of fiber breakdown. ×1,380.

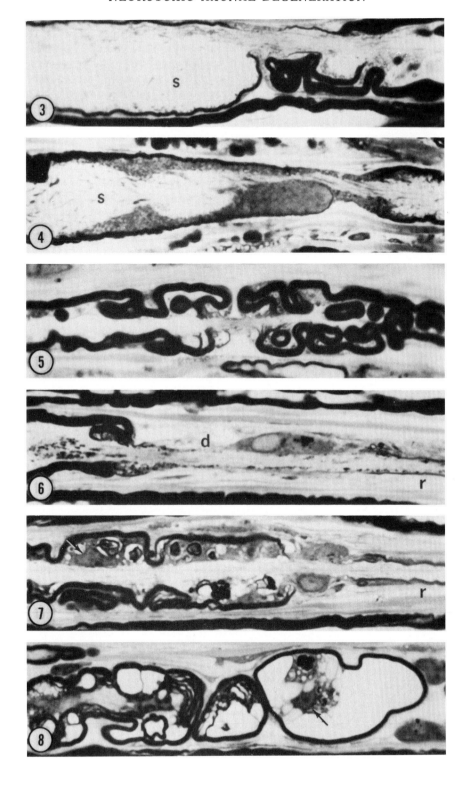

vivo, the evolution of peripheral nerve fiber damage in the hexacarbon model of slowly evolving distal axonopathy is clear (Figs. 3–8) (38). The initial morphological change occurs on the proximal sides of one or more nodes of Ranvier in the distal part of the axon, the more distally located swellings in the unbranched portion of a branching fiber usually developing before more proximal swellings. The paranodal swelling phase moves in the form of a wave up the nerve fiber, sequentially involving the proximal side of each node of Ranvier. Thus, the axon initially "dies back" in a saltatory fashion. During the swelling phase of each paranode, the associated myelin sheath loses its fluted indentations and later retracts away from the nodal region as the axon enlarges. (This leaves a demyelinated region which may shrink and undergo remyelination by the intercalation of a Schwann cell, which produces a short internode of thin myelin.) Axonal swellings may also appear focally or throughout the entire internode during the later phases of fiber change. Swellings sometimes develop on the distal sides of affected paranodes; but in contrast to the swellings on the juxtaposed proximal paranodes, these usually contain numerous mitochondria, vesicles, rather few neurofilaments, and profiles denoting ongoing Schwann cell sequestration (*vide infra*).

While this complex series of pathological events is slowly developing and spreading up the affected fiber, there develops at a certain position in the distal axon (probably a markedly swollen paranode) an irreversible condition which represents the committed step toward complete distal fiber breakdown. The sequence of events at this locus remains the subject of speculation (*vide infra*), but the result is clear—simultaneous, Wallerian-like breakdown of the entire length of distal axon. This portion of the fiber rapidly develops into a Schwann cell column punctuated by myelin ovoids and surrounded by the original basal lamina. Regenerating axon sprouts may later develop from the terminal preserved or newly created node, grow distally within the Schwann tube, and develop into a cluster of regenerating fibers displaying short internodes of thin myelin. Although the process has not been followed in detail, it is clear that regenerating axons may also undergo giant axonal swelling con-

current with the later pathological events in the original, more-proximal part of the fiber. The tissue culture studies, in which one is also examining short internodes, suggest that giant axonal swelling may cause the entire internode to undergo demyelination (40). Later in the disease process, it is assumed that a second committed step leading to distal fiber breakdown occurs at a more proximal position in the fiber, leading to repetition of the cycle of fiber breakdown and regeneration. As this process takes place in many fibers, and at ever more proximal sites, the affected nerve fiber tract appears to die back.

Role of the Node of Ranvier

The sequence of events occurring close to the affected nodes of Ranvier appears to hold the key to the process of fiber degeneration. The giant axonal swellings that develop on the proximal sides of distal nodes are composed of excessive numbers of normal-appearing neurofilaments arranged in a swirling array (Figs. 9 and 10). Trapped within this mass of neurofilaments are vesicles, mitochondria, smooth endoplasmic reticulum, and an apparently normal number of neurotubules. Frequently these organelles are clustered together and form channels which penetrate the swollen region and continue through an unswollen node. Although it has not been determined with certainty, it seems likely that the neurofilaments represent an accumulation of somatofugally moving material and not a local proliferation of neurofilaments. Their ability to accumulate in the paranode and not to invade the node may reflect the presence of circular collagen fibers which would tend to form a tight restricting collar around the nodal axon. A similar explanation would account for the focal swellings found at Schmidt–Lanterman incisures. Although this might explain how the swelling is held in the paranode, it does not explain its causation. In order to approach this question, it is necessary to determine why the filaments accumulate on the proximal side of the paranode and mitochondria on the distal side. One possibility is that a larger-than-normal number of neurofilaments move down the axon, a result of either excessive production or slowed turnover. This might

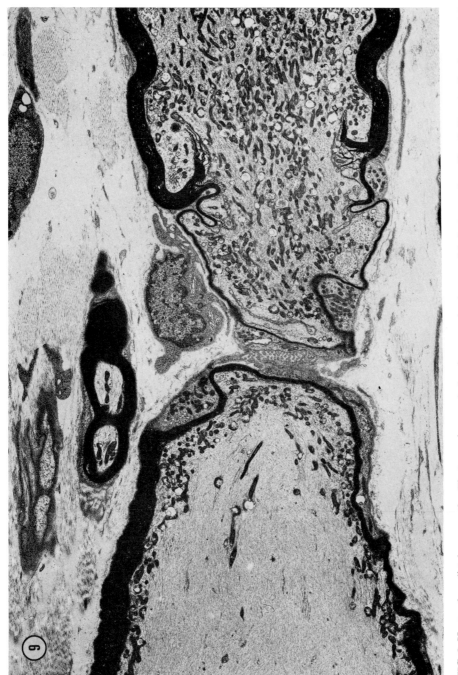

FIG. 9. Hexacarbon distal axonopathy. Electron micrograph showing a proximal paranodal giant axonal swelling (*left*) and a distal paranodal collection of axonal mitochondria (*right*). Longitudinal section. This figure and Figs. 10–12 are thin epoxy sections stained with uranyl acetate and lead citrate. Methyl-*n*-butyl ketone. ×6,000. (From ref. 38.)

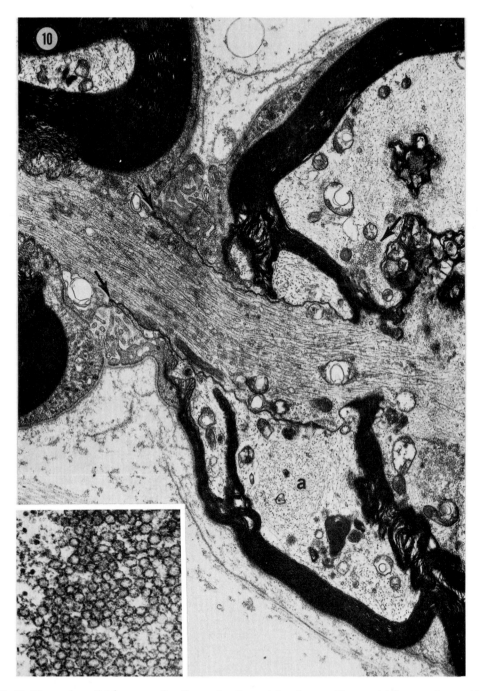

FIG. 10. Hexacarbon distal axonopathy. Paranode of a peripheral nerve fiber containing axoplasm with an abnormally large number of neurofilaments, clusters of clear-core vesicles (*arrowhead*) and scattered dense-core vesicles, several mitochondria, and a few dense bodies. Associated with these abnormal axonal organelles are protrusions of terminal Schwann cell tongues, some contributing to profiles engaged in sequestering axoplasm, others segregating pockets of abnormal axoplasm (a), and two extending into the adjacent node of Ranvier (*arrows*). ×14,400. **Inset:** An adjacent area of axoplasm containing numerous clear-core vesicles of synaptic vesicle proportions and dense particles resembling glycogen (*lower left*). ×53,000. (From ref. 42.)

produce an accumulation of neurofilaments on the proximal sides of paranodes, the attenuated nodal axon acting as a regulating valve, restricting the passage of abnormally large volumes of transported material. The large myelinated fibers would be most susceptible because nodal axonal attenuation is proportionately greater in these than in small fibers. However, this idea fails to account for the multifocal distribution of the swollen regions. A more plausible hypothesis, which takes into account the proximal paranodal swelling and adjacent, distal internodal attenuation, postulates the existence of deficient transportation of *slow*-moving filamentous protein across the nodal axon. This idea is consistent with recent experiments which have examined the fate of radioactive markers rapidly transported along the distal axons of animals with early pathological changes (11). Light and electron microscope autoradiography reveals a larger amount of transported label in the swollen paranodes relative to other parts of the distal axons. Transported label is located principally around the perimeter of the axon where the neurofilaments adopt a swirling array. This observation has been interpreted to indicate that fast-transported particles follow a corkscrew distal route around the edge of the swollen axon. This would delay the anterograde movement of materials and, since the swellings develop more proximally with time, would account for the observed progressive reduction in the rate of fast axonal transport (18).

Retrograde transport in affected axons is currently being investigated (12) using ^{125}I-labeled tetanospasmin injected into the leg muscles. Preliminary studies indicate accumulation of label principally on the swollen distal sides of affected distal paranodes. In summary, it is clear that abnormalities of antero- and retrograde transport occur in swollen paranodes, but whether this is related to the cause of the swellings remains to be determined.

Schwann Cell Sequestration

The Schwann cell plays an important role in sequestering and removing degenerate and effete axoplasmic organelles which accumulate in distal paranodes and at other inter-nodal sites in distal axonopathies (42). The phenomenon is sometimes seen in axons from control animals, especially within the perimeter of the paranodes where organelles sometimes accumulate. In the diseased axon, Schwann cell sequestration is a much more prominent feature, the degree of expression seemingly related to the number of organelles requiring sequestration. In order to perform its sequestering function, the Schwann cell first pushes a sheet of adaxonal cytoplasm *deep* into the axon surface, a coated region of the axolemma marking the locus for invagination. The sheet of cytoplasm envelops a group of axoplasmic organelles and, by dividing into multiple fronds, compartmentalizes small portions of abnormal axoplasm. Such sequestered areas of axoplasm are separated from each other by four membranes, an inner pair of apposed Schwann plasmalemmae separated by a variable amount of cytoplasm and, on the other sides of these membranes, an axolemma. The most common axonal organelles to be sequestered by the Schwann cell are clear-core vesicles of synaptic vesicle proportions. Whether these vesicles are moving retrograde from the nerve terminal has yet to be determined. Mitochondria and dense membranous bodies are also frequently involved in sequestration (Figs. 11–13).

The interpretation of this extraordinary phenomenon by which the Schwann cell interferes directly with the local economy of the axon is open to question. The answer may lie in the surprising fact that neurofilaments and neurotubules rarely appear in the sequestered portions of the axoplasm despite their abundance in the juxtaposed body of the axon. Instead, the sequestered organelles are associated with a floccular material. The breakdown of neurofilaments and neurotubules to a floccular state is known to be calcium-dependent (30). It is therefore conceivable that calcium levels are high in the sequestered axoplasm, perhaps from the breakdown of the trapped mitochondria and vesicles. In the event that the adaxonal Schwann cell cytoplasm failed to sequester sufficient degenerating mitochondria, intramitochondrial calcium might be released into the axon. This event would cause dissolution of the structural elements of the axon, concomitant failure of transport mecha-

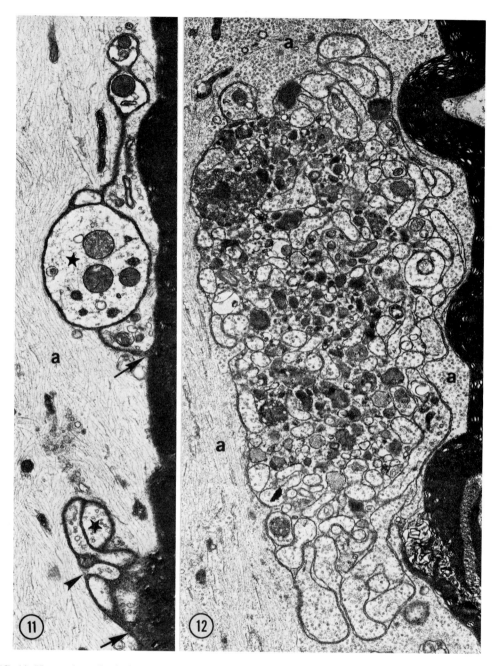

FIG. 11. Hexacarbon distal axonopathy. Internodal myelinated peripheral axon containing two groups of attenuated cytoplasmic profiles in continuity with adaxonal Schwann cell cytoplasm (*arrows*) and surrounding electron-lucent regions (*stars*), one of which shows continuity with the axon in this section (*arrowhead*). The largest portion of sequestered axoplasm (*upper star*) contains abnormal mitochondria, sparse neurofilaments, and neurotubules. Other areas of sequestered axoplasm (*lower star*) contain small, clear-core vesicles, also visible within the main axon (a). ×12,000. (From ref. 42.) **FIG. 12.** Hexacarbon distal axonopathy. Complex Schwann cell/axon network. Sequestered areas of axoplasm contain several types of abnormal organelles including rosette-shaped particles. (a) Axon. ×13,000. (From ref. 42.)

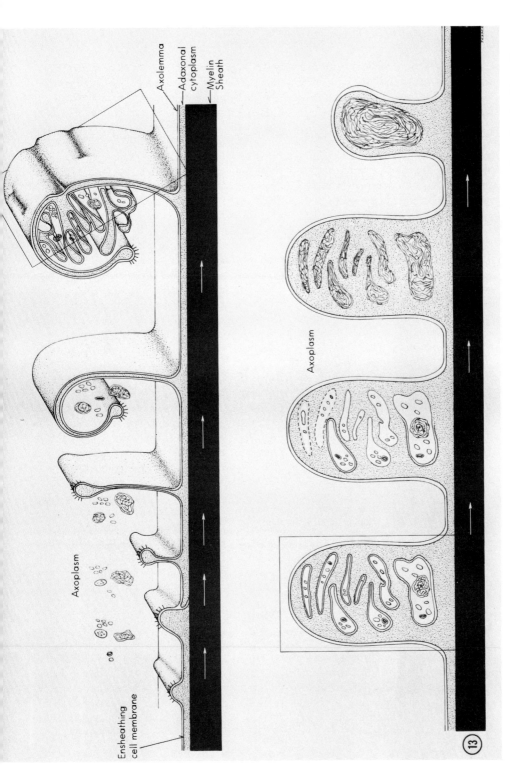

FIG. 13. Process of Schwann cell sequestration and phagocytosis of axonal debris. The process starts with the formation of a ridge of ensheathing cell cytoplasm adjacent to abnormal axoplasmic organelles and to an internally coated region of axolemma. The ridge of cytoplasm enlarges to form a thin sheet which indents the axon surface. The invaginating adaxonal cytoplasmic sheet surrounds the abnormal axonal organelles and segregates them from the remainder of the axon. The cytoplasmic sheet infolds on itself (*upper right*) and sequesters groups of axoplasmic organelles to form an interdigitated or honeycomb profile when viewed in section (*lower left*). The two membranes surrounding each portion of sequestered axoplasm become disrupted and are eventually lost. Axoplasmic material is then taken up by the surrounding Schwann cell cytoplasm, which subsequently retracts to its original, adaxonal position. (From ref. 42.)

nisms, and subsequent simultaneous degeneration of the entire distal axon. This concept is consistent with the paranodal accumulation of mitochondria during the early stage of Wallerian degeneration of a distal stump when organelles accumulate at paranodes but fail to become sequestered (2). By sequestering these organelles, the Schwann cell might provide a mechanism for the focal release of calcium without endangering the integrity of the axon.

After axonal organelles have been sequestered by the adaxonal cytoplasm, the membranes surrounding each axoplasmic compartment undergo dissolution, and the degenerating material enters the invaginated sheet of adaxonal Schwann cell cytoplasm. At this stage, the phagocytosed material adopts the character of dense membranous bodies. There are two possibilities regarding the fate of this material. One suggestion is that the material terminates as paranuclear Schwann cell lamellar bodies, but this would require movement from the adaxonal to the abaxonal cytoplasmic compartment. This hypothesis is currently being investigated using retrogradely transported axonal labels that have been identified in the sequestered portions of axoplasm (12). Another proposal is that material is deposited extracellularly between the axon and Schwann cell, an event which has been documented in the proximal stump of amputated nerves. This phenomenon is believed to be causally associated with the entry of foreign cells into the fiber at nodes of Ranvier and their phagocytic activity within the juxtanodal adaxonal space (Fig. 7). When the phagocyte withdraws from the fiber, the adaxonal space becomes edematous and bloated, and the fiber forms a myelin bubble (Spencer and Weinberg, *this volume*). This combination of changes—sequestration, phagocyte penetration, and myelin bubble formation—is rare in most distal axonopathies but is prominent in the very slowly evolving disease associated with sodium cyanate intoxication (44).

Oligodendrocytes and the Schwann cell-derived hemilamellar cells of the pacinian corpuscle also display the phenomenon of ensheathing cell axoplasmic sequestration and removal of debris in distal axonopathies (29,

42). In the pacinian corpuscle the hemilamellar cells penetrate the specialized polar regions of the elliptical axon where mitochondria and vesicles normally congregate. The degenerating organelles are engulfed by the hemilamellar cells and undergo intracytoplasmic dissolution. It seems likely that sequestration and phagocytosis might occur at other sites where the neuron and ensheathing cell also are intimately related, e.g., the satellite cell and sensory neuron, the motor end-plate, and other sensory terminals.

The inescapable conclusion from studying the phenomenon of sequestration is that the ensheathing cell and axon participate in a carefully orchestrated symbiotic relationship. The ensheathing cells—Schwann cell, oligodendrocyte, or hemilamellar cell—seem to police areas of axon under their domain, selectively removing stationary material from the axon which would endanger axonal integrity were this material allowed to disintegrate. This system operates at a low level under normal conditions in the fluted paranodal regions of large peripheral myelinated fibers where organelles probably become trapped in local eddy currents. In the diseased axon, however, where movement of axoplasmic components is known to be impaired, the ensheathing cells play a key role in determining the fate of the axon. In summary, it may be the failure of the ensheathing cell to respond adequately to the presence of ever-accumulating axonal mitochondria, which precipitates the committed step of fiber breakdown leading to distal, Wallerian-like degeneration.

Metabolic Lesion

Perhaps the greatest mystery underlying the dying-back process is how a large number of chemically unrelated substances can produce a similar pattern and distribution to that of axonal degeneration. Why, for example, should *n*-hexane and carbon disulfide each produce a giant axonal neuropathy? The answer to this question may be that these substances, or their active metabolites, act at nearby or related sites in intermediary metabolism, the net result being a common metabolic defect. If this idea is correct, then it should be possible to determine the specific metabolic lesions associated with any one neurotoxin and amend the metabolic problem by nutrient or enzyme replacement therapy. This approach has profound implications for certain human neurological conditions which display a progressive downhill course (polyneuropathies of inherited or metabolic origin, systematized degenerations) since it is likely that these represent naturally occurring examples of distal axonopathy (3,36).

An important problem associated with the use of toxic chemicals is to determine whether the parent compound or one of its metabolites is the active agent. With the hexacarbon compounds, our approach has been to test the water-soluble metabolites (2,5-hexanedione, and 2,5-hexanediol) determined *in vivo* for neurotoxic properties in the organotypic cord–ganglia–muscle tissue cultures referred to earlier. The advantage of this system is that the nutrient fluid, which provides the vehicle for the neurotoxin, is readily subjected to biochemical analysis before and after exposure to the nervous tissue. Any metabolites which appear in the nutrient fluid result from catabolic activity within the neuromuscular complex during the 2- to 3-day period of exposure to the tissue. By observing the degree of structural change over a period of many weeks, it is also possible to determine the relative potency of test agents. Using 2,5-hexanedione 300 μg/ml, distal axonopathy commences after approximately 4 weeks and no metabolites appear in the nutrient fluid. By contrast, 2,5-hexanediol is partly oxidized within the nutrient fluid to the dione and produces relatively minor neurotoxic damage over a similar period of time (33). The *in vitro* demonstration of the neurotoxic property of the dione, coupled with evidence that this compound is the major persistent metabolite of *n*-hexane and methyl-*n*-butyl ketone *in vivo*, provides support for the idea that 2,5-hexanedione represents the primary neurotoxic agent of the neurologically active hexacarbon compounds (9).

This conclusion led us to explore the toxic specificity of 2,5-hexanedione *in vivo*. Ten hydrocarbon derivatives were fed to young adult rats for periods of up to 6 weeks (Table 2). Animals intoxicated with 2,5-hexanedi-

TABLE 2. *Hydrocarbon derivatives tested for neurotoxic properties*

2-Heptanone	$CH_3COCH_2CH_2CH_2CH_2CH_3$
3,5-Heptanedione	$CH_3CH_2COCH_2COCH_2CH_3$
2,5-Hexanedione	$CH_3COCH_2CH_2COCH_3$
2,5-Hexanediol	$CH_3CHOH(CH_2)_2CHOHCH_3$
2,4-Hexanedione	$CH_3COCH_2COCH_2CH_3$
2,3-Hexanedione	$CH_3COCOCH_2CH_2CH_3$
1,6-Hexanediol	$HOCH_2CH_2CH_2CH_2CH_2CH_2OH$
Glutaraldehyde	$OCHCH_2CH_2CH_2CHO$
1,4-Butanediol	$CH_2OHCH_2CH_2CH_2OH$
Acetone	CH_3COCH_3

one or 2,5-hexanediol failed to gain weight normally; they slowly developed hindlimb weakness and displayed a characteristic distribution of giant axonal degeneration in the CNS and PNS. However, these clinical and pathological features of central–peripheral distal axonopathy failed to develop in rats drinking the closely related compounds. This study demonstrated the molecular specificity of hydrocarbon derivatives required for neurotoxic activity. Of the hexacarbon compounds tested, only 2,5-hexanedione and 2,5-hexanediol were neurotoxic, whereas 2,4-hexanedione, 2,3-hexanedione, and 1,6-hexanediol were neurologically inactive. Also inactive was acetone, which was examined because of its dimeric relationship to the putative primary neurotoxin 2,5-hexanedione (32).

These studies have provided test (2,5-hexanedione) and control (2,4- and 2,3-hexanedione) compounds with which to search for the metabolic basis of hexacarbon neurotoxicity. One metabolic locus which merits further study is the enzymatic conversion of dihydroxyacetone phosphate to L-α-glycerophosphate. It was postulated that the specific dehydrogenase might bind with the acetone dimer 2,5-hexanedione in preference to the natural compound dihydroxy*acetone* phosphate. *In vitro* studies have suggested that 2,5-hexanedione does inhibit the enzyme, but the specificity of this reaction and the biological significance, if any, has yet to be explored (19). Inhibition of metabolism at this site presumably would lead to excessive accumulation of dihydroxyacetone phosphate. Dihydroxyacetone phosphate is in equilibrium with D-glyceraldehyde-3-phosphate, but the kinetics of the reaction markedly favor accumulation of the former compound. A similar accumulation might also occur with impairment of enzymatic breakdown of D-glyceraldehyde-3-phosphate, a reaction known to be sensitive to disulfides. Such metabolic effects might back up the glycolytic pathway and favor the formation rather than the breakdown of glucose-6-phosphate as well as the production of glycogen. Such events occurring within the axon would be compatible with the observation of axonal glycogen accumulation in experimental hexacarbon neuropathy. More significant, perhaps, would be the profound effect on energy metabolism, which might account for both weight loss and the development of axonal degeneration, the disease being expressed initially in the nervous system because of the high energy requirements of this tissue.

A CONCISE WORKING HYPOTHESIS OF THE DYING-BACK PROCESS

One explanation of the dying-back phenomenon is that the neurotoxic agents progressively compromise the anabolic machinery of the neuronal perikaryon. This would result in a gradual reduction in the amount of materials exported to the axon, causing compromise of the most distal parts of large axons (those with the greatest demand for perikaryal supplies) and later affecting more proximal regions as the neuronal disease slowly developed. Cavanagh, the leading exponent of this theory of perikaryal disease, based the idea on histological observations of animals poisoned with *o*-cresyl phosphate and used the concept to explain a large number of neurotoxin-induced and naturally occurring distal axonopathies (3,4). By contrast, following the lead of Prineas, we suggested that the triad of early multifocal axonal change, late Wallerian-like distal degeneration, and axonal regeneration during intoxication was more consistent with an axonal locus of toxic action and *normal* perikaryal function (22). This idea, developed in a series of experimental studies on the dying-back process (29,38,39), discussed in detail elsewhere (34,36) and now also espoused by Shoental and Cavanagh (31), suggests that toxins inactivate substances in the axon required for the maintenance of axonal

integrity. The abnormally large total axonal demand for these substances in the intoxicated animal would outstrip the resupply from the neuronal perikaryon, causing the distal axon to become compromised.

An hypothesis can now be offered to explain why a focal, partial blockade of axonal transport might lead first to distal and subsequently, more proximal changes in those axons with the largest volume of axoplasm. This theory predicts that the toxin binds to enzymes distributed throughout the axon. These enzymes are required for the maintenance of normal axonal transport and can be resupplied only from the unaffected neuronal perikaryon. Their inactivation during intoxication would cause the total axonal demand for these enzymes to exceed the perikaryal supply. Such inactivated enzymes might be associated with production of energy needed to drive the transport systems and to convey the nerve impulse. The nodal region of the large fiber might then be the first to be affected (even before more-distal nodes of small branches of the same fiber) because of the probable high-energy demands in this area. Deficient nodal axonal transport would result. Eventually axonal transport would be altered in smaller fibers and in internodal regions. Axoplasmic organelles would accumulate at sites of transport failure and, if not sequestered and removed by the Schwann cell, would locally break down and release calcium into the axoplasm. This would disrupt the integrity of the axon and produce distal fiber breakdown. The disease would progress proximally with time because larger amounts of enzyme would be inactivated with maintained intoxication, allowing progressively shorter, more-proximal regions of the axon to be satiated. Eventually, a steady state would be reached whereby the rate of resupply of enzyme would be proportional to the rate of inactivation, thereby allowing the neuron to support a short, proximal length of axon and even permit some regeneration. This theory is not only consistent with many features of experimental distal axonopathy, it is also compatible with the available data regarding the biochemical action of the neurotoxic hexacarbons. Future experiments to test this hypothesis might include examination of the tissue-binding properties of the neurotoxins, biochemical and autoradiographic studies, and attempts to alter the course of the disease by dietary supplementation.

ACKNOWLEDGMENTS

The authors thank Drs. C. Moore, J. Griffin, D. Price, E. Koenig, and M. Sabri for discussion. Work was supported by USPHS grants OH 00535, NS 13106, NS 08952, and NS 03356, and a Joseph P. Kennedy, Jr. Fellowship in the Neurosciences to P.S.S.

REFERENCES

1. Allen, N., Mendell, J. R., Billmaier, D. J., Fontaine, R. E., and O'Neill, J. (1975): Toxic polyneuropathy produced by the industrial solvent methyl n-butyl ketone. *Arch. Neurol.*, 32:209–218.
2. Ballin, R. H. M., and Thomas, P. K. (1969): Changes at the node of Ranvier during wallerian degeneration: An electron microscope study. *Acta Neuropathol. (Berl)*, 14:237–249.
3. Cavanagh, J. B. (1964): The significance of the "dying-back" process in experimental and human neurological disease. *Int. Rev. Exp. Biol.*, 3:219–267.
4. Cavanagh, J. B. (1973): Peripheral neuropathy caused by chemical agents. *CRC Crit. Rev. Toxicol.*, 2:365–417.
5. Cho, E. S. (1977): Toxic effects of Adriamycin on the ganglia of the peripheral nervous system. *J. Neuropathol. Exp. Neurol. (in press).*
6. Cho, L., Schaumburg, H. H., and Spencer, P. S. (1977): Adriamycin produces ganglioradiculopathy in rats. *J. Neuropathol. Exp. Neurol.*, 36:597 (abstract).
7. Di Fronzo, G., Lenaz, L., and Bonadonna, G. (1973): Distribution and excretion of Adriamycin in man. *Biomedicine [Express]*, 19:169–171.
8. Di Marco, A. (1975): Adriamycin (NSC-123127): Mode and mechanism of action. *Cancer Chemother. Rep.*, 6:91–106.
9. DiVincenzo, G., Kaplan, C. J., and Dedinas, J. (1976): Characterization of the metabolites of methyl n-butyl ketone, methyl iso-butyl ketone, and methyl ethyl ketone in guinea-pig serum and their clearance. *Toxicol. Appl. Pharmacol.*, 36:511–522.
10. Duncan, I. (1976): Personal communication.
11. Griffin, J. W., Price, D. L., and Spencer, P. S. (1977): Fast axonal transport through giant axonal swellings in hexacarbon neuropathy. *J. Neuropathol. Exp. Neurol.*, 36:603 (abstract).
12. Griffin, J. W., Price, D. L., and Spencer, P. S. (1977): Unpublished data.
13. Herskowitz, A., Ishii, N., and Schaumburg, H. H. (1971): n-Hexane neuropathy: A syndrome occurring as a result of industrial exposure. *N. Engl. J. Med.*, 285:82–85.
14. Jacobs, J. M., Carmichael, N., and Cavanagh, J. B. (1975): Ultrastructural changes in the dorsal root and trigeminal ganglion of rats poisoned with methyl mercury. *Neuropathol. Appl. Neurobiol.*, 1:1–19.
15. Jacobs, J. M., Carmichael, N., and Cavanagh, J. B. (1977): Ultrastructural changes in the nervous system of rabbits poisoned with methyl mercury. *Toxicol. Appl. Pharmacol.*, 39:249–261.
16. Korobkin, R., Asbury, A. K., Sumner, A. J., and Nielsen, S. L. (1975): Glue sniffing neuropathy. *Arch. Neurol.*, 32:158–162.
17. Mendell, J. R., Saida, K., Ganansia, M. F., Jackson, D. B., Weiss, H., Gardier, R. W., Chrisman, C., Allen, N., Couri, D., O'Neill, J., Marks, B., and Hetland, L. (1974): Toxic polyneuropathy produced by methyl n-butyl ketone. *Science,* 35:787–789.
18. Mendell, J. R., Saida, K., Weiss, H. S., and Savage, R. (1976): Methyl n-butyl ketone-induced changes in fast axoplasmic transport. *Neurology (Minneap)*, 26:349 (abstract).
19. Moore, C., and Spencer, P. S. (1977): Unpublished data.
20. Philips, F. S., Gilladoga, A., Marquardt, H., et al. (1975): Some observations on the toxicity of Adriamycin (NSC-123–127) *Cancer Chemother. Rep.*, 6:177–181.
21. Pigram, W. J., Fuller, W., and Hamilton, L. D. (1972): Stereochemistry of interaction of daunomycin with DNA. *Nature [New Biol.]*, 235:17–19.
22. Prineas, J. B. (1969): The pathogenesis of dying-back polyneuropathies. 1. An ultrastructural study of experimental triorthocresyl phosphate intoxication in the cat. *J. Neuropathol. Exp. Neurol.*, 28:571–597.
23. Prineas, J. B. (1969): The pathogenesis of dying-back polyneuropathies. II. An ultrastructural study of experimental acrylamide intoxication in the cat. *J. Neuropathol. Exp. Neurol.*, 28:598–621.
24. Rosso, R., Esposito, M., Sala, R., et al. (1973): Distribution of daunomycin and adriamycin in mice: A comparative study. *Biomedicine [Express]*, 19:304–317.
25. Saida, K., Mendell, J. R., and Weiss, H. S. (1975): Peripheral nerve changes induced by methyl n-butyl ketone and potentiation by methyl ethyl ketone. *J. Neuropathol. Exp. Neurol.*, 35:204–225.
26. Schaumburg, H. H., and Spencer, P. S. (1977): Ultrastructural studies of the dying-back process. V. A systematic analysis of reversible and irreversible central nervous degeneration produced by neurotoxins. In preparation.
27. Schaumburg, H. H., and Spencer, P. S. (1977): Environmental hydrocarbons produce degeneration in cat hypothalamus and optic tract. *Science (in press).*

28. Schaumburg, H. H., and Spencer, P. S. (1976): Central and peripheral nervous system degeneration produced by pure n-hexane: An experimental study. *Brain,* 99:183–192.
29. Schaumburg, H. H., Wiśniewski, H., and Spencer, P. S. (1974): Ultrastructural studies of the dying-back process. 1. Peripheral nerve terminal and axon degeneration in systemic acrylamide intoxication. *J. Neuropathol. Exp. Neurol.,* 33:260–284.
30. Schlaepfer, W. W. (1974): Calcium-induced degeneration of axoplasm in isolated segments of rat peripheral nerve. *Brain Res.,* 69:203–215.
31. Schoental, R., and Cavanagh, J. B. (1977): Mechanisms involved in the 'dying-back' process—an hypothesis implicating coenzymes. *Neuropathol. Appl. Neurobiol.,* 3:145–147.
32. Spencer, P. S., Bischoff, M., and Schaumburg, H. H. (1977): Central-peripheral distal axonopathy: The specific molecular configuration of neurotoxic aliphatic hexacarbon compounds. *Toxicol. Appl. Pharmacol. (in press).*
33. Spencer, P. S., Peterson, E. R., DiVincenzo, and Schaumburg, H. H. (1977): Unpublished data.
34. Spencer, P. S., and Schaumburg, H. H. (1974): A review of acrylamide neurotoxicity. II. Experimental animal neurotoxicity and pathologic mechanisms. *Can. J. Neurol. Sci.,* 1:151–169.
35. Spencer, P. S., and Schaumburg, H. H. (1975): Experimental neuropathy produced by 2,5-hexanedione—a major metabolite of the neurotoxic industrial solvent methyl n-butyl ketone. *J. Neurol. Neurosurg. Psychiatry,* 8:771–775.
36. Spencer, P. S., and Schaumburg, H. H. (1976): Central-peripheral distal axonopathy —the pathology of dying-back polyneuropathies. *Prog. Neuropathol.,* 3:253–295.
37. Spencer, P. S., and Schaumburg, H. H. (1976): Feline nervous system response to chronic intoxication with commercial grades of methyl n-butyl ketone, methyl isobutyl ketone and methyl ethyl ketone. *Toxicol. Appl. Pharmacol.,* 37:301–325.
38. Spencer, P. S., and Schaumburg, H. H. (1977): Ultrastructural studies of the dying-back process. III. The evolution of experimental peripheral giant axonal degeneration. *J. Neuropathol. Exp. Neurol.,* 36:276–299.
39. Spencer, P. S., and Schaumburg, H. H. (1977): Ultrastructural studies of the dying-back process. IV. Differential vulnerability of PNS and CNS fibers in experimental central-peripheral distal axonopathies. *J. Neuropathol. Exp. Neurol.,* 36:300–320.
40. Spencer, P. S., Schaumburg, H. H., and Peterson, E. R. (1977): Ultrastructural studies of the dying-back process. VI. The spatial-temporal pattern of axonal degeneration in nerve fibers existing in vitro. In preparation.
41. Spencer, P. S., Schaumburg, H. H., Raleigh, R. L., and Terhaar, C. J. (1975): Nervous system degeneration produced by the industrial solvent methyl n-butyl ketone. *Arch. Neurol.,* 32:219–222.
42. Spencer, P. S., and Thomas, P. K. (1974): Ultrastructural studies of the dying-back process. II. The sequestration and removal by Schwann cells and oligodendrocytes of organelles from normal and diseased axons. *J. Neurocytol.,* 3:763–783.
43. Szendzikowski, S., Stetkiewicz, J., Wrónska-Nofer, T., and Karasek, M. (1974): Pathomorphology of the experimental lesion of the peripheral nervous system in white rats chronically exposed to carbon disulphide. In: *Structure and Function of Normal and Diseased Muscle and Peripheral Nerve,* edited by I. Hausmonowa-Petrusewicz and H. Jedrzejowska, pp. 319–326. Polish Medical Publishers, Warsaw.
44. Tellez-Nagel, I., Korthals, J. K., Vlassava, H. V., and Cerami, A. (1977): An ultrastructural study of chronic sodium cyanate-induced neuropathy. *J. Neuropathol. Exp. Neurol.,* 36:342–363.
45. Towfighi, J., Gonatas, N., Pleasure, D., Cooper, H., and McCrea, L. (1976): Glue-sniffer's neuropathy. *Neurology (Minneap),* 26:238–243.
46. Yamamura, Y. (1969): n-Hexane polyneuropathy. *Folia Psychiatr. Neurol. Jpn.,* 23:45–57.

Physiology and Pathobiology of Axons, edited by
S. G. Waxman. Raven Press, New York © 1978.

Pathology of Demyelination

Cedric S. Raine

Departments of Pathology (Neuropathology) and Neuroscience, Rose F. Kennedy Center for Research in Mental Retardation and Human Development, Albert Einstein College of Medicine, Bronx, New York 10461

In order to facilitate rapid conduction, nature has provided certain axons within the vertebrate nervous system with myelin sheaths, highly specialized ensheathments laid down in internodes between areas of the axon known as nodes of Ranvier, the effector centers for saltatory conduction (Cahalan, *this volume*). Each internode or myelin sheath is a flattened membrane formed by the compaction of a cellular process from a myelinating cell that is spirally wrapped along the segment of axon (analyzed more fully by Berthold, *this volume;* Hirano and Dembitzer, *this volume*). Myelin is one of the most characteristic elements of the vertebrate nervous system and exists in two forms according to topography—central nervous system (CNS) myelin and peripheral nervous system (PNS) myelin elaborated and maintained by oligodendrocytes and Schwann cells, respectively (20,34,57,74). Originally believed to be an inert element, biochemical studies on myelin have shown only certain of its components to be stable whereas others are metabolically active throughout life (47). Morphologically, myelin is a unique membrane and has specific biochemical and immunologic properties which readily distinguish it from other nervous system membranes (19,28,37, 51). These subjects are dealt with more fully in other chapters (Suzuki, *this volume;* Bornstein, *this volume*).

Contingent on its morphologic, biochemical, and immunologic peculiarities, myelin can be selectively vulnerable to a wide gamut of pathological stigmata. The specificity for myelin to be affected in certain CNS and PNS diseases has provided a scaffold for their classification, albeit tenuous in some cases. Superficially, the diseases in which myelin is primarily affected form a heterogenous group unrelated etiologically and pathologically, sharing only in their development the common denominator of a severe loss of myelin. These disorders of myelin were recently reappraised and classified according to contemporary dogma that took into account, in addition to the myelin anomalies, acquired and hereditary traits, toxic and nutritional factors, and traumatic features (50,83,88).

The subject of the present chapter, demyelination, has led to many semantic arguments. It is not sufficient to classify any CNS and PNS abnormality in which myelin is destroyed as *demyelinative.* Myelin loss is a common sequela of a vast multitude of states ranging from neoplasias, to selective loss of gray matter elements (neurons), to vascular problems. However, families of diverse CNS conditions do exist in which the lesions are expressed in the white matter and in which at some early stage in development myelin is depleted. Not all of these myelin disorders can be classed as purely demyelinative since frequently (e.g., in the hereditary metabolic states) extensive loss of other parenchymal elements, in particular axons, ensues. Although *demyelination as a process* is seen in many CNS and PNS conditions and involves the loss of myelin with relative sparing of axons, the term *demyelinating disease* is reserved for those conditions in which the myelin loss occurs amid a background of inflammation visualized by a preponderance of perivascular cuffing by hematogenous cells. This stringent application of the term demyelinating disease, as advocated by Adams and Sidman (2), inevitably restricts the term to the acquired inflammatory demyelinating states, of which multiple sclerosis (MS) is the paradigm.

HUMAN DEMYELINATING DISEASES

The human demyelinating diseases are:
1. Chronic MS
2. Variants of MS (e.g., acute MS, Devic's disease)
3. Acute disseminated encephalomyelitis (ADE)
4. Acute hemorrhagic leukoencephalopathy (AHLE)
5. Progressive multifocal leukoencephalopathy (PML)
6. Idiopathic polyneuritis
7. Diphtheritic neuropathy

Most of these human conditions are known or suspected to have an infectious etiology and, with the exception of PML and diphtheritic neuropathy, have pathogenetic mechanisms that reflect an immunologic component, evidenced by the presence of an inflammatory response in the nervous system. Whether the latter represents a primary or secondary phenomenon has been the subject of much research.

Due to a combination of factors related to chronicity, inability to biopsy affected areas, and poor preservation of autopsy material, the process of demyelination in MS and its related conditions still awaits analysis. Most studies on these diseases have been performed on biopsy or autopsy samples from chronically afflicted subjects; and although most of the myelin changes described were probably chronic and secondary to plaque formation (e.g., refs. 1,6,56,94), at least two studies concentrated on acute MS lesions (63,66). To compensate for these limitations, investigators were compelled to examine the more-available animal models of demyelination. In this regard, the present chapter, the backbone of which is the pathology of demyelination, analyzes in detail the patterns of myelin breakdown and repair in selected natural and experimental conditions considered to be of relevance to the human demyelinating diseases.

The following experimental and naturally occurring animal conditions represent the major analogs for the MS group of diseases:

1. Experimental allergic encephalomyelitis (EAE) (73)
2. Canine distemper encephalomyelitis (CDE) (106)
3. Mouse hepatitis virus (JHM strain) encephalomyelitis (42) } CNS
4. Theiler's virus encephalomyelitis (26)
5. Visna (55)
6. Goat leukoencephalopathy (24)
7. Experimental allergic neuritis (EAN) (9) } PNS
8. Marek's disease (68)
9. Coonhound paralysis (25)

PATHOGENETIC MECHANISMS IN THE DEMYELINATING DISEASES

From the abundance of evidence on the natural and experimental disorders of myelin, the following categories of myelin damage can be compiled:

1. Immunologic (antibody and/or cell-mediated)
2. Virologic (direct or indirect effects on myelin)
3. Genetic (enzyme anomalies affecting myelin production and/or maintenance)
4. Nutritional (mainly developmental effects)
5. Toxic (myelinotoxic compounds)
6. Traumatic (changes due to compression, etc.)

In most of the human demyelinating diseases, conventional and contemporary considerations have implicated an infectious etiology. However, an infectious agent alone cannot be deemed the sole factor responsible for the changes in the nervous system since the apparent absence of a demonstrable agent and the frequent invasion of the tissue by hematogenous, inflammatory cells (lymphocytes, plasma cells, and monocytes) appear to support a subsequent allergic type of reaction, perhaps of an autoimmune type. The distinction between those changes that might be due to a putative virus and those that might be due to a subsequent immunologic response is an unresolvable issue in the chronic MS lesion. Were cases of acute MS or acute lesions in chronic MS encountered more frequently, the pathologic events would be better dissected chronologically. To obviate the difficulties experienced during the study of these human demyelinating diseases, investigators have approached the exploration of possible pathogenetic mechanisms on a comparative basis by studying animal models in which demyelination is known to be linked to an immunologic or virologic complication, or both. Although not always possible *in situ* (since viral and immunologic events are usually highly synchronous), with the aid of well-established autoimmune models such as EAE and EAN, certain demyelinative phenomena have been dissected and attributed to immunologic events utilizing *in vivo* and *in vitro* techniques.

Immune-Mediated Demyelination

CNS Demyelination In Situ

The concept that MS might be the result of an immunologic response to a sequestered CNS antigen (viz., myelin) stemmed from comparative studies between acute EAE in monkeys, postrabies immunization encephalomyelitis in man (an iatrogenic form of ADE attributed to the presence of CNS tissue in the antirabies inoculum), and the acute form of MS (3,90,97). It is not the purpose of this chapter to reappraise yet again the justification for using EAE as a model for MS or to review the data on autosensitization to myelin antigens in MS versus EAE. This was the subject of several recent review articles (5,54,61,73,75), including one in this volume by Bornstein.

In EAE, cellular immunity to myelin basic protein (MBP) is readily demonstrable, and antibody to MBP has been shown on several occasions. In MS, suffice it to say that evidence exists from some (not all) reports, on different groups of subjects, that either cellular or antibody-mediated immunity (or both) to MBP is demonstrable in MS, and these are usually more prominent during acute phases of the disease than during chronic remissions (Bornstein, *this volume*). This putative autosensitization to MBP in MS might even have a genetic basis, since the prevalence of MS is being increasingly related to the possession of certain

determinants: histocompatibility antigens (HL-A) on the surface of leukocytes (49).

EAE, a model of autoimmune demyelination, can be induced in most species of laboratory animals (mice and cats are more difficult than other species) by (a) active sensitization with an emulsion of complete Freund's adjuvant (CFA) containing CNS white matter, purified CNS myelin, MBP, or encephalitogenic fragments of MBP; or (b) by passive transfer using lymphocytes from EAE-sensitized animals (43,53). Although not fully understood, it is believed that by effecting an overall stimulation in the number of lymphocytes during active sensitization the CFA serves to increase the clone of lymphocytes specifically sensitized to the CNS antigen.

Detailed morphological studies at the ultrastructural level on the process of CNS demyelination in acute EAE have shown that the loss of myelin is at least in part due to active phagocytosis by hematogenously derived macrophages. Lampert and Carpenter (40), the first to report myelin stripping by macrophages in EAE, showed that mononuclear cells entered the CNS parenchyma from the Virchow–Robin space, elaborated pseudopods around myelinated axons and between the layers of myelin, and then proceeded to divest the axons of their myelin sheaths (Fig. 1). This process has since been confirmed many times (73). The invasion of myelin sheaths in EAE occurred amid a background of inflammation, involving, as well as mononuclear cells, plasma cells and small lymphocytes. Within 24–48 hrs after the onset of signs, the actively phagocytosing cells have completed their task, leaving large groups of axons completely naked (Fig. 2); the cells probably leave the CNS parenchyma by returning to the bloodstream (Fig. 3). In hyperacute EAE lesions, polymorphonuclear leukocytes, extravasated red cells, fibrin, and plasma exudate are also seen (29,44). The process of CNS demyelination in EAE was invariably related to narrow rims of fibers surrounding the perivascular cuffs (Fig. 4).

The underlying reason for the selective cellular attack on myelin in EAE is not known. Whether it is effected by MBP-sensitized killer cells, nonspecifically sensitized lymphocytes recognizing an antigen opsonized by circulat-

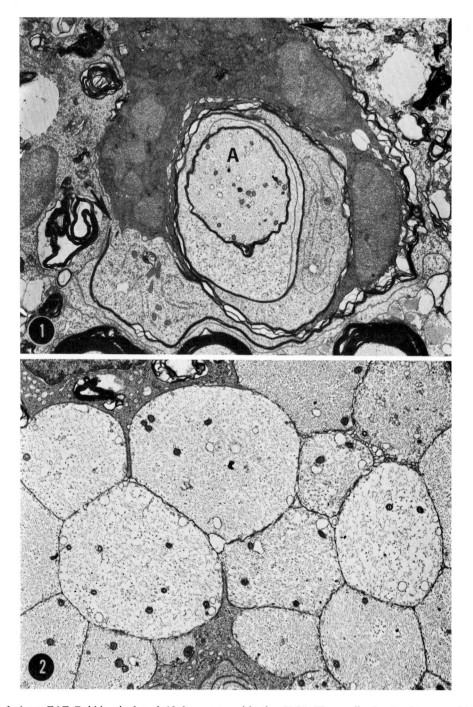

FIG. 1. Acute EAE. Rabbit spinal cord, 12 days postsensitization (P.S.). The myelin sheath of the axon (A) has been invaded by several macrophages that have extended processes between myelin lamellae. The broken outer layers of the myelin sheath are indicated by the arrows. ×6,200. (From ref. 67.)

FIG. 2. Acute EAE. Strain 13 guinea pig spinal cord, 17 days P.S. A group of tightly packed, naked axons is shown. ×11,000. (From ref. 84.)

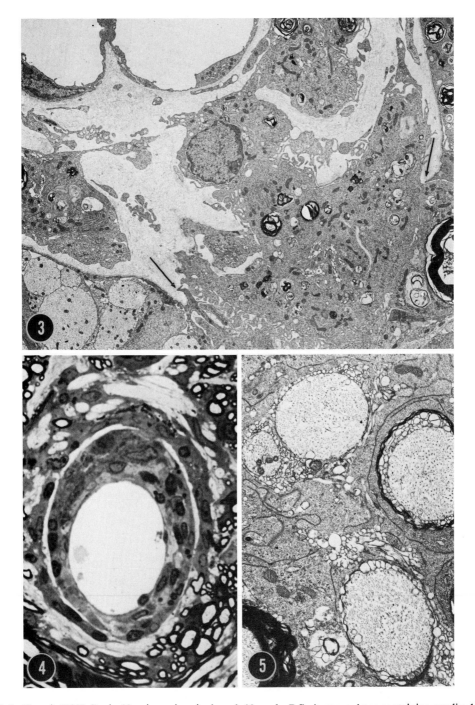

FIG. 3. Chronic EAE. Strain 13 guinea pig spinal cord, 13 weeks P.S. A macrophage containing myelin debris is seen entering an enlarged, fibrotic Virchow–Robin space through a gap in the glia limitans (*arrows*). Demyelinated axons can be seen at the lower left. ×2,800. (From ref. 84.)

FIG. 4. Acute EAE. Lewis strain rat spinal cord, 16 days P.S. A typical perivascular cuff is surrounded by a ring of naked axons. ×640. (From ref. 86.)

FIG. 5. Acute EAE. Strain 13 guinea pig spinal cord, 18 days P.S. A group of fibers shows extensive vesiculation of the myelin sheaths. ×10,000. (From ref. 84.)

ing serum factor, or macrophages interacting specifically with antibody–antigen (myelin) complexes [or nonspecifically, as was demonstrated recently in the myelinated retina of the rabbit (72) is not known, and these alternatives represent only a few of a number of possibilities.

Our current thinking on demyelination due to immunologic abnormalities is changing considerably in view of increasing evidence of a role for immunoglobulin in lesion development. Several previous studies on EAE lesions reported myelin disintegration apparently not immediately related to inflammatory cells (27, 38,79,104). This myelinolytic change was distinct from that shown above and involved the dissolution or vesiculation of the myelin away from the axon (Fig. 5); this debris was probably phagocytosed by local cells. Recent observations on acute MS lesions utilizing immunocytochemical techniques succeeded in localizing antibody to plasma cells, macrophages, and reactive astrocytes in the actively demyelinating margins of the lesions (66). This work appeared to implicate the astrocyte (as opposed to an hematogenous cell) as an early phagocyte in the disease process. That the phagocytic activity of this cell may be mediated by antibody can only be speculated from this work. That the presence of immunoglobulin in the CNS parenchyma resulted from an early change in the blood–brain barrier prior to cellular infiltration is a possibility.

CNS Demyelination In Vitro

Retrospectively, one can find support for the hypothesis on antibody-related myelin changes in EAE and MS by examining the results from ultrastructural studies on myelinated CNS cultures exposed to EAE sera (i.e., sera from animals sensitized with whole white matter in CFA) or to sera from some patients with MS (77,82). The application of organotypic CNS/PNS cultures affords the experimentalist an opportunity to manipulate the environment at will since blood–brain barrier and immune systems are lacking. For example, one can study selectively serum, lymphocyte, virus, toxic, and enzyme factors individually or together in the total absence of complications due to other host systems. When applied to the demyelinat-

ing diseases, this system showed that EAE and MS sera produced a specific damage to myelin (15,16). In the case of EAE, this serum factor was later characterized as a complement-dependent CNS-specific antibody (8). Within a few hours of exposure to an active EAE or MS serum sample, myelin disintegrates in a manner not unlike a melting process. The regular periodicity is replaced by "fingerprint" formations with a lamellar spacing of approximately 6nm (Fig. 6). One remarkable feature of this myelin damage was that the debris was actively phagocytosed by neighboring astrocytes, a previously unknown event in experimental demyelination (77) (Fig. 7). Although apparently de-emphasized for many years owing to the overwhelming evidence for T-cell mediation in EAE (73), experimental neuropathologists are now considering more and more that in the inflammatory demyelinating states, antibody and lymphocytes might operate together in the process of demyelination, or to quote one immunology wit: "It takes two to tango."

Of course, the problem of demonstrating the relative roles of antibody and lymphoid cells in EAE or MS lesions is a formidable task without a considerable amount of hindsight in determining what really represents the initial lesion. Tentative evidence from EAE (73) and acute MS (66) suggests that immunoglobulin deposition might precede cellular infiltration in the disease process, but this awaits further confirmation.

Initial Myelin Change in Serum-Induced Demyelination

One possible mechanism of demyelination involves a subtle tagging of the myelin sheath, with or without an accompanying structural alteration, by some diffusible humoral factor (e.g., immunoglobulin) which might precede overt myelin loss and cellular infiltration. As stated above, morphologic studies on immune-mediated demyelination in the CNS *in situ* failed to segregate convincingly the initial change in myelin configuration, an issue difficult to resolve *in situ*. In Bornstein's original descriptions of demyelination by EAE or MS serum factors *in vitro* (15,16), it was pointed out that prior to frank demyelination, myelin

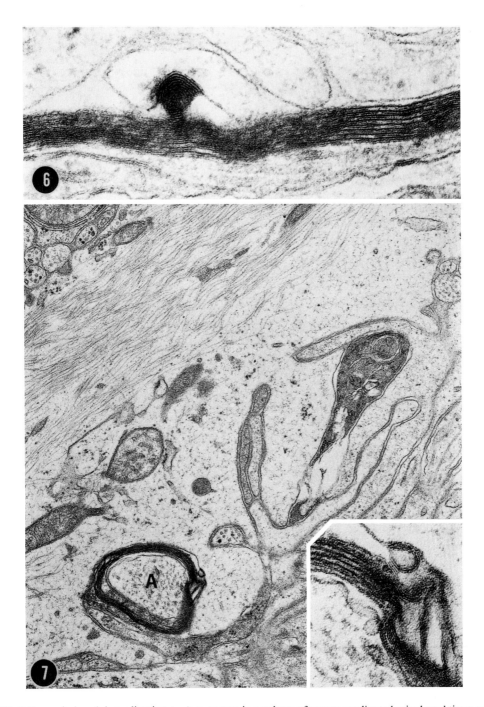

FIG. 6. Serum-induced demyelination *in vitro*, as seen in a culture of mouse myelinated spinal cord tissue which was exposed for 1 hr to MS serum. A small region of the myelin sheath of a longitudinally sectioned fiber (axon below) has been transformed into a fingerprint-like droplet with a periodicity of approximately 6 nm. This myelin figure has become dissociated from the main sheath and is becoming encompassed by an astroglial cell process. ×120,000. (From ref. 82.)

FIG. 7. Serum-induced demyelination *in vitro* in a preparation similar to that in Fig. 6. A swollen process of a fibrous astrocyte extends around a myelinated axon (A), which shows incipient myelin breakdown (**inset**) and some oligodendroglial cell fragments. Note the glial filaments (*upper left*). ×28,000. **Inset:** ×135,000. (From ref 82.)

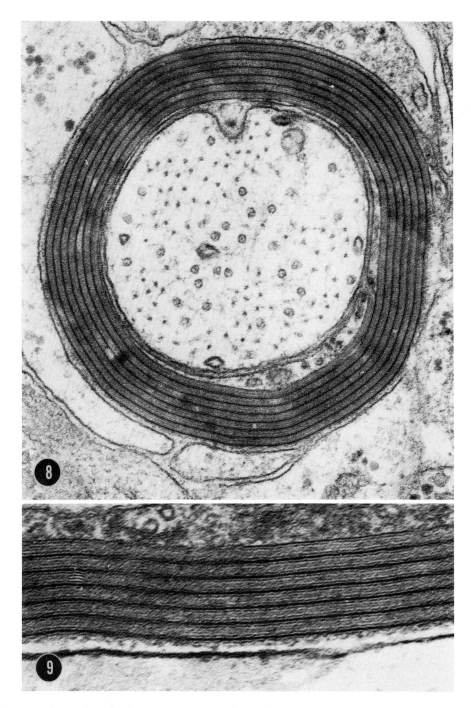

FIG. 8. Serum-induced myelin changes *in vitro*, as seen in a culture of mouse myelinated spinal cord tissue which was exposed for 20 hr to heated EAE serum from a rabbit. The myelin period is uniformly expanded from the normal 11 nm to 22 nm. Additional leaflets can be seen between each pair of major dense lines. ×75,000. (From ref. 17.)

FIG. 9. A preparation similar to that in Fig. 8, but exposed to heated EAE serum for 72 hr, shows detail of the changes during the myelin period. Note the presence of four leaflets in the space occupied normally by the two leaflets of the intraperiod line. ×200,000. (From ref. 17.)

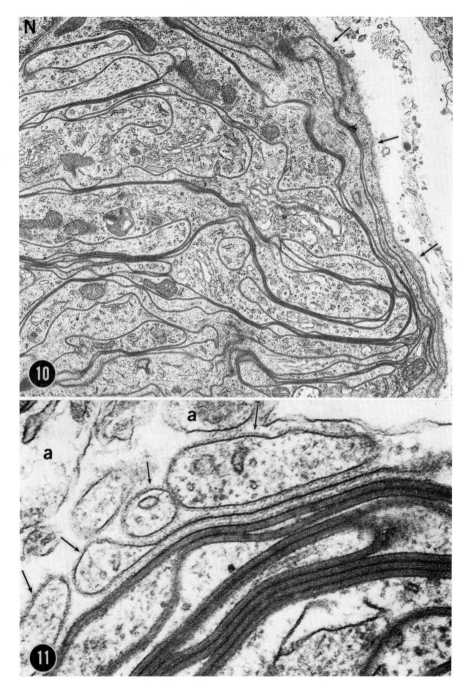

FIG. 10. Serum-induced myelin changes *in vitro* in a preparation similar to that in Fig. 8 but exposed for 9 days. A portion of an abnormal oligodendrocyte (nucleus at *upper left*) shows intense infolding of its cytoplasm which in places has compacted to form the same abnormal myelin as that seen in Figs. 8 and 9. Note the granular coating on the plasmalemma to the right (*arrows*). ×15,000. (From ref. 17.)

FIG. 11. Serum-induced myelin changes *in vitro* in a culture exposed for 20 hr to heated EAE serum. The periphery of an abnormal oligodendrocyte shows several of its processes coated with an additional granular material (*arrows*). One loop of cytoplasm (*second arrow from left*) extends toward the right as a compacted layer of myelin; between it and the compacted myelin below (all of which shows the four leaflets at the intraperiod line), there is a suggestion that the widened myelin is beginning to form. Astroglial cell processes (a) above show no membrane coating. ×70,000. (From ref. 17.)

sheaths displayed a transient brightening, after which they degenerated. During recent *in vitro* experiments attempting to purify the myelinotoxic factor, it was noticed that heat-inactivated sera (to remove complement) from several animals sensitized against whole white matter in CFA, induced an identical brightening or swelling in mature myelinated cultures. The myelin sheaths did not proceed to further degeneration (17). We therefore had apparently arrested the process of serum-induced demyelination in its initial phase, a phenomenon attributable to a factor presumably not dependent on complement. Total demyelination, on the other hand, is known to be complement-dependent in this same system (8). Ultrastructural analysis of these swollen myelin sheaths revealed a unique pattern of myelin pathology (Fig. 8). Without exception, every CNS myelin sheath displayed a periodicity of 22 nm instead of the usual 11 nm; and in the space occupied by the usually bilamellar intraperiod line, four distinct leaflets could be discerned (Fig. 9). Thus in this initial serum-induced myelin lesion, an additional pair of leaflets had been formed. The findings also suggested that the factor somehow diffused into the sheath in that the outermost myelin lamellae were affected first. Whether these changes are related to bound immunoglobulin or to the freeing of previously tightly incorporated membrane subunits, is not known. Equally intriguing in these cultures was the fact that the oligodendroglial cells had been stimulated to elaborate many cytoplasmic processes that compacted to form myelin within and around themselves. This myelin had the same aberrant 22 nm period as that seen around axons. Study of these cells gave some indication as to the origin of the extra intraperiod line. The plasmalemma of all affected oligodendroglia was covered by an amorphous, granular coating material (Figs. 10 and 11). Probably by the active folding of the cell processes on one another to produce compact myelin, this coating material either crept or became incorporated into the myelin period. This coating was highly specific for the oligodendroglial cell and the myelin sheath. The membranes of other cell types were not affected. This newly described myelin anomaly was found to be incompletely reversible in that

removal of the heated EAE serum for the culture medium resulted in a return to the normal period of the outermost lamellae only.

More recent studies on this myelin swelling factor showed that the initial formation of myelin is not prevented by the presence of heated EAE serum but that the CNS myelin that develops around axons is of the swollen type. Also, the oligodendroglia are stimulated to produce vast amounts of aberrant myelin, and many axons (probably as a result of the latter phenomenon) fail to acquire myelin sheaths (79). It therefore appears that we have in our hands a useful tool for studying some factors governing myelinogenesis.

The relevance of this myelin swelling factor to *in vivo* disease is not clear. A similar change has not been seen in MS, but this is not surprising since well-preserved confirmed acute lesions in MS have rarely been studied ultrastructurally. In EAE, however, a similar swelling was described on at least two occasions (38,67). In canine distemper encephalomyelitis (CDE), a virus-induced inflammatory demyelinating condition of dogs in which immune-mediated demyelination is thought to occur (7,71,106), a similar myelin swelling was described (71). The only human conditions in which a comparable change has been seen are some peripheral neuropathies associated with hypergammaglobulinemia (69,91). In these conditions PNS myelin was shown to have an increased period, and in the study by Sluga (91) a third leaflet was observed in the space occupied by the intraperiod line.

Oligodendroglial Cell Damage

One phenomenon poorly explored during the inflammatory demyelinating states is related to the fate of the myelinating oligodendroglial cell which is invariably lost from affected areas. It is important to analyze more fully the damage to the oligodendrocyte since it is possible that much of the myelin damage is secondary to the primary death of the cell, an interesting but difficult hypothesis to prove *in situ*. In MS, oligodendroglial cell lysis has been frequently suggested to be an early pathogenetic event, but the evidence has always been indirect. Ultrastructural evidence for a primary involvement of oligodendroglial cells

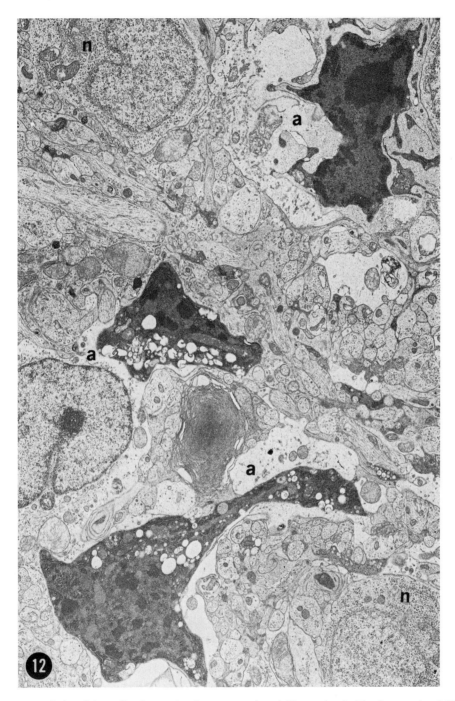

FIG. 12. Serum-induced demyelination *in vitro* in a preparation similar to that in Fig. 6 exposed to MS serum for 1 hr. Three oligodendrocytes (electron-dense cells) display necrotic changes. Each cell is becoming invested by clear cytoplasm (a) from adjacent astroglial cells. In time, the astroglia will phagocytose the cell debris. Adjacent neurons (n) show no changes. ×8,700. (From ref. 82.)

in MS or EAE is scant, although in both conditions a few degenerating cells have been identified in lesions as possibly being oligodroglial in origin. The demonstration of reactive astrocytes extending processes around neighboring oligodendrocytes in actively demyelinating lesions from a case of acute MS, as revealed by an immunoperoxidase technique (66), represented another, albeit indirect, piece of evidence of potential phagocytosis of the myelinating cell. Sensitization of animals with inocula containing purified preparations of oligodendroglial cells have failed to detect a specific encephalitogenic property of this cell type (86).

Stronger evidence for an antibody-mediated selective destruction of oligodendroglial cells comes from studies on myelinated CNS cultures exposed to actively demyelinating EAE or MS sera (77,82). Here, within hours of exposure, oligodendroglial cells were seen to undergo frank degeneration, a process occurring concomitantly with myelin changes (Fig. 12). Interestingly, the debris from the actively degenerating cells was phagocytosed by local astrocytes (82). Eventually, no myelin or oligodendroglial cells were present; and if the exposure to, for example, EAE serum was prolonged, the tissue went on to acquire a fibrous, demyelinated appearance (78) structurally reminiscent in some ways of a sclerotic, demyelinated MS plaque.

PNS Demyelination

Ranking most prominent among the human idiopathic neuropathies in which immune-mediated demyelination is implicated, is the Landry–Guillain–Barré syndrome (LGBS). This condition exists in a number of forms, ranging from an acute monophasic to a chronic relapsing disease (60). Indirect evidence indicates the involvement of an infectious agent (a herpes-type virus) in LGBS. Thus, a situation analogous to MS in the CNS is suspected. However, because of a less-complex organization in the PNS, more is known about demyelination in LGBS. Ultrastructural examinations have disclosed that the primary loss of myelin is related to an active invasion of PNS myelin sheaths by infiltrating lymphocytes and macrophages (23,62,65,107). Examination of au-

topsy or biopsy nerve tissue from LGBS revealed that the invading macrophages penetrate the basal laminae of myelinating Schwann cells at any level of the internode and push the cell cytoplasm aside. Cellular processes from the macrophages then break through the underlying layers of myelin (Figs. 13 and 14). These cellular fingers subsequently peel off and engulf the myelin sheath in a stripping fashion. Not infrequently, small lymphocytes invade the Schwann tubes; and although these cells do not themselves actively participate in the myelin stripping, their presence suggests they do have some role in the demyelination (62). Not uncommonly, the myelin in close contact with the invading cell is transformed into a vesicular network. Eventually, when the macrophages are laden with myelin debris or when the segment of axon is naked, the cells leave the Schwann tube to enter the endoneurium and eventually return to the circulation.

It is noteworthy that the process of phagocytosis and vascular response is highly efficient in the PNS and several weeks after an inflammatory episode, it is difficult to document evidence of inflammation. The same is not the case in the CNS, where macrophages and debris linger for many months after the onset of disease.

The above pattern of PNS demyelination in LGBS is identical morphologically to patterns occurring in the PNS of animals suffering from EAE, in which the PNS as well as the CNS can be involved (72,85,104) (Fig. 15), and from EAN (10,39). In animals successfully sensitized against peripheral nerve myelin, an acute often fatal syndrome (EAN) develops usually 12–16 days later. Although the clinical picture of EAN differs with that of LGBS (in which fatalities are rare today), the morphologic features of PNS demyelination are, as stated, indistinguishable (Fig. 16). In the above examples of PNS demyelination, there is remarkable sparing of axons and rapid remyelination of the affected internodes in surviving animals. This preservation of axons and restoration of myelin no doubt contribute to the rapid return of function to near normality after an acute attack. The tardiness (if present at all) of remyelination in the CNS, particularly in MS, and the loss of many of the naked fibers with time are possibly the under-

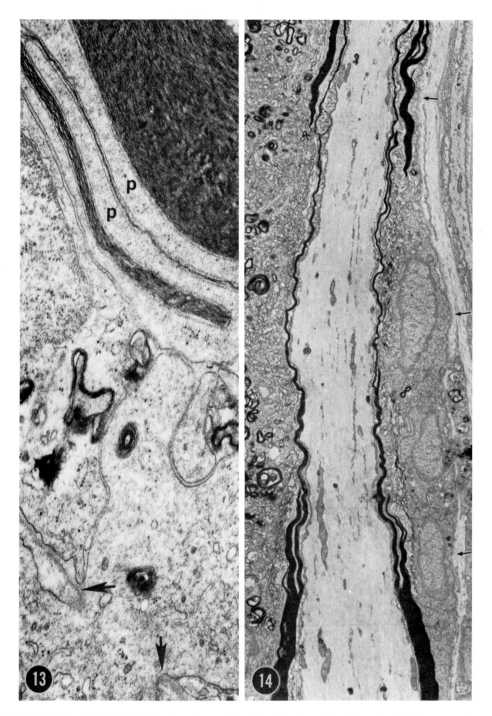

FIG. 13. Acute Landry–Guillain–Barré syndrome. A macrophage has extended a cytoplasmic process (*arrows*) through a gap in the basal lamina of a Schwann cell surrounding a myelinated PNS axon (*extreme upper right*). The same cell process has further divided into finger-like processes (p) which are separating groups of myelin lamellae from the main sheath. Elsewhere, phagocytosed myelin debris can be seen. ×27,000. (From ref. 62.)

FIG. 14. Acute Landry–Guillain–Barré syndrome. Mononuclear cells, including lymphocytes and macrophages, have penetrated the basal lamina (*arrows*) of a PNS fiber. These cells are associated with severe disruption of a segment of a myelin sheath some distance from a node of Ranvier. ×62,000. (From ref. 62.)

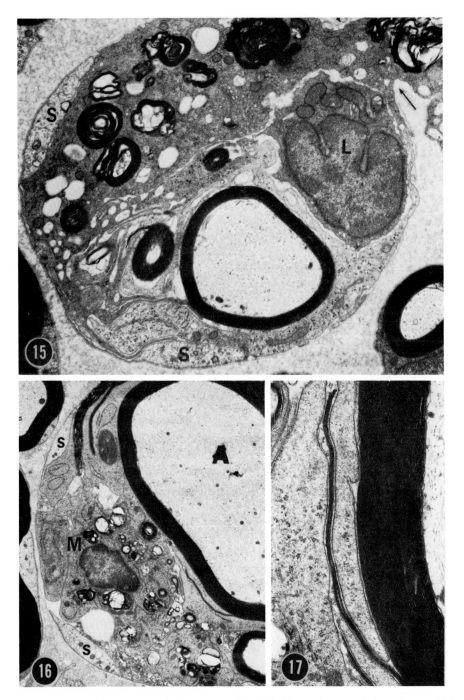

FIG. 15. Acute EAE. Rabbit posterior spinal nerve root from L7. Macrophages and a lymphocyte (L) have entered the basal lamina of a PNS fiber, pushing the Schwann cell cytoplasm (S) to the periphery. One macrophage contains myelin debris and extends a process through a gap in the basal lamina (*arrows*). ×8,400.

FIG. 16. Acute EAN. Rabbit sciatic nerve, 14 days P.S. A macrophage has invaded this PNS fiber, pushed the Schwann cell cytoplasm (S) aside, and extended processes between several layers of myelin around the axon (A). ×4,700.

FIG. 17. Detail from Fig. 16. Note how the process of the macrophage has separated several layers of myelin from the main sheath. ×34,000.

lying structural reasons for the less-promising prognosis in MS.

The fine structural features of CNS and PNS remyelination are similar regardless of the cause of the primary demyelination. For this reason, remyelination is dealt with in separate, more general sections later in this chapter.

Viral-Induced Demyelination

Mechanisms

Without exception, the CNS and PNS conditions with an infectious etiology and, as a hallmark in lesion formation demyelination, all belong to the inflammatory demyelinating conditions—the MS group. PML is the only viral-induced demyelinating condition in which inflammation is not prominent although on rare occasions one does encounter the odd case of PML that shows inflammatory cuffs in the CNS. In PML, the demyelination is regarded as the result of a primary infection and death of oligodendroglial cells by a papovavirus (36), and the myelin loss is secondary to this. The pathogenetic mechanisms in the human diseases with suspected virus-association (ADE, AHLE) are poorly studied, but extrapolation from naturally occurring animal counterparts (viz., CDE in the CNS and Marek's disease in the PNS) permits us to state that demyelinative events in these conditions are structurally similar to those in autoimmune conditions. However, the added complication of the presence of a viral antigen—in the case of CDE, the result of an antecedent, usually respiratory infection; and in the case of Marek's disease, an oncogenic herpesvirus—renders interpretation of the inflammatory response and the loss of myelin difficult. Several possibilities exist as to why myelin could be lost as a result of a viral infection, among them:

1. Selective infection and damage to the myelinating cell.

2. Damage to normal oligodendroglial cells and myelin resulting from a local immune response against a virus in which the local release of hydrolytic enzymes and/or cytotoxic lymphokines occurs.

3. Cross antigenic properties between the oligodendrocyte and its myelin sheath on the one hand and a virus on the other.

4. Selective immune-mediated destruction of oligodendroglia with expressed viral antigen on their surfaces.

5. Oligodendroglial cell death resulting from selective damage to other CNS components (neurons, astrocytes, etc.).

6. Physical disruption of the CNS or PNS environment by an immune response to a virus leading to impairment in normal transport mechanisms and damage to myelinating cells and their myelin sheaths.

7. A dying-back type of response by an oligodendroglial cell following its separation from a significant number of the many internodes of myelin it supports. The initial damage is viral-related whereas the second wave of myelin loss is due to the death of the cell.

As examples of CNS and PNS conditions displaying viral-induced demyelination, canine distemper encephalomyelitis (CDE) and Marek's disease (MD) have been selected.

Myelin Damage in CDE

Depending on location and severity, CDE lesions in the CNS have been classified as destructive or demyelinative. There is still some debate as to the specificity of the myelin damage in CDE and whether the demyelination represents an intermediary state of tissue destruction. Today most investigators agree that CDE is a primary demyelinating disease with an etiology related to an antecedent infection by canine distemper virus (CDV), a member of the Paramyxoviridae (7,48,71,106). CDE occurs in at least two forms: an acute, fulminant form affecting young animals, and a chronic, late-onset form occurring in adult animals. In both forms, CNS signs are usually preceded by an upper respiratory infection that resolves. Lesion formation in these two variants is believed to be similar. The destructive lesions in CDE probably represent the battlegrounds of particularly severe immune responses against the viral infection. A recent study of acute lesions in CDE (71) showed that the earliest change in the white matter is not always related to centers of inflammation but can involve the stripping of myelin sheaths from selected fibers by what have been interpreted as local cells, possibly astrocytes (Figs. 17 and 18). Such a finding conflicted some-

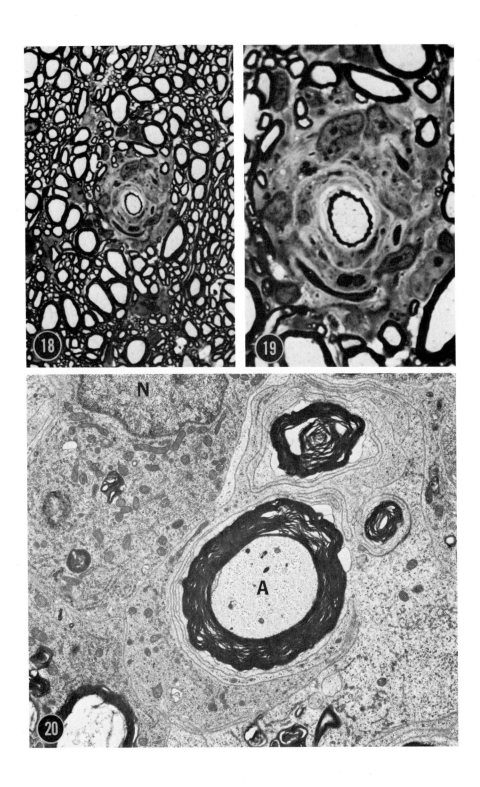

what with our previous observations (106), which tended to support a typical EAE type of stripping by invading cells (Fig. 19). It was concluded that the latter is highly relevant in CDE but is possibly not primary, the first change perhaps being independent of the immediate proximity of inflammatory cells. Thus as in EAE, it might be speculated that the initial alteration in the CNS parenchyma is related to a soluble factor (immunoglobulin), succeeded by a fulminant inflammatory response. Viral antigen in CDE is always found in lesion areas, more frequently in astrocytes than any other cell type. Chronically demyelinated areas in CDE are indistinguishable from those in any other CNS demyelinative state (Fig. 20) except that CDV can always be located (Fig. 21). That MS lesions share pathogenetic similarities with CDE cannot be stated definitively since in MS there is an absence of demonstrable viral antigen and no unequivocal ultrastructural evidence on the mechanism of myelin breakdown. One thing seems certain, however; that in areas of active demyelination in acute MS, an EAE-type of myelin stripping by hematogenous macrophages does not prevail (63,75), and at the growing, active edge of lesions, local cells are probably more involved in the myelin breakdown than was previously suspected.

Oligodendroglial Involvement

Although a frequently quoted concept in neuropathology, most of the evidence for a selective viral infection of oligodendroglia in the demyelinating diseases is indirect. In PML, papovavirus inclusions are frequently encountered within the nuclei of bizarre glial cells, including oligodendroglia. Since most of the material studied has been taken from lesions of undetermined age from patients, for example, with abnormalities of the reticuloendothial system who have been on immunosuppressive therapy for some time, to say whether the infection of the oligodendroglia was primary or secondary is open to question.

In mouse hepatitis virus encephalomyelitis, there is clear evidence of virus-induced oligodendroglial cell involvement manifested in chronic lesions displaying remyelination by the proliferation of myelin in a stimulated, abnormal fashion around axons situated close to the myelinating cell (59). In the same condition, selective damage to oligodendroglia during the acute stage of the disease has been proposed, and the demyelination is not dependent on the presence of an immune response. In this regard, immunosuppressed mice still showed glial infection and demyelination in the absence of inflammatory changes (36). The same is not the case, however, in Theiler's disease (26), where immunosuppression has been claimed to prevent demyelination (45), indicating perhaps that all viruses with a tropism for white matter do not behave alike.

In CDE the viral infection is pantropic, where all cell types can contain viral inclusions (7). The same has also been demonstrated in experimental subacute sclerosing panencephalitis (SSPE), a degenerative CNS condition related to a defective measles virus and in which some affinity for myelin loss is present (80,81).

PNS Myelin Damage in Marek's Disease

Among commercial chicken breeders, Marek's disease (MD) is a serious economic threat. MD is a lymphomatous condition, related to infection by a type B herpesvirus, which is occasionally associated with a periph-

←

FIG. 18. Acute canine distemper encephalomyelitis (CDE), 8 days after onset of signs. A CNS fiber in an otherwise unaffected area of an anterior column is surrounded by cells and debris which isolate it from other fibers. Toluidine blue-stained, 1-μm Epon section. ×480. (From ref. 71.)

FIG. 19. Higher magnification of Fig. 18. The partially demylinated fiber is in the center. The darker staining material, between the encircling cells, is myelin debris. ×1,200. (From ref. 71.)

FIG. 20. Acute CDE. An electron micrograph of the phenomenon seen in Figs. 18 and 19. The central fiber [axon (A)] is invested by processes from the surrounding cells, one of which (*upper left*) has the features of an astrocyte [nucleus (N)]. Myelin droplets lie between the cell processes and within the cytoplasm. ×7,500. (From ref. 71.)

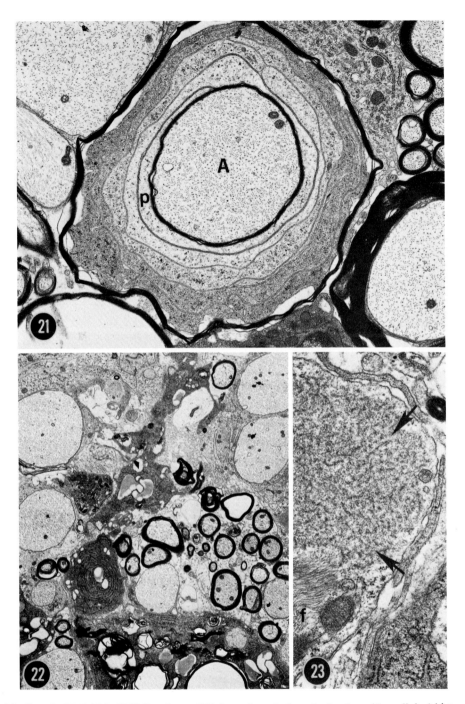

FIG. 21. Chronic CDE. This CNS fiber [axon (A)] from the spinal cord of a dog with a clinical history of 3 months has had its myelin sheath invaded by processes from macrophages, one of which (p) is stripping a layer of myelin from the remainder of the sheath. Naked axons lie at the upper left. ×10,200. (From ref. 106.)

FIG. 22. Chronic CDE, with a history similar to that of Fig. 21. Several naked axons are seen between normal fibers and myelin-laden macrophages. ×4,800.

FIG. 23. Chronic CDE. Viral nucleocapsid could be located in all lesions, usually within astrocytes. Here, a group of intracytoplasmic nucleocapsids is seen (*arrows*) within the process of a fibrous astrocyte. (f) Filaments. ×22,000.

eral neuropathy. Analysis of the mechanism of
PNS myelin breakdown in MD by Prineas and
Wright (68) disclosed a pattern which simu-
lates that seen in EAN and LGBS. Hematogenous macrophages entered the nerve
parenchyma and broke through the basal
laminae of myelinating Schwann cells, pushed
them aside, and went directly for the myelin
sheath (Fig. 24). Elsewhere, small lymphocytes and plasma cells could be seen. The relative roles of the immune system and the viral
infection were difficult to assess, but in view of
the absence of detectable virus in the PNS
(68), the process of demyelination has been
interpreted as perhaps being the result of an
autoimmune type of reaction.

Genetic Abnormalities of Myelin

Although not classed as demyelinating diseases, there exists in neuropathology a large
family of conditions in which hereditary factors lead to a breakdown of myelin, usually
during early or late infancy. Metachromatic
leukodystrophy (MLD), globoid leukodystrophy (GLD), adrenoleukodystrophy (ALD),
and Refsum's disease are conditions in which
a late abnormality (usually attributable to an
enzyme deficit) in myelin develops, whereas in
Pelizaeus–Merzbacher disease, Canavan's disease, Alexander's disease, and phenylketonurea,
the enzyme anomaly is usually expressed much
earlier, resulting in a paucity of myelination.
The reader is referred to two recent reviews on
this subject (83,88).

In most of these conditions, myelin is only
one of several elements lost during the disease
process, which is usually limited to white matter. Except for ALD, the conditions are non-
inflammatory. Although not entirely proved,
there is evidence to show that the enzymologic
anomaly primarily affects the behavior of the
myelinating cell. In GLD, for example, oligodendroglia have been shown to accumulate
GLD-specific inclusions. In the quaking
mouse, a hypomyelinating disease of relevance
to Pelizaeus–Merzbacher disease, abnormalities in both the oligodendrocyte and the
Schwann cell have been reported (95). These
changes are possibly reflected by the myelination abnormality (11,103). Also in this condition, large numbers of CNS axons never get

fully myelinated (Fig. 25). In the dystrophic
mouse, the lack of myelination from widespread areas of the PNS has been speculated to
be the result in a failure on the part of the
Schwann cell (18,100) (Fig. 26).

Nutritional Abnormalities of Myelin

In general, in experimental malnutrition
myelin damage is reflected by a reduction in
the amount of myelin produced and a reduction in brain weight. Demyelination *per se* has
not been documented in this condition. In man
the diseases linked to nutritional deprivation
include vitamin B_{12} deficiency, central pontine
myelinolysis, and Machiafava–Bignami disease
(83,88). In all three conditions, there is focal
loss of myelin from different areas of the CNS
white matter.

Toxic–Metabolic Myelin Abnormalities

Myelin is known to display degenerative
changes in response to a variety of toxic compounds. Included among these compounds are
triethyl tin sulfate (TETS) (4), hexachlorophene (41,58), lysolecithin (32), diphtheria
toxin (99,101,105), and 6-aminonicotinamide
(13). In TETS and hexachlorophene intoxication, myelin sheaths display focal edema (Fig.
27). In the case of TETS, this is a reversible
change. The swelling involves a splitting of the
intraperiod line with the subsequent accumulation of fluid, presumably water, in the swollen
regions. After local administration of lysolecithin, diphtheria toxin, and 6-aminonicotin-
amide, there is focal dissolution of myelin. The
debris from this lysis is phagocytosed largely
by local cells and after this, remyelination
ensues.

In man, myelin loss is a common consequence of vascular problems in which anoxic
anoxia and anemic anoxia occur (83,88). In
these conditions there can also be considerable
involvement of gray matter elements. The
mechanisms of myelin destruction in these
conditions are unknown.

Trauma-Induced Myelin Damage

Mechanical disturbances in the local CNS
or PNS environment are well-known factors
causing myelin perturbations. Chronically ap-

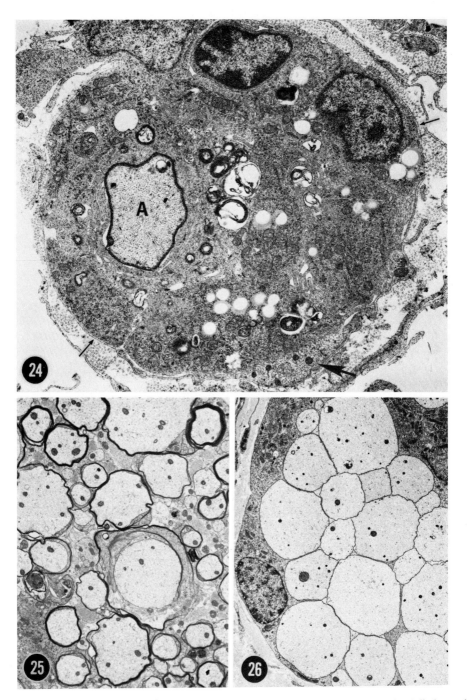

FIG. 24. Marek's disease in chicken sciatic nerve. Several hematogenous macrophages (*above*) lie beneath the basal lamina (*small arrows*) of a PNS fiber and have partially stripped the sheath from the axon (A). Schwann cell cytoplasm is seen at the large arrow. ×7,000. (From ref. 68.)

FIG. 25. Quaking mouse, spinal cord. A group of hypomyelinated CNS fibers is shown. Note disproportionately large axons and thin myelin sheaths (which, incidentally, are also features of remyelination. ×6,250. (Courtesy of Dr. K. Suzuki.)

FIG. 26. Dystrophic mouse, anterior spinal nerve root. A group of PNS axons which, judging from their large diameters, should have been well myelinated, have failed to acquire myelin sheaths. They also abut each other and are enclosed at the margin of the bundle by a ring of Schwann cells. ×3,400. (From ref. 100.)

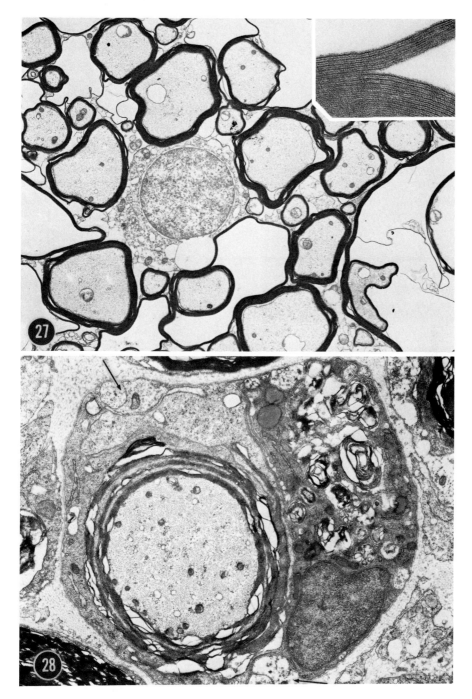

FIG. 27. Toxin-induced myelin changes by TETS, 24 hr after inoculation. This group of CNS fibers contain many myelin sheaths that show a type of edema characterized by the formation of clear, fluid-filled blebs, originating as splits at the intraperiod line **(inset).** An oligodendrocyte is also seen, apparently unaffected. This myelin change is reversible and does not lead to demyelination. ×6,000. **Inset:** ×140,000.

FIG. 28. Trauma-induced demyelination. Surgical opening of the perineurium leads to demyelination of the fibers, which herniate through the opening. This myelin destruction is effected by invading macrophages, as shown here. Schwann cell cytoplasm has become displaced peripherally (*arrow*). This type of cellular destruction of myelin differs from the autoimmune type in that lymphocytes and plasma cells do not participate. ×10,000 (Courtesy of Drs. J. W. Prineas, P. S. Spencer, and H. J. Weinberg.)

plied pressure on myelinated CNS tissue (e.g., in the vicinity of a tumor or an edematous area) and on PNS tissue (e.g., by the application of a tourniquet (52), or during the carpal tunnel syndrome), cause profound myelin abnormalities. In these states, focal pressure on myelinated fibers leads to axonal swelling, myelin slippage, and the thinning and/or loss of some myelin internodes. By performing cerebrospinal fluid (CSF) exchange, Bunge et al. showed that this transient change in the subarachnoid environment was sufficient to induce widespread subpial demyelination in the cat spinal cord (21).

Surgical rupture of the perineurium of the peripheral nerve leads to focal herniation of a number of underlying fibers, indicating that PNS fibers exist in an environment of positive pressure. This phenomenon provided the baseline for studying a relatively new model of demyelination, the perineurial window (92). Fibers in the herniated bleb of nerve tissue underwent a type of cell-related demyelination during the first week and then remyelinated. The process of demyelination involved a macrophagous cell, probably a monocyte, which invaded the myelin sheath by entering at the paranodal region. In cross section (Fig. 28), this cellular invasion is highly reminiscent of the process seen in EAN. However, since other lymphoid cell types were never present (i.e., small lymphocytes and plasma cells), the process was readily distinguishable from autoimmune demyelination. Similar active attack by cells on myelin sheaths has also been seen in other conditions in which immune mechanisms are not implicated.

REMYELINATION IN THE CNS

Before the advent of ultrastructural techniques, the loss of myelin in the CNS was regarded as an inexorable lesion. Study of the CSF barbotage lesion by Bunge et al. (22) and *in vitro* observations by Bornstein and Appel (16) on CNS explants, demonstrated unequivocally the ability of myelin to be regenerated in the CNS. This phenomenon has now been reported in a wide variety of conditions: chronic EAE (33,68,84,93), CDE (106), JHM virus infection (59), cyanide intoxication (35), x-irradiation (14), 6-amino-nicotinamide (13), cuprizone (12), diphtheria toxin (105), and occasionally MS (64), to mention a few. In the CNS, remyelinated axons are readily distinguished from the normal population by virtue of their disproportionately thin myelin sheaths in comparison to axon diameter (Fig. 29).

In general, the oligodendrocyte responds poorly after widespread primary demyelination, a property possibly related to its heavy myelinating commitment in that it is known that each oligodendrocyte is responsible for the upkeep of many myelin internodes (74). The above-reported examples of CNS remyelination usually involved narrow rims or small islands of fibers. In conditions characterized by grossly visible areas of demyelination and sclerosis (viz., MS and PML), the degree of remyelination is insignificant. It therefore appears that when the area of demyelination in the CNS is small, the oligodendrocyte is capable of total remyelination, but where lesions are large and scarring has occurred, recovery is poor. This observation suggests that previous fibrous astrogliosis has a deleterious effect on remyelination, a concept supported by *in vitro* studies on demyelination and sclerosis (78).

The perimeters of regions demonstrating CNS remyelination not infrequently display supernumerary oligodendrocytes, an observation suggestive of local mitotic activity and a conclusion arrived at following autoradiographic study of remyelination in JHM virus-infected mice (33).

Over the past few years, several reports have appeared in which chronically demyelinated regions of the CNS were apparently invaded and myelinated by Schwann cells (70). This phenomenon has now been described in a number of experimentally induced lesions (e.g., Refs. 13,14), chronic EAE (93), and MS (30,64,89). Although superficially an interesting phenomenon with great functional implication, the presence of PNS myelin in the CNS did not account for any clinical improvement. Although in these varied conditions it has been speculated that the Schwann cells enter the CNS from neighboring spinal nerve roots or along penetrating blood vessels, their existence in the normal CNS on rare occasions means that their presence is not always a pathologic sequela (70).

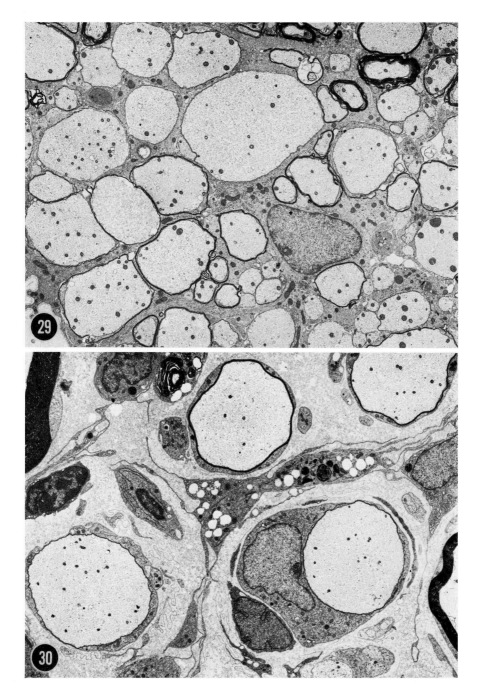

FIG. 29. CNS remyelination. An area of spinal cord from a guinea pig with chronic EAE shows large axons with thin myelin sheaths and some still naked. Normally, axons with such large diameters would be heavily myelinated. ×6,100. (From ref. 84.)

FIG. 30. PNS remyelination in the anterior spinal nerve root of a rabbit suffering from chronic EAE. Note the presence of thin rims of myelin around the four large-diameter axons. Part of a normal fiber with a thick myelin sheath can be seen at the upper left. ×22,000.

REMYELINATION IN THE PNS

The ability of peripheral axons to acquire new myelin after demyelination has been known for almost a century (31). The process of remyelination in the PNS is rapid, and all affected internodes acquire new myelin sheaths. These are distinguishable for several years after the disease by virtue of their being thinner than normal and the axons being smaller (Fig. 30). The manner in which the new myelin is wrapped around the axon appears identical to that seen during development. Ultrastructurally, PNS remyelination was first described by Webster et al. (99) during diphtheritic neuritis, and since that time it has been described in a wide variety of states, e.g., traumatic, toxic, and immunologic.

During an ultrastructural analysis of remyelination in the PNS in chronic EAE (87), an observation, first made by Lubinská (46) on regenerating nerve fibers, was confirmed and reappraised. This involved the occurrence of a marked decrease in axonal diameter during demyelination, a structural change which persisted even after fibers became remyelinated. This axonal reduction provides the morphologist with a ready index of demyelinative activity and may account for some deficiencies in conduction velocity. A later study on recurrent demyelination in the PNS (85) showed that with each subsequent episode of demyelination, remyelinated segments of axons could be repeatedly demyelinated, and such segments displayed a progressive reduction in axon diameter which may also be detectable physiologically. This subject was recently reviewed elsewhere (73). The propensity for axons to become smaller after demyelination caused us to speculate that a similar process could account for the minute axons seen in the center of onion-bulb formations in hypertrophic interstitial polyneuritis (96,98,102).

It is generally assumed that the rapid regeneration of myelin in the PNS is an innate property of the Schwann cell, which is committed to only a single myelin internode and which has enormous regenerative capacity. In our studies on chronic EAE, it was believed that the original Schwann cell might be responsible for the elaboration of new myelin, although some Schwann cell replacement was noted (87). In a recent study on early events during PNS remyelination in EAE (76), more evidence was accumulated that the original Schwann cell is replaced and that the new myelin might be elaborated by a new crop of cells. Whether after each episode of recurrent demyelination the old Schwann cells leave the Schwann tube and contribute to the formation of onion bulbs is an interesting but unsupported speculation in the immune-mediated conditions (76).

CONCLUSIONS AND PROSPECT

Taken in concert, the present chapter underscores the importance of the roles played by the myelinating cells of the CNS and PNS during development and disease, and serves to highlight the selective vulnerability of myelin in a wide spectrum of diseases of varied etiology. On the basis of the selectivity for myelin to be damaged in a variety of neurologic diseases and the multidisciplinary analysis of the myelin lesion, certain disorders can now be classified on the basis of the myelin changes. Chief among these are the acquired inflammatory demyelinating diseases.

The demyelinating diseases as such are those in which virologic and/or immunologic insults are operative and are epitomized by the human condition MS, a disease enigmatic both clinically and pathologically. The rapidity of the clinical worsenings (exacerbations) and their remission in MS are not matched by widespread lesion activity and repair, respectively. Thus it appears that the clinical and pathologic syndromes in MS might reflect two phenomena —perhaps with the clinical symptoms being related to a neuronal dysfunction, and the lesions to a slower, probably immunologic process. Although cell-mediated myelin damage in the demyelinating diseases was given great emphasis in the past, it is becoming increasingly apparent that humoral factors (immunoglobulins) are probably also involved in a cooperative manner, and that the role of antibody in these states may even be a primary event. Therefore one may postulate "that the areas of active inflammation in MS lesions might represent footprints of a disease process already passed by" (71). Although unlikely, it has been claimed that the inflammatory response visualized in the human demyelinating diseases might represent a healing rather than a destructive event such as is witnessed during clearance of a viral infection. However, comparative study of MS with experimental demyelinating diseases argues strongly against the inflammation seen during demyelination being a reparatory phenomenon.

Future avenues of research in the field of MS will continue to dissect the biochemical, immunologic, virologic, and morphologic substrata involved in demyelination. With the combination of *in vivo* and *in vitro* techniques and the virologic and immunopathologic tools available today, the pathogenetic mechanisms in the MS group of diseases are currently under heavy attack.

ACKNOWLEDGMENTS

I would like to thank a number of colleagues for their support and encouragement, especially Drs. R. D. Terry, M. B. Bornstein, J. Prineas, H. Wiśniewski, W. T. Norton, D. H. Snyder, S. H. Stone, and K. Suzuki; and Everett Swanson, Miriam Pakingan, and Howard Finch for their technical expertise. Mary Palumbo and Violet Hantz are thanked for their secretarial assistance.

Supported in part by a grant from the National Multiple Sclerosis Society (RG 1001-A-1); by USPHS grants NS 08952, NS 11920, and NS 70265; by a grant from the Kroc Foundation; and by a grant from the Alfred P. Sloan Foundation.

REFERENCES

1. Adams, C. W. M. (1977): Pathology of multiple sclerosis: Progression of the lesion. *Br. Med. Bull.*, 33:15–20.
2. Adams, R. D., and Sidman, R. L., editors (1968): *Introduction to Neuropathology.* McGraw-Hill, New York.
3. Adams, R. D. (1959): A comparison of the morphology of the human demyelinative diseases and experimental "allergic" encephalomyelitis. In: *"Allergic" Encephalomyelitis,* edited by M. W. Kies and E. C. Alvord, pp. 183–209. Charles C Thomas, Springfield, Ill.
4. Aleu, F. P., Katzman, R., and Terry, R. D. (1963): Fine structure and electrolyte analyses of cerebral edema induced by alkyl tin intoxication. *J. Neuropathol. Exp. Neurol.*, 22:403–413.
5. Alvord, E. C. (1970): Acute disseminated encephalomyelitis and "allergic" neuroencephalopathies. In: *Handbook of Clinical Neurology, Vol. 9: Multiple Sclerosis and Other Demyelinating Diseases,* edited by P. J. Vinken and G. W. Bruyn, pp. 500–571. North Holland, Amsterdam.
6. Andrews, J. M. (1972): The ultrastructural neuropathology of multiple sclerosis. In: *Multiple Sclerosis: Immunology, Virology and Ultrastructure,* edited by F. Wolfgram, G. W. Ellison, J. G. Stevens, and J. M. Andrews, pp. 23–52. Academic Press, New York.
7. Appel, M. J. G., and Gillespie, J. H. (1972): Canine distemper virus. *Virol. Monogr.*, 11:1–96.
8. Appel, S. H., and Bornstein, M. B. (1964): The application of tissue culture to the study of experimental "allergic" encephalomyelitis. II. Serum factors responsible for demyelination. *J. Exp. Med.*, 119:303–312.
9. Asbury, A. K., Arnason, B. W. G., and Adams, R. D. (1969): The inflammatory lesion in idiopathic polyneuritis. *Medicine (Balt)*, 48:173–215.
10. Ballin, R. H. M., and Thomas, P. K. (1969): Electron microscope observations on demyelination and remyelination in experimental allergic neuritis. I. Demyelination. *J. Neurol. Sci.*, 8:1–18.
11. Berger, B. (1971): Quelques aspects ultrastructuraux de la substance blanche chez la souris quaking. *Brain Res.*, 25:35–53.
12. Blakemore, W. F. (1973): Remyelination of the superior cerebellar peduncle in the mouse following demyelination induced by feeding cuprizone. *J. Neurol. Sci.*, 20:73–83.
13. Blakemore, W. F. (1975): Remyelination by Schwann cells of axons demyelinated by intraspinal injection of 6-aminonicotinamide in the rat. *J. Neurocytol.*, 4:745–757.
14. Blakemore, W. F., and Patterson, R. C. (1975): Observations on the interrelation of Schwann cells and astrocytes following x-irradiation of neonatal rat spinal cord. *J. Neurocytol.*, 4:573–585.
15. Bornstein, M. B. (1963): A tissue culture approach to demyelinative disorders. *Natl. Cancer Inst. Monogr.*, 11:197–214.
16. Bornstein, M. B., and Appel, S. H. (1961): The application of tissue culture to the study of experimental "allergic" encephalomyelitis. I. Patterns of demyelination. *J. Neuropathol. Exp. Neurol.*, 20:141–157.
17. Bornstein, M. B., and Raine, C. S. (1976): The initial structural lesion in serum-induced demyelination in vitro. *Lab. Invest.*, 35:391–401.
18. Bradley, W. B. G., and Jenkison, M. J. (1973): Abnormalities of peripheral nerves in murine muscular dystrophy. *J. Neurol. Sci.*, 18:227–247.
19. Brostoff, S. W. (1977): Immunological re-

sponses to myelin and myelin components. In: *Myelin*, edited by P. Morell, pp. 415–446. Plenum, New York.

20. Bunge, R. P. (1968): Glial cells and the central myelin sheath. *Physiol. Rev.*, 48:197–248.

21. Bunge, R. P., Bunge, M. B., and Ris, H. (1960): Electron microscopic study of demyelination in an experimentally induced lesion in adult cat spinal cord. *J. Biophys. Biochem. Cytol.*, 7:685–696.

22. Bunge, M. B., Bunge, R. P., and Ris, H. (1961): Ultrastructural study of remyelination in an experimental lesion in adult cat spinal cord. *J. Biophys. Biochem. Cytol.*, 10:67–74.

23. Carpenter, S. (1972): An ultrastructural study of an acute fatal case of the Guillain-Barré syndrome. *J. Neurol. Sci.*, 15:125–140.

24. Cork, L., and Davis, W. C. (1975): Ultrastructural features of viral leukoencephalomyelitis of goats. *Lab. Invest.*, 32:359–365.

25. Cummings, J. F., and Haas, C. D. (1967): Coonhound paralysis: An acute idiopathic polyradiculoneuritis in dogs resembling the Landry-Guillain-Barré syndrome. *J. Neurol. Sci.*, 4:51–81.

26. Dal Canto, M., and Lipton, H. (1975): Primary demyelination in Theiler's virus infection: An ultrastructural study. *Lab. Invest.*, 33:626–637.

27. Dal Canto, M., Wiśniewski, H. M., Johnson, A. B., Brostoff, S. W., and Raine, C. S. (1975): Vesicular disruption of myelin in autoimmune demyelination. *J. Neurol. Sci.*, 24:313–319.

28. Eylar, E. H., (1972): Experimental allergic encephalomyelitis and multiple sclerosis. In: *Multiple Sclerosis: Immunology, Virology and Ultrastructure*, edited by F. Wolfgram, G. W. Ellison, J. G. Stevens, and J. M. Andrews, pp. 449–486. Academic Press, New York.

29. Field, E. J., and Raine, C. S. (1969): Experimental allergic encephalomyelitis in the rhesus monkey—an EM study. *J. Neurol. Sci.*, 8:397–411.

30. Ghatak, N., Hirano, A., Doron, Y., and Zimmerman, H. M. (1973): Remyelination in MS with peripheral type myelin. *Arch. Neurol.*, 29:262–267.

31. Gombault, M. (1888): Contributions a l'étude anatomique de la nevrite parenchymateuse subaique et chronique: Nevrite segmentaire periaxiale. *Arch. Neurol. (Paris)*, 1:11–20.

32. Hall, S. (1972): The effect of injections of lysophosphatidyl choline into white matter of the adult mouse spinal cord. *J. Cell Sci.*, 10:535–546.

33. Herndon, R. M., Weiner, L. P., and Price, D. L. (1976): Thymidine labelling of glia during remyelination after JHM infection.

J. Neuropathol. Exp. Neurol., 35:108 (abstract).

34. Hirano, A., and Dembitzer, H. M. (1967): A structural analysis of the myelin sheath in the central nervous system. *J. Cell Biol.*, 34:555–567.

35. Hirano, A., Levine, S., and Zimmerman, H. M. (1968): Remyelination in the central nervous system after cyanide intoxication. *J. Neuropathol. Exp. Neurol.*, 27:234–245.

36. Johnson, R. T., and Weiner, L. P. (1972): The role of viral infections in demyelinating diseases. In: *Multiple Sclerosis: Immunology, Virology and Ultrastructure*, edited by F. Wolfgram, G. W. Ellison, J. G. Stevens, and J. M. Andrews, pp. 245–264. Academic Press, New York.

37. Kies, M. W. (1972): The biological activity of myelin basic proteins. In: *Multiple Sclerosis: Immunology, Virology and Ultrastructure*, edited by F. Wolfgram, G. W. Ellison, J. G. Stevens, and J. M. Andrews, pp. 429–444. Academic Press, New York.

38. Lampert, P. W. (1967): Electron microscopic studies on ordinary and hyperacute experimental allergic encephalomyelitis. *Acta Neuropathol. (Berl)*, 9:99–126.

39. Lampert, P. W. (1969): Mechanism of demyelination in experimental allergic neuritis. *Lab. Invest.*, 20:127–138.

40. Lampert, P. W., and Carpenter, S. (1965): Electron microscopic studies on the vascular permeability and the mechanisms of demyelination in experimental allergic encephalomyelitis. *J. Neuropathol. Exp. Neurol.*, 24:11–24.

41. Lampert, P., O'Brien, J., and Garrett, R. (1973): Hexachlorophene encephalopathy. *Acta Neuropathol. (Berl)*, 23:326–333.

42. Lampert, P. W., Sims, J. K., and Kniazeff, A. J. (1973): Mechanism of demyelination in JHM virus encephalomyelitis. *Acta Neuropathol. (Berl)*, 24:76–85.

43. Levine, S. (1974): Hyperacute, neutrophilic, and localized forms of experimental allergic encephalomyelitis: A review. *Acta Neuropathol. (Berl)*, 28:179–189.

44. Levine, S., Hirano, A., and Zimmerman, H. M. (1965): Hyperacute allergic encephalomyelitis: Electron microscopic observations. *Am. J. Pathol.*, 47:209–221.

45. Lipton, H. L., and Dal Canto, M. C. (1976): Theiler's virus induced demyelination—prevention by immunosuppression. *Science*, 192:62–64.

46. Lubinská, L. (1959): Region of transition between preserved and regenerating parts of myelinated fibers. *J. Comp. Neurol.*, 113:315–325.

47. Marks, N., Grynbaum, A., and Lajtha, A. (1976): The breakdown of myelin-bound proteins by intra- and extracellular proteases. *Neurochem. Res.*, 1:93–111.

48. McCullough, B., Krakowka, S., and

Koestner, A. (1974): Experimental canine distemper virus-induced demyelination. *Lab. Invest.*, 31:216–222.

49. McFarlin, D. E., and McFarland, H. F. (1976): Histocompatibility studies and multiple sclerosis. *Arch. Neurol.*, 33:395–398.

50. Morell, P., Bornstein, M. B., and Raine, C. S. (1976): Diseases involving myelin. In: *Basic Neurochemistry*, 2nd ed., edited by R. W. Albers, G. J. Siegel, R. Katzman, and B. W. Agranoff, pp. 581–604. Little Brown, Boston.

51. Norton, W. T. (1976): Formation, structure and biochemistry of myelin: In: *Basic Neurochemistry*, 2nd ed., edited by R. W. Albers, G. J. Siegel, R. Katzman, and B. W. Agranoff, pp. 74–99. Little Brown, Boston.

52. Ochoa, J., Fowler, T. J., and Gilliatt, R. W. (1972): Anatomical changes in peripheral nerves compressed by a pneumatic tourniquet. *J. Anat.*, 113:433–455.

53. Paterson, P. Y. (1960): Transfer of allergic encephalomyelitis in rats by means of lymph node cells. *J. Exp. Med.*, 111:119–136.

54. Paterson, P. Y. (1973): Multiple sclerosis: An immunologic reassessment. *J. Chronic Dis.*, 26:119–126.

55. Patursson, G., Nathanson, N., Georgsson, G., Pannitch, H., and Pallsson, P. A. (1976): Pathogenesis of visna. I. Sequential virologic, serologic and pathologic studies. *Lab. Invest.*, 35:402–412.

56. Périer, O., and Grégoire, A. (1965): Electron microscopic features of multiple sclerosis lesions. *Brain*, 88:937–952.

57. Peters, A., Palay, S. L., and Webster, H. de F., editors (1976): *The Fine Structure of the Nervous System. The Cells and Their Processes*. Harper & Row, New York.

58. Pleasure, D., Towfighi, J., Silberberg, D., and Parris, J. (1974): The pathogenesis of hexachlorophene neuropathy: In vivo and in vitro studies. *Neurology (Minneap)*, 24:1068–1075.

59. Powell, H. C., and Lampert, P. W. (1975): Oligodendrocytes and their myelin plasma membrane connections in JHM mouse hepatitis virus encephalomyelitis. *Lab. Invest.*, 33:440–445.

60. Prineas, J. W. (1970): Polyneuropathies of undetermined cause. *Acta Neurol. Scand.*, 46:7–72.

61. Prineas, J. W. (1970): The etiology and pathogenesis of multiple sclerosis. In: *Handbook of Clinical Neurology, Vol. 9: Multiple Sclerosis and Other Demyelinating Diseases*, edited by P. J. Vinken and G. W. Bruyn, pp. 107–160. North Holland Publishing, Amsterdam.

62. Prineas, J. W. (1971): Acute idiopathic polyneuritis: An electron microscope study. *Lab. Invest.*, 26:34–40.

63. Prineas, J. W. (1975): Pathology of the early lesions in multiple sclerosis. *Hum. Pathol.*, 6:531–554.

64. Prineas, J. W. (1976): Paramyxovirus-like particles in acute lesions in multiple sclerosis. In: *The Aetiology and Pathogenesis of the Demyelinating Diseases*, edited by H. Shiraki, T. Yonezawa, and Y. Kuroiwa. Japan Science Press.

65. Prineas, J. W., and McLeod, J. M. (1976): Chronic relapsing polyneuritis. *J. Neurol. Sci.*, 27:427–458.

66. Prineas, J., and Raine, C. S. (1976): Electron microscopy and immunoperoxidase studies of early multiple sclerosis lesions. *Neurology (Minneap) (Suppl.)*, 26:29–32.

67. Prineas, J., Raine, C. S., and Wisniewski, H. (1969): An ultrastructural study of experimental demyelination and remyelination. III. Chronic experimental allergic encephalomyelitis in the central nervous system. *Lab. Invest.*, 21:472–483.

68. Prineas, J. W., and Wright, R. G. (1972): The fine structure of peripheral nerve lesions in a virus-induced demyelinating disease in fowl (Marek's disease). *Lab. Invest.*, 26:548–557.

69. Propp, R. P., Means, E., Deibel, R., Sherer, G., and Barron, K. (1975): Waldenstraum's macroglobulinemia and neuropathy. *Neurology (Minneap)*, 25:980–988.

70. Raine, C. S. (1976): On the occurrence of Schwann cells in the normal central nervous system. *J. Neurocytol.*, 5:371–380.

71. Raine, C. S. (1976): On the development of lesions in natural canine distemper. *J. Neurol. Sci.*, 30:13–28.

72. Raine, C. S. (1976): Immune-mediated demyelination in the rabbit retina after intraocular injection of antigen. *Brain Res.*, 102:355–362.

73. Raine, C. S. (1976): Experimental allergic encephalomyelitis and related conditions. In: *Progress in Neuropathology*, Vol. 3, edited by H. M. Zimmerman, pp. 225–251. Grune & Stratton, New York.

74. Raine, C. S. (1977): Morphological aspects of myelin and myelination. In: *"Myelin,"* edited by P. Morell, pp. 1–49. Plenum Press, New York.

75. Raine, C. S. (1977): The etiology and pathogenesis of multiple sclerosis—recent developments. *Pathobiol. Annu. (in press)*.

76. Raine, C. S. Schwann cell responses during recurrent demyelination and their relevance to onion-bulb formation. *Neuropathol. App. Neurobiol. (in press)*.

77. Raine, C. S., and Bornstein, M. B. (1970); Experimental allergic encephalomyelitis: An ultrastructural study of experimental demyelination in vitro. *J. Neuropathol. Exp. Neurol.*, 29:177–191.

78. Raine, C. S., and Bornstein, M. B. (1970): Experimental allergic encephalomyelitis: A light and electron microscope study of remyelination and "sclerosis" in vitro. *J. Neuropathol. Exp. Neurol.*, 29:552–574.

79. Raine, C. S., Diaz, M., Pakingan, M., and Bornstein, M. B. Antiserum-induced dissociation of myelinogenesis in vitro: an ultrasound study. *Lab. Invest. (in press).*

80. Raine, C. S., Byington, D. P., and Johnson, K. P. (1974): Experimental subacute sclerosing panencephalitis in the hamster: Ultrastructure of the chronic disease. *Lab. Invest.,* 31:355–368.

81. Raine, C. S., Byington, D. P., and Johnson, K. P. (1975): Subacute sclerosing panencephalitis in the hamster: Ultrastructure of the acute disease in newborns and weanlings. *Lab. Invest.,* 33:108–116.

82. Raine, C. S., Hummelgard, A., Swanson, E., and Bornstein, M. B. (1973): Multiple sclerosis: Serum-induced demyelination in vitro: A light and electron microscope study. *J. Neurol Sci.,* 20:127–148.

83. Raine, C. S., and Schaumburg, H. H. (1977): The neuropathology of the diseases of myelin. In: *"Myelin,"* edited by P. Morell, pp. 271–323. Plenum Press, New York.

84. Raine, C. S., Snyder, D. H., Valsamis, M. P., and Stone, S. H. (1974): Chronic experimental allergic encephalomyelitis in inbred guinea pigs—an ultrastructural study. *Lab. Invest.,* 31:369–380.

85. Raine, C. S., Wiśniewski, H., Dowling, P. C., and Cook, S. D. (1971): An ultrastructural study of experimental demyelination and remyelination. IV. Recurrent episodes and peripheral nervous system plaque formation in experimental allergic encephalomyelitis. *Lab. Invest.,* 25:28–34.

86. Raine, C. S., Wiśniewski, H. M., Iqbal, K., Grundke-Iqbal, I., and Norton, W. T. (1977): Studies on the encephalitogenic effects of purified preparations of human and bovine oligodendroglia. *Brain Res.,* 120: 269–286.

87. Raine, C. S., Wiśniewski, H., and Prineas, J. (1969): An ultrastructural study of experimental demyelination and remyelination. II. Chronic experimental allergic encephalomyelitis in the peripheral nervous system. *Lab. Invest.,* 21:316–327.

88. Schaumburg, H. H., and Raine, C. S. (1977): The clinical neurology of the diseases of myelin. In: *"Myelin,"* edited by P. Morell, pp. 325–351. Plenum Press, New York.

89. Schoene, W. C., Leith, J. D., Behan, P. O., and Geschwind, N. (1974): Simultaneous occurrence of multiple sclerosis and hypertrophic neuropathy: Light, electron microscopic, immunologic and clinical study. *J. Neuropathol. Exp. Neurol.,* 33:190 (abstract).

90. Shiraki, H., and Otani, S. (1959): Clinical and pathological features of rabies postvaccinal encephalomyelitis in man: Relationship to multiple sclerosis and to experimental "allergic" encephalomyelitis in animals. In: *"Allergic" Encephalomyelitis,* edited by M. W. Kies and E. C. Alvord, pp. 59–129. Charles C Thomas, Springfield, Ill.

91. Sluga, E., (editor) (1974): Demyelinsieren des Neuropathie-syndrom mit Strukturveranderungen der Marklamellen. In: *Polyneuropathien Typen and Differenzierung Ergebnisse bioptischer Untersuchungen,* p. 51. Springer Verlag, Berlin.

92. Spencer, P. S., Weinberg, H. J., Raine, C. S., and Prineas, J. W. (1975): The perineurial window—a new model for the study of demyelination and remyelination. *Brain Res.,* 96:329–336.

93. Snyder, D. H., Valsamis, M. P., Stone, S. H., and Raine, C. S. (1975): Progressive and reparatory events in chronic experimental allergic encephalomyelitis. *J. Neuropathol. Exp. Neurol.,* 34:209–221.

94. Suzuki, K., Andrews, J. M., Waltz, J. M., and Terry, R. D. (1969): Ultrastructural studies of multiple sclerosis. *Lab. Invest.,* 20:444–454.

95. Suzuki, K., and Zagoren, J. (1977): Quaking mouse: An ultrastructural study of the peripheral nerves. *J. Neurocytol.,* 6:71–89.

96. Thomas, P. K., and Lascelles, R. G. (1967): Hypertrophic neuropathy. *Q. J. Med.,* 36: 223–238.

97. Uchimura, I., and Shiraki, H. (1957): A contribution to the classification and the pathogenesis of demyelinating encephalomyelitis with special reference to the central nervous system lesions caused by preventive inoculation against rabies. *J. Neuropathol. Exp. Neurol.,* 16:139–208.

98. Webster, H. deF., Schroeder, J. M., Asbury, A. K., and Adams, R. D. (1967): The role of Schwann cells in the formation of "onion bulbs" found in chronic neuropathies. *J. Neuropathol. Exp. Neurol.,* 26:276–299.

99. Webster, H. deF., Spiro, D., Waksman, B., and Adams, R. D. (1961): Phase and electron microscopic studies of experimental demyelination. II. Schwann cell changes in guinea pig sciatic nerves during experimental diphtheritic neuritis. *J. Neuropathol. Exp. Neurol.,* 20:5–21.

100. Weinberg, H. J., Spencer, P. S., and Raine, C. S. (1975): Aberrant PNS development in dystrophic mice. *Brain Res.,* 88:532–537.

101. Weller, R. O. (1965): Diphtheritic neuropathy in the chicken: An EM study. *J. Pathol.,* 89:591–598.

102. Weller, R. O. (1967): An electron microscope study of hypertrophic neuropathy of Déjèrine and Sottas. *J. Neurol. Neurosurg. Psychiatry,* 30:111–125.

103. Wiśniewski, H. M., and Morell, P. (1973): Quaking mouse: Ultrastructural evidence for arrest of myelination. *Brain Res.,* 29:63–73.

104. Wiśniewski, H., Prineas, J., and Raine, C. S. (1969): An ultrastructural study of experi-

mental demyelination and remyelination. I. Acute experimental allergic encephalomyelitis in the peripheral nervous system. *Lab. Invest.,* 21:105–118.

105. Wiśniewski, H., and Raine, C. S. (1971): An ultrastructural study of experimental demyelination and remyelination. V. Central and peripheral nervous system lesions caused by diphtheria toxin. *Lab. Invest.,* 25:73–80.

106. Wiśniewski, H., Raine, C. S., and Kay, W. J. (1972): Observations on viral demyelinating encephalomyelitis-canine distemper. *Lab. Invest.,* 26:589–599.

107. Wiśniewski, H., Terry, R. D., Whitaker, J. M., Cook, S. D., and Dowling, P. C. (1969): Landry-Guillain-Barré syndrome: A primary demyelinating disease. *Arch. Neurol.,* 21: 269–276.

Physiology and Pathobiology of Axons, edited by
S. G. Waxman. Raven Press, New York © 1978.

Immunobiology of Demyelination

Murray B. Bornstein

*Department of Neurology, Albert Einstein College of Medicine of Yeshiva University,
Bronx, New York 10461*

Many hypotheses have been advanced in attempts to understand the etiology and pathogenesis, and eventually to direct treatment of patients with multiple sclerosis (MS), the prototype of demyelinative diseases. Two have survived: one holding that the disease results from a latent, inapparent, or slow virus infection; and the other that autoallergic mechanisms are involved. The two are not mutually exclusive. This chapter emphasizes the immunological basis of demyelination in general and its effect on neuronal function in particular.

The possibility that MS, a chronic demyelinative disorder of the central nervous system (CNS), might result from an immunological attack first surfaced at the beginning of the century. The idea was generated by observations of patients who had received a series of injections of the Pasteur antirabies vaccine. A few of these patients developed a postinoculation encephalomyelitis. Since the inoculum consisted of an attenuated rabies virus and the brain tissue in which it had been passed, the causative agent might have been either the virus or the brain tissue. When the Semple-type vaccine was introduced during the 1920s, a vaccine which had been treated with phenol and therefore contained "killed" virus, the postinoculation neurological complications persisted. This suggested that the brain tissue and not the virus was the inciting agent. Here then was the germinal concept that an acute inflammatory disease of the nervous system might be caused by an immunological response to nerve tissue. A laboratory counterpart, experimental allergic encephalomyelitis (EAE), was developed during the period from approximately 1930 to 1950 and led to a complex series of experiments on which is based the present concept that an immunological pathogenetic mechanism plays a significant role in MS and its counterpart in the peripheral nervous system (PNS), the Guillain–Barré syndrome. In this chapter it is possible to present only a selected portion of the vast literature that has appeared during the past 50 years concerning EAE and its significance for the understanding of MS. For further references to the extensive literature, the reader may refer to Kies and Alvord (91), Pette and Bauer (135), Scheinberg et al. (157), Paterson (130–133), Porterfield (136), Shiraki et al. (168), and Brostoff (35).

The pioneering experiments of Witebsky and Steinfeld (200) and Brandt et al. (33) demonstrated that rabbits produce organ-specific complement-fixing antibrain antibodies in response to inoculations of brain tissue. The possibility of using an animal model for the investigation of human demyelinative diseases soon became established by Rivers and co-workers (150,151) and Ferraro and Jervis (63) who reported that a prolonged series of weekly injections of CNS tissue in saline into monkeys would eventually produce neurological signs and an acute inflammatory response of the CNS. The lesions were characterized by perivascular inflammation and demyelination with relative sparing of the axons. Freund et al. (67) discovered that a single injection of paraffin oil killed mycobacteria, and an emulsifying agent, a mixture which came to be called complete Freund's adjuvant (CFA), plus a suspension of brain tissue was capable of producing the CNS response within a few weeks. This technique was rapidly adopted by a number of investigators (87,120,201) whose early studies set the stage for the extensive utilization of EAE as a laboratory counterpart of MS. Kabat et al.'s (88) finding that the previously excised forebrain of a monkey in CFA could produce EAE when injected back into the same animal added significant support to the possibility that humans with MS might be affected by an autoimmune or autoallergic process. The impetus for the next 30 years of experimental studies derived from the facts that EAE could be produced in small laboratory animals, the acute response was obtainable within a relatively short period of time (2–3 weeks) after a single injection of brain tissue in CFA, and the CNS lesions bore a remarkable resemblance to those present in humans affected by acute disseminated encephalomyelitis (ADE). Shiraki and Otani (167) provided a significant correlative study in their description of the similar histological patterns observed in rabies postvaccinal encephalomyelitis, thus lending credence to EAE as a *bona fide* laboratory model for studying MS. A number of early articles compared the pathological patterns as observed in EAE-affected animals and ADE in humans, and discussed their relevance to MS (91). The model of acute EAE subsequently served an important role in the search for the responsible antigen(s) in CNS tissue and in the analysis of the immunological parameters involved in the production of the characteristic responses in animals and man (see sections on the antigen and the immunological response). Objections were voiced, however, concerning the significance and relevance of acute EAE to MS. These reservations had a certain validity since the laboratory model (EAE) consisted of a monophasic, frequently fatal response to a single inoculation, whereas MS is characteristically a chronic exacerbating and remitting or progressive illness. Moreover, the lesions in acute EAE resembled more the clinical types of ADE rather than those observed in MS. However, recent extensions of EAE into its chronic forms has greatly enhanced the use and substantiated the validity of the laboratory model as a proper instrument for examining both the immunological mechanisms and the tissue responses as they may relate to the pathogenesis of MS (114,144,145, 177,198).

Chronic EAE is most easily and reproducibly established in juvenile strain 13 guinea pigs, although other strains and other species (rabbits) may respond with similar patterns. The chronically affected animals do not develop a severe, rapidly lethal response. Instead, they may follow two clinical patterns. There may be a postinoculation delay of many weeks or months before any clinical manifestations are expressed. Examinations of the CNS tissues during the latent period from 2–3 weeks postinoculation nevertheless reveal histological lesions of acute EAE, i.e., perivascular inflammation and demyelination. With the onset of weakness, incontinence, etc., the clinical course may then follow a chronically progressive pattern, or it may proceed to a level of disability which is then maintained for long periods when it may again enter a period of active exacerbation (145). In the other clear pattern of response (198), the young animals develop overt clinical signs and symptoms approximately 2 weeks postinoculation. Most recover from this first episode and enter an interval of many weeks when they are free of any evidence of neurological illness. Most frequently, they then begin a second period of exacerbation. Some may recover and go on to repeat the pattern of exacerbation and remission. If the tissues of the chronically affected animals of either type are examined, they are found to contain areas of mild perivascular infiltration, demyelination in progress, totally denuded axons, remyelinating axons, and finally sclerosis—the identical lesion observed in patients with longstanding, active MS.

The evaluation of immunological factors (circulating antibodies and cell-associated activities) from animals with EAE and patients with MS by means of organotypic cultures of myelinated mammalian CNS tissues also yielded significant comparisons between the two and served to validate EAE in its acute and chronic forms as a proper model for studying MS (22,23,28,30). In this regard, it has been shown that sera obtained from animals responding to an inoculum of whole CNS white matter in CFA and those obtained from patients with MS produce a similar pattern of demyelination specifically directed against CNS tissues (32). Moreover, prolonged exposure to either the EAE or MS sera eventually leads to a state of sclerosis in the cultured tissues (141). These and other applications of organotypic cultures of nerve tissues to immunological and neuropathological aspects of myelin are presented in greater detail in following sections.

ANTIGEN(S) IN NERVE TISSUE

Since EAE is induced by exposure of laboratory animals to whole brain tissue (whether in saline as in the early experiments, or in CFA as currently applied in most laboratories), much study has been devoted to the isolation, characterization, analysis, and synthesis of the specific substance or substances that may be the antigen responsible for the immunological response (for details of the extensive literature on this subject, see refs. 43,58,60,90–92,115,131,146). The search for such an encephalitogenic substance was aided by the establishment of an assay system for evaluating the potencies of various fractions of CNS tissues (8). In this system, quantitation of the guinea pigs' involvement was expressed as an index of encephalitogenicity, de-

termined by the extent of manifest neurological signs and symptoms plus the severity of the histopathological lesions. Eventually, the major encephalitogenic component in brain tissue was identified as a myelin basic protein (MBP) with a molecular weight (MW) of approximately 18,000. A number of laboratories have been involved in determining the amino acid sequence of MBP and particularly in the evaluation of encephalitogenicity of the whole protein and some of its components. The complete sequences of amino acids in human and bovine basic protein were elucidated by Kibler et al. (89) and Eylar (54) and that of human MBP independently by Carnegie (40). The sequences of human and bovine MBP differ by only 11 amino acids, as shown in Fig. 1. At least eight loci for inducing a delayed hypersensitivity (DH) to MBP and three others active for antibody production have been reported (19).

There is general agreement that MBP is capable of producing EAE in most laboratory animals. It is also known that certain peptides derived from MBP can also retain encephalitogenic activity (35). There are, however, a

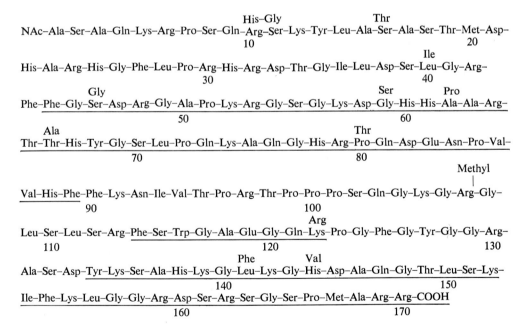

FIG. 1. Amino acid sequence of basic protein of bovine myelin. Substitutions in human basic protein are shown above the appropriate position of the bovine sequence. Between positions 10 and 11, a His–Gly dipeptide occurs in the human protein. (From ref. 54.)

number of species-specific differences to MBP and various peptide fractions of the MBP molecule (40,43,55–57,59,76,89,93,108,115, 116,182,192,193).

Therefore MBP has proved to be the major encephalitogenic component of the CNS. To date, no other CNS constituent has been clearly demonstrated to be capable of producing EAE. Yet there is evidence suggesting that MBP may not be the only agent and that other components may act in concert with the protein. A number of investigators have noted that the lesions found in animals exposed to MBP or some of its fractions in CFA may differ significantly from those observed after inoculations of whole white matter in CFA even though the animals' clinical manifestations are indistinguishable. Shapira et al. (161) actually failed to find any histological lesions in serially sectioned CNS of two EAE-affected monkeys inoculated with a peptide fragment of MBP (amino acids 45–90). In this regard, it should be recalled that the acute, demyelinating EAE lesions were first observed in monkeys after a series of injections with whole white matter in saline (63,120,150, 151). In guinea pigs MBP and synthesized EAE peptides do not produce the amount of demyelination found after exposure to whole tissue (77).

Seil et al. (159) made an interesting comparison between groups of guinea pigs inoculated with whole tissue or MBP in adjuvant. Both groups developed the classic signs of EAE approximately 2 weeks postinoculation. Those which had received whole tissue were shown to have circulating demyelinating factors in their sera but no anti-MBP antibodies, whereas the MBP-exposed animals were just the opposite, having circulating anti-MBP antibodies but no demyelinating activity.

The sera from rabbits immunized with cerebroside in adjuvant have been shown to be capable of demyelinating and inhibiting myelinogenesis in cultured CNS tissue (52, 70,78) in a manner identical to that found in antisera from EAE rabbits inoculated with whole tissue. Of the many rabbits used in the latter (70) studies, only one was observed to have signs of neurological dysfunction, moderate paraparesis. Examination of its lumbar spinal cord revealed small but definite loci of perivascular cellular infiltrates and demyelinated axons (Bornstein, Raine, and Lehrer, *unpublished observations*). Although exposure of animals to cerebroside in adjuvant does not usually induce EAE (124), the combination of MBP and cerebroside modifies the clinical manifestations and histological lesions of EAE in comparison to MBP alone (36).

Nagi et al. (121) recently demonstrated that rabbits immunized with total brain gangliosides, or GD_{1a} and GM, in CFA develop neurological signs and symptoms resembling EAE. Histological examinations of the GD_{1a}-immunized rabbits revealed extensive involvement of peripheral nerves, including a non-inflammatory breakdown of myelin and fragmentation of axis cylinders. The CNS, however, was affected only by mild perivascular cuffs localized primarily to periventricular areas.

Wray et al. (203) first described a useful *in vivo* model that is proving to be an interesting and valuable system, complementing that of the myelinated CNS tissues in culture, for the evaluation of antigenic and immunological factors in EAE. In the rabbit eye, myelinated axons of the optic nerve course over the retina. As a result, they are available for direct observation while exposed to various cell-associated, serum, or other migration inhibitory factors (MIF) that have been closely applied by injection into the vitreous overlying the optic nerve head. In the first application of this technique (202), lymph node cells were taken from rabbits exposed to guinea pig MBP in CFA. The injection of 10^6 cells in 0.2 ml of saline produced a passive transfer of EAE, as evidenced by an optic neuritis characterized by round-cell infiltration and myelin destruction.

In an extension of the rabbit eye model, Wiśniewski and Bloom (196) succeeded in producing the lesions of EAE without the involvement of nerve tissue of any kind. In this experiment, guinea pigs were first sensitized with CFA containing killed mycobacteria via inoculations into the footpads and nuchal muscles. At 4–8 weeks after sensitization, killed or living mycobacteria, purified protein derivative (PPD), or old tuberculin (OT) were injected into the ventricular system or the substance of the CNS or PNS. An acute inflammatory lesion appeared at the site of the injection characterized by perivascular inflammation and a proportional demyelination with preservation of axis cylinders. These responses bore a striking similarity to the pattern of response in acute EAE. Continuing this line of investigation (197), rabbits were similarly prepared with CNS white matter in CFA, basic protein (BP) in CFA, or CFA alone and were then challenged with injections of BP or PPD into the vitreous close to the retina. An extensive inflammatory reaction and primary demyelination of the optic nerve was induced by the intravitreous injection of PPD in those animals inoculated with white matter in CFA (WM/CFA) or CFA alone. The same response occurred in rabbits sensitized with CFA alone and challenged with PPD, but BP challenge produced no response in these animals. The retinas of nonsensitized animals injected with PPD or BP into the vitreous were normal. The production of segmental demyelination therefore may result from sensitization to a brain-specific antigen (BP) or an indifferent antigen (PPD). As in the previous study (196), the myelin may be affected as a "nonspecific" consequence of a specific delayed-type hypersensitivity reaction directed at a nonnervous tissue antigen. These data may be of signal importance in the understanding of MS when the neurological attack may be a response to either a specific or a nonspecific (viral or other) antigen.

In fact, Wiśniewski (*personal communication*) is currently demonstrating an identical response in the rabbit eye in animals preexposed to injections of common viruses and then challenged by intraocular injections of the same viruses. Finally, in regard to the possible involvement of virus in the pathogenesis of the autoallergic diseases of nerve tissues, one must mention the recent experience of the significant increase in incidence and severity of the Guillain–Barré syndrome in patients who had received swine flu inoculations.

Regardless of whether MBP represents the sole or primary antigen involved in the production of EAE, the nature of the immunological response in most instances has been demonstrated to bear a close relationship to a delayed hypersensitivity-type reaction. Animals with EAE respond with positive skin tests to CNS tissue or MBP (10,41,163,191). In addition, circulating lymphocytes in animals with EAE can be induced to respond to *in vitro* challenge with whole CNS tissue or various fractions with macrophage migratory inhibition and lymphocytic transformation (10,41,48, 163,191).

Not all investigators, however, agree that cellular immunity is necessarily correlated with the production of EAE. Spitler and her associates (173) suggested that there might be a dissociation between the two states. In a subsequent study (174) in guinea pigs, skin tests, lymphocyte DNA synthesis, and macrophage migration inhibition examinations 10 days postinoculation (DPI) of animals sensitized with human BP or tryptophan peptide failed to reveal cellular immunity to the disease-producing determinant of the BP molecule, thus supporting their previous conclusions.

The relationship between cell-bound and circulating antibody (AB) and MBP and the presence of histological EAE lesions has also been questioned (71) in experiments using horseradish peroxidase (HRP)-labeled and ^{125}I-labeled MBP to identify draining lymph nodes—probably B-cells (206) and circulating AB, respectively—in Lewis and Brown Norwegian rats challenged with high and low amounts of guinea pig and Lewis rat MBP in CFA. In Lewis rats high (500 μg) and low (5 μg) doses of antigen produced EAE, but the higher doses were associated with numerous MBP plasma cells correlating with high levels of circulating AB, whereas low doses were found to produce few or no AB-containing cells and significantly lower levels of circulating AB. Moreover, the EAE-resistant Brown Norwegian rats immunized with 500 μg MBP-CFA did not develop EAE in spite of a cell and AB response similar to that of Lewis rats similarly challenged.

In regard to MS, however, the evidence of involvement of MBP is much less certain (131,132; for a concise review, see ref. 94). Thus patients do not respond to injected CNS antigens with a delayed hypersensitivity skin reaction (175). A number of investigations have demonstrated macrophage migration inhibition in cells from MS patients treated with MBP (15,153,164,165), although some investigators report no migration inhibition with MS (17,105,179). Moreover, the specificity of the response in respect to MS is brought into question by demonstrations of the same reactions in neurological patients with diseases other than MS (17,41,105,165). Similar positive and negative reports have appeared concerning lymphocyte transformation in response to MBP. Although plasma cells in the nodes and CNS of rabbits with EAE specifically bind HRP-labeled MBP (84,86), similar examinations of plasma cells and CNS tissues, including active, longstanding plaques from MS patients, failed to reveal any such MBP-specific reactions (85,181).

It is of some interest, in relating EAE to the naturally occurring demyelinative disorders, that some studies employing proliferation lymphocyte responses (105) or skin tests (1) demonstrate a positive correlation to MBP in patients with acute disseminated encephalomyelitis but none in MS patients.

IMMUNE RESPONSE

Sensitized Cells

The suspected role of sensitized cells and cell-mediated immune responses in the production of EAE was firmly established by Paterson's (129) classic demonstration of passive transfer of EAE by sensitized lymphocytes. This key finding was soon confirmed (13,60, 176) and has been extended into numerous studies of delayed hypersensitivity-type reactions to MBP (for review, see refs. 10,131, 132,189,195). Definitive evidence for the T-cell requirement for the induction of EAE in the rat was recently afforded by Ortiz-Ortiz and co-workers (127,128). Both EAE and anti-BP ABs were induced in thymectomized, irradiated Lewis rats reconstituted with normal thymus and bone marrow cells and challenged with BP/CFA. If the specific T-cells were eliminated by treatment with BP heavily labeled with ^{125}I-BP, the recipients neither developed EAE nor produced antibody to BP. On the other hand, if the B-cell population had been eliminated and the T-cells were intact, EAE ensued but no antibodies were produced. Further evidence for the T-cell requirement was furnished by experiments with

thymectomized, irradiated rats reconstituted with lymphoid cells treated with antithymocyte serum (ATS). Injection with BP/CFA produced neither EAE nor circulating antibodies (127). In further experiments the same investigators transferred lymphoid cells from BP/CFA-sensitized rats into thymectomized, irradiated rats. If the lymphoid cells were from untreated donors, EAE resulted. If T-cell depletion of donor cells had been accomplished by previous ATS treatment, however, no EAE resulted, although the transfer recipients still produced anti-BP antibody. These experiments demonstrate an unequivocal requirement for T-cells in the induction of EAE. What they do not probe, however, is the possible interrelationships between sensitized cells and circulating antibody in the pathogenesis of the significant structural and functional lesions as they may occur in the response of a normal animal to a challenging inoculation and, more importantly, in the naturally occurring disease, MS.

The possible role of sensitized cells in MS, as determined by skin testing with CNS antigens, production of macrophage migration inhibition by an exposure of circulating lymphocytes to MBP, and lymphocyte transformation suggest that peripheral blood lymphocytes may be significant factors in the patient, but the specificity of the response to MBP as such is not convincing (94,134). Recently, circulating lymphocytes from MS patients were shown to produce a pattern of demyelination in cultured CNS tissue (156). This response is described in the section on cell–serum interactions.

Circulating Antibody

Although there is general agreement that cellular immunity (i.e., T-cell systems) is involved in EAE and possibly MS, the participation of circulating antibody in their pathogenesis has not been universally accepted. Yet there is no doubt that circulating factors are present in EAE and MS, and that they can reproduce characteristic and specific tissue responses in a number of laboratory model systems (41,134). The essential problem is not to pit one against the other, but to design and execute experiments that can demonstrate the individual and interacting capacities of T- and

B-cell systems as they may affect nerve tissues during the course of acute and chronic EAE as well as during periods of exacerbation and remission or chronic progression in MS patients.

The first evidence that demyelinating factors are present in the serum of EAE-affected rabbits challenged with whole rabbit or guinea pig CNS in CFA (unless otherwise stated, the term EAE serum is used to designate samples obtained from animals inoculated with and responding to whole tissue in CFA) was supplied through the use of organotypic, myelinated cultures of rat cerebellum (24). In the presence of antiserum and complement, but not control sera, the cultured tissues responded with a characteristic and specific pattern of demyelination, with sparing of the axis cylinders. Identical results were reported later (64, 107,108). Further examinations of EAE serum from guinea pigs, rats, and mice on myelinated cultures of spinal cord and cerebrum support the concept that the response is organ- and not species-specific (23).

A recent extension of these studies (32) examined the demyelinating activity of EAE rabbit and human (MS) sera on cultures that contain both CNS and PNS myelin. These sera destroyed the central sheaths within 24 hr of exposure, whereas the PNS myelin remained undisturbed during exposures to the same concentrations of demyelinating (EAE) sera for periods of time ranging up to 30 and 40 days. These results offer further evidence of the organ specificity of EAE and MS. In addition, the unresponsiveness of peripheral myelin argues against the possibility that the demyelination represents a nonspecific response to any noxious agent directed against nerve tissue. Of further interest in this regard is the response of similar spinal cord–dorsal root ganglion cultures to serum from animals with experimental allergic neuritis (EAN). In this instance, central and peripheral myelin were demyelinated, with the CNS responding a day or two earlier than the PNS (Bornstein, *unpublished observations*). These studies complement previously published reports of EAN by Winkler (194), Arnason et al. (12), and Yonezawa et al. (204).

After the consistent demonstration of demyelination by sera from EAE rabbits, further

analyses (11) characterized the circulating factors to be complement-dependent and present in the γ_2-globulin (7S) component of rabbit serum. The albumin and α-globulin (19S) fractions were inactive. Exposure of whole serum or its globulin component to rabbit or rat brain homogenates removed the myelinotoxic activity, but exposure to homologous or heterologous red blood cells, liver, lung, or kidney had no such effect. These studies provided the evidence that the myelinotoxic factors in EAE serum are antibodies.

The application of immunoperoxidase techniques (83,84) confirmed the immunofluorescent (11,166) localization of immunoglobulin on myelin sheaths in cultures exposed to EAE serum. Peroxidase-labeled anti-immunoglobulin antibodies, or Fab fragments, revealed reaction product on myelin and, with preliminary ultrastructural studies, on oligodendrocytic plasma membranes. However, in cultures incubated with MS sera of strong demyelinating activity and then exposed to antihuman immunoglobulins, no stained myelin was found.

Complement-dependent demyelinating antibodies, characterized as IgG_2 immunoglobulins, were recently (102) found in guinea pigs challenged with three CNS antigens. However, the immunoglobulins did not prove to be directed against either MBP or cerebroside. Seil et al. (159) also called into question the relationship between MBP, whole tissue, and EAE, as described previously.

Confirmatory evidence for the participation of circulating antibody in an immunological attack on the CNS in EAE has now been provided by a number of *in vivo* models. Jankovic et al. (80) first presented evidence that a series of intraventricular injections of antibrain antiserum into rabbits by means of an indwelling catheter produced structural changes resembling those found in EAE. The data were difficult to evaluate, however, without accompanying photographic evidence. Simon and Simon (170) recently reported clinical manifestations and structural changes, including perivascular infiltrates and myelin degeneration, in rabbits after a single intraventricular or intracisternal injection of rabbit antibrain antiserum. The injection of normal rabbit sera did not produce clinical or histological alterations.

Cell–Serum Interactions

The use of organotypic myelinated cultures has also begun to delineate the individual and interrelated roles that cell-associated and serum factors may play in production of the demyelinating lesion. This inquiry began with the examination of sequential samples of lymph node cells (LNCs) and serum from Lewis strain rats inoculated with whole CNS white matter in CFA (WM/CFA) (28). Both cells and serum produced the identical pattern of demyelination as had previously been noted to occur with sera from other species (24). By the third day postinoculation (DPI), the LNCs had already demonstrated a capacity to demyelinate the CNS axons. By the fifth DPI, both LNC and serum were potent and remained so in all samples up to the 16th DPI. A few later samples revealed the maintenance of demyelinating activity in the serum but its disappearance from the LNCs. Destroying the LNCs by freezing and thawing abolished their demyelinating capabilities. When LNCs were cultured in isolation for 3–5 days without further exposure to CNS tissue, the demyelinating activity was found in the nutrient medium. These data therefore revealed that both cell-associated and circulating factors were involved in the rat's EAE response to whole tissue in CFA. Current studies of a similar nature in Hartley strain guinea pigs demonstrate that LNCs, spleen cells, and circulating lymphocytes as well as serum develop demyelinating activities after WM/CFA inoculations (Bornstein, Salomon, and Sheppard, *unpublished observations*). These demonstrations are complemented in part by the *in vitro* studies of EAN by Winkler (194), Arnason et al. (12), and Yonezawa et al. (204).

One of the advantages of the tissue culture system as a model in which to examine factors that might operate in the demyelinative disorders is its availability as a common test object to compare EAE and MS. Thus one of the extensions of the examination of EAE serum was to introduce MS and control human sera into the complement-enriched nutrient medium and to note whether they also possessed demyelinating activity. The first study (22) demonstrated that a pattern of demyelination identical to that resulting from EAE

serum could be induced by human serum. Samples of serum from MS patients and normal or patient controls demonstrated demyelinating activity in approximately 65% in active MS patients and 10% in inactive patients, normal, and patient controls. Only patients with amyotrophic lateral sclerosis also demonstrated a high percentage of demyelinating sera, a fact later confirmed by Field and Hughes (64). With some variation in the percentage of active sera, the demonstration of demyelinating factors has since been confirmed in our own and other laboratories (27,79,107–109). Electron microscopic examinations (Raine, *this volume*) confirmed the similarity of the myelin-destructive actions of EAE and MS serum. As previously stated, the remarkable organ specificity of these antisera is shown by their inability to affect PNS myelin while simultaneously destroying the CNS myelin (32).

Currently, both serum and circulating lymphocytes from MS patients, obtained as single or serial samples, are being examined for their capacity to demyelinate CNS cultures (156). As previously reported, MS serum in the presence of complement demyelinates CNS axons. A consistent, but less potent demyelinating activity is noted when 10^6 circulating lymphocytes are introduced into the tissue culture nutrient medium. Complement is not required for this effect. These early data show that cells obtained from patients who are pursuing an active, demyelinating, and remitting course tend to have a greater demyelinating effect than do cells obtained from patients who are affected by a slowly progressive, chronic illness. The addition of MS serum to the lymphocyte-containing nutrient medium, without supplementary complement, increases the *in vitro* demyelinating effect.

The recent *in vivo* studies of Brosnan et al. (34) are of signal importance in regard to another role of circulating antibody in immunologically determined demyelination. Using the rabbit eye model (197,203), sera from rabbits immunized with homologous spinal cord in CFA were injected into the vitreous of normal rabbits either alone or admixed with an equal volume of supernatants from cultured activated lymphocytes. It had been shown by these investigators (178) that products of the activated lymphocytes alone injected into the vitreous of normal rabbits or those sensitized with lung, kidney, or CFA alone induced a monocytic infiltrate which did not, however, invade the retinal parenchyma or induce primary demyelination. However, in rabbits sensitized to homologous spinal cord, the injection of lymphocyte products induced a cellular infiltrate and demyelination resembling that found in animals with acute EAE. In the normal rabbit these injections of 0.1 ml EAE antiserum proved incapable of causing a primary demyelination, although it had previously been shown to be demyelinating when applied to cultured mouse spinal cord in 25% concentration and in the presence of complement. On the other hand, the injection of anti-CNS antiserum or antibodies plus the products of activated lymphocytes into normal rabbits induced an inflammatory response and focal primary demyelination in the vicinity of the invading cells. The factor was shown, by ammonium sulfate precipitation, to be present in the globulin fraction of the serum. It could be removed by an immunoadsorbent column of sheep antirabbit IgG; the adsorbed IgG, on elution, retained the activity. Thus this significant experiment establishes, for the first time, an antibody-dependent cell-mediated "cytotoxic" mechanism (ADCC) for primary demyelination in EAE.

Current preliminary experiments in tissue culture, essentially extensions of Brosnan's (34) EAE studies in the rabbit eye, appear to demonstrate a similar antibody-dependent cell-mediated demyelination (ADCD) in MS (Bornstein and Salomon, *unpublished observations*). In these experiments myelinated cultures are pre-exposed for 6 hr to 25% concentrations of serum from MS patients or normal individuals in nutrient medium with or without added complement. They are then washed free of the human serum-containing medium, which is replaced by a drop of medium containing 10^6 circulating lymphocytes from a normal human subject. The cultures previously exposed to MS sera will be demyelinated but not those pretreated with normal human serum. Patient controls from various nondemyelinating conditions are now being investigated. Thus the specificity of the reaction is still under investigation, but the ADCC re-

sponse to MS serum has been observed to occur in the cultures. These and other data from our tissue culture studies are discussed further in the section on the immunopathological response.

Histocompatibility Antigens

It is not possible to discuss the immunological involvement in pathological processes without referring to the genetic control of immunological responses. During the past 5 years, interest in histocompatibility antigens has spread into many fields of medicine. MS has been an area of particular interest, and the studies are assuming vast proportions. Indeed a supplementary issue of *Acta Neurologica Scandinavica* (65) is devoted entirely to the 1975 international symposium on the histocompatibility system in MS.

Batechelor (16) prepared a lucid, concise, scholarly review of the history and general principles of the histocompatibility complex of man and its particular relevance to MS. McFarlin and McFarlin (117) recently prepared a critical review of the various histocompatibility studies in MS, and Paterson (131,132) interrelated actual and theoretical considerations with details of immunological reactions in EAE and MS.

The major histocompatibility complex of man, the human leukocyte antigen (HLA) complex, was first demonstrated by serological means, the leukocyte agglutination and lymphocytotoxicity tests, and later by the interaction of mixtures of lymphocytes from different individuals, transforming some of the cells into blast cells—the mixed lymphocyte culture (MLC) reaction. Thus "the HLA complex consists of a series of closely linked genes, controlling the expression of antigens detectable by lymphocytotoxic antibodies and complement and another which determines the expression of MLC-activating factors" (16). Present terminology designates the lymphocytotoxic antibodies as A, B, and C (formerly LA, Four, and AJ), and the MLC factors as D. The identification of an individual's HLA antigens by lymphocytotoxicity tests are then designated by numbers: HLA-A1, HLA-B5, etc. The interest in the various antigens arises when one or more are associated in a given group of individuals (e.g., MS patients) more frequently than would be expected on the basis of their gene frequencies. In MS there is an association between HLA-A3, HLA-B7, and HLA-Dw2 (81). However, conflicting views have appeared concerning the levels of association of these antigens and MS. Nevertheless, it is possible that the susceptibility to an external agent, as suggested by epidemiological studies (97), may be influenced by a gene in the HLA region, and, secondly, that the severity and progression (i.e., the prognosis) may also be determined by a similar gene.

The possible relationship between immunogenetic factors, viral agents as either trigger mechanisms or ongoing slow or latent infections, and immunological responses has been suggested by a number of findings, particularly the increased measles antibody titers in the serum (5) and the CSF (125) of MS patients. The various comparative studies of histocompatibility antigens and the antibody titers to various viruses (117) may represent either a causal relationship between MS and the particular virus or simply an altered immunoresponsiveness in that particular group of patients.

Further studies relating the histocompatibility antigens to the cellular and humoral immune mechanisms discussed above and the sequential studies of their interrelationships in groups of MS patients may serve not only to clarify the associations but may also yield clues concerning the potential efficacy of treatments directed at various aspects of the immunological mechanisms.

Immunopathological Response

In the previous sections we have seen how the classic concept of EAE—and, by extension, MS as a delayed-type hypersensitivity reaction involving specifically sensitized cells —has gradually been expanded with data generated by *in vitro* (tissue culture) and *in vivo* (rabbit eye) models. It is now necessary to consider at least three other mechanisms: circulating antibody, products of activated lymphocytes (MIF), and antibody-dependent cell-mediated demyelination. In view of the invasion of the CNS by phagocytic cells as

well as the established phagocytic properties of astrocytes (4,22,142; Raine, *this volume*), this fifth mechanism must be considered as a possible contributing factor in the pathogenesis of the CNS lesion. How do these factors produce the significant lesion, and what are the significant lesions of the neural parenchyma in the demyelinating diseases? In the final analysis, from the point of view of MS, there is only one significant lesion: that which produces the dysfunction of the nervous system. The change in function, however, may involve a number of structural alterations (e.g., inflammation, demyelination, and sclerosis), although strictly speaking, inflammation *per se* is a mesodermal response and does not directly involve ectoderm, i.e., the neural parenchyma. The question of a strict causal relationship between structural change and dysfunction has been a subject of concern since the earliest descriptions of MS. Charcot, quoted by Taylor (185), regarded some symptoms as "conditioned by an altered resistance to conduction in the sclerotic area." This question continues to be a subject of concerned debate and inquiry (6,73,104,113,154,155).

Vascular Permeability and the Early Lesion

The sequence of events is of prime importance in attempting to establish the interrelationships and roles of the various immunological factors known to be present in the demyelinative disorders. The earliest changes are practically impossible to find in nerve tissues from MS patients, although with diligence early lesions may be found and examined in detail (137). For this reason, most of the information concerning the earliest events is derived from animals exposed to EAE-inducing inoculations.

A number of observations have established the occurrence of abnormal blood–brain (i.e., vascular) permeability in EAE with trypan blue, radioactive bovine albumin, or human serum albumin as markers (14,46,103,190). Oldstone and Dixon (126) reported the most pertinent information in their sequential immunohistochemical examinations of Lewis rats beginning on the first day after inoculation with guinea pig spinal cord or purified MBP in CFA and continuing for 14 days postinoculation. Immunologically specific rabbit antirat γ-globulin and fibrinogen and control globulins were fluoresceinated and applied to the frozen sections obtained from six sampled areas of brain and spinal cord. The late, 14-day lesions had well-developed perivascular and lymphoid infiltrates and predominantly a deposition of rat fibrinogen in the vessel wall and perivascular spaces. In addition, the cytoplasm of some perivascular mononuclear cells stained positively for γ-globulin. The γ-globulin also appeared to diffuse from the perivascular regions well into the brain parenchyma itself and, in 10–15% of the sections, to deposit in myelinated tracts without particular relation to the vessels. At earlier time points, however, there was a dissociation between the presence of minimal histological lesions and exudation of fibrinogen and γ-globulin. Only very rarely were histological lesions (i.e., perivascular infiltrates) detectable by 8 or 9 DPI, whereas by day 7 fibrinogen and γ-globulin were regularly observed. Adjacent and other sections at 7 DPI possessed no histologic lesions. Finally, examinations of the heart, kidney, liver, skeletal muscle, spleen, and testes failed to show any fibrinogen or γ-globulin. No immunopathological lesions were found in rats inoculated with kidney in CFA or CFA alone. Thus there is no doubt that the increased permeability of the blood vessels and the deposition of fibrinogen and γ-globulin occur several days before the appearance of infiltrating round cells, suggesting that a humoral factor(s) may initiate the sequence of pathological events in the disease.

Once the pathological process has become fully established, it is obviously no longer possible to distinguish cell-associated from circulating factors. However, the state of vascular permeability may still be a significant feature of the continuing process. For this purpose, the model of chronic relapsing EAE (144,198) has proved useful. Kristensson and Wisniewski (96) examined the vascular permeability in strain 13 and Hartley strain guinea pigs with chronic relapsing EAE produced by a sensitization with guinea pig spinal cord in CFA. A heavy leakage of protein tracers was noted in both recent and old demyelinating plaques, demonstrating disturbed permeability even in the older plaques in EAE. These investigators suggest that the demyelinating activity often observed at the edges of the plaques could therefore be mediated by the leaking antimyelin antibody.

The closest approximation of the naturally occurring lesion to that noted early in EAE-affected animals is Prineas' (137) presentation of the early lesion in MS. He refers to a number of investigators who disagree with previous authors that hypercellularity of the tissue is an important accompaniment of early myelin breakdown. Rather, they describe disintegration of myelin sheaths occurring in the absence of any local increase in the number of cells. In his own light and electron microscopic examinations of five brains of MS patients, two fixed by perfusion shortly after death, Prineas describes an unusual mechanism involving a progressive reduction in the number of myelin lamellae around nerve fibers in the vicinity of cells of uncertain origin, possibly altered oligodendroglia, containing filamentous and multilamellated cytoplasmic inclusions unlike the usual pleomorphic inclusions seen in myelin phagocytes. Lymphocytes were not directly involved in this process but were observed to contact the inclusion-containing material following its delivery to the Virchow–Robin spaces.

Adams (4) carefully examined the nature and progression of the lesions in MS and EAE, but these probably did not represent early lesions. The nature of the cells at the edge of active plaques remains an unresolved controversy. Some may be identified as oligodendrocytes and some as phagocytes of microglial or monocytic origin. However, demyelinating lesions may be observed in areas where no phagocytic attack can be discerned (180).

Demyelination

The demyelinating response of the CNS to serum and cell-associated factors in *in vitro* and *in vivo* models was presented in the preceding section on the immune mechanisms. The structural alterations associated with demyelination, as visualized in the light and electron microscope, are detailed by Raine (*this volume*). In general, the experimentally induced phenomena closely resemble changes found in MS plaques examined by the same techniques.

The presence of abnormal concentrations of lysosomal enzymes may represent biochemical mechanisms triggered by the immunological factors, which subsequently participate in the process of demyelination. MS tissues show an increase in such proteolytic activity as detected by histochemical and biochemical techniques (2–4,47,49,148). There is also a corresponding loss of MBP. One may speculate as to the involvement of such enzymes as an effect on MBP in the doubling of the periodicity of myelin lamellae and the changes in their intimate ultrastructure as the earliest structural event seen in EAE and MS antiserum-induced demyelination in culture (31) described in detail in Raine (*this volume*). Comparable changes have also been noted in canine distemper encephalomyelitis (140) and in the peripheral nervous system in human neuropathy associated with Waldenstraum's macroglobulinemia (139) and a patient with a polyneuropathy associated with a hypergammaglobulinemia who 5 years later developed multiple myeloma (171). Is there an antibody- or enzyme-induced release or a physicochemical alteration of MBP which secondarily affects the sheath's structure (147)? These possibilities are currently being examined in the tissue culture model. Adams (4) considers the source of the lysosomal enzymes to be phagocytic cells concerned with the breakdown of myelin, either as an initial or a secondary event. Direct evidence regarding this possibility may be obtained by the introduction of phagocytes from normal or EAE-sensitized animals in our current models (i.e., tissue culture or rabbit eyes) with and without serum or MIF factors. These experiments may also determine the participation of phagocytes from different origins (e.g., blood monocytes, microglia, astrocytes). It has already been established (21,141) that microglia and astrocytes may participate in the phagocytic breakdown of myelin in cultures affected by EAE and MS serum.

Remyelination

The capacity of the mammalian CNS to remyelinate following an immunologically in-

duced demyelinating experience was first observed in the tissue culture model system (21). Bunge et al. (38) had also demonstrated the ability of the adult cat spinal cord to remyelinate following a traumatically induced demyelination. Remyelination following an immunological insult has since been confirmed in animals with EAE (37,98,99,172) and in MS (61,62,180). However, the continued presence of low concentrations of EAE serum (29) or anticerebroside serum (69,70) plus complement is capable of inhibiting the differentiation of oligodendroglia and remyelination or, in fact, primary myelinogenesis in the CNS (29). Yonezawa et al. (205) reported that MS sera are also capable of inhibiting primary myelin formation. When the inhibiting antisera are removed, even after many weeks of exposure, oligodendroglia promptly differentiate and myelination proceeds normally. Immunobiological techniques may also serve to analyze and dissect normal biological processes, and this is one example of such an application. The capability of turning the process of myelinogenesis off and on at will is also serving as a useful immunological device to examine various biochemical parameters associated with myelin formation (68,70,101).

Sclerosis

A further comparison of the *in vitro* effects of EAE and MS serum is their capacity to produce a state of sclerosis following a prolonged exposure. In these experiments (141) cultures were continuously exposed to potent, demyelinating sera plus complement for periods of time ranging from 30 to 60 days. During this period, the astrocytic population was gradually transformed into a group of uniform cells whose cytoplasm was almost entirely occupied by masses of gliofibrils, hardly leaving room for mitochondria and glycogen granules. The neural parenchyma also lost its epithelial character, the usual close apposition of cell membranes being replaced by spaces of a micron or more separating neighboring cells. Thus the cultured tissues gradually assumed the structural configurations characteristic of the MS plaque (4) as well as the lesions that develop in the laboratory animal counterpart, chronic EAE (144,198). Concurrently with the development of the permanent structural changes in the neuroglial community, the CNS tissue lost its capacity to remyelinate.

Functional Alterations

The dramatic impact of a demyelinated plaque, as revealed by a sharply demarcated, clear area lying within a field of stained sheaths, understandably focused attention on the structural alteration as the cause of the neurological dysfunction in MS. Yet even Charcot (44) was not completely satisfied with a purely anatomical explanation. He noted the "apparent disproportion between the symptoms and the lesion constituting one of the most powerful arguments to show that the functional continuity of the nerve tubes is not absolutely interrupted, although these, in their course through the sclerosed patches, have been despoiled of their medullary sheaths and reduced to axis cylinders." Since then and until the present time, many concerned neurologists and investigators have been led by clinical or laboratory data to express dissatisfaction with a purely anatomical, demyelinated or sclerotic, lesion as the sole cause for the clinically manifest dysfunctions (6,7,113,155). These reservations are based on a number of considerations: the relatively rapid onset of, and recovery from, severe neurological deficits that frequently occur in acute exacerbations; the marked dissociation that may be found between the clinical findings and the structural involvement, with many patients possessing more extensive lesions than had been suspected (123). Indeed instances have been reported (112; McDonald, *personal communication*) in which routine postmortem examinations revealed multiple plaques in the CNS of patients who during their lifetimes had no known clinical evidence of a neurological disorder. Moreover, in particular areas of the nervous system (e.g., the optic nerve where there is no possibility for redundancy of functional units), there may be preservation of useful vision in optic nerves which at postmortem examination are shown to be totally lacking myelin sheaths (7) even for distances of 25–30 mm examined millimeter by millimeter (199). These observations led to the conclusion that factors in addition to morpho-

logically detectable myelin changes influence transmission.

In addition to the mounting evidence from clinical material, there are a number of laboratory findings from animal and tissue culture experiments that confirm the inadequacy of a purely structural explanation for the neuronal dysfunction. Moreover, they warrant further investigation into factors that may more directly affect the neuronal populations and their intimate functions in the propagation and transmission of the nervous impulse.

Still, many laboratory and clinical studies have demonstrated altered conduction in nerve fibers that were known or suspected of having been demyelinated. There are a number of excellent reviews of this aspect of the pathophysiology of MS (73,113,154; Rasminsky, *this volume*). In laboratory studies, demyelination has been produced by immunological techniques of experimental allergic neuritis as well as by a number of traumatic and metabolic or toxic insults. The resultant deficits in conduction of the nervous impulse have ranged from conduction block, with the most severe degrees of demyelination, through delayed or slowed transmission due to slowed conduction velocity, and inability to transmit rapidly repetitive impulses resulting from increased refractoriness. There is little doubt that bioelectrical dysfunctions are associated with the location and severity of the induced demyelinated areas. On the other hand, the possible involvement of the axons themselves may also contribute to the functional deficit. In many of these studies, particularly with the higher concentrations of diphtheria toxin, obvious damage to axis cylinders can be seen by light microscopy. One must wonder whether less obvious alterations in the integrity of the axon might not occur in many instances of experimentally induced primary demyelination. Axons may also be damaged in the vicinity of areas where cell-mediated immune reactions are occurring, as shown by axonal degeneration and segmental demyelination evolving in parallel in EAN-affected guinea pigs (118). Another aspect of the experimentally induced demyelinations and their relationship to bioelectrical functions is the reported recovery of function despite persistent demyelination. Thus in a lesion produced by repeated withdrawal and injection of CSF, Mayer (119) noted that "conduction velocities in the dorsal columns remained reduced 8 to 24 weeks after production of the lesion, but after 32 weeks the velocities recorded in six animals with persistent myelin changes were within normal limits."

Physiological studies and observations of patients with MS are contributing to the information that may be relevant to the laboratory data and, in some instances, assist in the diagnosis and evaluation of the disease process (73,75). For example, significant optic nerve dysfunction has been detected by visual evolved responses (VERs) in patients whose clinical signs and symptoms indicated only spinal cord involvement. Moreover, during the acute phase of optic neuritis, when vision is markedly affected or totally lost, VERs may be blocked (74). During clinical recovery, the block clears but delayed conduction remains. If, as is suggested, the slowed conduction velocity is due to demyelination, which also persists, one must then wonder what other factors were involved to produce total block. The well-known transient increase in disability that MS patients experience when they are exposed to stressful situations (e.g., raised body temperature) have been documented by objective studies such as critical fusion frequency (CFF) (122). These data not only demonstrate variations of neurological function in the presence of constant structural lesions but also reemphasize the fact that apparently normal function at the clinical level is possible in spite of probable histopathological involvement of the brain or spinal cord.

A number of studies of acute EAE-affected animals confirm the fact that pathological lesions may be present in the CNS in animals that show no overt evidence of disease. The following examples are pertinent in this regard: The largest available series (8) examined the clinical and pathological involvement of 439 guinea pigs injected with a "fully effective" and 413 with a "less effective" challenge. In the former group 42 (10%) and in the latter 98 (24%) animals were found to have pathological lesions in the absence of clinical involvement. In chronic EAE (144) in strain 13 guinea pigs, inflammatory changes and demyelination may be present 3–4 weeks

postinoculation, when the animals are still clinically normal.

Most guinea pigs affected by the chronic, relapsing form of EAE (198) show perivascular cuffs of hematogenous cells and demyelination if examined during the acute stage of the disease. However, some that died during the acute phase of EAE, having had severe paraparesis, displayed minimal if any morphological changes. Animals sacrificed during complete clinical remission showed large stretches of demyelination (198). During the relapse stage, however, both old and recent demyelinating plaques were present. Thus as in MS, the clinical involvement clears but the structural lesions remain. Finally, suppression of acute EAE with MBP may abort or prevent the onset of paraparesis, sphincter problems, weight loss, etc. in guinea pigs, but examinations of the CNS some weeks to months later may still show lesions (143). Thus adult guinea pigs suppressed with MBP in incomplete adjuvant from the 2nd DPI with whole CNS tissue in CFA developed no clinical signs and showed a few inflammatory cells in the meninges not associated with demyelination. Animals suppressed from the 7th or 10th DPI may have shown some early neurological signs (weight loss and slight weakness) from which they rapidly recovered, yet, when sacrificed at 14–21 DPI, had lesions indistinguishable from the acute EAE lesions seen in unsuppressed animals. Animals suppressed for more than 14 days had fewer inflammatory lesions, resembling the early stages of chronic EAE (138,144). Juvenile strain 13 guinea pigs inoculated for chronic EAE and suppressed from the 11th to the 38th DPI, failed to develop clinical signs over a 28-week period of study, yet displayed lesions identical to those seen during the latent period of nonsuppressed animals. These consisted of subpial demyelination and remyelination as well as chronic inflammation, but no acute inflammatory changes. Similarly, LNCs from Lewis rats rendered unresponsive to EAE by pretreatment with MBP markedly suppressed clinical but not histological EAE in normal recipients later challenged with an encephalitogenic emulsion (184). One must conclude, therefore, that many EAE-challenged animals, regardless of suppression, may show significant involvement (determined by histological examinations of their brains and spinal cords), but no clinical evidence of neurological involvement.

On the other hand, Wiśniewski and Keith's (198) observation of symptoms without lesions in EAE-affected animals, as mentioned above, has been reported in many previous studies. As early as 1934 Schwentker and Rivers (158) reported that some of their paralyzed EAE rabbits showed no pathological changes. A number of other reliable investigators noted symptoms in animals challenged with CNS tissue, oligodendroglia, MBP, or peptides with no evidence of histological involvement (95,143,152,161). Even in the published data of those who argue against the possibility that neurological signs can occur in EAE in the absence of inflammatory lesions in the CNS (104), there is ample evidence to the contrary. In the large series of guinea pigs already cited for instances of lesions without symptoms (8), 16 of the 439 (4%) guinea pigs injected with "fully effective" and 31 of 413 (8%) with "less effective" injections had symptoms but no lesions. In a companion publication designed to examine the early lesions in EAE (9), the earliest signs of leg weakness were found in "7 guinea pigs that had no histologic lesions." In the latest report by this group on the subject (104), the earlier findings are dismissed as unacceptable as "incontrovertible evidence of CNS damage." Yet in this latest study, 4 out of 30 guinea pigs were "considered weak or slow but had no lesions," whereas another animal had no clinical signs in the presence of histological involvement.

A direct correlation between observed areas of histological involvement and physiological evaluation of their functional capacities is an almost insurmountable technical problem in EAE. Yet attempts have been made (110); somatosensory evoked responses may be attenuated at low frequencies of stimulation, but there was no evident correlation between the severity of the electrophysiological effects and the histological lesions. Moreover, it is pertinent to the previous discussion to note that these investigators found that "positive electrophysiological alterations of EAE appear before the onset of familiar histological 'lesions,' that they are maximal before the histological infiltrates are maximal, and that they appear

to subside before they do." On the other hand, the tissue culture model is easily available for continuous monitoring of its histological appearance and, by extension, of its ultrastructural characteristics at any chosen instant while being exposed to experimental (e.g., immunological) manipulations of its environment. Thus it was useful not only for direct comparisons of structural responses to cell and serum factors in EAE and MS as outlined above, but also for evaluating bioelectrical functions under similar conditions. The first studies of the effects of EAE and MS sera on the functioning of cultured CNS tissue (25) showed a marked and frequently total block of both propagation and transmission of the nervous impulse by a complement-dependent factor. In these early studies as well as the confirmatory findings in a frog spinal cord preparation (42, 109), normal control sera did not produce similar blocking actions, a fact that has been challenged in more recent studies (see below). In early studies (25) describing the blocking of bioelectric functions, the phrase "polysynaptic activity" was used. This term was meant to describe the fact that multineuronal interrelationships were affected. The choice of words was unfortunate, however, since it has been interpreted to mean that the blocking effect was thought to occur at the synapse. Although this is one possible site of action of the immunological or other factors, this meaning was not intended, and we recognize that neuronal function may be affected by an immunological attack anywhere along the axon, at its termination, or for that matter on surrounding neuroglia. Actually, changes in the content and the uptake of GABA in the lumbar cord of guinea pigs during EAE can be detected before the onset of motor dysfunction (72), suggesting a possible involvement of synapses.

Since the first description of the blocking effect, similar actions have been found in many sera from apparently normal laboratory animals (45,160). Seil et al. (160) did not distinguish the active factors as either complement-dependent or heat-labile and, moreover, used considerably higher concentrations of sera. In examining these other parameters, Crain et al. (45) still find blocking activity in EAE and normal rabbit sera, but suggest that the former are less heat-labile and active at relatively low concentrations (5–10%) whereas the normal sera require concentrations higher than 10% to be effective. Further experiments are in progress in attempts to determine the significance of the blocking factors in normal sera and the specificity of factors in EAE and MS.

In reference to the possible relationship between neuronal blocking effects and structural alterations produced by exposure to antisera, the data from the culture system tends to deny a significant correlation between the bioelectrical parameters tested (which admittedly do not include conduction velocities) and the histological lesions (26). In the first place, the functional block may occur within minutes after exposure to the serum, hours before any effective demyelination can be demonstrated. Second, a totally demyelinated culture washed free of antiserum and returned to normal nutrient medium is normally responsive to electrical stimuli within a day, whereas remyelination may not begin before another 3 days or more. Finally, totally demyelinated and sclerosed cultures, which are incapable of remyelination, may return to apparently normal (bioelectric) activity when they are eventually removed from the influence of the antiserum.

Lumsden et al. (111) recently reported that only myelinated cultures are capable of responding to the blocking action of EAE, and therefore that the effect must result in some way from the demyelinating activity. We (Bornstein and Crain, *unpublished observations*) have been unable to confirm this result in three *in vitro* systems (nonmyelinated versus myelinated cerebellum, normally myelinated spinal cord versus that in which myelinogenesis had been inhibited, and hippocampus that had not yet myelinated). All cultures, regardless of whether myelin was present, displayed neuroelectric blocking effects when exposed to EAE sera in the presence of complement.

Considering all these data, one must voice serious doubts that neurological dysfunction is solely dependent on structural alterations in the demyelinative disorders. Whether perivascular infiltrates are present may in fact be irrelevant. The significant question must be concerned with the means by which immunological factors, whether produced *in situ* or at a distance, directly and indirectly affect

axonal functions. Moreover, in MS and chronic EAE one could consider that there are essentially two kinds of neuronal dysfunction: (a) the temporary, transient, or changeable; and (b) the permanent. It is possible that different mechanisms may contribute to the total manifest dysfunction at any particular moment.

Treatment of Multiple Sclerosis

The increasing weight of evidence that MS may involve an immunopathogenetic mechanism has led to a number of attempts to treat patients by techniques that alter immunological responsiveness. Consequently, four types of therapeutic agents have been proposed and are being examined: steroids and/or ACTH; immunosuppressive drugs; transfer factor; and MBP, or synthetic peptide copolymers. A historical review as well as other aspects of therapeutic attempts (e.g., anti-infectious agents and dietary regimens, immunosuppressant drugs, and transfer factor) were recently published by Liversedge (106).

He reports the application of ACTH or steroids, which by now have been widely examined. In general, these applications have led to the opinion that a brief course of these drugs may decrease the severity and duration of an acute exacerbation but that their long-term use does not decrease the frequency or severity of attacks. Moreover, their chronic use is more likely to produce undesirable side reactions.

The immunosuppressive drugs have been receiving more attention recently in attempts at treating acute exacerbations even though some brief clinical trials appeared to be unpromising (50,169). However, feasibility trials of intense immunosuppression (as in the combination of azothiaprine, prednisone, and antilymphocyte globulin) appeared to produce some favorable results in exacerbating and remitting forms of MS (100), and immunosuppression is currently being submitted to a blinded clinical trial. Ring et al. (149) also reported the use of massive immunosuppressant therapy in attempts to treat exacerbating forms of MS.

The use of dialyzable transfer factor from human blood leukocytes is based on the assumption that MS patients may possess a deficient immune system incapable of overcoming a persistent slow virus (measles) infection. By supplying the factors, the patients would presumably be rendered capable of eliminating the infection and therefore the MS. However, reports of the results to date have not demonstrated any significant favorable effect of transfer factor in the course of MS (18,66,82,207).

The most promising avenue of approach to the treatment of MS has developed from the use of MBP, its fragments, or synthetic peptide polymers to suppress the course of EAE in experimental animals (20,51,53,57,162,183). Some of this work was presented in previous sections. A preliminary application (39) of MBP to MS patients apparently had no unfavorable effects, although in view of present plans for a blinded clinical trial (Eylar, *personal communication*) the dosage used may not have been sufficient to produce favorable results. The clinical application of synthetic polypeptide was recently reported (1) following a series of laboratory studies on small laboratory animals and nonhuman primates (186–188). The results in this preliminary application of copolymer I in physiological saline to four patients with MS and three with acute disseminated encephalomyelitis show considerable promise. One can expect that a number of controlled clinical trials will soon be implemented for the critical evaluation of MBP and the synthetic copolymers in the definitive treatment of MS.

ACKNOWLEDGMENT

Research on the demyelinative disorders in the author's laboratory is currently supported by grant NS 11920 from the NINCDS and a grant from the Sloan Foundation.

REFERENCES

1. Abramsky, O., Teitelbaum, D., and Arnon, R. (1977): Effect of synthetic polypeptide (COP I) on patients with multiple sclerosis and with acute disseminated encephalomyelitis: A preliminary report. *J. Neurol. Sci.,* 31:433–438.
2. Adams, C. W. M. (1967): The histochemistry of proteolytic enzymes and lipoproteins in the normal and diseased nervous system. In: *Macromolecules and the Function of the Neuron,* edited by Z. Lodin and S. P. R. Rose, p. 111. Excerpta Medica, Amsterdam.
3. Adams, C. W. M., (editor) (1972): *Research on Multiple Sclerosis,* pp. 35–41, 80–90, 96–110. Charles C Thomas, Springfield, Ill.
4. Adams, C. W. M. (1977): Pathology of multiple sclerosis. *Br. Med. Bull.,* 33:15–20.
5. Adams, J. W., and Imagawa, D. T. (1962): Measles antibodies in multiple sclerosis. *Proc. Soc. Exp. Biol. Med.,* 111:562–566.
6. Adams, R. D. (1959): A comparison of the morphology of the human demyelinative diseases and experimental "allergic" encephalomyelitis. In: *"Allergic" Encephalomyelitis,* edited by M. W. Kies and E. C. Alvord, Jr., pp. 183. Charles C Thomas, Springfield, Ill.
7. Adams, R. D., and Sidman, R. L. (1968): *Introduction to Neuropathology.* McGraw-Hill, New York.
8. Alvord, E. C., Jr., and Kies, M. W. (1959): Clinico-pathologic correlations in experimental allergic encephalomyelitis. II. Development of an index for quantitative assay of encephalitogenic activity. *J. Neuropathol. Exp. Neurol.,* 18:447–457.
9. Alvord, E. C., Jr., Magee, K. R., Kies, M. W., and Goldstein, N. P. (1959): Clinico-pathologic correlations in experimental "allergic" encephalomyelitis. I. Observations in the early lesion. *J. Neuropathol. Exp. Neurol.,* 18:442–446.
10. Alvord, E. C., Jr., Shaw, C-M., Hruby, S., Peterson, R., and Harvey, F. H. (1975): In: *The Nervous System, Vol. I: The Basic Neurosciences,* edited by D. B. Tower, pp. 647–653. Raven Press, New York.
11. Appel, S. H., and Bornstein, M. B. (1964): The application of tissue culture to the study of experimental allergic encephalomyelitis. II. Serum factors responsible for demyelination. *J. Exp. Med.,* 119:303–312.
12. Arnason, B. G. W., Winkler, G. F., and Hadler, N. M. (1969): Cell-mediated demyelination of peripheral nerve in tissue culture. *Lab. Invest.,* 21:1–10.
13. Aström, K. E., and Waksman, B. H. (1962): The passive transfer of experimental allergic encephalomyelitis and neuritis with living lymphoid cells. *J. Pathol.,* 83:89–106.
14. Barlow, C. F. (1956): A study of abnormal blood-brain permeability in experimental allergic encephalomyelitis. *J. Neuropathol. Exp. Neurol.,* 15:196–207.
15. Bartfeld, H., and Atoynatan, T. (1970): In vitro delayed (cellular) hypersensitivity in multiple sclerosis to central nervous system antigens. *Int. Arch. Allergy Appl. Immunol.,* 39:361–367.
16. Batchelor, J. R. (1977): Histocompatability antigens and their relevance to multiple sclerosis. *Br. Med. Bull.,* 33:72–77.
17. Behan, P. O., Behan, W. M. H., Feldman, R. G., and Kies, M. W. (1972): Cell-mediated hypersensitivity to neural antigens: Occurrence in human patients and non hu-

man primates with neurological diseases. *Arch. Neurol.,* 27:145–152.

18. Behan, P. O., Melville, I. D., Durward, W. F., McGeorge, A. P., and Behan, W. M. F. (1976): Transfer-factor therapy in multiple sclerosis. *Lancet,* 1:988–990.

19. Bergstrand, H. (1972): *Studies on the Localization of Antigenic Determinants for Cell-Mediated Immunity on Bovine Encephalitogenic Protein,* pp. 5–71. Institute of Biochemistry and the Turnblad Institute, University of Lund, Sweden.

20. Bernard, C. A., Mackay, I. R., Whittingham, S., and Brous, P. (1976): Durability of immune protection against experimental autoimmune encephalomyelitis. *Cell. Immunol.,* 22:297–310.

21. Bornstein, M. B. (1963): A tissue culture approach to the demyelination disorders. *Natl. Cancer Inst. Monogr.,* 11:197–214.

22. Bornstein, M. B. (1963): Phagocytic activities of cultured neuroglia. *J. Neuropathol. Exp. Neurol.,* 22:253.

23. Bornstein, M. B. (1973): The immunopathology of demyelinative disorders examined in organotypic cultures of mammalian central nerve tissues. In: *Progress in Neuropathology,* Vol. II, edited by H. Zimmerman, pp. 69–90. Grune & Stratton, N.Y.

24. Bornstein, M. B., and Appel, S. H. (1961): The application of tissue culture to the study of experimental "allergic" encephalomyelitis. I. Patterns of demyelination. *J. Neuropathol. Exp. Neurol.,* 20:141–157.

25. Bornstein, M. B., and Crain, S. M. (1965): Functional studies of cultured mammalian CNS tissues as related to "demyelination disorders." *Science,* 148:1242–1244.

26. Bornstein, M. B., and Crain, S. M. (1965) *Structural and Functional Studies of Cultured Mammalian CNS Tissues as Related to Demyelinative Disorders,* pp. 253–256. International Congress Series 100. Excerpta Medica, Amsterdam.

27. Bornstein, M. B., and Hummelgard, A. (1976): Multiple sclerosis: serum-induced demyelination in tissue culture. In: *The Aetiology and Pathogenesis of the Demyelinating Diseases,* edited by H. Shiraki, T. Yonezawa, and Y. Kuroiwa, pp. 341–350. Japan Science Press, Tokyo.

28. Bornstein, M. B., and Iwanami, H. (1971): Demyelinating activity of serum and sensitized lymph node cells on cultured nerve tissue. *J. Neuropathol. Exp. Neurol.,* 30:240–248.

29. Bornstein, M. B., and Raine, C. S. (1970): Experimental allergic encephalomyelitis: Antiserum inhibition of myelination in vitro. *Lab. Invest.,* 25:536–542.

30. Bornstein, M. B., and Raine, C. S. (1976): Central nervous system. In: *Textbook of Immunopathology,* edited by P. A.

Miescherand and H. J. Muller-Eberhard, pp. 701–714. Grune & Stratton, New York.

31. Bornstein, M. B., and Raine, C. S. (1976): The initial structural lesion in serum-induced demyelination in vitro. *Lab. Invest.,* 35:391–401.

32. Bornstein, M. B., and Raine, C. S. (1977): Multiple sclerosis and experimental allergic encephalomyelitis: Specific demyelination of CNS in culture. *Neuropathol. Appl. Neurobiol.,* 36:594.

33. Brandt, R., Gutt, H., and Muller, R. (1926): Zur frage der Organspezifität Von Lipoidantikörpen. *Klin. Wochenschr.,* 5:655.

34. Brosnan, C. F., Stoner, G. L., Bloom, B. R., and Wiśniewsky, H. M. (1977): Study on demyelination by activated lymphocytes in the rabbit eye. II. Antibody-dependent cell-mediated demyelination. *J. Immunol.* 118:2103–2110.

35. Brostoff, S. W. (1977): Immunological responses to myelin and myelin components. In: *Myelin,* edited by P. Morell, pp. 415–446. Plenum, New York.

36. Brostoff, S. W., and Powers, J. M. (1975): Allergic encephalomyelitis: Modification of the response by synthetic membrane structures containing bovine myelin basic protein and cerebroside. *Brain Res.,* 93:175–181.

37. Bubis, J. J., and Luse, S. A. (1964): An electron microscopic study of experimental allergic encephalomyelitis in the rat. *Am. J. Pathol.,* 44:299–317.

38. Bunge, M. B., Bunge, R. P., and Ris, H. (1961): Ultrastructural study of remyelination in an experimental lesion in adult cat spinal cord. *J. Biophys. Biochem. Cytol.,* 10:67–94.

39. Campbell, B. Vogel, P. J., Fisher, E., and Lorenz, R. (1973): Myelin basic protein administration in multiple sclerosis. *Arch. Neurol.,* 29:10–15.

40. Carnegie, P. R. (1971): Amino acid sequence of the encephalitogenic basic protein from human myelin. *Biochem. J.,* 123:57–67.

41. Caspary, E. A. (1977): Humoral factors involved in immune processes in multiple sclerosis and allergic encephalomyelitis. *Br. Med. J.,* 33:50–53.

42. Cerf, J. A., and Carels, G. (1966): Multiple sclerosis: Serum factor producing reversible alterations in bioelectric responses. *Science,* 152:1066–1068.

43. Chao, L-P., and Einstein, E. R. (1970): Physical properties of the bovine encephalitogenic protein: Molecular weight and conformation. *J. Neurochem.,* 17:1121–1131.

44. Charcot, J. M. (1879): *Lectures on the Diseases of the Nervous System.* Translated from the second edition by G. Sigerson. Lea, Philadelphia.

45. Crain, S. M., Bornstein, M. B., and Lennon, V. A. (1975): Depression of complex bio-

electric discharges in cerebral tissue cultures by thermolabile complement-dependent serum factors. *Exp. Neurol.*, 49:330–335.

46. Cutler, R. W. P., and Barlow, C. F. (1967): Alterations in brain vascular permeability in allergic encephalomyelitis. *J. Neuropathol. Exp. Neurol.*, 26:558–571.

47. Cuzner, M. L., Barnard, R. O., and MacGregor, B. J. L. (1976): Myelin composition in acute and chronic MS in relation to cerebral lysosomal activity. *J. Neurol. Sci.*, 29:323–334.

48. David, J. R., and Paterson, P. Y. (1965): In vitro demonstration of cellular sensitivity in allergic encephalomyelitis. *J. Exp. Med.*, 122:1161–1171.

49. Davison, A. N., and Cuzner, M. L. (1977) Immunochemistry and biochemistry of myelin. *Br. Med. Bull.*, 33:60–66.

50. Drachman, D. A., Paterson, P. Y., Schmidt, R. T., and Spehlman, R. F. (1975): Cyclophosphamide in exacerbations of multiple sclerosis: Therapeutic trial and a strategy for pilot studies. *J. Neurol. Neurosurg. Psychiatry*, 38:592–597.

51. Driscoll, B. F., Kies, M. W., and Alvord, E. C., Jr. (1975): Adoptive transfer of experimental allergic encephalomyelitis: Prevention of successful transfer by treatment of donors with myelin basic protein. *J. Immunol.*, 114:291–292.

52. Dubois-Dalcq, M., Niedieck, B., and Buyse, M. (1970): Action of anti-cerebroside sera on myelinated nervous tissue cultures: Demyelination of cerebellum cultures. *Pathol. Eur.*, 5:331–347.

53. Einstein, E. R., Chao, L. P., and Czejtey, J. (1972): Suppression of experimental allergic encephalomyelitis by chemically modified encephalitogens. *Immunochemistry*, 9:1013–1019.

54. Eylar, E. H. (1970): Amino acid sequence of the basic protein of the myelin membrane. *Proc. Natl. Acad. Sci. USA*, 67:1425–1431.

55. Eylar, E. H., Brostoff, S., Jaclson, J., and Carter, H. (1972): Allergic encephalomyelitis in monkeys induced by a peitide from the A_1 protein. *Proc. Natl. Acad. Sci. USA*, 69:617–619.

56. Eylar, E. H., and Hashim, G. A. (1968): Allergic encephalomyelitis: The structure of the encephalitogenic determinant. *Proc. Natl. Acad. Sci. USA*, 61:644–650.

57. Eylar, E. H., Jackson, J., Rothenberg, B., and Brostoff, S. W. (1972): Suppression of the immune response: Reversal of the disease state with antigen in allergic encephalomyelitis. *Nature (Lond)*, 236:74–76.

58. Eylar, E. H., Salk, J., Beveridge, G. C., and Brown, L. V. (1969): Experimental allergic encephalomyelitis: An encephalitogenic basic protein from bovine myelin. *Arch. Biochem.*, 132:34–48.

59. Eylar, E. H., Westall, F. C., and Brostoff, S. (1971): Allergic encephalomyelitis: An encephalitogenic peptide derived from the basic protein of myelin. *J. Biol. Chem.*, 246:3418–3424.

60. Falk, G. A., Kies, M. W., and Alvord, E. C., Jr. (1968): Delayed hypersensitivity to myelin basic protein in the passive transfer of experimental allergic encephalomyelitis. *J. Immunol.*, 101:638–644.

61. Feigin, I., and Ogata, J. (1971): Schwann cells and peripheral myelin within human central nervous tissues: The mesenchymal character of Schwann cells. *J. Neuropathol. Exp. Neurol.*, 30:603–612.

62. Feingin, I., and Popoff, N. (1966): Regeneration of myelin in multiple sclerosis: The role of mesenchymal cells in such regeneration and in myelin formation in the peripheral nervous system. *Neurology (Minneap)*, 16:364–372.

63. Ferraro, A., and Jervis, G. A. (1940): Experimental disseminated encephalopathy in the monkey. *Arch. Neurol. Psychiatry*, 43:195–209.

64. Field, E. J., and Hughes, P. (1965): Toxicity of motor neurone disease serum for myelin in tissue culture. *Br. Med. J.*, 2:1399–1401.

65. Fog, T., (editor) (1977): The international symposium on the histocompatibility system in multiple sclerosis, Copenhagen, 1975. *Acta Neurol. Scand. [Suppl. 63]*, 55.

66. Fog, T., Jersild, C., Dupont, B., Platz, P. J., Svejgaard, A., Thomsen, M., Midholm, S., Raun, N. E., and Grob, P. (1975): Transfer factor treatment in multiple sclerosis. *Neurology (Minneap)*, 25:489–490.

67. Freund, J., Stern, E. R., and Pisani, T. M. (1947): Isoallergic encephalomyelitis and radiculitis in guinea pigs after one injection of brain and mycobacteria in water-in-oil emulsion. *J. Immunol.*, 57:179–194.

68. Fry, J. M., Lehrer, G. M., and Bornstein, M. B. (1972): Sulfatide synthesis: Inhibition by experimental allergic encephalomyelitis serum. *Science*, 175:192–194.

69. Fry, J. M., Lehrer, G. M., and Bornstein, M. B. (1973): Experimental inhibition of myelination in spinal cord tissue cultures: Enzyme assays. *J. Neurobiol.*, 4:453–459.

70. Fry, J. M., Weissbarth, S., Lehrer, G. M., and Bornstein, M. B. (1974): Cerebroside antibody inhibits sulfatide synthesis and myelination and demyelinates in cord tissue culture. *Science*, 183:540–542.

71. Gonatas, N. K., Gonatas, J. O., Stieber, A., Lisak, R., Suzuki, K., and Martinson, R. E. (1974): The significance of circulating and cell-bound antibodies in experimental allergic encephalomyelitis. *Am. J. Pathol.*, 76:529–544.

72. Gottesfield, H., Teitelbaum, D., Webb, C., and Arnon, R. (1976): Changes in the GABA system in experimental allergic en-

cephalomyelitis-induced paralysis. *J. Neurochem.*, 27:695–699.

73. Halliday, A. M., and McDonald, W. I. (1977): Pathophysiology of demyelinating disease. *Br. Med. Bull.*, 33:21–27.

74. Halliday, A. M., McDonald, W. I., and Mushin, J. (1972): Delayed visual evoked responses in optic neuritis. *Lancet,* 1:982–985.

75. Halliday, A. M., McDonald, W. I., and Mushin, J. (1973): The visual evoked response in the diagnosis of multiple sclerosis. *Br. Med. J.,* 4:661–664.

76. Hashim, G. A. (1977): Experimental allergic encephalomyelitis in Lewis rats: Chemical synthesis of disease-inducing determinants. *Science,* 196:1219–1221.

77. Hoffman, P. M., Gaston, D. D., and Spitter, L. E. (1973): Comparison of experimental allergic encephalomyelitis induced with spinal cord, basic protein and synthetic encephalitogenic peptide. *Clin. Immunol. Immunopathol.,* 1:364–371.

78. Hruby, S., Alvord, E. C., Jr., and Seil, F. (1977): Synthetic galactocerebrosides evoke myelination-inhibiting antibodies. *Science,* 195:173–175.

79. Hughes, D., and Field, E. J. (1967): Myelotoxicity of serum and spinal fluid in multiple sclerosis: A critical assessment. *Clin. Exp. Immunol.,* 2:95–309.

80. Jankovic, D., Draskoci, M., and Janjic, M. (1965): Passive transfer of "allergic" encephalomyelitis with antibrain serum injected into the lateral ventricle of the brain. *Nature (Lond),* 207:428–429.

81. Jersild, C., Dupont, B., Fog, T., Platz, P. J., and Svejgaard, A. (1975): Histocompatibility determinants in multiple sclerosis. *Transplant. Rev.,* 22:148–163.

82. Jersild, C., Platz, P., Thomsen, M., Dupont, B., Svejgaard, A., Ciongoli, A. K., Fog, T., and Grob, P. (1976): Transfer factor treatment of patients with multiple sclerosis. I. Preliminary report of changes in immunological parameters. *Scand. J. Immunol.,* 5:141–148.

83. Johnson, A. B., and Blum, N. R. (1972): Peroxidase-labelled antigens in light and electron immunohistochemistry and their utilization in studies of experimental allergic encephalomyelitis. *J. Histochem. Cytochem.,* 20:841.

84. Johnson, A. B., Blum, N. R., and Bornstein, M. B. (1977): Immunoperoxidase studies on allergic encephalomyelitis and multiple sclerosis in tissue culture. *J. Neuropathol. Exp. Neurol. (in press).*

85. Johnson, A. B., and Dal Canto, M. C. (1976): Multiple sclerosis, Guillain-Barré syndrome and myelin basic protein-specific cellular antibody. *Nature (Lond),* 264:453–454.

86. Johnson, A. B., Wiśniewski, H. M., Raine, C. S., Eylar, E. H., and Terry, R. D. (1971): Specific binding of peroxidase labelled myelin basic protein in allergic encephalomyelitis. *Proc. Natl. Acad. Sci. USA,* 68:2694–2698.

87. Kabat, E. A., Wolf, A., and Bezer, H. (1947): The rapid production of acute disseminated encephalomyelitis in rhesus monkeys by injection of heterologous and homologous brain tissue with adjuvants. *J. Exp. Med.,* 85:117–130.

88. Kabat, E. A., Wolf, A., and Bezer, H. (1949): Studies on acute disseminated encephalomyelitis produced experimentally in rhesus monkeys. IV. Disseminated encephalomyelitis produced in monkeys with their own brain tissue. *J. Exp. Med.,* 89:395–398.

89. Kibler, F. R., Shapira, R., McKneally, S., Jenkins, J., Selden, P., and Chou, F. (1969): Encephalitogenic protein structure. *Science,* 164:577–580.

90. Kies, M. W. (1975): Immunology of myelin basic proteins. In: *The Nervous System, Vol. 1: The Basic Neurosciences* edited by D. B. Tower, pp. 637–646. Raven Press, New York.

91. Kies, M. W., and Alvord, E. C., Jr., editors (1959): *"Allergic" Encephalomyelitis.* Charles C Thomas, Springfield, Ill.

92. Kies, M. W., Alvord, E. C., Jr., and Robuz, E. (1958): Production of experimental allergic encephalomyelitis in guinea pigs with fractions isolated from bovine spinal cord and killed tubercle bacilli. *Nature (Lond),* 182:104–106.

93. Kies, M. W., Driscoll, B. F., Lisak, R. P., and Alvord, E. C., Jr. (1975): Immunologic activity of myelin basic protein in strain 2 and strain 13 guinea pigs. *J. Immunol.,* 115:75–79.

94. Knight, S. C. (1977): Cellular immunity in multiple sclerosis: Role of nervous tissue antigens. *Br. Med. Bull.,* 33:45–49.

95. Kopeloff, L. M., and Kopeloff, N. (1947): Neurologic manifestations in laboratory animals produced by organ (adjuvant) emulsions. *J. Immunol.,* 57:229–237.

96. Kristensson, K., and Wisniewski, H. M. (1976): Chronic relapsing experimental allergic encephalomyelitis—studies in vascular permeability. *Acta Neuropathol. (Berl)* 36:307–314.

97. Kurtzke, J. F. (1976): An overview of the epidemiology of multiple sclerosis. In: *The Etiology and Pathogenesis of the Demyelinating Diseases,* edited by H. Shiraki, T. Yonezawa, and Y. Kuroiwa, pp. 59–94. Japan Science Press, Tokyo.

98. Lampert, P. W. (1965): Demyelination and remyelination in experimental allergic encephalomyelitis: Further electric microscopic observations. *J. Neuropathol. Exp. Neurol.,* 24:371–385.

99. Lampert, P. (1967): Electron microscopic studies on ordinary and hyperacute experi-

mental allergic encephalomyelitis. *Acta Neuropathol. (Berl)*, 9:99–126.

100. Lance, E. M., Kremer, M., Abbosh, J., Jones, V. E., Knight, S., and Medawar, P. B. (1975): Intensive immunosuppression in patients with disseminated sclerosis. I. Clinical response. *Clin. Exp. Immunol.*, 21:1–12.

101. Latovitzky, N., and Silberberg, D. H. (1975): Ceramide glycosyltransferases in cultured rat cerebellum; changes with age with demyelination and with inhibition of myelination by 5-bromo-2'-deoxyuridine or experimental allergic encephalomyelitis serum. *J. Neurochem.*, 24:1017–1021.

102. Lebar, R., Boutry, J-M., Vincent, C., Robineaux, R., and Voisin, G. A. (1976): Studies on autoimmune encephalomyelitis in the guinea pig. II. An in vitro investigation on the nature, properties and specificity of the serum-demyelinating factor. *J. Immunol.*, 116:1439–1446.

103. Leibowitz, S. (1969): Cerebral vascular permeability in experimental allergic encephalomyelitis. *Neuropat. Pol.*, 7:303–309.

104. Levine, S., Sowinski, R., Shaw, C-M., and Alvord, E. C., Jr. (1975): Do neurological signs occur in experimental allergic encephalomyelitis in the absence of inflammatory lesions of the central nervous system? *J. Neuropathol. Exp. Neurol.*, 34:501–506.

105. Lisak, R. P., Behan, P. O., Zweiman, B., and Shetty, T. (1974): Cell-mediated immunity to myelin basic protein in acute disseminated encephalomyelitis. *Neurology (Minneap)*, 24:560–564.

106. Liversedge, L. A. (1977): Treatment and management of multiple sclerosis. *Br. Med. Bull.*, 33:78–83.

107. Lumsden, C. E. (1965): The clinical pathology of multiple sclerosis. In: *Multiple Sclerosis: A Re-appraisal*, edited by D. McAlpine, C. E. Lumsden, and E. D. Acheson, p. 376. Livingstone, Edinburgh.

108. Lumsden, C. E. (1971): The immunogenesis of the multiple sclerosis plaque. *Brain Res.*, 28:365–396.

109. Lumsden, C. E. (1972): The clinical immunology of multiple sclerosis. In: *Multiple Sclerosis*, edited by D. McAlpine, C. E. Lumsden, and E. D. Acheson, pp. 309–621. Churchill Livingstone, London.

110. Lumsden, C. E., Howard, L., and Aparicio, S. R. (1975): Antisynaptic antibody in allergic encephalomyelitis: Neurophysiological studies in guinea pigs on the exposed cerebral cortex and peripheral nerves following immunological challenges with myelin and synaptosomes. *Brain Res.*, 93:267–282.

111. Lumsden, C. E., Howard, L., Aparicio, S. R., and Bradbury, B. (1975): Antisynaptic antibody in experimental allergic encephalomyelitis. II. The synapse-blocking effects in tissue culture of demyelinating sera from experi-

mental allergic encephalomyelitis. *Brain Res.*, 93:283–299.

112. Mackay, R. P., and Hirano, A. (1967): Forms of benign multiple sclerosis. *Arch. Neurol.*, 17:588–600.

113. McDonald, W. I. (1974): Pathophysiology in multiple sclerosis. *Brain*, 97:179–196.

114. McFarlin, D. E., Blank, S. E., and Kibler, R. F. (1974): Recurrent experimental allergic encephalomyelitis in the Lewis rat. *J. Immunol.*, 113:712–715.

115. McFarlin, D. E., Blank, S. E., Kibler, R. F., McKneally, S., and Shapira, R. (1973): Experimental allergic encephalomyelitis in the rat: Response to encephalitogenic proteins and peptides. *Science*, 179:478–480.

116. McFarlin, D. E., Hsu, C-L. S., Slementa, B., Chou, C-H. F., and Kibler, R. F. (1975): The immune response against myelin basic protein in the strains of rat with different genetic capacity to develop experimental allergic encephalomyelitis. *J. Exp. Med.*, 141:72–81.

117. McFarlin, D. E., and McFarlin, H. F. (1976): Histocompatibility studies and multiple sclerosis. *Arch. Neurol.*, 33:395–398.

118. Madrid, R. E., and Wisniewski, H. M. (1977): Axonal degeneration in demyelinating disorders. *J. Neurocytol.*, 6:103–117.

119. Mayer, R. F. (1971): Conduction velocity in the central nervous system of the cat during experimental demyelination and remyelination. *Int. J. Neurosci.*, 1:287–308.

120. Morgan, I. M. (1947): Allergic encephalomyelitis in monkeys in response to injection of normal monkey nervous tissue. *J. Exp. Med.*, 85:131–140.

121. Nagai, Y., Momoi, T., Saito, M., Mitsuzawa, E., and Ohtani, S. (1976): Ganglioside syndrome, a new autoimmune neurologic disorder experimentally induced with brain gangliosides. *Neurosci. Lett.*, 2:107–111.

122. Namerow, N. S. (1971): Temperature effect on critical flicker fusion in multiple sclerosis. *Arch. Neurol.*, 25:269–275.

123. Namerow, N. S., and Thompson, L. R. (1969): Plaques, symptoms and the remitting course of multiple sclerosis. *Neurology (Minneap)*, 19:765–774.

124. Niedieck, B. (1975): On a glycolipid hapten of myelin. *Prog. Allergy*, 18:353–422.

125. Norby, E., Link, H., and Olsson, J. E. (1974): Measles virus antibodies in multiple sclerosis: Comparison of antibody titers in cerebrospinal fluid and serum. *Arch. Neurol.*, 30:285–292.

126. Oldstone, M. B. A., and Dixon, F. J. (1968): Immunohistochemical study of allergic encephalomyelitis. *Am. J. Pathol.*, 52:251–257.

127. Ortiz-Ortiz, L., Nakamura, R. M., and Weigle, W. O. (1976): T cell requirement for experimental allergic encephalomyelitis induction in the rat. *J. Immunol.*, 117:576–579.

128. Ortiz-Ortiz, L., and Weigle, W. O. (1976): Cellular events in the induction of experimental allergic encephalomyelitis in rats. *J. Exp. Med.*, 144:604–616.

129. Paterson, P. Y. (1960): Transfer of allergic encephalomyelitis in rats by means of lymph node cells. *J. Exp. Med.*, 111:119–136.

130. Paterson, P. Y. (1966): Experimental allergic encephalomyelitis and autoimmune disease. *Adv. Immunol.*, 5:131–208.

131. Paterson, P. Y. (1977): Autoimmune neurologic disease: experimental animal systems and implications for multiple sclerosis. In: *Autoimmunity*, edited by N. Tolal. Academic Press, New York (*in press*).

132. Paterson, P. Y. (1977): Clinical, histopathologic, and immunovirologic aspects of experimental animal autoimmune disease models and neurologic disorders of man. In: *Introduction to Clinical Immunology*, edited by W. J. Irvine. Blackwell, Edinburgh (*in press*).

133. Paterson, P. Y. (1977): The demyelinating diseases: clinical and experimental studies in animals and man. In: *Immunological Diseases*, 3rd ed., edited by M. Samter, N. Alexander, B. Rose, W. B. Sherman, D. W. Talmadge, and J. H. Vaughn. Little Brown, Boston (*in press*).

134. Paterson, P. Y. (1977): Neurological diseases. In: *Introduction to Clinical Immunology*, edited by W. J. Irvine. Blackwell, Edinburgh (*in press*).

135. Pette, E., and Bauer, H., editors (1964): Experimental contributions to the pathogenesis of the demyelinating encephalomyelitides. *Z. Immunitaetsforsch.*, 126:1–248.

136. Porterfield, J. S. (1977): Multiple sclerosis. *Br. Med. Bull.*, 33.

137. Prineas, J. (1975): Pathology of the early lesion in multiple sclerosis. *Hum. Pathol.*, 6:531–554.

138. Prineas, J., Raine, C. S., and Wisniewski, H. (1969): An ultrastructural study of experimental demyelination and remyelination. III. Chronic and experimental allergic encephalomyelitis in the central nervous system. *Lab. Invest.*, 21:472–483.

139. Propp, R. P., Means, E., Deibel, R., Sherer, G., and Barron, K. (1975): Waldenstraum's macroglobulinemia and neuropathy. *Neurology (Minneap)*, 25:980–988.

140. Raine, C. S. (1976): On the development of lesions in natural canine distemper. *J. Neurol. Sci.*, 30:13–28.

141. Raine, C. S., and Bornstein, M. B. (1970): Experimental allergic encephalomyelitis: A light and electron microscope study of remyelination and "sclerosis" in vitro. *J. Neuropathol. Exp. Neurol.*, 29:552–574.

142. Raine, C. S., Hummelgard, A., Swanson, E., and Bornstein, M. B. (1973): Multiple sclerosis: serum-induced demyelination in vitro: A light and electron microscope study. *J. Neurol. Sci.*, 20:127–148.

143. Raine, C. S., Snyder, D. H., Stone, S. H., and Bornstein, M. B. (1977): Suppression of acute and chronic experimental allergic encephalomyelitis in strain 13 guinea pigs. *J. Neurol. Sci.*, 31:355–367.

144. Raine, C. S., Snyder, D. H., Valsamis, M. P., and Stone, S. H. (1974): Chronic experimental allergic encephalomyelitis in inbred guinea pigs. *Lab. Invest.*, 31:369–380.

145. Raine, C. S., Wiśniewski, H. M., and Dowling, P. C. (1971): An ultrastructural study of experimental demyelination and remyelination. IV. Recurrent episodes and peripheral nervous system plaque formation in experimental allergic encephalomyelitis. *Lab. Invest.*, 25:28–34.

146. Rauch, H. C., and Einstein, E. R. (1974): Specific brain proteins: a biochemical and immunological review. In: *Reviews of Neuroscience*, Vol. I, edited by S. Ehrenpreiss and I. Kopin, pp. 283–343. Raven Press, New York.

147. Rauch, H. C., Einstein, E. R., and Csejtey, J. (1973): Enzymatic degradation of myelin basic protein in central nervous system lesions of monkeys with experimental allergic encephalomyelitis. *Neurobiology*, 3:195–205.

148. Riekkinen, P. J., Rinne, U. K., Arstila, A. U., and Frey, A. (1970): Enzymic changes in the white matter of multiple sclerosis brains. In: *VIth International Congress of Neuropathology*, p. 490. Masson, Paris.

149. Ring, J., Lob, M., Augstwurum, M., Brass, B., Backmund, H., Seifert, J., Coulin, K., Frich, E., Mertin, J., and Brendel, W. (1974): Intense immunosuppression in the treatment of multiple sclerosis. *Lancet*, 2:1093–1099.

150. Rivers, T. M., and Schwentker, F. F. (1935): Encephalomyelitis accompanied by myelin destruction experimentally produced in monkeys. *J. Exp. Med.*, 61:689–702.

151. Rivers, T. M., Sprunt, D. H., and Berry, G. P. (1933): Observations on attempts to produce acute disseminated encephalomyelitis in monkeys. *J. Exp. Med.*, 58:39–53.

152. Robson, G. S. M., McPherson, T. A., and Mackay, I. R. (1971): A histological dose-response effect in guinea pigs injected with graded amounts of basic protein and peptides from human brain. *Br. J. Exp. Pathol.*, 52:338–344.

153. Rocklin, R. E., Sheramata, W. A., Feldman, R. G., Kies, M. W., and David, J. R. (1971): The Guillain-Barré syndrome and multiple sclerosis. *N. Engl. J. Med.*, 284:803–808.

154. Rogart, F. B., and Ritchie, J. M. (1977): Pathophysiology of conduction in demyelinated nerve fibers. In: *Myelin*, edited by P. Morell, pp. 353–382. Plenum Press, New York.

155. Rose, A. S. (1963): *Mechanisms of De-*

myelination, edited by A. S. Rose and C. M. Pearson, p. 215. McGraw-Hill, New York.

156. Salomon, R. M., Doyle, A., Sheppard, R., and Bornstein, M. B. (1977): Demyelinating activities of peripheral lymphocytes and serum from MS patients examined in tissue culture. *J. Neuropathol. Exp. Neurol.,* 36: 627.

157. Scheinberg, L. C., Kies, M. W., and Alvord, E. C., Jr., editors (1965): Research in demyelinating disease. *Ann. NY Acad. Sci.,* 122.

158. Schwentker, F. F., and Rivers, J. M. (1934): The antibody response of rabbits to injections of emulsions and extracts of homologous brain. *J. Exp. Med.,* 60:559–574.

159. Seil, F. J., Falk, C. A., Kies, M. W., and Alvord, E. C., Jr. (1968): The in vitro demyelinating activity of sera from guinea pigs sensitized with whole CNS and with purified encephalitogen. *Exp. Neurol.,* 22:545–555.

160. Seil, F. J., Smith, M. E., Leiman, A. L., and Kelly, J. M., III (1975): Myelination inhibition and neuroelectric blocking factors in experimental allergic encephalomyelitis. *Science,* 187:951–953.

161. Shapiro, R., Chou, C-H., McKneally, S., Urban, E., and Kibler, R. F. (1971): Biological activity and synthesis of an encephalitogenic determinant. *Science,* 173:736–738.

162. Shaw, C. M., Alvord, E. C., Jr., Fahlberg, W. J., and Kies, M. W. (1962): Specificity of encephalitogen-induced inhibition of experimental allergic encephalomyelitis in the guinea pig. *J. Immunol.,* 89:54–61.

163. Shaw, C., Alvord, E. C., Jr., Kaku, J., and Kies, M. W. (1965): Correlation of experimental allergic encephalomyelitis with delayed-type skin sensitivity to specific homologous encephalitogen. *Ann. NY Acad. Sci.,* 122:318–331.

164. Sheramata, W., Cosgrave, J. B. R., and Eylar, E. H. (1974): Cellular hypersensitivity to basic myelin (A₁) protein and clinical multiple sclerosis. *N. Engl. J. Med.,* 291: 14–17.

165. Sheramata, W., Cosgrove, J. B. R., and Eylar, E. R. (1976): Multiple sclerosis and cell-mediated hypersensitivity to myelin A₁ protein. *J. Neurol. Sci.,* 27:413–425.

166. Sherwin, L. A., Richter, M., Cosgrove, J. B., and Rose, B. (1961): Myelin-binding antibodies in experimental "allergic" encephalomyelitis. *Science,* 134:1370–1372.

167. Shiraki, H., and Otani, S. (1959): Clinical and pathological features of rabies postvaccinal encephalomyelitis in man. In: *Allergic Encephalomyelitis,* edited by M. W. Kies and E. C. Alvord, Jr., p. 58. Charles C Thomas, Springfield, Ill.

168. Shiraki, H., Yonezawa, T., and Kuroiwa, Y., editors (1976): *The Aetiology and Pathogenesis of the Demyelinating Diseases.* Japan Science Press, Tokyo.

169. Silberberg, D., Lisak, B. P., and Zweiman, B. (1973): Multiple sclerosis unaffected by azothiaprine in pilot study. *Arch. Neurol.,* 28: 210–212.

170. Simon, J., and Simon, O. (1975): Effect of passive transfer of anti-brain antibodies to a normal recipient. *Exp. Neurol.,* 47:523–534.

171. Sluga, E. (1974): In: *Polyneuropathien typen und differenzierung ergebnisse bioptischer untersuchiengen,* p. 51. Springer Verlag, Berlin.

172. Snyder, D. H., Valsamis, M. P., and Stone, S. H. (1975): Progressive and reparatory events in chronic experimental allergic encephalomyelitis. *J. Neuropathol. Exp. Neurol.,* 34:209–221.

173. Spitler, L. E., Von Muller, C. M., Fudenberg, H. H., and Eylar, E. H. (1972): Experimental allergic encephalomyelitis: Dissociation of cellular immunity to brain protein and disease production. *J. Exp. Med.,* 136:156–174.

174. Spitler, L. E., Von Muller, C. M., and Young, J. D. (1975): Experimental allergic encephalomyelitis: Study of cellular immunity to the encephalitogenic component. *Cell. Immunol.,* 15:143–151.

175. Stauffer, R. E., and Waksman, B. H. (1954): Dermal and serological reactions to nervous tissue antigens in multiple sclerosis. *Ann. NY Acad. Sci.,* 58:520–524.

176. Stone, S. H. (1961): Transfer of allergic encephalomyelitis by lymph node cells in inbred guinea pigs. *Science,* 134:619–620.

177. Stone, S. H., and Lerner, E. M. (1965): Chronic disseminated allergic encephalomyelitis in guinea pigs. *Ann. NY Acad. Sci.,* 122:227–241.

178. Stoner, G. L., Brosnan, C. F., Wisniewski, H. M., and Bloom, B. R. (1977): Studies on demyelination by activated lymphocytes in the rabbit eye. I. Effects of a mononuclear cell infiltrate induced by products of activated lymphocytes. *J. Immunol.* 118:2094–2102.

179. Strandgaard, S., and Jorgensen, P. N. (1972): Delayed hypersensitivity to myelin antigen in multiple sclerosis investigated with the leucocyte migration method. *Acta Neurol. Scand.,* 48:243–248.

180. Suzuki, K., Andrews, J. M., Waltz, J. M., and Terry, R. D. (1969): Ultrastructural studies of multiple sclerosis. *Lab. Invest.,* 20:444–454.

181. Suzuki, K., Kamushita, S., Eto, Y., Tourtellotte, W. W., and Gonatas, J. O. (1973): Normal amounts of MBP in myelin from normal white matter in MS. *Arch. Neurol.,* 28:293–297.

182. Swanborg, R. H. (1970): The effect of selective modification of tryptophan, lysine and arginine residues of basic protein on encephalitogenic activity. *J. Immunol.,* 105: 865–871.

183. Swanborg, R. (1972): Antigen-induced inhibition of experimental allergic encephalitis.
I. Inhibition in guinea pigs with non-encepha-
litogenic modified myelin basic protein. *J.
Immunol.*, 109:540–546.
184. Swierkosz, J. E., and Swanborg, R. H.
(1975): Suppressor cell control of unresponsiveness to experimental allergic encephalomyelitis. *J. Immunol.*, 115:631–633.
185. Taylor, E. W. (1922): In: *Multiple Sclerosis,*
Vol. II, Chap. 4. Hoeber, New York.
186. Teitelbaum, D., Meshorer, T., Hirschfeld,
P., Arnon, R., and Sela, M. (1971): Suppression of experimental allergic encephalomyelitis by a synthetic polypeptide. *Eur. J.
Immunol.*, 1:242–248.
187. Teitelbaum, D., Webb, C., Bree, M., Meshorer, A., Arnon, R., and Sela, M. (1974):
Suppression of experimental allergic encephalomyelitis in rhesus monkeys by a
synthetic basic copolymer. *Clin. Immunol.
Immunopathol.*, 3:256–262.
188. Teitelbaum, D., Webb, C., Meshorer, A.,
Arnon, R., and Sela, M. (1972): Suppression
by several synthetic polypeptides of experimental allergic encephalomyelitis induced in
guinea pigs and rabbits with bovine and human encephalitogen. *Eur. J. Immunol.*, 3:
273–279.
189. Thompson, E. J. (1977): Multiple sclerosis:
Immunological and biochemical aspects. *Br.
Med. Bull.*, 33:28–33.
190. Volpe, M., Hawkins, A., and Roziditsky, B.
(1960): Permeability of cerebral blood vessels in experimental allergic encephalomyelitis studied by radioactive iodinated bovine
albumin. *Neurology (Minneap)*, 10:171–177.
191. Waksman, B. H., and Morrison, L. P.
(1951): Tuberculin type sensitivity to spinal
cord antigen in rabbits with isoallergic encephalomyelitis. *J. Immunol.*, 66:421–444.
192. Westall, F. C., Robinson, A. B., Caccam, J.,
Jackson, J., and Eylar, H. E. (1971): Essential chemical requirements for induction of
allergic encephalomyelitis. *Nature (Lond)*,
229:22–24.
193. Williams, R. M., and Moore, M. J. (1973):
Linkage of susceptibility to experimental allergic encephalomyelitis to the major histocompatibility focus in the rat. *J. Exp. Med.*,
138:775–783.
194. Winkler, G. F. (1965): In vitro demyelination of peripheral nerve induced with sensitized cells. *Ann. NY Acad. Sci.*, 122:287–
296.
195. Wiśniewski, H. (1977): Immunopathology
of demyelination in autoimmune diseases and
virus infections. *Br. J. Med.*, 33:54–59.
196. Wiśniewski, H. M., and Bloom, B. R.
(1975): Primary demyelination as a nonspecific consequence of cell mediated immune reaction. *J. Exp. Med.*, 141:346–359.
197. Wiśniewski, H. M., and Bloom, B. R.
(1975): Experimental allergic optic neuritis
(EAON) in the rabbit. *J. Neurol. Sci.*, 24:
257–263.
198. Wiśniewski, H. M., and Keith, A. B. (1976):
Chronic relapsing experimental allergic encephalomyelitis: An experimental model of
multiple sclerosis. *Ann. Neurol.*, 1:144–148.
199. Wiśniewski, H., Oppenheimer, D., and Mc-
Donald, W. I. (1976): Relation between
myelination and function in MS and EAE.
J. Neuropathol. Exp. Neurol., 35:327.
200. Witebsky, E., and Steinfeld, J. (1928): Untersuchungen über spezifische: Antigen-funk-
tionen von organen. *Z. Immunitaetsforsch.*,
58:271–296.
201. Wolf, A., Kabat, E. A., and Bezer, H.
(1947): The pathology of acute disseminated
encephalomyelitis produced experimentally
in the rhesus monkey and its resemblance to
human demyelinating diseases. *J. Neuropathol. Exp. Neurol.*, 6:333–357.
202. Wray, S. H., Cogan, D. G., and Arnason,
B. G. W. (1974): Experimental allergic optic neuritis (EAON) in the rabbit. *J. Neurol.
Sci.*, 24:257–263.
203. Wray, S. H., Cogan, D. G., and Arnason,
B. G. W. (1976): Experimental allergic encephalomyelitis: Passive transfer by the intraocular injection of sensitized cells. *Arch.
Neurol.*, 33:183–185.
204. Yonezawa, T., Ishihara, Y., and Matsuyama,
H. (1968): Studies on experimental allergic
peripheral neuritis. I. Demyelinating patterns
studied in vitro. *J. Neuropathol. Exp.
Neurol.*, 27:453–463.
205. Yonezawa, T., Saida, T., and Hasegawa, M.
(1976): Myelination inhibition factor in experimental allergic encephalomyelitis and demyelinating diseases. In: *The Etiology and
Pathogenesis of the Demyelinating Diseases,*
edited by H. Shiraki, T. Yonezawa, and
Y. Kuroiwa, pp. 255–263. Japan Science
Press, Tokyo.
206. Yung, L. L. I., Diener, E., McPherson, T. A.,
Barton, M. A., and Hyde, H. A. (1973):
Antigen-binding lymphocytes in normal man
and guinea pig to human encephalitogenic
protein. *J. Immunol.*, 110:1383–1387.
207. Zabriskie, J. B., Utermohlen, V., Espinoza,
L. R., Plank, C. R., and Collins, R. C.
(1975): Immunologic studies with transfer
factor in multiple sclerosis patients. *Neurology (Minneap)*, 25:490.

Physiology and Pathobiology of Axons, edited by
S. G. Waxman. Raven Press, New York © 1978.

Biochemistry of Myelin Disorders

Kunihiko Suzuki

*Saul R. Korey Department of Neurology, Department of Neuroscience, and the Rose F. Kennedy
Center for Research in Mental Retardation and Human Development, Albert Einstein College
of Medicine, Bronx, New York 10461*

The myelin sheath, both central and peripheral, is histologically and biochemically affected in various pathological conditions. Since myelin is a specialized extension of the plasma membrane of the oligodendroglia in the central nervous system (CNS) and of the Schwann cell in the peripheral nerve, destruction of myelin can occur by any mechanisms that interfere with the normal metabolic process of myelin maintenance. They include abnormalities in the chemical architecture or the metabolism of myelin itself, exogenous agents (e.g., infections, or toxins) for which myelin is the target tissue, disorders affecting its parent cell, the oligodendroglia and/or the Schwann cell, and disorders or destruction of the axon, which normally maintains a specific and still poorly understood relationship with the myelin sheath.

The term "demyelinating disease" has a relatively narrow and specific meaning for neuropathologists. For example, Raine and Schaumburg (43) state, "the majority of neuropathologists and neurologists now reserve the term 'demyelinating' to include only the acquired inflammatory demyelinating diseases such as multiple sclerosis in which there is loss of myelin with striking sparing of axons." This definition naturally excludes a large number of pathological conditions that affect myelin. Furthermore, this etiological and morphological classification does not always divide various biochemical processes of myelin destruction into proper groups. For example, multiple sclerosis is the prototype of the demyelinating disease, whereas Wallerian degeneration is not a "demyelinating disease" and myelin destruction is merely secondary to axonal degeneration. Despite the obvious differences in what triggers myelin breakdown and in pathology (sparing of the axon in multiple sclerosis and its loss in Wallerian degeneration), there is no evidence at the present time to indicate that the biochemical process of myelin destruction is in any way different between the two pathological conditions.

It seems feasible, therefore, to examine the pathological conditions of myelin from a biochemist's view, unencumbered by the traditional definitions of what is primary or secondary demyelination. Objections from neuropathologists are anticipated. If the focus of the chapter is not on how myelin destruction is initiated biochemically but largely on the process of myelin breakdown *after* it was initiated, it only points to the present limit of our knowledge on biochemistry of myelin breakdown. Biochemists have been studying mostly the *phenomena* as they occur in the course of myelin breakdown. We cannot yet talk intelligently, in biochemical terms, about the loss of the axonal "signal" essential for normal maintenance of the myelin sheath that must occur initially in Wallerian degeneration, or about the initial biochemical events in either myelin itself or in oligodendroglia that lead to demyelination in multiple sclerosis. It should also be pointed out that we know practically nothing about the biochemistry of the axon in diseases involving myelin.

The following, then, comprises a rather personal view of one neurochemist looking at the present knowledge on biochemistry of myelin in pathological conditions. All pathological conditions involving myelin abnormalities are included, rather than the traditional "demyelinating" diseases. Attempts are made to present a systematic, unified perspective without going into detailed cataloguing of facts for individual diseases.

PERSPECTIVE OF BIOCHEMICAL ABNORMALITIES OF MYELIN

Within the present limited knowledge, biochemical abnormalities of the myelin sheath can be divided into two major categories: specific and nonspecific. The specific abnormalities include the group of metabolic disorders which involve some of the important constituents of myelin. Such pathological conditions result in either production of compositionally abnormal myelin which are chemically or metabolically unstable, or they affect the metabolism of oligodendroglia. In either case, the end result is abnormal myelination or destruction of myelin. These conditions are often referred to as "dysmyelination," implying intrinsic abnormalities of the myelin sheath, rather than destruction of intrinsically normal myelin.

Normal myelin, on the other hand, appears to have a limited repertoire of reactions to a multitude of extrinsic insults—trauma, loss of axons, infections, toxic agents—and undergoes a biochemically nonspecific process of destruction. In this type of myelin abnormality, the trigger mechanisms that initiate myelin destruction are certainly different in different diseases and are likely to be specific at least for certain disease conditions. However, once the process of myelin breakdown is initiated, degenerating myelin shows similar abnormalities irrespective of the initiating events. The nonspecific myelin breakdown is commonly accompanied by esterification of cholesterol which results in histologically demonstrable sudanophilia. In some instances the myelin sheath is nonspecifically degraded without cholesterol ester formation.

In the following sections we examine briefly what is known biochemically about the myelin sheath in pathological conditions. For this purpose, it is obviously important to know the morphology of myelin in normal and pathological conditions, as well as the biochemistry of normal myelin and myelination. Because of space limitation, readers are referred to recent review articles (36,42; Berthold, *this vol-*

ume; Hirano and Dembitzer, *this volume*). There are excellent recent reviews which cover more factual details of biochemistry of pathological myelin that are omitted from this chapter (35,37).

MYELIN BREAKDOWN CAUSED BY SPECIFIC METABOLIC ABNORMALITIES

Biochemically specific forms of myelin disorders occur as the result of specific metabolic abnormality involving one or more myelin constituents. This category includes metachromatic leukodystrophy, globoid cell leukodystrophy (Krabbe's disease), adrenoleukodystrophy, and Refsum's disease. In addition, Pelizaeus–Merzbacher disease and spongy degeneration of the white matter (Canavan's disease) are hereditary metabolic disorders which primarily affect the white matter. However, the specific biochemical abnormalities underlying these two disorders are not yet known.

Metachromatic Leukodystrophy

Metachromatic leukodystrophy (MLD) is an autosomal recessive genetic disorder that occurs as the result of mutation(s) of a lysosomal hydrolytic enzyme, arylsulfatase A, which normally hydrolyzes one of the important myelin constituents, sulfatide (galactosylceramide sulfate) (8,33,34). Because of the normally high concentration of sulfatide in the myelin sheath, there is a severe loss of central and peripheral myelin. The degree of myelin loss varies according to the stage of the disease, but almost total loss of myelin may result at the terminal stage. This is not the primary demyelination in the neuropathological sense. The axons also degenerate in severely involved areas. Sudanophilic droplets or inflammatory changes are not a part of the regular pathology.

The presence of abnormal granules in the white matter and the peripheral nerve is the most characteristic feature of the disease. These granules stain metachromatically with acidic cresyl violet. The metachromatic reaction and positive staining for the periodic acid-Schiff reagent (PAS) and for sudan black indicate the presence of an acidic glycolipid. These abnormal granules are present intracellularly in the oligodendroglia or in Schwann cells (4,25, 46,62). Ultrastructural localization of acid phosphatase activities within these abnormal bodies suggest their lysosomal origin (45). Similar metachromatic granules are often found in moderate numbers also in the renal tubules, the mucosal cells of the gallbladder, and rarely in other systemic organs.

Positive analytical proof for excess storage of sulfatide was provided during the late 1950s by two laboratories (5,28). The white matter and the peripheral nerve show abnormally increased amounts of sulfatide with concomitant decreases in galactosylceramide (galactocerebroside). Consequently, the normal cerebroside/sulfatide ratio of approximately 4 becomes reversed (60). Because of the large amounts of these galactolipids normally present in the myelin sheath, the chemical abnormality is most prominent in the white matter and the peripheral nerve. The characteristic abnormal metachromatic granules have been isolated from the brain of a patient and were shown to contain a large excess of sulfatide (56,57).

Metachromatic leukodystrophy was the first disorder in which the composition of myelin was shown to be specifically abnormal, reflecting the fundamental metabolic defect of the disease (39,41). When myelin was isolated postmortem from brains of patients, it appeared ultrastructurally normal, although the yield was, as expected, much lower than normal. Isolated myelin contained very high sulfatide and low galactosylceramide. It is a matter of conjecture, then, that the myelin with such grossly abnormal composition might be structurally unstable. It should be noted that sulfatide, present in a large excess in MLD myelin, is a highly charged acidic molecule. The analytical data are summarized in Table 1. The sulfatide content of whole white matter is even higher than that of myelin or the MLD granules. Therefore sulfatide in the metachromatic granules and the myelin sheath can account for only a very small proportion of the total sulfatide content of the white matter. It is likely that other membrane structures in the white matter also contain abnormally high sulfatide. Normal myelinated axons were recently found to be relatively rich in galactosylceramide and sulfatide, in contrast to the earlier view that these galactolipids are specific for myelin (12,13,38). Although direct evidence is lacking, the MLD axons probably also contain a large amount of sulfatide. This might be at least a contributing cause to the severe axonal degeneration seen in MLD.

Refsum's Disease

Refsum's disease (heredopathia atactica polyneuritiformis) is another metabolic disorder in which the fundamental metabolic de-

TABLE 1. *Lipid composition of MLD brain fractions*

Constituents	White matter[a]		Myelin[a]		MLD granules[b]
	MLD	Control	MLD	Control	
Total lipid (% dry wt.)	34.2	52.7	63.2	70.0	53.1
Cholesterol	16.2	26.8	21.2	25.6	18.7
Galactolipids	50.1	25.0	37.4	28.2	46.1
Galactosylceramide	5.9	19.5	9.0	24.7	7.0
Sulfatide	44.2	5.5	28.4	3.5	39.1
Total phospholipid	32.9	49.4	36.1	42.8	35.3
Ethanolamine phospholipid	5.5	17.1	8.1	15.6	9.2
Lecithin	12.1	14.6	10.7	10.1	14.1
Sphingomyelin	8.8	7.6	7.1	7.0	5.8
Serine phospholipid	3.3	7.4	3.8	5.1	4.0
Monophosphoinositide	1.1	1.1	3.1	0.9	0.8
Plasmalogen	3.0	11.2	5.3	11.7	—

Values are expressed as percent of total lipid, except for total lipid.
[a] Data from Norton (37).
[b] Data from Suzuki et al. (57).

fect is reflected in the abnormal composition of the myelin sheath. The disease is characterized neurologically by severe polyneuropathy, retinal degeneration, and cerebellar ataxia. The disease is caused by defective phytanic acid α-hydroxylase, which normally initiates the degradation of phytanic acid (10). Phytanic acid (3,7,11,15-tetramethylhexadecanoic acid), which is of dietary origin, is present in patients' plasma and tissue lipids at greatly increased concentrations (31).

Myelin was isolated from the brain and spinal cord of a patient (32). Glycerophospholipids, particularly lecithin, in isolated myelin contained a substantial amount of phytanic acid at the 1-position. Lecithin of the whole sciatic nerve contained 24% phytanic acid at the 1-position. To what extent the presence of this unusual fatty acid in the myelin membrane influences its structural stability remains a matter of speculation. One interesting finding by MacBrinn and O'Brien (32) was the normal α-hydroxy fatty acid content in galactosylceramide and sulfatide in myelin. This indicated a genetically distinct α-hydroxylase for phytanic acid.

Globoid Cell Leukodystrophy (Krabbe's Disease)

Globoid cell leukodystrophy (GLD) is biochemically closely related to MLD. Each is an autosomal recessive disorder caused by a mutation of a lysosomal hydrolytic enzyme at adjacent degradative steps of a single series of glycosphingolipids both of which are highly enriched in the myelin sheath (Fig. 1). The enzyme involved is galactosylceramidase, which normally hydrolyzes galactosylceramide to galactose and ceramide (54).

As expected, there are similarities in the clinical, morphological, and analytical manifestations between MLD and GLD (for recent detailed reviews, see refs. 52,53,55). As in MLD, GLD manifests almost exclusively as a disease of the white matter and the peripheral nerve. The main pathological features are an almost complete lack (or disappearance) of myelin and oligodendroglia, severe astrocytic gliosis, and the presence of numerous abnormal globoid cells, which are probably of mesodermal origin. The peripheral nerve is less severely affected, but segmental demyelination is found consistently, associated with delayed conduction velocity. Two types of abnormal inclusion are found in the globoid cell. The first, more common type of inclusion is a straight or curved, hollow, tubular structure with irregular crystalloid cross sections (50). The second type of inclusion, first described by Yunis and Lee (66), has the structure of right-handed twisted tubules.

Analytical abnormalities in GLD show interesting dissimilarities to MLD. Unlike the sulfatide accumulation in MLD, galactosylceramide is always much less than normal in the brain. The analytical findings of the white matter simply reflects the almost total loss of myelin. In 1963 Austin (7) and Svennerholm (60) independently reported the important finding that, although decreased galactosylceramide was expected, the galactosylceramide/sulfatide ratio was abnormally high. In view of the almost total lack of myelin, this abnormal ratio appears to be due to a disproportionate preservation of galactosylceramide. Thus despite the degradative block, abnormal accumulation of galactosylceramide is limited only to the globoid cells (6).

Unlike in MLD, myelin in GLD is composi-

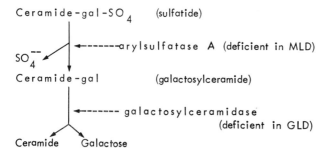

FIG. 1. Degradative pathway of the two galactolipids characteristic of myelin, and the two hydrolytic enzymes involved in genetic leukodystrophies.

tionally normal (19). The low overall level of galactosylceramide and the normal composition of the myelin sheath can be explained by the early and rapid death of the oligodendroglial cells. Since these are the cells which normally synthesize galactosylceramide, their disappearance terminates any further accumulation of galactosylceramide and any further myelin formation, abnormal or otherwise. The assumption here is that myelin is produced only in early stages of the disease by the oligodendroglial cells which are still relatively healthy, and therefore the myelin composition does not reflect the genetic defect.

Extensive axonal degeneration occurs in GLD. Since galactosylceramide has been found at a surprisingly high concentration in the myelinated axons (12,13,38), axonal involvement can be expected. In this regard, MLD and GLD appear analogous.

Adrenoleukodystrophy

There has long been a somewhat ambiguously defined disease entity characterized by progressive and often massive myelin destruction. It has been called sudanophilic leukodystrophy or Schilder's disease. It has also been recognized that some cases of Schilder's disease occur as an X-linked genetic trait and are associated with adrenal insufficiency. Recent work by Schaumburg, Powers, Richardson, and co-workers has made it clear that most if not all cases of so-called Schilder's disease or sudanophilic leukodystrophy are in fact X-linked genetic disorders, and that the adrenals of patients consistently show characteristic pathology (47). Since it is logically impossible to exclude the existence of sudanophilic leukodystrophy which is not adrenoleukodystrophy (ALD), it is difficult to determine whether the cases recorded in the literature as sudanophilic leukodystrophy or Schilder's disease are all ALD. Schaumburg, however, was unable to identify a single case in the literature in which absence of the adrenal lesions was definitively documented (*personal communication*).

This present status creates a difficult problem in interpretation of earlier biochemical studies on "Schilder's disease" (26,48) or on "sudanophilic leukodystrophy" (22,44,61), except for those instances in which the cases were identified as ALD by retrospective pathological examination (14,59).

Unlike the other genetic leukodystrophies already discussed, the myelin destruction in ALD is associated with prominent sudanophilia. General analytical findings reflect severe myelin loss in the white matter—increased water content, decreased lipids (particularly galactolipids), and varying amounts of esterified cholesterol. Although the fundamental genetic defect of ALD is not yet known, what appears to be a unique biochemical abnormality was reported by Igarashi et al. (27). They identified that the characteristic birefringent material found in the brain and the adrenal of patients is cholesterol esterified with unusually long-chain saturated fatty acids, ranging from C_{22} to C_{30}. Such long-chain fatty acids were also found in the ganglioside fraction.

Since cholesterol esters are not constituents of myelin, myelin in ALD brain does not share this fatty acid abnormality. In fact, the composition of myelin isolated from ALD brains showed abnormalities characteristic of the nonspecific changes of degenerating myelin, which is discussed later (21,59). Although the fundamental cause of the myelin destruction in ALD must be specific and the specific chemical abnormality is known, they are not reflected in the composition or the mode of degeneration of myelin. Thus in ALD the distinction of specific and nonspecific biochemical abnormalities becomes blurred.

When we turn our attention to other genetic diseases affecting myelin (e.g., Pelizaeus–Merzbacher's disease or spongy degeneration of the white matter), the picture gets murkier. Although their genetic nature indicates specific underlying causes for the myelin destruction, no specific metabolic or compositional abnormalities are known; and, at least in the spongy degeneration, isolated myelin showed only nonspecific changes.

NONSPECIFIC ABNORMALITIES OF MYELIN

As already remarked for myelin isolated from brains of patients with ALD, there is a

TABLE 2. *Nonspecific lipid abnormality of degenerating human myelin*

Constituents	Control[a]	SSPE[a]	Spongy degeneration[b]	ALD[c]	G_M-ganglio-sidosis[d]
Total lipid (% dry wt.)	70.0	73.7	63.8	63.1	68.0
Cholesterol	27.7	43.7	58.0	33.4	44.5
Galactolipids	26.5	21.6	10.0	16.4	12.4
Galactosylceramide	22.7	18.8	8.0	11.4	9.5
Sulfatide	3.8	2.8	2.0	3.4	2.9
Total phospholipid	43.1	36.6	33.4	48.2	35.4
Ethanolamine phospholipid	15.6	9.7	9.8	13.6	7.9
Lecithin	11.2	10.4	11.3	14.5	12.3
Sphingomyelin	7.9	8.8	5.9	7.1	7.0
Serine phospholipid	4.8	4.6	5.5	6.9	6.5
Monophosphoinositide	0.6	1.4	0.8	1.3	1.7
Plamalogen	12.3	9.1	—	11.3	—

Values are expressed as percent of total lipid, except for total lipid.
[a] Data from Norton et al. (40).
[b] Data from Kamoshita et al. (30).
[c] Data from Suzuki et al. (59).
[d] Data from Suzuki et al. (58).

set of abnormal composition of myelin that is found in many pathological conditions of diverse etiology. The concept of the nonspecific process of myelin breakdown, first pointed out in 1971 (49), suggests that when maintenance of normal myelin is no longer possible it follows a stereotyped route to complete destruction, irrespective of the initiating causes. The etiological factors can be neuronal loss (Wallerian degeneration), infections, mechanical pressure, or any number of other causes. This type of myelin abnormality was first reported in subacute sclerosing panencephalitis (SSPE) (40) and has subsequently been found in experimental Wallerian degeneration (9), ALD (59), spongy degeneration of white matter (30), triethyltin edema (20), gangliosidoses (58), Niemann–Pick disease (29), and at least one case of multiple sclerosis (65).

Despite diverse etiology, myelin isolated from these diseases exhibits similar chemical abnormalities, although in varying degrees. Usually the proportion of total protein and total lipid is not dramatically altered, but proportions of individual lipids are abnormal (Table 2). The amount of cholesterol is increased, often strikingly so, constituting more than half the total lipid in contrast to approximately 25% in normal myelin. No esterified cholesterol is found in the myelin sheath, even though some of these disorders exhibit sudanophilic myelin destruction with abundant cho-

lesterol esters in the whole tissue. Total galactolipids may be decreased to one-half to one-third of normal, and galactosylceramide is usually much more severely affected than sulfatide. In addition, moderate decreases of ethanolamine phospholipid are common. Such abnormal myelin is likely to represent an intermediate from normal myelin to complete degradation. It is interesting to note that similar abnormalities are noted in diseases in which myelin is degraded by invading phagocytic cells with associated cholesterol ester formation or in those instances in which no evidence for inflammation or phagocytic activity exists.

Multiple Sclerosis

It would be a heresy for neuropathologists to call myelin destruction in multiple sclerosis nonspecific. However, except for the justifiable *a priori* notion for an initiating mechanism specific for multiple sclerosis, there is no definitive biochemical evidence that indicates specific chemical abnormalities of either myelin or the process of myelin breakdown in multiple sclerosis. It is the most common and most important among demyelinating diseases, and consequently voluminous literature exists concerning the biochemistry, histochemistry, and some enzymatic studies on the plaques, the areas surrounding the plaques, normal-appearing white matter, and isolated myelin (for a recent review, see ref. 37). Analytical results for pathologically affected areas are consistent with the histological changes. Minor abnormalities have been reported also in grossly normal-appearing white matter. Such abnormalities can be explained on the basis of the possible presence of microscopic or diffuse lesions undetectable by the naked eye, a possibility that is practically impossible to exclude. Minor and often contradictory abnormalities have also been reported with respect to the composition of isolated myelin from the normal-appearing white matter. A critical examination of the data published by 1972 led Wolfgram (64) to the conclusion that myelin from normal-appearing white matter in multiple sclerosis is normal, a conclusion supported by a subsequent detailed study (51). The nonspecific compositional abnormality of myelin isolated from affected areas in one case was mentioned above (65). It appears reasonably certain that in multiple sclerosis the biochemical process of myelin degeneration, once initiated, is fundamentally the same as in many other pathological conditions, e.g., Wallerian degeneration. The crucial question concerns the series of events that make normal maintenance of myelin no longer possible. This question remains almost totally unanswered at present.

Cholesterol Esters

In many diseases in which myelin breaks down nonspecifically, formation of abnormal amounts of cholesterol esters takes place. Normal brain characteristically contains very little esterified cholesterol. The increased cholesterol ester in demyelinating conditions is the chemical counterpart of the sudanophilic droplets observed histologically, and it appears to indicate the presence of phagocytic activity. Thus increased cholesterol esters are seen in multiple sclerosis, ALD, SSPE, and myelin breakdown secondary to neuronal loss (Wallerian-type degeneration). Even among the conditions of nonspecific myelin breakdown, no accumulation of cholesterol esters is seen in spongy degeneration of the white matter, or in triethyltin-induced edema. Once cholesterol is esterified, it is no longer a part of the myelin sheath and is recovered by the conventional

subcellular fractionation procedure as a very light, abnormal "floating fraction." This was first reported in SSPE (40) and has since been observed repeatedly. The fatty acid composition of this esterified cholesterol is different from that of the minute amount of cholesterol esters in normal brain or from that of cholesterol esters in plasma. It is, however, very similar to fatty acids at the 2-position in phosphatidylcholine in the white matter (14,44).

The precise biochemical steps of cholesterol ester formation in sudanophilic myelin breakdown are not yet clear. It is assumed that both cholesterol and fatty acids derive from myelin, but the conclusive evidence is lacking. From the fatty acid composition, two possible pathways can be considered. One possibility is the direct transfer of the 2-position fatty acid of phosphatidylcholine to cholesterol by lecithin-cholesterol acyltransferase (23,24). The enzyme is known to be active in plasma, playing the key role in cholesterol ester formation in atherosclerotic plaques. This would have neatly explained the striking similarity of the fatty acid composition. However, Eto and Suzuki were unable to detect activity of lecithin-cholesterol acyltransferase not only in normal rat brain (15) but also in an experimental condition in which sudanophilia and macrophage infiltration were present following heat lesions of the cerebral cortex (Eto and Suzuki, *unpublished*). Another possibility would be activation of phospholipase A_2 which then provides the source of free fatty acids from the 2-position of glycerophospholipids. Examination of the white matter of patients with various sudanophilic myelinoclastic conditions failed to show specific activation of phospholipase A_2 (Eto and Suzuki, *unpublished*).

A series of studies on the enzymes of cholesterol ester metabolism in rat brain have revealed at least four enzymes (15–18). There appears to be only one cholesterol-esterifying enzyme which uses free cholesterol and free fatty acid, rather than acyl-CoA, as the substrates. On the other hand, there are three distinct cholesterol ester hydrolases in rat brain. The subcellular distributions and developmental changes indicate that each of the four enzymes is distinct from the others, and particularly that the esterifying enzyme is not one of the three hydrolases catalyzing the reverse reaction. Of particular interest is that one cholesterol ester hydrolase is localized almost exclusively in the myelin sheath. Its functional significance with respect to the metabolism of myelin is not yet clear.

ROLE OF AXONS IN DEMYELINATION

As is perhaps clear by now, the neurochemical approach has been quite successful in describing the biochemical phenomena associated with the multitude of pathological conditions in which normal formation or maintenance of the myelin sheath is disturbed. However, we have been far less successful in the more mechanistic aspect of the problem, particularly with respect to the events that initiate myelin breakdown. There is little question that the axon plays a crucial role in formation and maintenance of myelin. Wallerian degeneration is the classic model to show the dependence of normal myelin maintenance on the axons. Weinberg and Spencer (63) and Aguayo et al. (2,3) showed that the Schwann cells originally associated with unmyelinated fibers can be induced to form myelin if provided with the axons of another nerve which is normally myelinated. At the same time, in a study with a mutant mouse, trembler, Aguayo et al. (1) showed that, even when provided with normal axons, the Schwann cells derived from the mutant mouse retain their abnormal myelination characteristics. The interaction therefore must be mutual. This is an important and promising area for study.

Some analytical studies were carried out on the axons isolated from myelinated tract of the CNS (12,13,38). A few surprises were in store. The isolated axons from bovine or rat brain were shown to contain substantial amounts of galactosylceramide and sulfatide, previously thought to be highly enriched only in myelin. Their concentrations in axons were similar to those in myelin on the basis of lipid, although the total content was less in the axons because the myelin sheath was richer in lipids. Furthermore, Costantino-Ceccarini and DeVries (11) recently showed that not only galactosylceramide but the enzyme which catalyzes the last step of its synthesis, UDP-galactose:ceramide galactosyltransferase,

is also present in the axons. Although the functional significance of these findings is not yet clear, they require close attention. Unfortunately it is not known whether unmyelinated axons also contain high concentrations of the galactolipids because the limitation of the present technology dictates that the only axons from myelinated fibers can be isolated. At least it appears that the high galactolipid content is acquired by the axons during myelination, because the white matter prior to myelination contains very little galactolipids. The interactions between the axons and myelin, the nature of the mutual signals, and their disturbance in pathological states would be fruitful areas for study.

REFERENCES

1. Aguayo, A. J., Attiwell, M., Trecarten, J., Perkins, S., and Bray, G. M. (1977): Abnormal myelination in transplanted trembler mouse Schwann cells. *Nature (Lond)*, 265:73–75.
2. Aguayo, A. J., Charron, L., and Bray, G. M. (1976): Potential of Schwann cells from unmyelinated nerves to produce myelin. A quantitative ultrastructural and radiographic study. *J. Neurocytol.*, 5:565–573.
3. Aguayo, A. J., Epps, J., Charron, L., and Bray, G. M. (1976): Multipotentiality of Schwann cells in cross-anastomosed and grafted unmyelinated nerves—quantitative microscopy and radioautography. *Brain Res.*, 104:1–20.
4. Aurebeck, G., Osterberg, K., Blaw, M., Chou, S., and Nelson, E. (1964): Electron microscopic observations on metachromatic leucodystrophy. *Arch. Neurol.*, 11:273–288.
5. Austin, J. H. (1959): Metachromatic sulfatides in cerebral white matter and kidney. *Proc. Soc. Exp. Biol.*, 100:361–364.
6. Austin, J. H. (1963): Studies in globoid (Krabbe) leukodystrophy. II. Controlled thin-layer chromatographic studies of globoid body fractions in seven patients. *J. Neurochem.*, 10:921–940.
7. Austin, J. H. (1963): Studies in globoid (Krabbe) leukodystrophy. I. The significance of lipid abnormalities in white matter in eight globoid and thirteen control patients. *Arch. Neurol.*, 9:207–221.
8. Austin, J., Armstrong, D., and Shearer, L. (1965): Metachromatic form of diffuse cerebral sclerosis. V. The nature and significance of low sulfatase activity: a controlled study of brain, liver and kidney in four patients with metachromatic leukodystrophy (MLD). *Arch. Neurol.*, 13:593–614.

9. Bignami, A., and Eng, L. F. (1973): Biochemical studies of myelin in Wallerian degeneration of rat optic nerve. *J. Neurochem.,* 20:165–173.

10. Blass, J. P., and Steinberg, D. (1973): Disorders of fatty acids. In: *Biology of Brain Dysfunction,* Vol. 2, edited by G. E. Gaull, pp. 225–264. Plenum Press, New York.

11. Costantino-Ceccarini, E., and DeVries, G. H. (1976): UDP-galactose:ceramide galactosyltransferase in rat axon. *Trans. Am. Soc. Neurochem.,* 7:196.

12. DeVries, G. H., Hadfield, M. G., and Cornbrooks, C. (1976): The isolation and lipid composition of myelin-free axons from rat CNS. *J. Neurochem.,* 26:725–731.

13. DeVries, G. H., Norton, W. T., and Raine, C. S. (1972): Axons: Isolation from mammalian central nervous system. *Science,* 175:1370–1372.

14. Eto, Y., and Suzuki, K. (1971): Cholesterol esters in demyelination: Fatty acid composition of cholesterol esters in brains of patients with Schilder's disease, G_{M1}-gangliosidosis and Tay-Sachs disease, and its possible relationship to the β-position fatty acids of lecithin. *J. Neurochem.,* 18:1007–1016.

15. Eto, Y., and Suzuki, K. (1971): Cholesterol ester metabolism in the brain: Properties and subcellular distribution of cholesterol esterifying enzyme and cholesterol ester hydrolase in adult rat brain. *Biochim. Biophys. Acta,* 239:293–311.

16. Eto, Y., and Suzuki, K. (1972): Cholesterol esters in developing rat brain: Enzymes of cholesterol ester metabolism. *J. Neurochem.,* 19:117–121.

17. Eto, Y., and Suzuki, K. (1973): Cholesterol ester metabolism in rat brain: A cholesterol ester hydrolase specifically localized in the myelin sheath. *J. Biol. Chem.,* 248:1986–1991.

18. Eto, Y., and Suzuki, K. (1973): Developmental changes of cholesterol ester hydrolases localized in myelin and microsomes of rat brain. *J. Neurochem.,* 20:1475–1477.

19. Eto, Y., Suzuki, K., and Suzuki, K. (1970): Globoid cell leukodystrophy (Krabbe's disease): Isolation of myelin with normal glycolipid composition. *J. Lipid Res.,* 11:473–479.

20. Eto, Y., Suzuki, K., and Suzuki, K. (1971): Lipid composition of rat brain myelin in triethyltin-induced edema. *J. Lipid Res.,* 12:570–579.

21. Eviatar, L., Harris, D. R., and Menkes, J. H. (1973): Diffuse sclerosis and Addison's disease: Biochemical studies in gray matter, white matter and myelin. *Biochem. Med.,* 8:268–279.

22. Gerstl, B., Rubinstein, L. J., Eng, L. F., and Tavaststjerna, M. (1966): A neurochemical study of a case of sudanophilic leukodystrophy. *Arch. Neurol.,* 15:603–614.

23. Glomset, J. A. (1962): The mechanism of the plasma cholesterol esterification reaction: Plasma fatty acid transferase. *Biochim. Biophys. Acta,* 65:128–135.

24. Glomset, J. A. (1968): The plasma lecithin:cholesterol acyltransferase reaction. *J. Lipid Res.,* 9:155–167.

25. Grégoire, A., Périer, O., and Dustin, P. (1966): Metachromatic leucodystrophy, an electron microscopic study. *J. Neuropathol. Exp. Neurol.,* 25:617–636.

26. Hogan, E. L., Joseph, K. C., Hurt, J. P., and Krigman, M. R. (1972): Schilder's diffuse sclerosis: A biochemical and ultrastructural study of myelinoclastic demyelination. *Acta Neuropathol. (Berl),* 20:85–95.

27. Igarashi, M., Schaumburg, H. H., Powers, J., Kishimoto, Y., Kolodny, E. H., and Suzuki, K. (1976): Fatty acid abnormality in adrenoleukodystrophy. *J. Neurochem.,* 26:851–860.

28. Jatzkewitz, H. (1958): Zwei Typen von Cerebrosid-schwefelsäureestern als sog: "Prälipoide" und Speichersubstanzen bei der Leukodystrophie, Typ Scholtz (metachromatische Form der diffusen Sklerose). *Z. Physiol. Chem.,* 311:279–282.

29. Kamoshita, S., Aron, A. M., Suzuki, K., and Suzuki, K. (1969): Infantile Niemann-Pick disease: A chemical study with isolation and characterization of membranous cytoplasmic bodies and myelin. *Am. J. Dis. Child.,* 117:379–394.

30. Kamoshita, S., Rapin, I., Suzuki, K., and Suzuki, K. (1968): Spongy degeneration of the brain: A chemical study of two cases including isolation and characterization of myelin. *Neurology (Minneap),* 18:975–985.

31. Klenk, E., and Kahlke, W. (1963): Über das Vorkommen der 3,7,11,15-Tetra-methylhexadecansäure (Phytansäure) in den Cholesterinestern und anderen Lipoid-fraktionen der Organe bei einem Krankheitsfall unbekannter Genese (Verdacht auf Heredopathia atactica polyneuritiformis [Refsum-Syndrom]). *Z. Physiol. Chem.,* 333:133–139.

32. MacBrinn, M. C., and O'Brien, J. S. (1968): Lipid composition of the nervous system in Refsum's disease. *J. Lipid Res.,* 9:552–561.

33. Mehl, E., and Jatzkewitz, H. (1965): Evidence for the genetic block in metachromatic leukodystrophy (ML). *Biochem. Biophys. Res. Commun.,* 19:407–411.

34. Mehl, E., and Jatzkewitz, H. (1968): Cerebroside 3-sulfate as a physiological substrate of arylsulfatase A. *Biochim. Biophys. Acta,* 151:619–627.

35. Morell, P., Bornstein, M. B., and Raine, C. S. (1976): Diseases involving myelin. In: *Basic Neurochemistry,* edited by G. J. Siegel, R. W. Albers, R. Katzman, and B. W. Agranoff, pp. 581–604. Little Brown, Boston.

36. Norton, W. T. (1977): Isolation and characterization of myelin. In: *Myelin,* edited by P. Morell, pp. 161–199. Plenum Press, New York.

37. Norton, W. T. (1977): Chemical pathology of diseases involving myelin. In: *Myelin,* edited by P. Morell, pp. 383–413. Plenum Press, New York.

38. Norton, W. T., Abe, T., Poduslo, S. E., and DeVries, G. H. (1975): The lipid composition of isolated brain cells and axons. *J. Neurosci. Res.,* 1:57–75.

39. Norton, W. T., and Poduslo, S. E. (1966): Metachromatic leukodystrophy: chemically abnormal myelin and cerebral biopsy studies of three siblings. In: *Variation in the Chemical Composition of the Nervous System,* edited by G. B. Ansell, p. 82. Pergamon, Oxford.

40. Norton, W. T., Poduslo, S. E., and Suzuki, K. (1966): Subacute sclerosing leukoencephalitis. II. Chemical studies including abnormal myelin and an abnormal ganglioside pattern. *J. Neuropathol. Exp. Neurol.,* 25:582–597.

41. O'Brien, J. S., and Sampson, L. E. (1966): Myelin membrane: A molecular abnormality. *Science,* 150:1613–1614.

42. Raine, C. S. (1977): Morphologic aspects of myelin and myelination. In: *Myelin,* edited by P. Morell, pp. 1–49. Plenum Press, New York.

43. Raine, C. S., and Schaumburg, H. H. (1977): The neuropathology of myelin diseases. In: *Myelin,* edited by P. Morell, pp. 271–323. Plenum Press, New York.

44. Ramsey, R. B., and Davison, A. N. (1974): Steryl esters and their relationship to normal and diseased human central nervous system. *J. Lipid Res.,* 15:249–255.

45. Résibois, A. (1969): Electron microscopic study of metachromatic leucodystrophy. III. Lysosomal nature of the inclusions. *Acta Neuropathol. (Berl),* 13:149–156.

46. Résibois-Grégoire, A. (1967): Electron microscopic studies of metachromatic leucodystrophy. II. Compound nature of the inclusions. *Acta Neuropathol. (Berl),* 9:244–253.

47. Schaumburg, H. H., Powers, J. M., Raine, C. S., Suzuki, K., and Richardson, E. P., Jr. (1975): Adrenoleukodystrophy: A clinical and pathological study of 17 cases. *Arch. Neurol.,* 33:577–591.

48. Smith, J. K., Gerstl, B., Tavaststjerna, M., and Porter, W. R. (1961): A case of sudanophilic diffuse sclerosis with study of the brain lipids. *Neurology (Minneap),* 11:395–401.

49. Suzuki, K. (1971): Lipid composition of purified myelin in various white matter diseases: A hypothesis of chemical abnormality of myelin in nonspecific demyelination. *Riv. Patol. Nerv. Ment.,* pp. 87–95.

50. Suzuki, K., and Grover, W. D. (1970): Krabbe's leukodystrophy (globoid cell leukodystrophy: An ultrastructural study. *Arch. Neurol.,* 22:385–396.

51. Suzuki, K., Kamoshita, S., Eto, Y., Tourtellotte, W. W., and Gonatas, J. O. (1973): Myelin in multiple sclerosis: Composition of myelin from normal-appearing white matter. *Arch. Neurol.,* 28:293–297.

52. Suzuki, K., and Suzuki, K. (1973): Disorders of sphingolipid metabolism. In: *Biology of Brain Dysfunction,* Vol. 2, edited by G. E. Gaull, pp. 1–73. Plenum Press, New York.

53. Suzuki, K., and Suzuki, K. (1973): Globoid cell leukodystrophy (Krabbe's disease). In: *Lysosomes and Storage Diseases,* edited by H. G. Hers and F. van Hoof, pp. 395–410. Academic Press, New York.

54. Suzuki, K., and Suzuki, Y. (1970): Globoid cell leukodystrophy (Krabbe's disease): Deficiency of galactocerebroside β-galactosidase. *Proc. Natl. Acad. Sci. USA,* 66:302–309.

55. Suzuki, K., and Suzuki, Y. (1977): Galactosylceramide lipidosis: globoid cell leukodystrophy (Krabbe's disease). In: *Metabolic Basis of Inherited Disease,* 4th ed., edited by J. B. Stanbury, J. B. Wyngaarden, and D. S. Fredrickson. McGraw-Hill, New York (*in press*).

56. Suzuki, K., Suzuki, K., and Chen, G. C. (1966): Metachromatic leucodystrophy: Isolation and chemical analysis of metachromatic granules. *Science,* 151:1231–1233.

57. Suzuki, K., Suzuki, K., and Chen, G. C. (1967): Isolation and chemical characterization of metachromatic granules from a brain with metachromatic leukodystrophy. *J. Neuropathol. Exp. Neurol.,* 26:537–550.

58. Suzuki, K., Suzuki, K., and Kamoshita, S. (1969): Chemical pathology of G_{M1}-gangliosidosis (generalized gangliosidosis). *J. Neuropathol. Exp. Neurol.,* 28:25–73.

59. Suzuki, Y., Tucker, S. H., Rorke, L. B., and Suzuki, K. (1970): Ultrastructural and biochemical studies of Schilder's disease. II. Biochemistry. *J. Neuropathol. Exp. Neurol.,* 29:405–419.

60. Svennerholm, L. (1963): Some aspects of the biochemical changes in leucodystrophy. In: *Brain Lipids and Lipoproteins and the Leukodystrophies,* edited by J. Folch-Pi and H. Bauer, pp. 104–119. Elsevier, Amsterdam.

61. Tsuchiya, Y., Numabe, T., and Yokoi, S. (1970): Neuropathological and neurochemical studies of three cases of sudanophilic leukodystrophy. *Acta Neuropathol. (Berl),* 16:353–366.

62. Webster, H. deF. (1962): Schwann cell alterations in metachromatic leucodystrophy: Preliminary phase and electron microscopic observations. *J. Neuropathol. Exp. Neurol.,* 21:534–554.

63. Weinberg, H. J., and Spencer, P. S. (1976): Studies on the control of myelinogenesis. II. Evidence for neuronal regulation of myelin production. *Brain Res.,* 113:363–378.

64. Wolfgram, F. (1972): Chemical theories of the demyelination in multiple sclerosis. In: *Multiple Sclerosis, Immunology, Virology and*

Ultrastructure, edited by F. Wolfgram, G. W. Ellison, J. G. Stevens, and J. M. Andrews, pp. 173–182. Academic Press, New York.

65. Wolfgram, F., Fewster, M. E., and Mead, J. F. (1971): Lipids and amino acids of mul-

tiple sclerosis myelin. *Riv. Patol. Nerv. Ment.,* pp. 96–100.

66. Yunis, E. J., and Lee, R. E. (1969): The ultrastructure of globoid (Krabbe) leukodystrophy. *Lab. Invest.,* 21:415–419.

Physiology and Pathobiology of Axons, edited by
S. G. Waxman. Raven Press, New York © 1978.

Physiology of Dying-Back Neuropathies

Austin Sumner

Department of Neurology, University of Pennsylvania, Philadelphia, Pennsylvania 19104

In 1896 Seymour J. Sharkey, Physician to
St. Thomas Hospital, made the following observations in a lecture delivered in London
(37): "It is somewhat remarkable that in
multiple neuritis the terminal portion of the
nerves are nearly always first affected. Why
is this? May it be partly that they are so delicate in structure, partly because in their peripheral ramifications they cover a much larger
area than they do when collapsed into bundles,
and so are more exposed to the poison circulating in the capillaries; partly perhaps because
they are farthest removed from the nerve cells,
on the energy radiating from which their
health certainly depends."

More than 80 years later we are still quite
ignorant of the cause of this stereotyped response of neurons to a wide variety of toxic
and metabolic insults. The term "dying-back
reaction" was introduced to describe a characteristic pattern of peripheral nerve fiber pathology in which the earliest degeneration occurs in the distal portion of axons and, in time,
spreads slowly more proximally (7,39). In the
case of primary sensory neurons, degenerative
changes occur terminally at both peripheral
and central extensions of axons (33–35,38).
The polyneuropathies associated with chronic
alcoholism, uremia, multiple myeloma, carcinoma, malnutrition, diabetes, heavy metal
poisoning, and certain toxic chemicals and
drugs are generally accepted as examples of
dying-back neuropathies. It is usually assumed
that an effect on the cell body itself results in
a failure to maintain the integrity of the most
distant portions of the cell cytoplasm, i.e., the
terminal axon. Abnormalities in the perikaryon
synthesis (1) and slowing of axoplasmic transport (32) were postulated mechanisms whereby

such a change could be effected, but both of
these observations have been challenged (3),
and to date there is insufficient evidence to
conclude that a primary somal defect is responsible for the dying-back reaction.

The pattern of nerve terminal degeneration
appears to be essentially the same as Wallerian
degeneration and as such is clearly distinguished from those types of polyneuropathy in
which the Schwann cell and myelin sheath are
primarily involved. As our understanding of
the pathophysiology of dying-back neuropathies is based in large measure on our more
complete understanding of Wallerian degeneration, it is appropriate at the onset to review
the neurophysiological changes associated with
classical Wallerian degeneration as studied in
experimental animals and man.

NERVE CONDUCTION IN WALLERIAN DEGENERATION

The concomitant destruction of axon and
myelin was originally described by Waller (46)
in the distal stump of the sectioned glossopharyngeal and hypoglossal nerves of the frog.
It is not proposed to review the sequence of
morphological changes in detail. Suffice it to
say that the earliest degenerative changes are
visible in the terminal arborization of the
motor axon and in the endplates themselves
(14,17,30). These changes are followed by
disintegration of axons setting in more or less
simultaneously at different points along their
length.

Conduction ceases altogether in a sectioned
peripheral nerve after a few days. The time to
conduction failure varies considerably in different species (14). Conduction failure is pre-

ceded by a progressive reduction in the size of the whole nerve action in the distal part of the nerve stump (6). The maximum conduction velocity and distal motor latency do not change until almost all nerve fibers have ceased to conduct. At this stage distal latency is increased and conduction velocity is often mildly decreased. Whether this reduction is due to a change in individual fiber conduction or simply to the longer survival of axons with a relatively slow velocity is not known. There is failure of neuromuscular transmission before conduction fails in peripheral nerve trunks (14).

Alterations in conduction have also been described in nerve trunks *proximal* to lesions. Cragg and Thomas (8) used four kinds of lesion—crush, constriction, section followed by end-to-end suture of the cut ends, and section with avulsion of the distal stump—to investigate proximal conduction velocity changes in the rabbit peroneal nerve. With the former three types of lesion, maximum conduction velocity was reduced slightly to 80–90% of normal for some 150 days but had virtually returned to normal by 200 days. By contrast, in those animals in which the distal stump was avulsed, the velocity continued to decrease and at 400 days was 60% of normal. Cragg and Thomas were able to relate these conduction velocity changes to axon diameter. Axons decreased in size proximal to nerve section but returned to normal if reinnervation was successful. When reinnervation was prevented, axon diameter continued to decrease, although this may not be the only explanation for the decreased conduction velocity. Some decrease may be due to large-fiber degeneration. In rats a diminution of the number of nerve cells by 16% is seen 24 months after nerve section if regeneration is obstructed (45). There is no convincing evidence of significant proximal degeneration after nerve section in man.

In man an apparent decrease in maximum conduction velocity was reported in the proximal nerve trunk after traumatic section and suture of the median and ulnar nerves at the wrist (13), after compression of the deep branch of the ulnar nerve in the hand (9), and in the carpal tunnel syndrome (44). The significance of these findings is open to question, however, because the recording sites in these observations were distal to the lesion. Thus conduction block in the fast-conduction fibers at the level of the lesion could account for this apparent slowing (44). In carpal tunnel syndrome ascending nerve action potential velocities in the forearm are usually normal.

NERVE CONDUCTION IN DYING-BACK NEUROPATHY

Following the observations of Lambert and colleagues (18,24) that nerve conduction velocities were strikingly slowed in some forms of human polyneuropathy, the technique of nerve conduction velocity measurement has found widespread application in the assessment of patients with peripheral nerve disease. It was soon clearly established that marked slowing of nerve conduction velocities was associated with segmental demyelination af axons. In the dying-back axonal type of polyneuropathies, conduction velocity changes were less impressive, and it was generally concluded that in this situation if a fiber is capable of conducting impulses at all it does so normally. The most striking changes from an electrophysiological point of view is a diminution in the number of functioning fibers rather than a change in conduction velocity.

In line with the concept of dying-back response being analogous to Wallerian degeneration, Kaeser and Lambert (22) compared the findings in experimental thallium poisoning with those following nerve section. In both instances velocity showed very little change until no response could be elicited by nerve stimulation. Thallium poisoning, however, does not prove to be a very convenient experimental model of a dying-back neuropathy. Large doses killed a high proportion of animals, and small doses did not affect the peripheral nerves at all.

EXPERIMENTAL ACRYLAMIDE NEUROPATHY

Although there is a number of neurotoxins available to produce an axonal-type polyneuropathy in animals, acrylamide neuropathy has many advantages that have resulted in it becoming the most closely studied experimental model. It produces a relatively pure axonal-type degeneration, and animals generally remain well, maintaining body weight, general health, and grooming until the neuropathy is well advanced.

Acrylamide ($CH_2 = CHOCNH_2$) is a low-molecular-weight monomer which itself has very little industrial use. The polymer, however, is extensively employed by industry. It is used as a soil groating agent in tunneling operations, as a flocculator for improving the dry strength of chipboard, as coating for paper, and by biochemists for polyacrylamide gel electrophoresis. The polymer is nontoxic, but cases of polyneuropathy occurring in those handling the monomer have been reported from many countries (2,12). It is neurotoxic to all laboratory animals in which it has been studied (mice, rats, cats, baboons, and rhesus monkeys), but a biochemical basis for its neurotoxicity remains obscure.

Fullerton and Barnes (11) and Hopkins and Gilliatt (19) studied the electrophysiological changes in acrylamide neuropathy in rats and baboons, respectively. In rats with severe clinical neuropathy, motor conduction velocity in the nerve to the hind paw was reduced to approximately 80% of the control value. When paralyzed animals were no longer given acrylamide, they recovered from their weakness and conduction velocities returned to normal values. In baboons the observed decline in motor conduction velocities was somewhat greater. In some animals the anterior tibial velocity fell to 51% of the control value. In both studies histological evidence of selective large-fiber degeneration was found, and it was concluded that the conduction velocity slowing was a consequence of this large-fiber loss, with presumably normal conduction being preserved in intact smaller-diameter axons. In baboons some motor axons normally conduct at as little as 55% of the maximum (15).

SINGLE-FIBER STUDIES IN ACRYLAMIDE NEUROPATHY

Electrophysiological observations on the whole nerve population have not clarified the effects of a dying-back neuropathy on the function of individual axons. Does physiological function fail in the terminal portions of the axon? Do individual axons conduct at nor-

mal velocities? Are axons of certain size or function selectively affected? It should be possible to answer these questions in a dying-back neuropathy by studying the responses of single units isolated in fine dorsal and ventral root filaments in animals with acrylamide neuropathy. (40,42).

Figure 1 illustrates compound action potentials elicited from stimulation of the nerve to medial gastrocnemius and recorded from the whole L7 dorsal root. The upper recording is from a control animal, the lower from a cat with acrylamide neuropathy demonstrating moderately severe hind limb ataxia, weakness and loss of tendon jerks. In spite of the obvious clinical deficit in the neuropathic animal, these recordings indicate that muscle afferent fibers were normally excitable and conducted at normal rates. The dorsal root filaments were then teased apart until a number of the single axons making up the compound action potential were systemically sampled. Each unit had a conduction velocity and could be tested for physiological responsive-

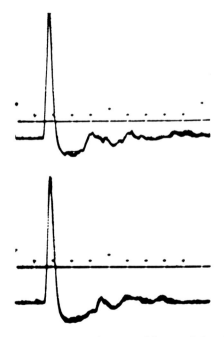

FIG. 1. Compound action potentials recorded at the same gain from the whole L7 dorsal root in a control animal (*top*) and an animal with moderately severe acrylamide neuropathy: acrylamide 10 mg/kg for 38 days (*bottom*). Timer 1 and 5 meters/sec.

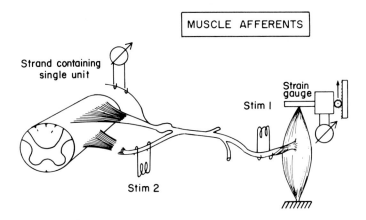

FIG. 2. Recording arrangement for studying the responses of single stretch afferents from the medial gastrocnemius.

ness. The recording arrangement is illustrated in Fig. 2. In cat medial gastrocnemius, almost all group I (> 72 meters/sec) and group II (24–72 meters/sec) afferents arise from muscle stretch receptors. These are either muscle spindles (groups IA and II) or tendon organs (group IB). The responses of these two types of muscle stretch receptor can be easily distinguished by their classic patterns of response to muscle stretch or muscle contraction (20,25) (Fig. 3). It soon became clear that in neuropathic animals many single units were isolated that conducted at velocities which indicated that they supplied stretch receptors; yet muscle stretch or muscle contraction failed to elicit any physiological response. These nonresponsive units are believed to result from terminal failure of conduction in neuropathic fibers, as would be predicted by the dying-back concept. When the pooled samples of single units isolated from animals with mild, moderate, or severe neuropathy are compared (Fig. 4), there is a sharp increase in the proportion of nonresponsive stretch afferents, rising from only 10% of the sample from mildly affected

animals to 89% of the sample of severely disabled animals. Single units that remained responsive continued to conduct within their normal velocity range. Thus the two surviving tendon organ afferents in Fig. 4C still conduct at greater than 72 meters/sec, in sharp contrast with the findings in a demyelinative type polyneuropathy (27). Study of these histograms also confirms what other investigators had suspected: that large-diameter fibers seem more prone to fail than fibers of smaller size.

Cutaneous afferent fiber responses from the sural nerve can be studied by a similar technique (41). In Fig. 5 is illustrated the sural compound action potentials recorded from the S1 root from a control animal, an animal with severe acrylamide neuropathy, and one with a similar clinical disability resulting from administration of diphtheria toxin (28). In the diphtheritic neuropathy it is obvious that the very low amplitude response indicates failure of conduction in many axons of those units making up the dispersed response; it is also clear that conduction velocities are very slow. These findings characterize the demyelinative

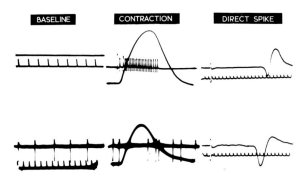

FIG. 3. Identification of single stretch afferents by responses of tendon stretch (baseline) and muscle contraction. A tendon organ response is illustrated above and a muscle spindle below. The conduction velocity of each axon is calculated from the response latency and the nerve length measured at the end of each experiment.

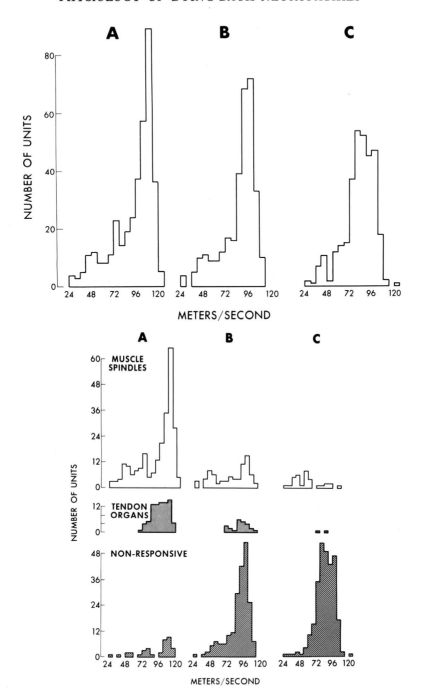

FIG. 4. Histograms of single stretch afferents accumulated by systematically teasing dorsal root filaments in cats with mild (A), moderate (B), and severe (C) neuropathy. The total populations (**top**) are subdivided (**bottom**) into functioning muscle spindles, tendon organ afferents, or nonresponsive afferents. (From ref. 42.)

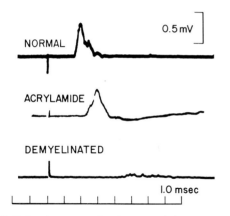

FIG. 5. Sural compound action potentials recorded in the S1 dorsal root from normal (*top*), acrylamide (*center*), and diphtheria-intoxicated animals (*bottom*). (The demyelinated response is from ref. 28.)

type of polyneuropathy. By contrast, in an equally disabled acrylamide animal, the compound action potential is of near-normal amplitude and velocity. However, when the responsiveness of these axons is tested by physiological stimulation of the skin, it is again apparent that many are nonresponsive. Almost 80% of A-alpha fibers (Fig. 6) in this population were nonresponsive. In the case of A-delta fibers (i.e., those conducting at less than 36 meters/sec), the percentage of nonresponsive fibers was much lower. If allowance is made for nociceptor afferents, which would not be activated by the physiological stimulation used in these experiments (5), only approximately one-third of these small fibers were nonresponsive. It seems clear both in the case of the muscle afferents and cutaneous afferents that large-diameter fibers are two to three times more likely to be neuropathic than small-diameter fibers of the same length.

Again, the distinctive difference in the effects of axonal degeneration and demyelination is illustrated by comparing the histograms of hair units (Fig. 7) and touch units (Fig. 8) between normals, acrylamide, and diphtheria neuropathies. In the dying-back neuropathy, functioning units retain their normal conduction properties, whereas in the demyelinative

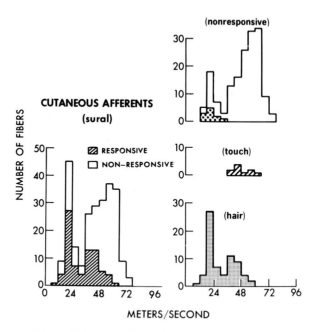

FIG. 6. Histogram of a sampled population of single sural cutaneous afferents in cats with acrylamide neuropathy. The solid line (*left*) illustrates the whole population. The shaded portion shows those axons which responded to skin stimulation. The population is further subdivided into nonresponsive, touch, and hair units (*right*). Allowance must be made for nociceptor afferents (*checked, right*), which would not be activated by the physiological stimulation used in these experiments.

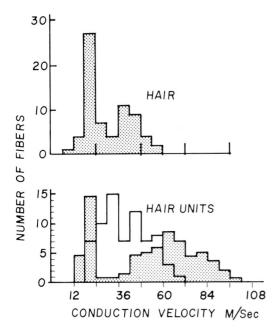

FIG. 7. Distribution of responsive hair units in acrylamide neuropathy (*shaded, top*) is compared with distribution of hair units in normals (*shaded, below*) and in diphtheritic neuropathy (*unshaded, below*). Note that the distribution of units remains bimodal in acrylamide neuropathy but with a loss of the faster-conducting fibers. In diphtheritic neuropathy the distribution of these units is shifted to the left. (Normal hair units and diphtheritic units are from refs. 21 and 28, respectively.)

neuropathy functioning units are isolated that conduct at much slower velocities than those found in normal animals.

Peripheral fiber size, however, is not the only determinant of susceptibility to the neurotoxic effects of acrylamide. The response of single motor axons teased from ventral root filaments can also be assessed by these methods (40,42). Figure 9 illustrates that the functional responses of motor axons can be determined by measuring the tension produced in the medial gastronemius following single-unit stimulation. Nonresponsive axons were those which produced measurable tension in the muscle. The histogram of the population of single motor axons is illustrated in Fig. 10.

Note that none of the axons conducting at less than 48 meters/sec produced muscle tension. This is a normal finding, as these fibers are the fusimotor supply to the muscle

spindles. Surprisingly, however, of the 201 α-motor fibers, only 10% failed to produce tension at a time when afferent fibers of the same size to the same muscle were more than 80% nonresponsive. In the cat at least, sensory fibers are much more susceptible to the neurotoxic effects of acrylamide than are motor fibers. The reason for this is obscure, but it is tempting to speculate that it too relates to cell size. Sensory neurons of course have both peripheral and central extensions and therefore have much more cytoplasm than motor neurons which have but a single peripheral axon. The ability of a large cell to maintain itself against a toxic insult may be less than that of a small cell. With sensory neurons it is quite apparent that this cell size susceptibility holds true.

Schaumberg et al. (36), in an elegant ultrastructural study of acrylamide neuropathy, demonstrated that the primary endings of muscle spindles degenerate before secondary ends, and these both before there is any evidence of breakdown in adjacent motor endplates. They noted incidentally that the earliest ultrastructural changes occurred in the Pacinian corpuscles of the cat's hindpaw. The peripheral axon subserving these receptors is smaller than that from the primary spindle ending, but the central extensions of these footpad receptor axons are the fastest conducting fibers in the dorsal columns (4). Thus it appears likely that these are among the largest sensory neurons in the cat when both peripheral and cen-

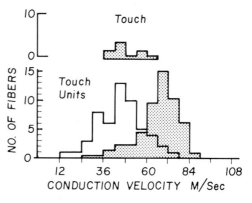

FIG. 8. As in Fig. 7, the distribution of sural touch afferents in acrylamide neuropathy (*shaded, above*), diphtheritic neuropathy (*open, below*), and normals (*shaded, below*) is compared.

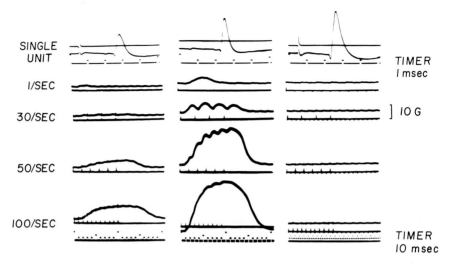

FIG. 9. Responses of three single motor fibers (conductive velocities 72.8, 87.5, and 86.5 meters/sec, respectively in a cat with acrylamide neuropathy. The first two units produce a twitch or tetanic response in medial gastrocnemius when electrically excited. The third unit, a nonresponsive motor axon, does not.

tral portions of the cell are considered, and observations to date are consistent with the cell size hypothesis.

REGENERATION IN A DYING-BACK NEUROPATHY

With a cessation of the administration of acrylamide, neuropathy usually progresses for some weeks and then often recovers completely. In contrast to peripheral nerve regeneration after nerve section, motor conduction velocities return to normal. This rapid recovery and complete restoration of axon size is probably a consequence of the axon dying-back but a short distance from its end-organ.

If nerve regeneration proceeds so effectively after withdrawal of the toxin, is the regenerative ability of the nerve impaired during the administration of acrylamide? Regeneration in the peripheral nervous system appears to depend first on the initial outgrowth of the axon and second on the supply of axoplasmic proteins from the cell body. Little is known about

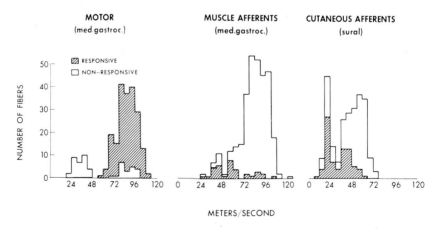

FIG. 10. Histograms of the populations of single muscle efferents, muscle afferents, and cutaneous afferents are compared. Note that the relative portion of responsive units (*shaded*) is much higher for motor fibers than sensory fibers of comparable conduction velocity.

the factors responsible for the outgrowths of the axon, but it seems clear that the supply of axoplasm is essential for the normal maturation of regenerating nerve fibers (47,48). If current ideas about the dying-back process are correct—that there is a primary biochemical lesion in the cell body—then the process of regeneration and maturation might be expected to be abnormal. Morgan-Hughes et al. (31) studied regeneration following nerve crush in rats with acrylamide neuropathy. The pattern of peripheral nerve regeneration was profoundly affected. In some fibers regeneration was completely inhibited, whereas in others the rate of growth was delayed and fibers remained immature. In spite of this, a proportion of fibers did successfully re-establish functional contact with their end-organs, but this took at least twice as long as in control animals. Because regenerative motor fibers were hypoplastic in acrylamide animals, motor conduction velocities were lower than those recorded in regenerated fibers in normal animals. Hypoplastic regenerating fibers may be the explanation for the prolonged distal latencies that are sometimes recorded in *chronic* as opposed to *acute* axonal neuropathies in man (10,26). Morgan-Hughes et al. (31) concluded that this altered pattern of nerve regeneration was compatible with the hypothesis of either a defect in the synthesis of axoplasmic protein by the neuron or a defect in their transport along the fiber. In addition, they were impressed by the number of fibers that showed no evidence of regeneration at all. Instead, these fibers terminated in bulbous axonal swellings concentrated over a 2-cm segment of sciatic nerve immediately around the site of crush. In these fibers it was suggested that acrylamide may have inhibited the initial outgrowth of the axon.

AXOPLASMIC FLOW IN DYING-BACK NEUROPATHIES

Studies of axoplasmic flow in dying-back neuropathy provided rather conflicting results. Pleasure et al. (32) found that the slow phase ceased in the dorsal roots of cats with acrylamide neuropathy but that protein transport was normal in animals poisoned with triorthocresyl phosphate (TOCP). Bradley and Williams (3) studied fast and slow transport

rates and were unable to confirm these findings. They concluded that flow rates were not significantly altered in acrylamide neuropathy. A more recent study (43) demonstrated a small (10%) reduction in the rate of fast axoplasmic transport, while confirming Bradley and Williams' observation that slow transport was normal. Direct injections of small amounts of acrylamide into the dorsal root ganglion resulted in a sharp reduction in the amount of labeled protein that was transported by fast flow (43). These authors speculate that acrylamide alters the *amount* rather than the *rate* of protein transported to the periphery.

In a study designed to elucidate the role of axonal transport in the impaired regeneration of a dying-back neuropathy Griffin et al. (16) showed that the terminal bulbs of unregenerated axons were heavily labeled by transported radioactivity. They concluded that the impaired regeneration was the result of failure of utilization, rather than the failure of delivery of transport materials.

CONCLUSIONS

It is probably a correct assumption that the many axonal neuropathies encountered in neurological practice due to alcoholism, uremia, multiple myeloma, carcinoma, vitamin deficiency, drug toxicity, and other toxic chemicals are of the dying-back type. However, only the neuropathies produced by acrylamide, *n*-hexane and its analogs methyl-*n*-butyl ketone (MBK) and 2,5-hexanedione, triorthocresylphosphate, and thiamine deficiency have been studied in sufficient detail to justify this conclusion. Others claim that Friedreich's ataxia, the neuronal type of Charcot-Marie-Tooth and even amyotrophic lateral sclerosis are examples of the dying-back phenomenon, but in these conditions the neurons themselves degenerate and there is no firm evidence available that the pattern of peripheral nerve degeneration in these diseases is of the dying-back type.

The essential histological features of the dying-back response is the demonstration of axonal degeneration, often beginning multifocally, in the terminal portions of axons both peripherally and centrally, without neuronal degeneration. In clinical practice nerve conduction studies are extremely helpful. In axonal neuropathies velocities may be normal or mildly reduced. Most of the conduction velocity reduction in acute axonal neuropathies is due to selective degeneration of the larger-diameter fibers. In more chronic or intermittent neuropathies like alcoholism or uremia, greater degrees of conduction slowing may be found, especially in the terminal portion of nerves, owing to slowed conduction in hypoplastic regenerating axons. The axonal neuropathies produced by the aliphatic hydrocarbons form an exception to this general rule (23). There, axonal swelling at nodes results in marked paranodal retraction, and this secondary demyelination is associated with marked conduction slowing. It is indistinguishable by electrodiagnosis from a primary demyelinative neuropathy.

Because degeneration begins so terminally, conventional sensory and motor conduction studies may not be the most sensitive ways of detecting early disease. Experimental studies indicate that function is interrupted well before axonal degeneration is visible in nerve trunks. A modification of McLeod's (29) technique of eliciting a sensory action potential by mechanical stimulation of the nail bed is likely to prove valuable in clinical practice.

ACKNOWLEDGMENT

This work was supported in part by USPHS grants N.S. 121301-01 and N.S. 08075–09.

REFERENCES

1. Asbury, A. K., Cox, S. C., and Kanada, D. (1973): ^{3}H-Leucine incorporation in acrylamide neuropathy in the mouse. *Neurology (Minneap)*, 23:406 (abstract).
2. Auld, R. B., and Bedwell, S. F. (1967): Peripheral neuropathy with sympathetic overactivity from industrial contact with acrylamide. *Can. Med. Assoc. J.*, 96:652–654.
3. Bradley, W. C., and Williams, M. H. (1973): Axoplasmic flow in axonal neuropathies. I. Axoplasmic flow in cats with toxic neuropathies. *Brain*, 96:235–246.
4. Brown, A. G. (1968): Cutaneous afferent fiber collaterals in the dorsal column of the cat. *Exp. Brain Res.*, 5:293–305.
5. Burgess, P. R., and Perl, E. R. (1967): Myelinated afferent fibers responding specifically to noxious stimulation of the skin. *J. Physiol. (Lond)*, 190:541–562.
6. Causey, G., and Stratmann, C. J. (1953): The spread of failure of conduction in degenerating mammalian nerve. *J. Physiol. (Lond)*, 121:215–223.
7. Cavanaugh, J. B. (1964): The significance of the "dying-back" process in experimental and human neurological disease. *Int. Rev. Exp. Pathol.*, 3:219–267.
8. Cragg, B. G., and Thomas, P. K. (1961): Changes in conduction velocity and fiber size proximal to peripheral nerve lesions. *J. Physiol. (Lond)*, 157:315–327.
9. Ebeling, P., Gilliatt, R. W., and Thomas, P. K. (1960): A clinical and electrical study of ulnar nerve lesions in the hand. *J. Neurol. Neurosurg. Psychiatry*, 23:1.
10. Fullerton, P. M. (1969): Electrophysiological and histological observations in peripheral nerves in man. *J. Neurol. Neurosurg. Psychiatry*, 23:186–192.
11. Fullerton, P. M., and Barnes, J. M. (1966): Peripheral neuropathy in rats produced by acrylamide. *Br. J. Ind. Med.*, 23:210–221.
12. Garland, T. O., and Patterson, M. W. H. (1967): Six cases of acrylamide poisoning. *Br. Med. J.*, 4:134–138.
13. Gilliatt, R. W. (1961): In: *Electrodiagnosis and Electromyography*, edited by S. Licht. Waverly Press, Baltimore.
14. Gilliatt, R. W., and Hjorth, R. J. (1972): Nerve conduction during wallerian degeneration in the baboon. *J. Neurol. Neurosurg. Psychiatry*, 35:335–341.
15. Gilliatt, R. W., Hopf, H. C., Rudge, P., and Baraitser, M. (1976): Axonal velocities of motor units in the hand and foot muscle of the baboon. *J. Neurol. Sci.*, 29:249–258.
16. Griffin, J. W., Price, D. L., and Drachman, D. B. (1976): Impaired regeneration in acrylamide neuropathy: Role of axoplasmic transport. *Neurology (Minneap)*, 26:350.
17. Gutmann, E., and Holubar, J. (1952): Degeneration in terminal organs in cross striated and smooth muscle. *Physiol. Bohemoslov.*, 1:168 (in Russian).
18. Henriksen, J. D. (1956): Conduction velocity of motor nerves in normal subjects and patients with neuromuscular disorders. M.S. thesis, University of Minnesota.
19. Hopkins, A. P., and Gilliatt, R. W. (1971): Motor and sensory nerve conduction velocity in the baboon: Normal values and changes during acrylamide neuropathy. *J. Neurol. Neurosurg. Psychiatry*, 34:415–426.
20. Hunt, C. C. (1954): Relation of function to diameter in afferent fibers of muscle nerves. *J. Gen. Physiol.*, 38:117–131.
21. Hunt, C. C., and McIntyre, A. K. (1960): Analysis of fiber diameter and receptor characteristics of myelinated cutaneous afferent fibers in the cat. *J. Physiol. (Lond)*, 153:99–112.
22. Kaeser, H. E., and Lambert, E. H. (1962): Nerve function studies in experimental poly-

neuritis. *Electroencephalogr. Clin. Neurophysiol.* (*Suppl.*), 22:29–35.

23. Korobkin, R., Asbury, A. K., Sumner, A. J., and Nielsen, S. L. (1975): Glue-sniffing neuropathy. *Arch. Neurol.*, 32:158–162.

24. Lambert, E. H. (1956): Electromyography and electrical stimulation of peripheral nerves in muscle. In: *Clinical Examination in Neurology.* Mayo Clinic, Philadelphia.

25. Matthews, B. H. C. (1933): Nerve endings in mammalian muscles. *J. Physiol.* (*Lond*), 78:1.

26. Mawdsley, C., and Mayer, R. F. (1965): Nerve conduction in alcoholic polyneuropathy. *Brain*, 88:335.

27. McDonald, W. I. (1962): Conduction in muscle afferent fibers during experimental demyelination in cat nerve. *Acta Neuropathol.* (*Berl*), 1:425–432.

28. McDonald, W. I. (1963): The effects of experimental demyelination in conduction in peripheral nerve: a histological and electrophysiological study. II. Electrophysiological observations. *Brain*, 86:501–524.

29. McLeod, J. G. (1966): Digital nerve conduction in the carpal tunnel syndrome after mechanical stimulation of the finger. *J. Neurol. Neurosurg. Psychiatry*, 29:12–22.

30. Miledi, R., and Slater, C. R. (1970): On the degeneration of rat neuromuscular junctions after nerve section. *J. Physiol.* (*Lond*), 207:507–528.

31. Morgan-Hughes, J., Sinclair, S., and Durston, J. H. J. (1974): The pattern of peripheral nerve regeneration induced by crush in rats with severe acrylamide neuropathy. *Brain*, 97:232–250.

32. Pleasure, D. E., Mischler, K. C., and Engel, W. K. (1969): Axonal transport of proteins in experimental neuropathies. *Science*, 166:524.

33. Prineas, J. (1969): The pathogenesis of dying-back polyneuropathies. I. An ultrastructural study of experimental tri-orthocresyl phosphate intoxication in the cat. *J. Neuropathol. Exp. Neurol.*, 28:571–597.

34. Prineas, J. (1969): The pathogenesis of dying-back polyneuropathies. II. An ultrastructural study of experimental acrylamide intoxication in the cat. *J. Neuropathol. Exp. Neurol.*, 28:598–621.

35. Prineas, J. (1970): Peripheral nerve changes in thiamine deficient rats. *Arch. Neurol.*, 23:541–548.

36. Schaumberg, H. H., Wiśneiwski, H. M., and Spencer, P. S. (1974): Ultrastructural studies of the dying-back process. I. Peripheral nerve terminal degeneration in acrylamide intoxication. *J. Neuropathol. Exp. Neurol.*, 33:260–284.

37. Sharkey, S. J. (1896): On peripheral neuritis. *Br. Med. J.*, 1:456–458.

38. Spencer, P. S., and Schaumberg, H. H. (1977): IV. Ultrastructural studies of the dying-back process. *J. Neuropathol. Exp. Neurol.*, 36:300–320.

39. Swank, R. L. (1940): Avian thiamine deficiency. *J. Exp. Med.*, 71:683–702.

40. Sumner, A. J. (1975): Early discharge of muscle afferents in acrylamide neuropathy. *J. Physiol.* (*Lond*), 246:277–288.

41. Sumner, A. J., and Asbury, A. K. (1974): Acrylamide neuropathy: Selective vulnerability of sensory fibers. *Arch. Neurol.*, 30:419 (abstract).

42. Sumner, A. J., and Asbury, A. K. (1975): Physiological studies of the dying-back phenomenon. I. Effects of acrylamide on muscle stretch afferents. *Brain*, 98:91–100.

43. Sumner, A. J., Pleasure, D., and Ciesielka, K. (1976): Slowing of fast axoplasmic transport in acrylamide neuropathy. *J. Neuropathol. Exp. Neurol.*, 35:319.

44. Thomas, P. K. (1960): Motor nerve conduction in the carpal tunnel syndrome. *Neurology* (*Minneap*), 10:1045–1050.

45. Turner, R. S. (1943): Chromatolysis and recovery of efferent neurons. *J. Comp. Neurol.*, 79:73.

46. Waller, A. (1850): XX. Experiments on the section of the glossopharyngeal and hypoglossal nerves of the frog, and observations of the alterations produced thereby in the structure of their primitive fibers. (Communicated by Professor Owen, F.R.S.) *Philos. Trans.*, 140:423–429.

47. Weiss, P. (1969): Neuronal dynamics and neuroplasmic ("axonal") flow. In: *Cellular Dynamics of the Neuron*, vol. 8. Edited by S. H. Barondes. Academic Press, New York.

48. Weiss, P., and Hiscoe, H. B. (1948): Experiments on the mechanism of nerve growth. *J. Exp. Zool.*, 107:315.

Physiology and Pathobiology of Axons, edited by
S. G. Waxman. Raven Press, New York © 1978.

Physiology of Conduction in Demyelinated Axons

Michael Rasminsky

*Division of Neurology, Montreal General Hospital, Montreal, Quebec, H3G 1A4 Canada; and
Department of Neurology and Neurosurgery, McGill University, Montreal, Quebec, Canada*

A major function of nerve fibers is to transmit information reliably from one site to another. When an axon is severed this function is lost. If the axon of a myelinated fiber remains in continuity despite alterations or local absence of its myelin sheath, the fiber may retain its ability to conduct nervous impulses, but the information the fiber transmits may reach its destination in a distorted form. This chapter reviews what is currently known about conduction of nervous impulses in axons with abnormalities of the myelin sheath.

The term demyelination embraces a spectrum of abnormalities ranging from minimal changes in paranodal morphology to complete absence of myelin over entire internodes. Conduction in demyelinated nerve has been studied in a variety of experimental preparations in the peripheral and central nervous systems. These include nerve compression (4,24,31,32,61); diphtheritic neuropathy, both systemic (44, 62,64,72) and focal in the peripheral (82,86) and central (69,70) nervous systems; experimental allergic neuritis (EAN) (17,19,36); experimental granuloma of nerve (54); and lead neuropathy (30). Despite marked differences in morphology in the various types of demyelination (78), no physiological findings appear to be unique to any type or site of demyelination. In particular, no findings unique to central nervous system (CNS) demyelination have been reported. In discussions of the functional implications of demyelination, it is conventionally assumed that physiological findings in peripheral demyelinated fibers are also applicable to CNS demyelination (64,65, 68,82).

Conduction has also been studied in the nerves of dystrophic (39,85) and trembler

(57,58) mice, two genetic strains with congenital deficiencies of myelination (2,13,15,-55,56). The physiological findings in these mice are similar to those reported in demyelinated nerves.

Some properties of demyelinated fibers (e.g., decreased conduction velocity, conduction block, and increased refractory period) are explicable solely (but not necessarily exclusively) in terms of alterations in fiber geometry and are reproduced in computer simulations of demyelinated nerve. Other properties lend themselves less readily to explanation exclusively in terms of altered structure. For example, the distribution of electrical excitability in demyelinated or bare axons may reflect changes in axonal properties caused by disruption of the normal intimate relationship between axons and their enveloping glial cells.

This chapter is primarily concerned with the electrophysiological abnormalities of demyelinated nerve fibers and the mechanisms underlying these abnormalities, but also includes a brief discussion of the possible relationships of certain clinical findings in demyelinating disease to the various physiological phenomena characteristic of demyelinated nerve fibers.

CONDUCTION BLOCK AND DECREASED CONDUCTION VELOCITY

The earliest studies of the physiological properties of demyelinated nerve were performed during World War II by Denny-Brown and Brenner (24), who produced focal demyelinating lesions in cat nerves with tourniquet compression or percussion. Electrical stimulation distal to the site of a demyelinating lesion caused a normal muscle contraction which was not evoked when the same nerve was stimulated proximal to the site of the lesion. This provided the first inferential evidence for conduction block at the site of a demyelinating lesion. Direct recordings of compound action potentials from focally demyelinated nerves subsequently established that conduction proceeded normally along the morphologically normal portion of the nerve and that conduction block (as manifested by the disappearance of the compound action potential) did indeed occur at the junction of normal and demyelinated parts of the same nerve (61,64).

Conduction block is the extreme consequence of demyelination; in less severe lesions conduction is preserved. The compound action potential recorded from demyelinated nerve is characteristically delayed, dispersed, and reduced in amplitude (17,54,61,64). These findings are compatible with blockage of conduction and decreased conduction velocity in fibers contributing to the compound action potential. By comparing the frequency distribution of conduction velocities of various types of afferent receptors in cats with systemic diphtheritic neuritis and normal cats, McDonald (62,64) established that conduction velocity was reduced in single nerve fibers as a result of demyelination. Hall (36) reported similar findings for guinea pigs with EAN. McDonald and Gilman (67) showed that conduction velocity was reduced in single nerve fibers in the area of demyelination and normal in the morphologically normal portion of the same nerve.

Demyelination in the CNS caused by focal microinjection of diphtheria toxin has similar consequences. In severe lesions there is conduction block at the site of the lesion (69,70); in less severe lesions conduction velocity in single fibers is decreased within the zone of demyelination (70).

MODE OF CONDUCTION IN DEMYELINATED NERVE FIBERS

The methods originally used to establish that conduction velocity was reduced in single demyelinated fibers did not permit any conclusions regarding the mechanism responsible for conduction slowing. Conduction of nervous impulses is saltatory in peripheral (41,99) and central (11,98) myelinated nerve fibers. During excitation each node generates inward membrane current, which in turn stimulates the adjacent node to activity; the intervening internodal axon membrane remains inactive, generating no inward membrane current. It has been unclear whether the internodal axon membrane is inactive because it is inherently inexcitable or simply because it is insulated with the myelin sheath (86). In unmyelinated nerve fibers the axon membrane is uniformly excitable, and conduction is continuous; during transmission of a nervous impulse, each patch of axon membrane generates inward membrane current, which in turn stimulates the adjacent patch of membrane to activity. Conduction in unmyelinated fibers proceeds relatively slowly because of the large capacitance of uninsulated axon membrane.

Decreased conduction velocity in demyelinated nerve fibers could in principle be due to: (a) preservation of saltatory conduction with increased delay between excitation of successive nodes, or (b) reversion to continuous conduction along demyelinated internodal axon. Both mechanisms have now been observed in peripheral demyelinated fibers (12, 86) using the preparation developed by Rasminsky and Sears (86) to study conduction in single fibers of undissected rat spinal roots.

Saltatory Conduction

In normal myelinated fibers the time course of external longitudinal current is abruptly displaced at each successive node of Ranvier (41,86), average internodal conduction time being 20 μsec in normal rat fibers of internodal lengths 0.75–1.45 mm (86). In most rat ventral root fibers demyelinated with focal application of diphtheria toxin, the time course of external longitudinal current also undergoes repeated abrupt displacements at intervals appropriate to internodal length as the impulse advances along the fiber (Fig. 1a), but the delay in transmission across successive internodes is greatly increased (Fig. 1b and c). Internodal conduction times in demyelinated nerve fibers range from normal to several hundred microseconds, and there is usually great variation in internodal conduction time at successive internodes of a given single fiber. In severely affected fibers conduction block oc-

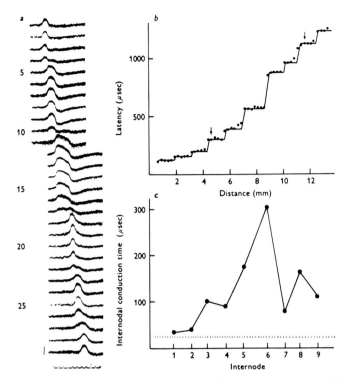

FIG. 1. Saltatory conduction in a demyelinated rat ventral root fiber. **a:** Successive records (*top to bottom*) of external longitudinal current recorded from two wires approximately 350 μm apart which were moved along the ventral root in 0.2-mm steps. Time scale: 100 μsec/small division. **b:** Latency to initial peak of external longitudinal current as a function of distance along the fiber. Zero time and distance are arbitrary. Arrows indicate first and last records illustrated in **a**. **c:** Data of **b** replotted as internodal conduction time for each of the nine successive internodes examined. Dotted line indicates normal internodal conduction time. (From ref. 86).

curs and the site of the block can be identified (82,86) (Fig. 2).

Preservation of saltatory conduction in demyelinated fibers does not necessarily imply that the spatially separated sites of excitable membrane retain all of the characteristics of nodal membrane. In normal myelinated fibers inward membrane current flows only at nodes of Ranvier, presumably across the portion of the axon membrane bounded on either side by the paranodal apparatus. It is possible that some of the spatially separated sites of excitable membrane observed in demyelinated fibers have a linear extent that is greater than the dimensions of a normal node of Ranvier, perhaps corresponding to the short lengths of bare axon exposed during paranodal demyelination (6,8). Present recording techniques for single mammalian nerve fibers are inadequate to distinguish between excitable membrane confined to a node of Ranvier and that distributed over lengths of as much as 2–300 μm (12,85). Insofar as saltatory conduction is preserved, such spatially separated sites or short lengths of excitable membrane function as nodes and for convenience are occasionally designated as such in the ensuing discussion.

The delay between excitation of successive nodes of Ranvier in *normal* fibers is substantially due to capacitive and resistive losses of current through the internodal myelin and at nodes of Ranvier. This delay will be exaggerated by: (a) increased leakage of current between nodes, or (b) depression of excitable properties of nodal membranes, i.e., decreased current-generating capacity or increased threshold for excitation. Excessive current leakage and depression of excitability may contribute to the decreased conduction velocity and conduction block observed in demyelinated fibers. The safety factor of transmission is defined as [current available to stimulate a node to activity/current required to stimulate the node to activity (99)]. Conduction fails at a given

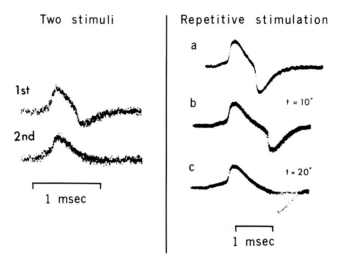

FIG. 2. External longitudinal current recordings illustrating conduction and conduction failure across severely affected internodes of demyelinated single fibers at the refractory period of transmission and during repetitive activity. The initial upward deflection reflects current flowing toward the node proximal to the recording site during excitation (i.e., opposite to the direction of propagation); the subsequent downward deflection reflects current flowing in the opposite direction toward the node distal to the recording site. Each record is approximately 20 superimposed traces. **Left:** The fiber is stimulated twice, the second impulse following 4.3 msec after the first. At this interstimulus interval biphasic external longitudinal current becomes monophasic, indicating failure of excitation of the distal node. **Right:** (a) Another fiber is stimulated at 3 Hz and then (b) at 100 Hz. After 10 sec internodal conduction time is increased (increased separation of upward and downward deflection). (c) After 20 sec there is a further increase in the internodal conduction time, and excitation of the distal node has become intermittent. (Adapted from ref. 86.)

node if the safety factor falls below 1. Reference to the safety factor is a simplistic but nonetheless useful way to indicate the complex conditions that must be fulfilled for propagation of electrical excitation from one part to another of any excitable cell.

Current Leakage

There is some evidence that capacitive and resistive leakage of current is greatest in the paranodal portion of fibers demyelinated with diphtheria toxin (86). Local thinning of axons seen in demyelinating neuropathies (63,79) would also cause decreased conduction velocity because of increased resistance to axial current flow and consequent diversion of longitudinal current transversely through the myelin.

Depression of Excitability

The spatially separated sites of excitable membrane in fibers demyelinated with diphtheria toxin appear to generate currents that are roughly similar in magnitude to those generated by the nodes of normal fibers (86), but no data are yet available explicitly comparing the electrical properties of axon membranes in normal and demyelinated fibers. During repetitive activity, an increase in internodal conduction time (decrease in conduction velocity) is associated with a decrease in membrane current generation at the spatially separated sites of excitable membrane (nodes) of demyelinated fibers (86) (Fig. 2).

Continuous Conduction

Although it originally appeared that conduction in demyelinated fibers invariably remained saltatory to the point of conduction block (86), Bostock and Sears (12) subsequently demonstrated that continuous conduction may occur over short lengths (approximately 0.5 mm) of demyelinated fibers with diameters less than 6 μm (Fig. 3). The conduction velocity in the continuously conducting segments is approximately 5% of that expected

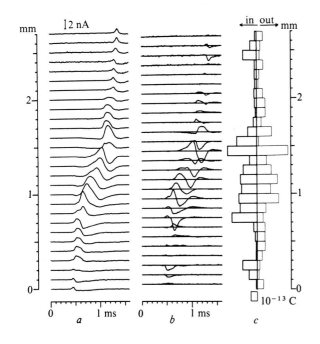

FIG. 3. Action currents in partially demyelinated rat ventral root fiber, showing stretch of continuous conduction and resumption of saltatory conduction. (a) Successive (*bottom to top*) longitudinal currents (1,024 sweeps) recorded from two platinum wires 130 μm apart which were slid 100 μm along the root between averages. (b) Membrane current (inward current downward) obtained by subtracting adjacent records of longitudinal current. Conduction in the middle of the illustrated portion of the fiber is termed continuous because there is a continuous change in latency of the longitudinal currents from one position to the next, and each 100 μm of nerve in turn becomes a source of inward current, indicating a continuous progression of excitation. (c) Inward (*thick line*) and outward (*thin line*) current integrals calculated from (b). (From ref. 12.)

for normal stretches of the same fiber (12). Continuous conduction at greatly reduced conduction velocity also occurs over much longer lengths (at least 4 mm) of the bare portion of large diameter ($\leq 7\mu$m) spinal root axons of dystrophic mice (85). These observations establish that electrical excitability is not invariably confined to nodes of Ranvier in myelinated nerve fibers.

Continuous conduction of a nervous impulse can occur in a bare or demyelinated axon only if the voltage–time-dependent membrane conductances are appropriately matched to the cable properties of the fiber. For example, Cooley and Dodge (16) have shown that propagation fails in computer-simulated squid axon if maximum membrane conductances for sodium and potassium ($\bar{g}_{Na}$ and $\bar{g}_K$) are reduced to 26.1% of normal. This is formally equivalent to reducing the density of sodium and potassium channels in the membrane. Below a critical level of sodium channel density, continuous conduction cannot occur.

On the basis of binding experiments with ^{3}H-saxitoxin (STX), Ritchie and Rogart (89) estimate that the density of sodium channels in internodal axon membrane of normal myelinated fibers from rabbit sciatic nerve is less than $25/\mu$m^2 in comparison to a sodium chan-

nel density of $12,000/\mu$m^2 at nodal membranes of the same nerve. The estimated density of sodium channels in unmyelinated axons of rabbit nerve based on STX binding is approximately $110/\mu$m^2 (90). This density of sodium channels must be adequate to sustain propagation in small-diameter unmyelinated fibers. It is not known whether the much lower sodium channel density of $<25/\mu$m^2 would be sufficient to sustain propagation in the larger-diameter fibers were they not insulated by myelin; it is possible that a precondition for continuous conduction following demyelination is a redistribution of sodium channels within axon membrane. Such redistribution would be expected to occur following demyelination if maintenance of high concentrations of sodium channels at nodes of Ranvier and very low concentrations of sodium channels in internodes were dependent on local interactions between glial cells and axons.

There are tentative morphological indications that glial cells may indeed be responsible for the striking difference between nodal and internodal sodium channel concentrations. Freeze-fracture studies of the outer lamella of nodal membranes in the frog brain reveal a high density of particles of diameter slightly less than 200 Å which may be sodium ionophores (91). These particles are seen in much lower concentration in internodal axon membrane, and Rosenbluth (91) suggested a mechanism for their accumulation at nodes of Ranvier and in the paranodal region that is contingent on the close apposition of axonal and glial membranes in the paranodal region. These morphological studies suggest the possibility that disruption or absence of paranodal structures would lead to a more even distribution of sodium channels along the axon membrane, their concentrations in demyelinated axons (12) or the bare axons of dystrophic mice (85) giving rise to sufficiently large $\bar{g}_{Na}$ to sustain continuous conduction. Redistribution of sodium channels following demyelination may be a process requiring time, just as the spread of acetylcholine sensitivity from the endplate region after muscle denervation requires several days (89).

The observations that both continuous conduction and conduction block can occur in demyelinated nerve are not mutually inconsistent. Geometrical considerations will influence whether the mode of transmission in a demyelinated fiber can be successively saltatory, continuous, and saltatory. For example, computer simulations (88) show that invasion of an unmyelinated terminal by an impulse originating in a myelinated fiber will occur only if the last internode is shorter than that appropriate to fiber diameter, and there are certainly similar restrictions on whether an impulse can emerge from a continuously conducting portion of a fiber to stimulate the first node of the portion of the fiber where saltatory conduction is resumed. The sodium channel density of the continuously conducting membrane is obviously of crucial importance. It would not be surprising if the necessary conditions for successful transmission *through* a region of continuous conduction were only infrequently met.

OTHER PROPERTIES OF DEMYELINATED NERVE FIBERS

The ability of a nerve fiber to function effectively as a conduit of information depends not only on its conduction velocity but also on its reliability of performance within a normal range of metabolic conditions and during repetitive activity. In these respects the performance of demyelinated fibers varies greatly from that of normal myelinated fibers.

Refractory Period

The refractory period of a nerve fiber is the minimal interval at which the fiber responds to the second of two stimuli at the stimulus site. In the context of conduction of impulses in a fiber, the term "refractory period of transmission" refers to the minimum interval at which the second of two impulses can enter but not traverse an abnormal portion of a nerve fiber (70). Both multifiber (49,51) and single-fiber (70,86) studies have shown an increase in the refractory period of transmission of demyelinated nerve fibers. In cat dorsal column fibers demyelinated with diphtheria toxin, refractory periods of transmission were as high as 4.2 msec, in comparison with a normal refractory period of 0.5–1.0 msec (70).

During the second of two closely spaced impulses conducted along a normal myelinated fiber, the threshold for excitation of each node is increased and each node generates less current than in the resting state (99). This causes a reduction in the safety factor of transmission which may be of critical importance at internodes where the safety factor of transmission is already so low that any further reduction may lead to conduction block. In a demyelinated fiber in which conduction is saltatory, the internode with the lowest safety factor is least able to tolerate any further decrease in the safety factor, and blockage of conduction of the second of two closely spaced impulses occurs at the most severely affected internode traversed by the impulse (Fig. 2). The interval between impulses at which the second impulse fails to be propagated across a critically affected internode is greatest for the most severely affected internode (86). It is worth emphasizing that the refractory period of transmission of a given fiber is a reflection of the safety factor of transmission of the most severely affected internode in the fiber and thus bears no necessary relationship to the conduction velocity of the fiber, which is determined by the properties of all the internodes.

The mechanism described for the increased refractory period of transmission of demyelinated fibers applies to fibers in which conduction remains saltatory. The refractory period of transmission across continuously conducting segments of demyelinated nerve fibers has not been explicitly studied.

Conduction of Trains of Impulses

Demyelinated nerve fibers have an impaired ability to transmit trains of impulses (19,50, 52,53,70,86); the frequencies at which conduction becomes intermittent [as low as 80 Hz (86)] are well within the normal physiological range. Just as for the refractory period of transmission, intermittent conduction block during transmission of trains occurs at internodes with markedly increased internodal conduction times where the safety factor is low (86). However, the interstimulus interval corresponding to the frequency at which conduction ultimately becomes intermittent or fails in demyelinated fibers is considerably greater than the refractory period of transmission (70,86); thus the increased refractory period of transmission cannot be accepted as the explanation for conduction failure during trains of impulses.

The mechanism of intermittent conduction block has been examined in demyelinated fibers in which saltatory conduction is preserved (86). At appropriate frequencies of stimulation, there is a *progressive* increase in the internodal conduction time during repetitive transmission across severely affected internodes, which may eventuate in conduction failure (Fig. 2). The progressive increase in internodal conduction time is associated with a progressive decrease in current generation by the node proximal to the affected internode (86) and may also reflect decreased responsiveness of the node distal to the affected internode. Possible mechanisms for these phenomena include intracellular sodium accumulation at the nodal region during the tetanus (86), changes in potassium concentration gradients (70,86), and as yet unspecified changes in axonal excitability that are known to occur at normal nodes during repetitive activity (87).

Post-Tetanic Depression

Following repetitive stimulation of nerves demyelinated with EAN, the compound action potential recorded in response to a single stimulus is decreased (17,19). The higher the frequency of the conditioning volley, the more marked is the post-tetanic depression (19). Post-tetanic depression in demyelinated fibers is seen after frequencies of stimulation as low as 10 Hz (19). The phenomenon has not been studied in single-fiber preparations; its explanation is presumably similar to those suggested for conduction block during repetitive stimulation.

Effects of Temperature and Metabolic Changes

Increases in temperature cause reversible blockage of conduction in demyelinated fibers (21,82) and in nerves of trembler mice (58) at temperatures within the physiological range (Fig. 4). Failure of saltatory conduction occurs at internodes with substantially increased internodal conduction time; as temperature increases, blockage of conduction occurs at the most severely affected internode of a given fiber (82). The lowest blocking temperature

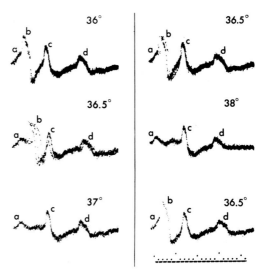

FIG. 4. Effect of changes in temperature on conduction in four single fibers from a demyelinated rat ventral root. All external longitudinal current records are from the same position on the fibers. Time scale: 100 μsec/small division. Conduction in fiber b is reversibly blocked at 37°C. At 38°C the external longitudinal current record for fiber d becomes monophasic, indicating that blockage in this fiber has occurred at the node just distal to the recording electrodes. (From ref. 82.)

observed in single fibers demyelinated with diphtheria toxin was 30.5°C. Blocking temperature falls with anoxia (82).

A likely explanation for temperature-reversible conduction block is a decrease in axon membrane current generation with increased temperature, with a consequent reduction of the safety factor of transmission (82). In principle, blocking temperature should be an index of the severity of demyelination of the blocked fiber (22,92), more specifically of the most severely affected internode (82). A more severe conduction abnormality should be associated with a lower blocking temperature. Compound action potential studies suggest that this is indeed the case (22), but this hypothesis has not been tested with single-fiber studies. It is not known whether reversible blockage of conduction occurs in the continuously conducting portion of demyelinated fibers within the physiological range of temperature.

Any metabolic factor that affects the properties of excitable membranes would be expected to influence the safety factor of transmission for demyelinated fibers. Reducing external calcium concentration reduces the threshold for excitation of excitable membranes (29). This should enhance transmission across regions of nerve with low safety factor and has been shown to do so in pressure-injured frog nerves (21).

Ectopic Impulse Generation in Demyelinated Fibers

Nervous impulses entering a zone of focal demyelination may be reflected to travel backward in the same axon (38). Such reflections are seen at regions of marked local slowing of conduction in simulated axons with local inhomogeneities (34,80). In addition to serving as points of reflection of impulses, areas of focal demyelination may act as local generators of impulses, especially when stimulated by pressure (38). Spontaneous impulses arise in midroot of spinal root axons of dystrophic mice and propagate in both directions (83); some of these spontaneous impulses are due to ephaptic interactions (cross-talk) between adjacent bare axons (39,84). Such ephaptic interactions are occasionally invoked in the literature of demyelinating disease as an ex-

planation for certain clinical phenomena (see below); ephaptic interactions between demyelinated nerve fibers have not yet been experimentally demonstrated.

STRUCTURE–FUNCTION RELATIONSHIPS IN DEMYELINATION

So far, the discussion has as much as possible deliberately avoided questions of structure. These questions are now addressed with two objectives: first, to consider the relationship between morphology and conduction velocity in demyelinated nerve and, secondly, to consider the relationship between morphology and electrical excitability of axon membrane.

Conduction Velocity and Conduction Block

Teased-fiber studies show that there is a variation in the extent of myelin loss or damage at successive internodes of single demyelinated fibers (100). This is reflected in the variation in internodal conduction time across successive internodes of single demyelinated fibers (86). No statement can currently be made concerning the amount of demyelination or myelin damage necessary to give rise to a given degree of conduction slowing or conduction block. There is experimental (72) and theoretical (45) evidence that slight changes in nodal morphology, such as occur in the early stages of demyelinating neuropathies, are not associated with significant changes in conduction velocity. Conduction velocity is substantially reduced in certain metabolic neuropathies in the absence of significant morphological changes (94,95), but in other situations conduction velocity may be relatively normal in the face of obvious morphological changes in myelin. For example, although conduction velocity in peripheral nerves of rats is reduced in the early stages of triethyltin intoxication, it returns to normal when vacuolization of myelin is still present (35).

Conduction velocity is a function not only of fiber geometry but also of properties of excitable membranes (rate constants and magnitudes of voltage–time-dependent membrane conductances); ion concentration gradients; capacitivity of myelin and axolemma; resistivity of myelin, axolemma, and axoplasm; and resistance of extracellular pathways to current flow (e.g., refs. 42,43). Many of these properties could change in the absence of striking morphological alterations in nerve, whether the mode of conduction is saltatory or continuous. It is clear that great difficulty is to be anticipated in any attempt to establish a precise relationship between morphological and physiological findings in demyelinated nerve fibers, even if it ultimately becomes possible to make physiological and morphological observations on the same single fiber.

Conduction in Remyelinated Axons

Serial studies of conduction in guinea pigs with diphtheritic neuritis (72) and EAN (46) show a return toward normal conduction velocity during recovery from demyelination. This is presumably due to the remyelination which occurs in both diphtheritic neuritis and EAN (7). Following demyelination and remyelination, the spacing of nodes of Ranvier is much less regular than that found in normal nerve (100); the relocation of nodes of Ranvier has been clearly illustrated for the compression lesion in primate nerve (74). New nodes are also formed in regenerating nerve in which internodal lengths are short (103); conduction velocity in regenerated nerve ultimately reaches approximately 75% of normal (18). The normal or only moderately reduced conduction velocity in remyelinated and regenerated nerve must reflect normal or near-normal physiological functioning of such newly formed nodes and constitutes further evidence of the mobility of sodium channels within axon membrane and their ability to be concentrated at new nodal sites.

Continuous Conduction

In normal peripheral myelinated nerve fibers, Schwann cell terminal loops are closely apposed to axon membrane in the paranodal region (47). Detachment of terminal myelin loops from the axolemma, as occurs in the early stages of demyelinating neuropathies (8,9), may expose internodal axolemma to the extracellular space; this might open a relatively low resistance pathway external to axolemma

but beneath the myelin for local circuit currents during propagation of a nervous impulse. It is not yet clear whether such damage to the paranodal apparatus is an adequate pathological substrate for continuous conduction or if continuous conduction requires complete absence of the Schwann cell and myelin sheath, as in the dystrophic mouse spinal root fibers (13,14).

Morphological and Histochemical Correlates of Excitable Membranes

Since the demonstration of dense bodies immediately underlying the nodal axolemma (25), interest has centered on possible structural correlates of axon membrane excitability; these dense bodies are similar to those underlying the initial axon segment (76), which is thought to be the most excitable part of the nerve cell. As noted above, more recent freeze-fracture studies have revealed high concentrations of particles, which may be sodium ionophores, in the outer face of nodal membranes (91).

Histochemical studies have disclosed other features unique to nodal membranes. Ferric ion and ferrocyanide stain the inner surface of nodal membranes but not the internodes of rat peripheral nerves; in the electric organs of *Sternarchus albifrons,* narrow nodes of Ranvier which exhibit spike electrogenesis are stained with ferric ion and ferrocyanide, whereas the larger nodes, which do not generate spikes but rather function as a series capacitance, are unstained (77).

The polyanionic matrix of the nodal gap substance may have an important role in maintaining the ionic environment of normal nodes of Ranvier (47,48). During demyelination in the perineurial window (97), normal nodal and paranodal cuprous ion binding activity is lost, indicating loss of the paranodal polyanionic matrix, and reappears coincident with reappearance of nodes of Ranvier during remyelination (23). Conduction has not been studied in axons demyelinated in the perineurial window, but the fact that continuous conduction occurs in axons demyelinated with diphtheria toxin (12) and in the spinal root axons of dystrophic mice (85) indicates the necessity for caution in interpreting specific morphological and histochemical properties of nodes of Ranvier as definitive markers of electrical excitability. STX binding studies suggest that the sodium channel densities of mammalian nodal axon membrane are approximately two orders of magnitude greater than those of unmyelinated axon membrane (89); any specific morphological or histochemical marker for excitable membrane might thus be present in much lower concentration in nonnodal excitable membrane than in nodal membrane. As Quick and Waxman (77,106) recognized, apparent qualitative histochemical differences between nodal and nonnodal axon membranes may in fact reflect only quantitative differences in membrane composition.

COMPUTER SIMULATIONS OF CONDUCTION IN DEMYELINATED NERVE FIBERS

Computer simulations of propagated action potentials in amphibian myelinated fibers show excellent agreement with experimental findings (33,40); these simulations have been modified to simulate conduction in demyelinated fibers (45,92,96). The simulations of demyelinated fibers have assumed that (a) excitability remains confined to nodes of Ranvier during demyelination; (b) the nodal membrane properties are unchanged in demyelinated fibers; and (c) demyelination can be represented by changes in the cable properties of internodal myelin. As noted above, there is recent experimental evidence that the first of these assumptions is not always correct (12), and no experimental evidence is yet available concerning the second. The simulations have in general represented demyelination as an increase in internodal myelin capacitance and a decrease in internodal myelin resistance. Simulation of concomitant axonal constriction by increasing axonal resistance would have similar effects on conduction (45,92). Because there are only fragmentary data available concerning both active membrane properties (37) and cable properties (26) of mammalian myelinated nerve fibers, simulations of conduction in demyelinated fibers have, of necessity, been simulations of conduction in demyelinated amphibian myelinated axons. Although the published simulations must not be understood as accurate

quantitative descriptions of conduction in demyelinated fibers, they do provide some useful qualitative insights into conduction in such fibers.

A surprising degree of demyelination is tolerated before conduction block ensues (45,96); if demyelination is confined to a single internode of the model fiber, conduction occurs across this internode, albeit with a substantial delay until the myelin thickness is reduced to less than 2.7% of normal (45) (Fig. 5). Paranodal demyelination is more effective in slowing conduction than the equivalent change in cable properties distributed evenly over entire internodes; a given amount of paranodal demyelination slows conduction more if it is located symmetrically on both sides of the node rather than lateralized to the proximal or

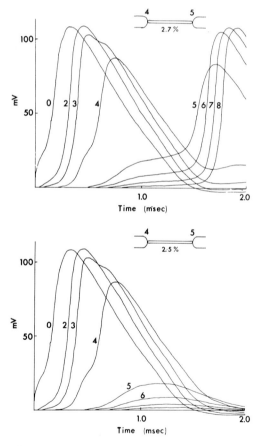

FIG. 5. Propagated action potential in a simulated demyelinated fiber at nodes 0 and 2–8. Internode 4–5 is demyelinated to 2.7% (*top*) and 2.5% (*bottom*) of normal myelin thickness. (From ref. 45.)

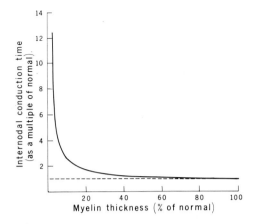

FIG. 6. Variation of internodal conduction time with myelin thickness for demyelination of a single internode in a computer-simulated demyelinated fiber. (Recalculated from ref. 45.)

distal side of the node (45). Propagation of an impulse through a zone of demyelination is a function not only of the severity of demyelination but also of the number of internodes involved. In the model fiber an impulse successfully traverses one but not two adjacent internodes with myelin thickness 4% of normal (45).

Internodal conduction time increases (i.e., conduction velocity decreases) with decreasing myelin thickness much more precipitously as myelin becomes thinner (Fig. 6). Propagation across internodes with very thin myelin is sensitive not only to small further changes in myelin thickness but also to small changes in the metabolic environment of the fiber and to changes in nodal properties. For example, increases in internal sodium concentration which have a trivial effect on conduction in normal fibers may cause blockage of conduction in demyelinated fibers (45). Increased temperature also blocks conduction in simulated demyelinated fibers at temperatures much lower than the blocking temperature for normal fibers (45,92). Factors that raise the blocking temperature of simulated demyelinated nerve are those which enhance propagation across demyelinated internodes such as a decrease in external calcium concentration and an increase in the sodium inactivation time constant τ_h; the blocking temperature is lowered by decreasing the maximum sodium permeability (92).

The refractory period of transmission is in-

creased in simulated demyelinated fibers, more demyelination being associated with a greater increase in refractory period (92).

The computer simulations of demyelinated fibers are thus in qualitative agreement with experimental results in demonstrating a wide range of possible internodal conduction times before conduction block, increased refractory period of transmission, and blockage of conduction at physiological temperatures.

CLINICAL IMPLICATIONS

Blockage of conduction in a large enough proportion of demyelinated fibers in either the peripheral or central nervous system will be associated with a neurological deficit. The various transient neurological deficits that hyperthermia may provoke in patients with multiple sclerosis are thought to be due to reversible blockage of conduction in demyelinated fibers (21,82). Transient improvements in neurological function in patients with multiple sclerosis occur following procedures which lower serum calcium concentration (10,20); this is thought to reflect resumption of conduction in previously blocked fibers. The safety factor of transmission in demyelinated nerve is enhanced by factors which prolong the action potential; for this reason Schauf and Davis (92) suggested that drugs which delay sodium inactivation or potassium activation should be of value in patients with demyelinating disease. Successful clinical trials of drugs with such effects have not been reported.

It is worth re-emphasizing that although a given nerve fiber may be several hundred internodes in length, blockage of conduction at any one of these internodes removes the functional contribution of the whole fiber (82,105). For every demyelinated fiber, there exists in principle a critical site (demyelinated internode) at which conduction is most susceptible to blockage with changes in temperature or metabolic conditions. For each critical site, a temperature and/or metabolic condition at which blockage will occur can be specified. For a large group of fibers there will be a continuum of critical blocking conditions, and it is intuitively obvious that relatively small changes in temperature or metabolic environment can be expected to have dramatic effects on the proportion of functioning fibers within an entire nerve or tract. A similar argument is more formally presented by Waxman et al. (105), who demonstrate how the proximodistal gradient of sensory deficit in peripheral neuropathies is predicted by the precipitous increase in probability of conduction failure with increased fiber length for any fixed probability of conduction failure at a single internode.

The effect on clinical function of slowing of conduction in demyelinated fibers remains speculative. Waxium (104) discussed mechanisms by which axons act as precisely timed delay lines in the CNS. Reduced conduction velocity in a large proportion of fibers in a peripheral nerve or CNS tract would give rise to temporal distortions in the pattern of arrival at their destination(s) of impulses in a group of fibers. McDonald (65) illustrated how this might adversely influence neurological functions, e.g., critical flicker fusion frequency in patients with multiple sclerosis. Functions less dependent on the strict temporal sequence of impulses (e.g., muscle strength) would be less affected by conduction slowing (68). During recovery from acute demyelinating neuropathies and in some chronic peripheral neuropathies, there is an impressive discrepancy between decreased nerve conduction velocities and the paucity of clinical findings. Possible explanations for this discrepancy are discussed by McDonald and Kocen (68).

Functions like sensory coding (104,105) for which the temporal pattern of impulses is critical, will also be affected by the decreased ability of demyelinated nerve to transmit trains of impulses and by ectopic generation of impulses. Intermittent conduction block with repetitive activity has been advanced as an explanation for muscle fatigue in demyelinating disease (70).

Spontaneous generation of impulses from pathological regions of nerve (38,83) has been suggested as the explanation for paresthesias which some patients with cervical cord lesions experience on neck flexion (5). The various paroxysmal symptoms of multiple sclerosis (e.g., tic douloureux, paroxysmal dysarthria, and painful tonic seizures) (for review see refs. 60,71,75) may also be caused by ectopic impulse generation, perhaps due to ephaptic interactions between adjacent fibers

within plaques of demyelination (60,75). It is interesting that such paroxysmal symptoms are prevented by treatment with carbamazepine (27,28), which depresses nerve excitability (93), and are provoked by hyperventilation (60,75,101). The paradox that hyperventilation can both improve (20) and provoke neurological symptoms in demyelinating disease may be more apparent than real. The increased nerve excitability induced by hyperventilation, perhaps mediated by reduction in serum ionized calcium, would be expected to increase the safety factor and thus enhance transmission across severely affected internodes of certain fibers (20,92) as well as to promote spontaneous discharge and ephaptic excitation of others (81). If symptoms in demyelinating disease are thought of in the Jacksonian sense as either negative (e.g., paralysis or sensory loss) or positive (e.g., tic douloureux or paroxysmal attacks), increasing nerve excitability would be expected to alleviate negative symptoms and exacerbate positive symptoms.

A persistent theme in the literature of multiple sclerosis is the poor correlation between pathological and clinical findings. Extensive lesions may be associated with little or no clinical deficit (59,73). As noted above, computer simulations suggest that saltatory conduction can be preserved even in the face of very severe demyelination; it is also possible that impulses may traverse some fibers in plaques of demyelination by reversion to continuous conduction. No matter what the mode, conduction through a plaque of demyelination would be locally slowed but not necessarily blocked; it appears that such local slowing does not necessarily give rise to clinical deficits.

There are a number of possible explanations for recovery of function in demyelinating lesions. Remyelination is an important factor in recovery from peripheral nervous system demyelination; although remyelination may occur in the CNS, it is less extensive than in the peripheral nervous system (66). Edema could cause blockage of conduction through regions of low safety factor; conduction might resume with the resolution of edema. Recovery of function might also reflect continuous conduction in previously blocked fibers; the delay frequently seen in recovery from new deficits in demyelinating disease might represent the time required for redistribution of sodium channels in demyelinated nerve (89). Finally, recovery of function does not necessarily demand changes in conduction in demyelinated fibers; it could also reflect adaptation within the CNS to different patterns of input (64,68).

CONCLUSION

In normal myelinated nerve fibers, the intimate relationship between axons and glial cells manifests itself in a number of ways. Axons provide a mitogenic stimulus to Schwann cells (108) and direct the Schwann cells either to produce or not to produce myelin (3,107). Axonal diameter influences internodal length and myelin thickness (see ref. 47 for review); Schwann cells in turn can influence axonal diameter (1). Schwann cells are also thought to have a major role in maintaining the metabolic environment of the node of Ranvier (47). Further aspects of the symbiotic relationship between axons and glial cells are reviewed elsewhere (102).

In sum, the function of the myelin-producing glial cell is much more complex than simply to act as a source of insulation to increase the conduction velocity of myelinated nerve fibers. The electrophysiological, morphological, and STX-binding studies reviewed here suggest that a further important function of glial cells is to control the distribution of electrical excitability within axons.

Failure of development or loss of the normal intimate relationship between glial cells and axons results in the abnormalities in transmission properties of nerve fibers which have been the subject of this chapter.

ACKNOWLEDGMENTS

Supported by the Medical Research Council of Canada.

REFERENCES

1. Aguayo, A. J., Attiwell, M., Trecarten, J., Perkins, S., and Bray, G. M. (1976): Schwann cell transplantation: Evidence for a primary disorder of myelination in trembler mouse nerves. *Clin. Res.*, 24:688A.
2. Aguayo, A. J., Attiwell, M., Trecarten, J., Perkins, S., and Bray, G. M. (1977): Abnormal myelination in transplanted trembler mouse Schwann cells. *Nature (Lond)*, 265: 73–74.
3. Aguayo, A. J., Epps, J., Charron, L., and Bray, G. M. (1976): Multipotentiality of Schwann cells in cross anastomosed and grafted myelinated and unmyelinated nerves: Quantitative microscopy and radioautography. *Brain Res.*, 104:1–20.
4. Aguayo, A. J., Nair, C. P. V., and Midgeley, R. (1971): Experimental progressive compression neuropathy in the rabbit. *Arch. Neurol.*, 24:358–364.
5. Alajouanine, T., Thurel, R., and Papaioanou, C. (1949): La douleur à type de décharge électrique provoquée par la flexion de la tête et parcourant le corps de haut en bas. *Rev. Neurol. (Paris)*, 81:89–97.
6. Allt, G. (1969): Repair of segmental demyelination in peripheral nerves: An electron microscopic study. *Brain*, 92:639–646.
7. Allt, G. (1976): Pathology of the peripheral nerve. In: *The Peripheral Nerve*, edited by D. N. Landon, pp. 666–739. Chapman and Hall, London.
8. Allt, G., and Cavanagh, J. B. (1969): Ultrastructural changes in the region of the node of Ranvier in the rat caused by diphtheria toxin. *Brain*, 92:459–468.
9. Ballin, R. H. M., and Thomas, P. K. (1968): Electron microscopic observations on demyelination and remyelination in experimental allergic neuritis. 1. Demyelination. *J. Neurol. Sci.*, 8:1–18.
10. Becker, F. O., Michael, J. A., and Davis, F. A. (1974): Acute effects of oral phosphate on visual function in multiple sclerosis. *Neurology (Minneap)*, 24:601–607.
11. Bement, S. L., and Ranck, J. B. (1969): A quantitative study of electrical stimulation of central myelinated fibers. *Exp. Neurol.*, 24:147–170.
12. Bostock, H., and Sears, T. A. (1976): Continuous conduction in demyelinated mammalian nerve fibers. *Nature (Lond)*, 263: 786–787.
13. Bradley, W. G., and Jenkison, M. (1974): Abnormalities of peripheral nerve in murine muscular dystrophy. *J. Neurol. Sci.*, 18:227–247.
14. Bray, G. M., and Aguayo, A. J. (1975): Quantitative ultrastructural studies of the axon–Schwann cell abnormality in spinal nerve roots from dystrophic mice. *J. Neuropathol. Exp. Neurol.*, 34:517–530.
15. Bray, G. M., Perkins, S., Peterson, A. C., and Aguayo, A. J. (1977): Schwann cell multiplication deficit in nerve roots of newborn dystrophic mice: A radioautographic and ultrastructural study. *J. Neurol. Sci.* 32: 203–212.
16. Cooley, J. W., and Dodge, F. A. (1966): Digital computer solutions of excitation and propagation of the nerve impulse. *Biophys. J.*, 6:583–599.

17. Cragg, B. G., and Thomas, P. K. (1964): Changes in nerve conduction in experimental allergic neuritis. *J. Neurol. Neurosurg. Psychiatry,* 27:106–115.

18. Cragg, B. G., and Thomas, P. K. (1964): The conduction velocity of regenerated peripheral nerve fibers. *J. Physiol. (Lond),* 171:164–75.

19. Davis, F. A. (1972): Impairment of repetitive impulse conduction in experimentally demyelinated and pressure injured nerves. *J. Neurol. Neurosurg. Psychiatry,* 35:537–544.

20. Davis, F. A., Becker, F. O., Michael, J. A., and Sorenson, E. (1970): Effect of intravenous sodium bicarbonate, disodium edetate (Na₂EDTA), and hyperventilation on visual and oculomotor signs in multiple sclerosis. *J. Neurol. Neurosurg. Psychiatry,* 33:723–732.

21. Davis, F. A., and Jacobson, S. (1971): Altered thermal sensitivity in injured and demyelinated nerve: A possible model of temperature effects in multiple sclerosis. *J. Neurol. Neurosurg. Psychiatry,* 34:551–561.

22. Davis, F. A., Schauf, C. L., Reed, B. J., and Kesler, R. L. (1976): Experimental studies of the effects of extrinsic factors on conduction in normal and demyelinated nerve. 1. Temperature. *J. Neurol. Neurosurg. Psychiatry,* 39:442–448.

23. De Baecque, C., Raine, C. S., and Spencer, P. S. (1976): Copper binding at PNS nodes of Ranvier during demyelination and remyelination in the perineurial window. *Neuropathol. Appl. Neurobiol.,* 6:459–470.

24. Denny-Brown, D., and Brenner, C. (1944): Paralysis of nerve induced by direct pressure and by tourniquet. *Arch. Neurol. Psychiatry,* 51:1–26.

25. Elvin, L-G. (1961): The ultrastructure of the nodes of Ranvier in cat sympathetic nerve fibers. *J. Ultrastruct. Res.,* 5:374–387.

26. Eliasson, S. V. (1969): Properties of isolated nerve fibres from alloxanized rats. *J. Neurol. Neurosurg. Psychiatry,* 32:525–529.

27. Espir, M. L. E., and Millac, P. (1970): Treatment of paroxysmal disorders in multiple sclerosis with carbamazepine. *J. Neurol. Neurosurg. Psychiatry,* 33:528–531.

28. Espir, M. L. E., Watkins, S. M., and Smith, H. V. (1966): Paroxysmal dysarthria and other transient neurological disturbances in disseminated sclerosis. *J. Neurol. Neurosurg. Psychiatry,* 29:323–330.

29. Frankenhaeuser, R., and Hodgkin, A. L. (1957): The action of calcium on the electrical properties of squid axons. *J. Physiol. (Lond),* 137:218–244.

30. Fullerton, P. M. (1966): Chronic peripheral neuropathy produced by lead poisoning in guinea-pigs. *J. Neuropathol. Exp. Neurol.,* 25:214–236.

31. Fullerton, P. M., and Gilliatt, R. W. (1967): Pressure neuropathy in the hind foot of the guinea-pig. *J. Neurol. Neurosurg. Psychiatry,* 30:18–25.

32. Fullerton, P. M., and Gilliatt, R. W. (1967): Median and ulnar neuropathy in the guinea-pig. *J. Neurol. Neurosurg. Psychiatry,* 30:393–402.

33. Goldman, L., and Albus, J. S. (1968): Computation of impulse conduction in myelinated fibers: Theoretical basis of the velocity diameter relation. *Biophys. J.,* 8:596–607.

34. Goldstein, S. S., and Rall, W. (1974): Changes of action potential shape and velocity for changing core conductor geometry. *Biophys. J.,* 14:731–757.

35. Graham, D. I., deJesus, P. V., Pleasure, D. E., and Gonatas, N. K. (1976): Triethyltin sulfate-induced neuropathy in rats: Electrophysiologic, morphologic, and biochemical studies. *Arch. Neurol.,* 33:40–48.

36. Hall, J. I. (1967): Studies on demyelinated peripheral nerves in guinea-pigs with experimental allergic neuritis, a histological and electrophysiological study. II. Electrophysiological observations. *Brain,* 90:313–332.

37. Horáckova, M., Nonner, W., and Stämpfli, R. (1968): Action potentials and voltage clamp currents of single rat Ranvier nodes. *Int. Physiol. Congr. XXIV,* 7:198.

38. Howe, J. F., Calvin, W. H., and Loeser, J. D. (1976): Impulses reflected from dorsal root ganglia and from focal nerve injuries. *Brain Res.,* 116:139–144.

39. Huizar, P., Kuno, M., and Miyata, Y. (1975): Electrophysiological properties of spinal motoneurones of normal and dystrophic mice. *J. Physiol. (Lond),* 248:231–246.

40. Hutchinson, N. A., Koles, Z. J., and Smith, R. S. (1970): Conduction velocity in myelinated nerve fibres of Xenopus laevis. *J. Physiol. (Lond),* 208:279–289.

41. Huxley, A. F., and Stämpfli, R. (1949): Evidence for saltatory conduction in peripheral myelinated nerve fibres. *J. Physiol. (Lond.),* 108:315–339.

42. Jack, J. J. B. (1975): Physiology of peripheral nerve fibres in relation to their size. *Brit. J. Anaesth.* 47:175–182.

43. Jack, J. J. B. (1976): Electrophysiological properties of peripheral nerve. In: *The Peripheral Nerve,* edited by D. N. Landon, pp. 740–818. Chapman and Hall, London.

44. Kaeser, H. E. and Lambert, E. H. (1962): Nerve function studies in experimental polyneuritis. *Electroencephalog. Clin. Neurophysiol.,* Suppl. 22:29–35.

45. Koles, Z. J. and Rasminsky, M. (1972): A computer simulation of conduction in demyelinated nerve fibres. *J. Physiol. (Lond),* 227:351–364.

46. Kraft, G. H. (1975): Serial nerve conduction and electromyographic studies in ex-

perimental allergic neuritis. *Arch. Phys. Med. Rehabil.*, 56:333–340.

47. Landon, D. N. and Hall, S. (1976): The myelinated nerve fibre. In: *The Peripheral Nerve,* edited by D. N. Landon, pp. 1–105. Chapman and Hall, London.

48. Landon, D. N. and Langley, O. K. (1971): The local chemical environment of nodes of Ranvier: a study of cation binding. *J. Anat.,* 108:419–432.

49. Lehmann, H. J. (1967): Zur Pathophysiologie der Refractär-periode peripherer Nerven. *Dtsch. Z. Nerv Heilk,* 192:185–192.

50. Lehmann, H. J., Lehmann, G. and Tackmann, W. (1971): Refraktärperiode und Übermittlung von Serien impulsen im N. tibialis des Meerschw einchens bei experimentaller allergischer Neuritis. *Z. Neurol.* 199:67–85.

51. Lehmann, H. J. and Pretschner, D. P. (1966): Experimentelle Untersuchungen zum Engpassyndrom peripherer Nerven. *Dtsch. Z. Nerv Heilk.,* 188:308–330.

52. Lehmann, H. J., and Tackmann, W. (1970): Die Übermittlung frequenter Impulserien in demyelinisierten und in degenerietenden Nerven Fasern. *Arch. Psychiatr. Nervenkr.,* 213:215–227.

53. Lehmann, H. J., Tackmann, W., and Lehmann, G. (1971): Funktionsänderung markhaltiger Nervenfasern im N. tibialis des Meerschweinchens bei post diphtherischer Polyneuritis. *Z. Neurol.,* 199:86–104.

54. Lehmann, H. J., and Ule, G. (1964): Electrophysiological findings and structural changes in circumspect inflammation of peripheral nerves. *Prog. Brain Res.,* 6:169–173.

55. Low, P. A. (1976): Hereditary hypertrophic neuropathy in the trembler mouse. 1. Histopathological studies: light microscopy. *J. Neurol. Sci.,* 30:327–341.

56. Low, P. A. (1976): Hereditary hypertrophic neuropathy in the trembler mouse. 2. Histopathological studies: electron microscopy. *J. Neurol. Sci.,* 30:343–368.

57. Low, P. A., and McLeod, J. G. (1975): Hereditary demyelinating neuropathy in the trembler mouse. *J. Neurol. Sci.,* 26:565–574.

58. Low, P. A., and McLeod, J. G. (1977): The refractory period, conduction of trains of stimuli, and effect of temperature on conduction in chronic hypertrophic neuropathy: Electrophysiological studies on the trembler mouse. *J. Neurol. Neurosurg. Psychiatry* 40:434–447.

59. Mackay, R. P., and Hirano, A. (1967): Forms of benign multiple sclerosis. *Arch. Neurol.,* 17:588–600.

60. Matthews, W. B. (1975): Paroxysmal symptoms in multiple sclerosis. *J. Neurol. Neurosurg. Psychiatry,* 38:617–623.

61. Mayer, R. F., and Denny-Brown, D. (1964): Conduction velocity in peripheral nerve dur-

ing experimental demyelination in the cat. *Neurology (Minneap),* 14:714–726.

62. McDonald, W. I. (1962): Conduction in muscle afferent fibres during experimental demyelination in cat nerve. *Acta Neuropathol. (Berl),* 1:425–432.

63. McDonald, W. I. (1963): The effects of experimental demyelination on conduction in peripheral nerve: a histological and electrophysiological study. I. Clinical and histological observations. *Brain,* 86:481–500.

64. McDonald, W. I. (1963): The effects of experimental demyelination on conduction in peripheral nerve: a histological and electrophysiological study. II. Electrophysiological observations. *Brain,* 86:501–524.

65. McDonald, W. I. (1974): Pathophysiology in multiple sclerosis. *Brain,* 97:179–196.

66. McDonald, W. I. (1974): Remyelination in relation to clinical lesions of the central nervous system. *Br. Med. Bull.,* 30:186–189.

67. McDonald, W. I., and Gilman, S. (1968): Demyelination and muscle spindle function: Effect of diphtheritic polyneuritis on nerve conduction and muscle spindle function in the cat. *Arch. Neurol.,* 18:508–519.

68. McDonald, W. I., and Kocen, R. S. (1975): Diphtheritic neuropathy. In: *Peripheral Neuropathy,* edited by P. J. Dyck, P. K. Thomas, and E. H. Lambert, pp. 1281–1300. Saunders, Philadelphia.

69. McDonald, W. I., and Sears, T. A. (1969): Effect of demyelination on conduction in the central nervous system. *Nature (Lond),* 221:182–183.

70. McDonald, W. I., and Sears, T. A. (1970): The effects of experimental demyelination on conduction in the central nervous system. *Brain,* 93:583–598.

71. Miley, C. E., and Forster, F. M. (1974): Paroxysmal signs and symptoms in multiple sclerosis. *Neurology (Minneap),* 24:458–461.

72. Morgan-Hughes, J. A. (1968): Experimental diphtheritic neuropathy, a pathological and electrophysiological study. *J. Neurol. Sci.,* 7:157–175.

73. Namerow, N. S., and Thompson, L. R. (1969): Plaques, symptoms and the remitting course of multiple sclerosis. *Neurology (Minneap),* 19:765–774.

74. Ochoa, J., Fowler, T. J., and Gilliatt, R. W. (1972): Anatomical changes in peripheral nerves compressed by a pneumatic tourniquet. *J. Anat.,* 113:433–455.

75. Osterman, P. O., and Westerberg, C-E. (1975): Paroxysmal attacks in multiple sclerosis. *Brain,* 98:189–202.

76. Palay, S. L., Sotelo, C., Peters, A., and Orkand, P. M. (1968): The axon hillock and the initial segment. *J. Cell Biol.,* 38:193–201.

77. Quick, D. C., and Waxman, S. G. (1977): Specific staining of the axon membrane at

nodes of Ranvier with ferric ion and ferrocyanide. *J. Neurol. Sci.,* 31:1–11.

78. Raine, C. S. (1977): *This volume.*

79. Raine, C. S., Wiśniewski, H., and Prineas, J. (1969): An ultrastructural study of experimental demyelination and remyelination. II. Chronic experimental allergic encephalomyelitis in the peripheral nervous system. *Lab. Invest.,* 21:316–327.

80. Ramón, F., Joyner, R. W., and Moore, J. W. (1975): Propagation of action potentials in inhomogeneous axon regions. *Fed. Proc.,* 34:1357–1363.

81. Ramón, F., Joyner, R., and Moore, J. W. (1976): Ephaptic transmission in squid giant axons. *Biophys. J.,* 16:26a.

82. Rasminsky, M. (1973): The effects of temperature on conduction in demyelinated single nerve fibers. *Arch. Neurol.,* 28:287–292.

83. Rasminsky, M. (1976): Nervous impulses arising in mid root of spinal root axons of dystrophic mice. *Neurosci. Abstr.,* 2:417.

84. Rasminsky, M. (1977): Cross talk between single fibers in spinal roots of dystrophic mice. *Neurology (Minneap)* 27:394.

85. Rasminsky, M., Kearney, R. E., Aguayo, A. J., and Bray, G. M. (1977): Conduction of nervous impulses in spinal roots and peripheral nerves of dystrophic mice. *Brain Res. (in press).*

86. Rasminsky, M., and Sears, T. A. (1972): Internodal conduction in undissected demyelinated nerve fibres. *J. Physiol. (Lond),* 277:323–350.

87. Raymond, S. A., and Pangaro, P. (1975): Mediation of impulse conduction in axons by threshold changes. *Neurosci. Abstr.,* 1:609.

88. Revenko, S-V., Timin, Y. N., and Khodorov, B. I. (1973): Special features of the conduction of nerve impulses from the myelinized part of the axon into the nonmyelinated terminal. *Biophysics,* 18:1140–1145.

89. Ritchie, J. M., and Rogart, R. B. (1977): Density of sodium channels in mammalian myelinated nerve fibers and nature of the axonal membrane under the myelin sheath. *Proc. Natl. Acad. Sci. USA,* 74:211–215.

90. Ritchie, J. M., Rogart, R. B., and Strichartz, G. R. (1976): A new method for labelling saxitoxin and its binding to non-myelinated fibres of the rabbit vagus, lobster walking leg, and garfish olfactory nerves. *J. Physiol. (Lond),* 261:477–494.

91. Rosenbluth, J. (1976): Intramembranous particle distribution at the node of Ranvier and adjacent axolemma in myelinated axons of the frog brain. *J. Neurocytol.,* 5:731–745.

92. Schauf, C. L., and Davis, F. A. (1974): Impulse conduction in multiple sclerosis: A theoretical basis for modification by temperature and pharmacological agents. *J. Neurol. Neurosurg. Psychiatry,* 37:152–161.

93. Schauf, C. L., Davis, F. A., and Marder, J. (1974): Effects of carbamazepine on the ionic conductances of Myxicola giant axons. *J. Pharmacol. Exp. Ther.,* 189:538–543.

94. Sharma, A. K., and Thomas, P. K. (1974): Peripheral nerve structure and function in experimental diabetes. *J. Neurol. Sci.,* 23:1–15.

95. Sharma, A. K., Thomas, P. K., and Baker, R. W. R. (1976): Peripheral nerve abnormalities related to galactose administration in rats. *J. Neurol. Neurosurg. Psychiatry,* 39:794–802.

96. Smith, R. S., and Koles, Z. J. (1970): Myelinated nerve fibers: Computed effect of myelin thickness on conduction velocity. *Am. J. Physiol.,* 219:1256–1258.

97. Spencer, P. S., Weinberg, H. J., Raine, C. S., and Prineas, J. W. (1975): The perineurial window—a new model of focal demyelination and remyelination. *Brain Res.,* 96:323–329.

98. Tasaki, I. (1952): Properties of myelinated fibres in frog sciatic nerve and in spinal cord as examined with microelectrodes. *Jpn. J. Physiol.,* 3:73–94.

99. Tasaki, I. (1953): *Nervous Transmission.* Charles C Thomas, Springfield, Ill.

100. Thomas, P. K., and Lascelles, R. G. (1965): Schwann cell abnormalities in diabetic neuropathy. *Lancet,* 1:1355–1357.

101. Toyokura, Y., Sakuta, M., and Nakanishi, T. (1976): Painful tonic seizures in multiple sclerosis. *Neurology (Minneap),* 26:No. 6, part 2, 18–19.

102. Varon, S. (1975): Neurons and glia in neural cultures. *Exp. Neurol.,* 48:No. 3, part 2, 93–134.

103. Vizoso, A. D., and Young, J. Z. (1948): Internode length and fibre diameter in developing and regenerating nerves. *J. Anat.,* 82:110–134.

104. Waxman, S. G. (1975): Integrative properties and design principles of axons. *Int. Rev. Neurobiol.,* 18:1–40.

105. Waxman, S. G., Brill, M. H., Geschwind, N., Sabin, T. D., and Lettvin, J. (1976): Probability of conduction deficit as related to fiber length in random-distribution models of peripheral neuropathies. *J. Neurol. Sci.,* 29:39–53.

106. Waxman, S. G., and Quick, D. C. (1977): Cytochemical differentiation of the axon membrane in A- and C-fibres. *J. Neurol. Neurosurg. Psychiatry,* 40:379–386.

107. Weinberg, H. J., and Spencer, P. S. (1976): Studies on the control of myelinogenesis. II. Evidence for neuronal regulation of myelin production. *Brain Res.,* 113:363–378.

108. Wood, P. M., and Bunge, R. P. (1975): Evidence that sensory axons are mitogenic for Schwann cells. *Nature (Lond),* 256:662–664.

Physiology and Pathobiology of Axons, edited by
S. G. Waxman. Raven Press, New York © 1978.

Physiology of Sensation After Peripheral Nerve Injury, Regeneration, and Neuroma Formation

P. D. Wall and M. Devor

Cerebral Functions Research Group, Department of Anatomy and Embryology, University College London, London, W.C. 1E 6BT, England; and Neurobiology Unit, Institute of Life Sciences, The Hebrew University of Jerusalem, Jerusalem, Israel

The most pressing questions about the sensory consequences of peripheral nerve injury arise from the signs and symptoms reported in the clinic. In some conditions (e.g., causalgia, phantom limb, and amputation stump pain) there are bizarre sensations which sometimes spread far beyond the region of injury itself and are often resistant to therapy. For this reason there has been a tendency to transfer the cause of the continuing pain into the central nervous system (CNS) (14,77). Here we wish to emphasize that it is necessary first to consider a wide variety of disordered states of peripheral nerves, including changes of their central connections before abandoning a peripheral explanation. A major reason for our reticence to resort prematurely to the depths of the CNS is that the mechanism of central disorders is often hypothetical, unpalpable, and unamenable to treatment. In contrast, there are more and more techniques available for analysis of peripheral disorders in man and for their simulation in animals.

We must presume that what is sensed as a result of nerve activity is a function of the central connections of the axons involved. The peripheral receptor end is a filter that ensures that the real world stimulus that excites the fiber is appropriate to what will be sensed during activity in it. Normally this correspondence is brought about by developmental mechanisms as yet poorly understood. Following injury, however, the correspondence can be upset.

In considering the consequences of damage to peripheral nerve, we must extend our viewpoint to recognize that even local damage to an axon produces reactions in all parts of the cell of which the axon is one extension. Furthermore, a peripheral nerve cell is in dynamic relationship with neighboring nervous and nonnervous elements. Thus injury to one neuron could affect the functioning of intact neighbors. Figure 1 shows a peripheral nerve cell whose axon has been cut or damaged at the point marked with a cross. We must consider 12

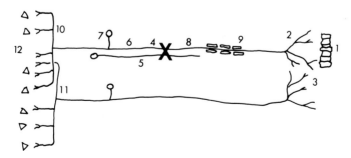

FIG. 1. When a nerve is damaged (X), physiological changes at any of a number of points can result in abnormalities of sensation. Twelve such points are discussed in the text.

points at which there may be physiological changes as a result of the damage. These can be grouped into three zones: the receptor end of the nerve, its course through the periphery, and the nerve's distribution in the spinal cord.

RECEPTOR END

Peripheral Receptor

The excitability of the transduction elements of an axon can be raised or lowered by damage in their vicinity (7). Following local injury (e.g., sunburn), weak, otherwise innocuous stimuli can excite pain (primary hyperalgesia). We do not know what happens to the receptor endings if an axon is only partly damaged. It may be presumed, however, that they are not unaffected.

In some places the axon ends in close association with nonneural cells that play a crucial role in sensory transduction. Examples of such structures are taste buds in the tongue and type I receptor domes (Haarscheibe) (75) in mammalian hairy skin. Following nerve section or crush, the distal part of the affected axons and their receptor arborizations undergo Wallerian degeneration. In many cases the integrity of organization of the nonneural cells is dependent on the presence of the sensory nerve fiber just as muscle requires motor axons. Following denervation they degenerate and disappear (9). If the skin in reinnervated the specializations return. Burgess et al. (10) made detailed maps of the distribution of type I domes on a region of rump skin in the cat. Following reinnervation after crushing the nerve, an injury that preserves the continuity of the endoneurial tubes, there was nearly complete restitution of the original map. Restitution was only partial following nerve section, probably because this injury interrupts the endoneurial tube, permitting the escape of axons from their normal channels. Even so, reinstated domes tended to be at sites previously occupied by domes.

Reinnervation of Skin by Homotypic Nerves

More important than precise distribution is the question of whether fibers regain their original receptor transduction characteristics

following reinnervation. Can a fiber with central connections signifying an intense tissue-damaging event reinnervate a low-threshold mechanoreceptor, and will the stimulus be felt as pain on light touching?

Burgess and Horch (11) argued that there is a remarkable degree of specificity in homotypic reinnervation; only fibers that formerly innervated dome receptors return to them, and likewise with other receptor types. In their experiments the sural nerve in cats was severed. Following regeneration, all receptor types were represented in approximately their normal proportions and with stimulus properties indistinguishable from normal. One wants to know, however, the original properties of the fibers. This was accomplished by characterizing fibers with particular response properties according to their peripheral and central (dorsal column) conduction velocity and according to their presence or absence at high cervical levels (C_2) in the spinal cord (11,41). In normal animals, for example, fibers with high threshold receptors (nociceptors) conduct at low velocity and do not project as far as C_2. The guard hair system has rapidly conducting axons, nearly all of which do achieve C_2. Following severance of the sural nerve, only 87% of the fibers succeeded in re-establishing functional peripheral connections. In these, axon conduction velocity and level of central projection continued to bear the normal relation to response property. This indeed suggests that particular fibers return to their original receptor type.

Unfortunately the data describe populations of axons and therefore do not rule out the possibility of moderate numbers of exceptions. For example, as in intact cats, none of the regenerated fibers with high threshold receptors projected as far as C_2. This population did have an increased mean peripheral conduction velocity, however (27–40 meters/sec; $p < 0.05$), indicating either a real retrograde increase in velocity (71) or contamination with fibers of higher velocity that also do not project to C_2—D hair or type I receptors, for example. Another possibility not definitely excluded is that both the conduction velocity and central projection level of a fiber are changed as a result of its having formed a particular type of peripheral receptor. The respecification of central connections by peripheral ones has been claimed in a number of nonmammalian systems (e.g., refs. 46,92) but has never been convincingly demonstrated in mammals. Horch (40) further argued against this hypothesis on the grounds that he found no gross shifts in the spinal cord level to which fibers ascend during the progress of regeneration. Again, however, this is a population study, and small or counterbalanced changes may have been missed. That fibers regain the same receptor function after regeneration as they had before would seem to be a strong tendency in the case of return of a nerve to its original territory. It may or may not be an absolute rule.

Reinnervation of Skin by Heterotypic Nerves

The reinnervation of skin by alien nerves—either by collateral sprouting, direction of a particular nerve into territory it does not normally innervate, or grafting of skin into a foreign region—has not been examined extensively in mammals. Such heterotypic reinnervation has been examined to a greater extent in nonmammals and in other systems, e.g., the reinnervation of taste buds (45,91). Two main points concern us here: (a) Sensory, but not motor or autonomic, fibers can induce the regeneration of receptor specializations in foreign skin. When they do, the specializations are typical of the skin innervated rather than the nerve itself. In a classic example, duck bill skin was grafted onto the duck's leg (21). Following invasion by local cutaneous nerves, Grandry corpuscle receptors returned to the transplanted skin. These receptors are typical of duck bill skin but are not found in leg skin. In a similar experiment, Kadanoff (47) demonstrated reinnervation of hair follicles transplanted to hairless skin on the soles of the feet of mice and guinea pigs. (b) It is not clear whether axons that have occupied heterotypical receptors take on the response characteristics of the new receptor. In the taste system, this appears to be the case (65,70,95).

In the absence of much needed data, we might conclude that fibers exercise a remarkable degree of selectivity when reinnervating homotypical skin under relatively favorable conditions but can, if forced, make (functional?) connections with heterotypic receptors. The problem is to clarify the meaning of the term "forced." In a common sort of peripheral nerve injury a major trunk may be severed and its cut ends approximated with more-or-less fascicular mismatch. Will those errant fibers that proceed into endoneurial tubes leading to heterotypic receptor loci form functional connections there, or will/can they continue on to seek the receptor type appropriate to their central connections? Does it matter whether the fiber is led to the same general area it formerly innervated? Does it matter how many other normal or errant fibers are in competition with it and restricting its freedom of choice. The reinnervation of low-threshold receptor specializations by fibers with central connections of nociceptors could account for some features of hyperesthetic sensation.

Generation of Afferent Activity by Nonreceptor Mechanisms

Immediately after axons have been cut across or crushed they fire off a high-frequency repetitive volley, or "injury discharge." This can best be explained by the sudden depolarization of the axon due to current leakage through the cut end. In a matter of seconds or at most minutes, however, the fibers fall silent, although they can still be excited by electrical stimulation (50,87). Apparently the cut end self-seals, and adequate membrane potential is restored. During the next few days and weeks the axons die back a short distance (up to a few millimeters) and then emit one or more (commonly a number of) sprouts. Some sprouts curve centrally whereas others reach out. For those that fail to find the substrate of the distal peripheral nerve, continued growth is aborted and the sprouts form a tangled mass, the neuroma, the morphology of which has been extensively reviewed (13,19,26,38,77). The physiology of spike generation in the sprouts differs fundamentally from that in normal fiber endings (1).

Beginning as early as 3.5 hr after injury, severed sensory fibers take on a sustained spontaneous activity (50,85,86). We do not know yet if all fibers are involved or only selected classes. Motor fibers with sprouts do not fire spontaneously. The anomalous activity may persist for an unlimited period if regeneration is prevented and a nerve end neuroma forms.

On the other hand, following crush injury spontaneous activity ceases when peripheral connections are reformed and impulse generation again comes under the control of the peripheral receptor transduction process. The mechanisms generating the spontaneous activity have not been investigated closely. Kirk (50) argued that it originates in dorsal root ganglion cells rather than at the nerve end (86).

Electrical stimulation of a nerve with a neuroma sends spikes orthodromically toward the spinal cord and antidromically into the neuroma. A single antidromic volley silences the spontaneous activity for approximately 20 msec. A continuous stimulation train can silence spontaneous activity entirely. Even more surprising, a brief high-frequency tetanus can reduce the spontaneous spike rate for an hour or more (86). We proposed that these effects of antidromic invasion may be one of the mechanisms accounting for pain relief by transcutaneous electrical stimulation, particularly in cases where the relief long outlasts the stimulation (83,86). If this were the whole explanation, however, the activity aroused by counterstimulation should be no less painful than the spontaneous activity it blocks. Other mechanisms such as central inhibition must be invoked.

Axon sprouts in a neuroma are unmyelinated and therefore may resemble normal C-fibers. Relatively high frequency activity in C-fibers results in their hyperpolarization probably because of sodium pump activation (66, 69). This could account for the silencing of spontaneous activity of a neuroma by antidromic volleys. One might ask whether activity and therefore hyperpolarization of one sprout in a neuroma tends to hyperpolarize and silence its immediate neighbors. This seems not to be the case. In recordings of spontaneous activity in dorsal rootlets whose axons originate in a neuroma, stimulation of the remainder of the root had no effect on recorded spontaneous activity (86).

Granit et al. (34,35) demonstrated a substantial amount of cross-talk between adjacent axons in a nerve immediately following injury (crush or section). For example, a volley of impulses is recorded on dorsal roots on stimulation of ventral roots that share the same injured nerve. We recently confirmed this phenomenon in both rat and cat following crush or section of the sciatic nerve. The coupling begins to fail within seconds after the injury, however, and lasts at most approximately 30 min. If such interaction returned it could have important implications for altered sensation in damaged nerves. For example, anomalous afferent activity could be generated by intended movements or by dorsal root reflexes (81). In experiments using Nembutal-anesthetized or decerebrate rats in which a neuroma had formed on the severed sciatic nerve, we sought interaction between the peripheral part of dorsal and ventral roots and between adjacent dorsal roots. Recordings were made from whole roots and single fibers on stimulation of the remaining roots or the sciatic nerve itself. In no case have we been able to demonstrate cross-talk between adjacent myelinated or unmyelinated fibers. Impulse interaction has been described among segmentally demyelinated spinal root fibers in a strain of dystrophic mice (8,44,68).

Howe et al. (42) proposed another source of internally generated afferent activity in injured nerves. When a spike conducted along a large-diameter fiber approaches a region of geometric or electrical inhomogeneity (a sudden narrowing branch point, perhaps a zone of segmental demyelination), it may become prolonged. If its duration extends beyond the refractory period of the membrane it has just passed, a second impulse ("reflection potential") is generated and conducted back along the parent axon (32). Although the chance of reflection at each such point is small, if there were enough of them a single antidromic impulse (e.g., a dorsal root reflex) could in principle generate a cascade of orthodromic impulses. The proposal remains hypothetical. What is more, it seems more likely that afferent activity would be blocked by collision than overexcited by such a mechanism.

In addition to their generation of spontaneous impulses, axonal sprouts progressing successfully or arrested in a neuroma are unusually sensitive to mechanical disturbances (53,63). Percussion of an outgrowing nerve produces a tingling or frankly painful sensation (Tinel sign). Palpation of a neuroma can cause pain for years after the original nerve damage (77). In spinal nerves severed experimentally, palpation of the nerve end generates a vigorous afferent volley (50,85,86). This mechanical sensitivity is abolished by local anesthesia of the nerve end.

Dorsal root ganglia are also sensitive to mechanical disturbance and emit prolonged spike trains to maintained distortion (43). Finally, axon sprouts are unusually sensitive to the application of norepinephrine (86) and acetylcholine (20). It is not known if these sensitivities are universal or restricted to special axonal classes.

Sympathetic Efferents

In normal tissue the sympathetic system is thought to play little role in determining peripheral sensitivity. However, in certain types of nerve damage (e.g., causalgia and Sudek's atrophy), severe pain can be relieved by sympathectomy (23,73,77). The explanation generally offered is that in the area of the injury sympathetic and sensory fibers are coupled electrically and so sympathetic volleys generate afferent volleys (23). As described above, this hypothesis has not held up under experimental testing. Another possibility is chemical coupling. Since sprouts of sensory axons are sensitive to norepinephrine, they could become excited by norepinephrine leakage from damaged sympathetic fibers.

CHANGES ALONG THE COURSE OF AN AXON

Retrograde Shrinkage

Not only do injured nerves undergo peripheral degeneration followed by sprouting at the cut end, but there is also a series of complex retrograde changes that have been collectively termed "the axon reaction" (reviewed in ref. 55). Prominent among these changes is a reduction in fiber diameter and a consequent reduction in conduction velocity. The extent of retrograde shrinkage has been reported to be on the order of 20% (2), with corresponding slowing of spike conduction (15). Unless precise timing of impulse conduction across the fiber spectrum is an important component of

sensory coding, however, such shrinkage alone should not cause major sensory anomalies.

Differential Cell Death

A more important consideration is selective loss of certain components of the fiber spectrum. Small-diameter axons of the $A\delta$ and C groups include all fibers with high-threshold receptors (nociceptors) (12,96). Furthermore, it has been proposed that activity along large-diameter, low-threshold fibers impedes the forward conduction of nociceptive volleys by means of a spinal gate mechanism (59,62). Thus differential loss of large-diameter axons might be expected to cause pain. The compound action potential recorded on dorsal roots associated with a spinal nerve with a neuroma is slower and smaller than normal. Axon counts made just proximal to traumatic nerve injury, however, usually reveal increased numbers of axons along with a strong shift in their spectrum toward smaller diameters. This is a result of retrograde growth of some sprouts and retrograde shrinkage of parent fibers (2, 39,77). In fact, the number of parent fibers represented proximal to the point of injury can fall substantially due to retrograde degeneration of dorsal root ganglion cells (55,67). In addition, some of the remaining DRG cells may be sufficiently affected as to lose their ability to conduct centrally. Such functional blockade could be maintained for an extended period of time without frank morphological degeneration of the fibers (18,93).

There has recently been a great increase of our knowledge about the fiber spectrum in peripheral neuropathies (26,79). Unfortunately it is no longer possible to make generalizations about the expected symptomatology associated with a particular fiber spectrum. Large fibers are preferentially lost in postherpetic neuralgia, an unusually painful condition (64), but there is a loss of large fibers without pain in Friedreich's ataxia (24) and in uremic neuropathy (80). At the other end of the spectrum, Fabry's disease is associated with loss of small myelinated fibers and pain (52), but a hereditary sensory neuropathy described by Schoene et al. (72) has a loss of myelinated fibers (preserving C-fibers) and is associated with analgesia. In an attempt to make sense of this chaos, Dyck et al. (25) introduced the dynamic factor of the presence of ongoing degeneration as being an important predictor of pain. It does seem reasonable to conclude that fiber diameter alone is not enough or is completely irrelevant to explain the origin of pain in neuropathies. The reasons for this include the possibility that the area of significant change has not been examined. It might be that the important changes are central or peripheral to the biopsy site. Furthermore, anatomy does not necessarily predict physiology. The fibers may have abnormal sensitivities or central terminals, or may have lost inhibitory effects. The fibers may be in a state of change that is not revealed by a single static biopsy. Only when the anatomy and physiology of the entire length of the fiber is understood will it be possible to pinpoint the nature of the sensory defect in peripheral neuropathies.

Differential Sprouting

A sectioned axon usually emits a number of sprouts (13,39,74,90,91). Thus in the early stages of regeneration many more fibers appear distal to the lesion than proximal to it. With maturation the number of distal fibers declines until it is close to matching the number proximally. It has thus been presumed that only one of the sprouts is maintained and that the rest degenerate. This statistical argument is very much open to question, however, particularly in view of the fact that some proximal fibers may not contribute any sprouts at all. The possibility that certain regenerating fibers

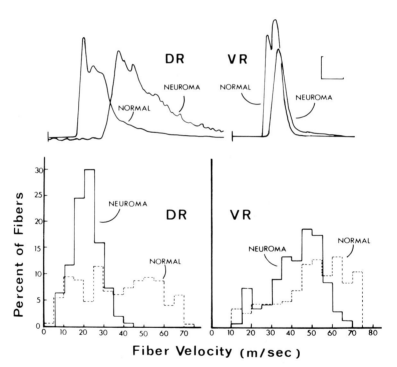

FIG. 2. Differential slowing of nerve conduction proximal to a chronic injury (neuroma). **Top:** Compound action potential recorded on dorsal roots (DR) and ventral roots (VR) L_4–L_6 on stimulation of a normal sciatic nerve or one with a neuroma of 83 days' standing. All four traces are from the same rat, comparing the intact side with the lesioned side. Note the differences in vertical calibration. Horizontal: 1.0 msec. Vertical: DR normal 1.0 mV, DR neuroma 0.2 mV, VR normal 5.0 mV, VR neuroma 2.0 mV. **Bottom:** Histograms of single fibers ($N = 141$–165) sampled from dorsal and ventral roots originating in normal sciatic nerve and in neuromas of 81–85 days' standing. Each fiber was driven by stimulation on the neuroma or the corresponding point on normal nerve, but fiber velocity was measured from a point 10–15 mm proximally and thus represents the velocity of the parent fiber.

maintain multiple distal branches has not been convincingly excluded (29). If this did occur, a number of interesting physiological consequences might be expected. For instance, afferent input entering the common parent fiber from one of the branches would interfere, by collision, with input approaching along its sister branches (56). The branch point itself might act as a spike frequency filter (37). The maintenance of multiple distal branches would have important implications for sensory localization and referred sensations.

Regenerating sprouts are not necessarily contributed equally by all members of the parent fiber population. Some classes may sprout more successfully than others. We examined the conduction velocity of those parent fibers that respond to electrical stimulation distal to a crush injury in the rat sciatic nerve. Single fiber recordings were made from small sheds of L_4–L_6 dorsal rootlets, and the conduction velocity from a point proximal to the crush was found for all responding fibers. At short survival times (up to 100 days) small-diameter parent fibers were underrepresented. By 150 days after the crush, however, the distribution of parent fiber velocities had become normal. We conclude that, given time, parent fibers of all classes emit successful sprouts and in approximately their normal representation in the nerve. The same result was obtained after sciatic nerve section and resuture.

Using similar means, we examined the parent axons whose sprouts are activated by electrical stimulation of a neuroma (17). Only parent fibers with slowly conducting axons were activated, and the slowing was more pronounced among dorsal root than ventral root fibers (Fig. 2). Interestingly, this relationship is reversed if the lesion is performed at an early age (78). It would seem that among sensory fibers participating in a neuroma either (a) small-diameter axons sprout selectively, (b) large-diameter fibers sprout but are blocked, or (c) large-diameter sensory fibers undergo more severe retrograde shrinkage and/or degeneration than has thus far been reported.

Fibers that end in a neuroma have a number of anomalous physiological properties: spontaneous activity, mechanical and chemical sensibility, and lasting retrograde changes. One or all of these peculiarities may account for the clinical symptoms of neuroma formation. We have preliminary evidence that the same properties may hold for those fibers in a severed nerve that fail to cross the gap and reinnervate skin. A partially damaged nerve that appears normal on palpation or even exploration may nevertheless behave physiologically like a neuroma by virtue of the scattered presence within it of fibers with sprouts that have come to a dead end.

Schwann Cells and Other Surrounding Tissue

These cells react to damage of axons and to degeneration (3). Since the myelin sheath depends on them, and presumably they also influence the chemical and ionic environment and supply of the axons, changes in surrounding cells might change the excitability and transmission properties of axons in their neighborhood.

CHANGES WITHIN THE SPINAL CORD

Severed axons undergo retrograde change. It has long been thought, however, that the effect is limited to the dorsal root ganglion and peripheral nerve, and does not influence spinal cord physiology or anatomy. Recent evidence suggests at least three mechanisms by which it might.

Changes in Primary Afferent Distribution

Retrograde change of neurons whose peripheral axon has been severed may subtly effect the intracord axon of the neuron. Horch et al. (40) sought the most rostral position in the dorsal columns from which dorsal root fibers could be driven by antidromic stimulation. Peripheral nerve injury did not affect the limits of fiber distribution as measured by this method, although the conduction velocity of the axonal segment within the dorsal columns was reduced. Within these limits, however, fine terminal arbors of primary afferents do undergo degenerative changes (33,51,94). Correlated with this is the reduction of acid phosphatase activity, a histochemical marker of some primary afferent endings in the substantia gelatinosa (4,51). In cases where the nerve injury is sufficiently severe to lead to death of ganglion cells, of course, the central axonal process degenerates completely. This mode of degeneration can be delayed by several weeks from the time of nerve injury (36). In sufficiently young animals injury in the periphery can lead to a failure of central and even cortical end-stations to elaborate (6,82).

Changes in Neighboring Primary Afferents

The central distribution and/or effectiveness of intact afferents may be changed by injury of adjacent fibers peripheral to the ganglion. A number of authors have claimed, but not unanimously, that following section of dorsal roots in adult cats, fibers of neighboring roots undergo collateral sprouting and expand their distribution in the cord at the expense of the degenerated fibers (31,48,49,57,58). Such collateral sprouting has not been reported as a consequence of injury peripheral to the ganglion, although such a possibility cannot be excluded. Biochemical changes have been detected in dorsal root ganglion cells following division of neighboring roots distal to the ganglion (89). Similarly, the terminal branches of Ia afferents in the ventral horn are affected by peripheral axotomy of their target motoneurons (30,60).

Basbaum and Wall (5) severed all dorsal roots caudal to L_3 in the cat except for S_1, which was spared. Immediately after the lesion they found that dorsal horn cells in the zone bordering L_4–L_5 were unresponsive to peripheral stimulation of any kind. Approximately a month later, however, cells in this zone began to show receptive fields in the skin innervated by the nearest intact roots, L_3 and/or S_1. These responses may reflect the invasion of collateral sprouts. On the other hand, it was recently demonstrated that even in normal animals the L_3 and S_1 roots in fact have distal axonal branches in the L_4–L_5 segments (88). Most of the synapses formed by these branches, however, are relatively ineffective in driving the cells after natural stimulation of the skin (16, 61) and therefore do not participate in their receptive fields. The appearance of responses in the previously nonresponsive zone may therefore indicate the uncovering or strength-

ening of previously existing connections. Dostrovsky et al. (22) demonstrated a similar unmasking in the dorsal column nuclei immediately after blocking primary afferent conduction, thus ruling out sprouting as an explanation. The absence of activity in neighboring fibers may well be stimulus enough to bring about a shift in the effective drive of the postsynaptic cell. It remains to be determined if these unmasking phenomena also occur following peripheral nerve injury.

Changes in Spinal Cord Cells Receiving Peripheral Afferents

The excitability of central cells is partially determined by the sum total of arriving impulses. If an axon is damaged, the central cell receives the injury discharge followed by silence and accordingly adjusts its excitability and ongoing discharge. If the damaged nerve develops its own abnormal afferent activity, the central cells again react (30,84).

Eccles and his collaborators (27,28) argued that disuse of an afferent channel leads to a reduction in its transmission capacity. In their strongest experiments they severed the nerve leading to a hindlimb muscle and after several weeks noted a reduction in motoneuron excitatory postsynaptic potentials (EPSPs) generated by stimulation of this nerve as compared to that generated by stimulation of the nerve to a synergistic muscle. Their conclusion is complicated by a number of factors. Among them is the fact that severance of a nerve does not in fact silence it for long, and such injury can cause changes in primary afferent terminals within the cord. In fact the opposite conclusion —that disuse sensitizes a synaptic channel— has stronger support. Afferent activity to Clarke's column neurons can be effectively silenced without degeneration by unloading the muscle spindles involved. This has been done for the gastrocnemius and soleus by severing the Achilles tendon, tenotomy in combination with muscle de-efferentation and fracture of the os calcis (54,76). In each instance, the result was an increased postsynaptic volley from the Clarke's column neurons after electrical stimulation of the silenced peripheral nerve.

We must remember that the normal afferent

barrage delivers an interacting complex of inhibitory and excitatory signals. An imbalance of these counterbalanced inputs caused by peripheral nerve injury may produce unusual and unpleasant sensations. It is not always simple to locate the origin of the abnormal discharge which agonizes the patient. In causalgia where local partial damage to a nerve has occurred or in pain associated with a herniated intervertebral disc, the pain ceases if the fibers central to lesion are blocked with local anesthetic. However, pain may also be relieved by blocking peripheral to the damage. It is not at all certain if this means that there are abnormal firings induced peripherally or if the pain requires the sustaining effect of the normal afferent barrage.

Finally, in certain rare cases of phantom limb pain, the pain persists when the amputation stump is completely anesthetized. It is not obvious in such a case whether some central mechanism now endlessly repeats the memory of the past injury, or if the axons and spinal cord cells central to the lesion are reacting to the nerve section. In an individual case of pain associated with peripheral nerve disease or damage, it is necessary to be able to lay aside the 12 factors discussed here before moving to the CNS in search of an explanation.

SUMMARY

Before resorting to the depths of the CNS for an explanation of the dysesthesia and pain that sometimes follow peripheral nerve injury, one must consider at least 12 sorts of physiological abnormality that may occur in the primary afferents themselves:

1. Modifications of receptor properties
2. Axon–receptor mismatch following regeneration
3. Mismatch in heterotypic reinnervation
4. Generation of afferent activity by non-receptor mechanisms
5. Sympathetic involvement
6. Retrograde cell reaction
7. Death of primary afferent neurons
8. Differential sprouting
9. Changes in supporting cells
10. Changes in axonal distribution in the spinal cord
11. Adjustment of neighboring fibers.

12. Changes in the efficacy of synapses on secondary sensory neurons

ACKNOWLEDGMENT

Prepared with support from the Medical Research Council, the National Institutes of Health, the Thyssen Foundation, and the Foundations' Fund for Research in Psychiatry.

REFERENCES

1. Aguayo, A. J., and Bray, G. M. (1975): Pathology and pathophysiology of unmyelinated nerve fibers. In: *Peripheral Neuropathy*, edited by P. J. Dyck, P. K. Thomas, and E. H. Lambert. Saunders, Philadelphia.
2. Aitken, J. T., and Thomas, P. K. (1962): Retrograde changes in fiber size following nerve section. *J. Anat.*, 96:121–129.
3. Asbury, A. K. (1975): The biology of Schwann cells. In: *Peripheral Neuropathy*, edited by P. J. Dyck, P. K. Thomas, and E. H. Lambert. Saunders, Philadelphia.
4. Barron, K. D., and Tuncbay, T. O. (1962): Phosphatase in cuneate nuclei after brachial plexectomy. *Arch. Neurol.*, 7:203–210.
5. Basbaum, A. I., and Wall, P. D. (1976): Chronic changes in the response of cells in adult cat dorsal horn following partial deafferentation: The appearance of responding cells in a previously non-responsive region. *Brain Res.*, 116:181–204.
6. Belford, G., and Killackey, H. P. (1976): The consequence of neonatal vibrissae removal on trigeminal pathways in rat. II. Development of anomalous brain stem pathways (primary and secondary afferents). *Neurosci. Abstr.*, 2:902.
7. Bessou, P., and Perl, E. R. (1969): Response of cutaneous sensory units with unmyelinated fibers to noxious stimuli. *J. Neurophysiol.*, 32:1025–1043.
8. Bray, G. M., and Aguayo, A. J. (1975): Quantitative ultrastructural studies of the axon–Schwann cell abnormalities in spinal nerve roots from dystrophic mice. *J. Neuropathol. Exp. Neurol.*, 34:517–530.
9. Brown, A. G., and Iggo, A. (1963): The structure and function of cutaneous 'touch corpuscles' after nerve crush. *J. Physiol. (Lond)*, 165:28–29P.
10. Burgess, P. R., English, K. B., Horch, K. W., and Stensaas, L. J. (1974): Patterning in the regeneration of type I cutaneous receptors. *J. Physiol. (Lond)*, 236:57–82.
11. Burgess, P. R., and Horch, K. W. (1973): Specific regeneration of cutaneous fibers in the cat. *J. Neurophysiol.*, 36:101–114.
12. Burgess, P. R., and Perl, E. R. (1973): Cutaneous mechanoreceptors and nociceptors.

In: *Handbook of Sensory Physiology, Vol. 2: Somatosensory System,* edited by A. Iggo. Springer-Verlag, Berlin.

13. Cajal, S. R. Y. (1928): *Degeneration and Regeneration in the Nervous System.* Translated and edited by R. M. May. Reprinted 1959. Hafner, New York.

14. Carlen, P. L., Wall, P. D., Nadvorna, H., and Steinbach, T. (1977): A study of phantom limbs and related phenomena in recent traumatic amputations. *In press.*

15. Cragg, B. G., and Thomas, P. K. (1961): Changes in conduction velocity and fiber size proximal to peripheral nerve lesions. *J. Physiol. (Lond),* 157:315–327.

16. Devor, M., Merrill, E. G., and Wall, P. D. (1977): Dorsal horn cells that respond to stimulation of distant dorsal roots. *J. Physiol. (Lond),* 270:519–532.

17. Devor, M., and Wall, P. D. (1976): Type of sensory nerve fibre sprouting to form a neuroma. *Nature (Lond),* 262:705–708.

18. Denny-Brown, D., and Brenner, C. (1944): Paralysis of nerve induced by direct pressure and by tourniquet. *Arch. Neurol. Psychiatry,* 51:1–26.

19. Denny-Brown, D., and Brenner, C. (1944): The effect of percussion of nerve. *J. Neurol. Neurosurg. Psychiatry,* 7:76–95.

20. Diamond, J. (1959): The effects of injecting acetylcholine into normal and regenerating nerves. *J. Physiol. (Lond),* 145:611–629.

21. Dijkstra, C. (1933): Die De-und Regeneration der sensiblen Endkörperchen des Entenschnabels (Grandry-und Herbst-Körperchen) nach Durchschneidung des Nerven, nach Fortnahme der ganzen Haut und nach Transplantation des Hautstückchens. *Z. Mikrosk. Anat. Forsch.,* 34:75–158.

22. Dostrovsky, J. O., Millar, J., and Wall, P. D. (1976): The immediate shift of afferent drive of dorsal column nucleus cells following deafferentation: A comparison of acute and chronic deafferentation in gracile nucleus and spinal cord. *Exp. Neurol.,* 52:480–495.

23. Doupe, J., Cullen, C. H., and Chance, G. Q. (1944): Post-traumatic pain and causalgic syndrome. *J. Neurol. Neurosurg. Psychiatry,* 7:33–48.

24. Dyck, P. J., Lambert, E. H., and Nichols, P. (1971): Sensation related to compound action potentials and number and size of myelinated and unmyelinated fibers of sural nerve in health, Friedreich's ataxia, hereditary sensory neuropathy and tabes dorsalis. In: *Handbook of EEG and Clinical Neurophysiology, Vol. 9,* edited by A. Remond. Elsevier, Amsterdam.

25. Dyck, P. J., Lambert, E. H., and O'Brien, P. C. (1976): Pain in peripheral neuropathy related to rate and kind of fiber degeneration. *Neurology (Minneap),* 26:466–471.

26. Dyck, P. J., Thomas, P. K., and Lambert, E. H., editors (1974): *Peripheral Neuropathy.* Saunders, Philadelphia.

27. Eccles, J. C., Krnjevic, K., and Miledi, R. (1959): Delayed effects of peripheral severance of afferent nerve fibers on the efficacy of their central synapses. *J. Physiol. (Lond),* 145:204–220.

28. Eccles, J. C., and McIntyre, A. K. (1953): The effects of disuse and of activity on mammalian spinal reflexes. *J. Physiol. (Lond),* 121:492–516.

29. Fullerton, P. M., and Gilliatt, R. W. (1965): Axon reflex in human motor nerve fibers. *J. Neurol. Neurosurg. Psychiatry,* 28:1–11.

30. Gelfan, S. (1975): Denervation and neuronal interdependence. In: *Advances in Neurology, Vol. 12* edited by G. W. Kreutzberg. Raven Press, New York.

31. Goldberger, M. E., and Murray, M. (1974): Restitution of function and collateral sprouting in the cat spinal cord: The deafferented animal. *J. Comp. Neurol.,* 158:37–54.

32. Goldstein, S. S., and Rall, W. (1974): Changes of action potential shape and velocity for changing core conductor geometry. *Biophys. J.,* 14:731–757.

33. Goode, G. E. (1976): The ultrastructural identification of primary and suprasegmental afferents in the marginal and gelatinous layers of lumbar spinal cord following central and peripheral lesions. *Neurosci. Abstr.,* 2:975.

34. Granit, R., Leksell, L., and Skoglund, C. R. (1944): Fibre interaction in injured or compressed region of nerve. *Brain,* 67:125–140.

35. Granit, R., and Skoglund, C. R. (1945): Facilitation, inhibition and depression at the 'artificial synapse' formed by the cut end of a mammalian nerve. *J. Physiol. (Lond),* 103:435–448.

36. Grant, G., and Arvidsson, J. (1975): Transganglionic degeneration in trigeminal primary sensory neurons. *Brain Res.,* 95:265–279.

37. Grossman, Y., Spira, M. E., and Parnas, I. (1973): Differential flow of information into branches of a single axon. *Brain Res.,* 64:327–386.

38. Guth, L. (1956): Regeneration in the mammalian peripheral nervous system. *Physiol. Rev.,* 36:441–478.

39. Gutmann, E., and Sanders, F. K. (1943): Recovery of fiber numbers and diameters in the regeneration of peripheral nerves. *J. Physiol. (Lond),* 101:489–518.

40. Horch, K. W. (1976): Ascending collaterals of cutaneous neurons in the fasciculus gracilis of the cat during peripheral nerve regeneration. *Brain Res.,* 117:19–32.

41. Horch, K. W., Burgess, P. R., and Whitehorn, D. (1976): Ascending collaterals of cutaneous neurons in the fasciculus gracilis of the cat. *Brain Res.,* 117:1–17.

42. Howe, J. F., Calvin, W. H., and Loeser, J. D. (1976): Impulses reflected from dorsal root ganglia and from focal nerve injuries. *Brain Res.,* 116:139–144

43. Howe, J. F., Loeser, J. D., and Calvin, W. H.

(1977): Mechanosensitivity of dorsal root ganglia and chronically injured axons: A physiological basis for the radicular pain of nerve root compression. *Pain*, 3:25–41.

44. Huizar, P., Kuno, M., and Miyata, Y. (1975): Electrophysiological properties of spinal motoneurons of normal and dystrophic mice. *J. Physiol. (Lond)*, 248:231–246.

45. Jacobson, M. (1971): Formation of neuronal connections in sensory systems. In: *Handbook of Sensory Physiology, Vol. 1: Principles of Receptor Physiology*, edited by W. R. Loewenstein. Springer-Verlag, Berlin.

46. Jacobson, M., and Baker, R. E. (1969): Development of neuronal connections with skin grafts: Behavioral and electrophysiological studies. *J. Comp. Neurol.*, 137:121–142.

47. Kadanoff, D. (1925): Untersuchungen über die Regeneration der sensiblen Nervenendigungen nach Vertauschen verschieden innervierten Hautstucke. *Arch. Entw. Mech. Organ.*, 106:249–278.

48. Kerr, F. W. L. (1975): Neuroplasticity of primary afferents in the neonatal cat and some results of early deafferentation of the trigeminal spinal nucleus. *J. Comp. Neurol.*, 163:305–328.

49. Kerr, F. W. L. (1972): The potential of cervical primary afferents to sprout in the spinal nucleus of V following long term trigeminal denervation. *Brain Res.*, 43;547–560.

50. Kirk, E. J. (1974): Impulses in dorsal spinal nerve rootlets in cats and rabbits arising from dorsal root ganglia isolated from the periphery. *J. Comp. Neurol.*, 2:165–176.

51. Knyihar, E., and Csillik, B. (1976): Effect of peripheral axotomy on the fine structure and histochemistry of the Rolando substance: Degenerative atrophy of central processes on pseudounipolar cells. *Exp. Brain Res.*, 26:73–87.

52. Kocen, R. S., and Thomas, P. K. (1970): Peripheral nerve involvement in Fabry's disease. *Arch. Neurol.*, 22:81–89.

53. Konorski, J., and Lubinska, L. (1946): Mechanical excitability of regenerating nerve fibers. *Lancet*, 250:609–610.

54. Kozak, W., and Westerman, R. A. (1961): Plastic changes of monosynaptic responses from tenotomized muscles in cats. *Nature (Lond)*, 189:753–755.

55. Lieberman, A. R. (1971): The axon reaction: A review of the principle features of perikaryal responses to axon injury. *Int. Rev. Neurobiol.*, 14:49–124.

56. Lindblom, U. F. (1958): Excitability and functional organization within a peripheral tactile unit. *Acta Physiol. Scand. [Suppl. 153]*, 44.

57. Liu, C. N., and Chambers, W. W. (1958): Intraspinal sprouting of dorsal root axons. *Arch. Neurol. Psychiatry*, 79:46–61.

58. McCouch, G. P., Austin, G. M., Liu, C. N., and Liu, C. Y. (1958): Sprouting as a cause of spasticity. *J. Neurophysiol.*, 21:205–216.

59. Melzack, R., and Wall, P. D. (1965): Pain mechanisms: A new theory. *Science*, 150:971–979.

60. Mendell, L. M., Munson, J. B., and Scott, J. G. (1974): Connectivity changes of Ia afferents on axotomized motoneurons. *Brain Res.*, 73:338–342.

61. Merrill, E. G., and Wall, P. D. (1972): Factors forming the edge of a receptive field: The presence of relatively ineffective afferents. *J. Physiol. (Lond)*, 226:825–846.

62. Meyer, G. A., and Fields, H. L. (1972): Causalgia treated by selective large fiber stimulation of peripheral nerve. *Brain*, 95:163–168.

63. Nathan, P. W., and Rennie, A. M. (1946): Value of Tinel's sign. *Lancet*, 250:610–611.

64. Noordenbos, W. (1959): *Pain*. Elsevier, Amsterdam.

65. Oakley, B. (1967): Altered temperature and taste responses from cross-regenerated sensory nerves in the rats' tongue. *J. Physiol. (Lond)*, 188:353–371.

66. Rang, H. P., and Ritchie, J. M. (1968): On the electrogenic sodium pump in mammalian non-myelinated nerve fibers and its activation by various external cations. *J. Physiol. (Lond)*, 196:183–221.

67. Ranson, S. W. (1906): Retrograde degeneration in the spinal nerves. *J. Comp. Neurol.*, 16:265–293.

68. Rasminsky, M., and Kierney, R. E. (1976): Continuous conduction in large diameter bare axons in spinal roots of dystrophic mice. *Neurology (Minneap)*, 26:367.

69. Ritchie, J. M., and Staub, R. W. (1957): The hyperpolarization which follows activity in mammalian non-medullated fibers. *J. Physiol. (Lond)*, 136:80–97.

70. Robbins, N. (1967): Peripheral modification of sensory nerve responses after cross-regeneration. *J. Physiol. (Lond)*, 192:493–504.

71. Sanders, F. K., and Whitteridge (1946): Conduction velocity and myelin thickness in regenerating nerve fibers. *J. Physiol. (Lond)*, 105:152–174.

72. Schoene, W. C., Asbury, A. L., Astrom, K. E., and Masters, R. (1970): Hereditary sensory neuropathy. *J. Neurol. Sci.*, 11:463–472.

73. Seddon, H. J. (1972): *Surgical Disorders of the Peripheral Nerves*. Williams & Wilkins, Baltimore.

74. Shawe, G. D. H. (1955): On the number of branches formed by regenerating nerve-fibers. *Br. J. Surg.*, 42:474–488.

75. Smith, K. R. (1967): The structure and function of the Haarscheibe. *J. Comp. Neurol.*, 131:459–474.

76. Spencer, W. A., and April, R. S. (1972): Plastic properties of monosynaptic pathways in mammals. In: *Short-Term Changes in Neural Activity and Behavior*, edited by

G. Horn and R. A. Hinde. (C.U.P. 1970).

77. Sunderland, S. (1972): *Nerves and Nerve Injuries.* Churchill Livingstone, London.

78. Szentagothai, J., and Rajkovits, K. (1955): Die Ruckwirkung der Spezifischen Funktion auf die Struktur der Nervenelemente. *Acta Morphol. Hung.,* 253–274.

79. Thomas, P. K. (1975): The anatomical substratum of pain. *Can. J. Neurol. Sci.,* 1:92–97.

80. Thomas, P. K., Hollinrake, K., Lascelles, R. G., O'Sullivan, D. J., Baillod, R. A., Moorhead, J. F., and Mackenzie, J. C. (1971): The polyneuropathy of chronic renal failure. *Brain,* 94:761–780.

81. Toennies, J. F. (1938): Reflex discharge from the spinal cord over the dorsal roots. *J. Neurophysiol.,* 1:378–390.

82. Van der Loos, H., and Woolsey, T. A. (1973): Somatosensory cortex: Structural alterations following early injury to sense organs. *Science,* 179:395–397.

83. Wall, P. D. (1977): The gate control theory of pain mechanisms: A critique of a critical review. *In press.*

84. Wall, P. D. (1964): Presynaptic control of impulses at the first central synapse in the cutaneous pathway. In: *Progress in Brain Research, Vol. 12: Physiology of Spinal Neurons,* edited by J. C. Eccles and J. P. Schade. Elsevier, Amsterdam.

85. Wall, P. D., and Gutnick, M. (1974): Properties of afferent nerve impulses originating from a neuroma. *Nature (Lond),* 248:740–743.

86. Wall, P. D., and Gutnick, M. (1974): Ongoing activity in peripheral nerves: The physiology and pharmacology of impulses originating from a neuroma. *Exp. Neurol.,* 43:580–593.

87. Wall, P. D., Waxman, S., and Basbaum, A. I. (1974): Ongoing activity in peripheral nerve: Injury discharge. *Exp. Neurol.,* 45:576–589.

88. Wall, P. D., and Werman, R. (1976): The physiology and anatomy of long ranging afferent fibers within the spinal cord. *J. Physiol. (Lond),* 255:321–334.

89. Watson, W. E. (1973): Some responses of neurons of dorsal root ganglia to axotomy. *J. Physiol. (Lond),* 231:41–42P.

90. Weddell, G. (1942): Axonal regeneration in cutaneous nerve plexuses. *J. Anat.,* 77:49–62.

91. Weddell, G., Guttman, L., and Gutman, E. (1941): The local extension of nerve fibers into denervated areas of skin. *J. Neurol. Psychiatry,* 4:206–225.

92. Weiss, P. (1936): Selectivity controlling the central-peripheral relations in the nervous system. *Biol. Rev.,* 11:494–531.

93. Weiss, P., and Davis, H. (1943): Pressure block in nerves provided with arterial sleeves. *J. Neurophysiol.,* 6:269–286.

94. Westrum, L. E., Canfield, R. C., and Black, R. G. (1976): Transganglionic degeneration in the spinal trigeminal nucleus following removal of tooth pulps in adult cats. *Brain Res.,* 101:137–140.

95. Zalewski, A. A. (1973): Regeneration of taste buds in tongue grafts after reinnervation by neurons in transplanted lumbar sensory ganglia. *Exp. Neurol.,* 40:161–169.

96. Zimmerman, M. (1976): Neurophysiology of nociception. *Int. Rev. Physiol.,* 10:179–222.

Physiology and Pathobiology of Axons, edited by
S. G. Waxman. Raven Press, New York © 1978.

Axonal Specification of Schwann Cell Expression and Myelination

Peter S. Spencer and Harold J. Weinberg

Departments of Neuroscience and Pathology, Rose F. Kennedy Center for Research in Human Development and Mental Retardation, Albert Einstein College of Medicine, Bronx, New York 10461

The purpose of this chapter is to explore the concept that the neuron plays the dominant role in regulating the function and metabolic activity of the cells which ensheath its axon, notably in regard to their property of myelination. The evidence for this statement is drawn almost exclusively from investigations of the mammalian peripheral nervous system (PNS). Nevertheless, given the conservative nature of biological evolution, it would be surprising if the principles of organizational control which operate in the mammalian central nervous system (CNS) differ fundamentally from those which exist in the periphery. The need for brevity precludes review of the vast literature pertaining to peripheral nerve biology and pathology (13,23,41,42). Instead, we have chosen to presume the reader's familiarity with the subject, while attempting to erect a speculative theory of axon–Schwann cell interaction based on communication between putative surface membrane molecules.

Several features of the biology of peripheral nerve fibers betray the existence of a controlled interdependence between the neuron and the Schwann cells which ensheath its axon. For example, consider the proportional relationship found between the volume of the neuronal soma, the diameter of the axon, the territorial (internodal) length of the ensheathing Schwann cells, and the thickness of the myelin sheath. Note also the regular spacing of Schwann cells along myelinated and unmyelinated fibers and the 1:1 relationship of axon and Schwann cell required for myelination. Other features of the cellular interrelationship

become evident in pathological states: the consistent attenuation of the axon during focal demyelination, the formation of shortened internodes of myelin during remyelination and regeneration, and the mitotic responses of Schwann cells to axonal degeneration *in vivo* and axonal regeneration *in vitro* (50). A vivid illustration of the mutual interdependence of axon and myelinating cell may be gleaned from heterogenous grafting experiments utilizing nerves obtained from normal mice and the myelin-deficient trembler mutant (1). Abnormally small trembler regenerating axons enlarge and become well myelinated when presented to normal Schwann cells; conversely, normal regenerating axons presented to trembler Schwann cells become attenuated and myelin-deficient. Such evidence indicates that it would be a mistake to deny the role of the Schwann cell in regulating axonal size and perhaps other aspects of axonal and neuronal biology. However, it is the thesis of this chapter that the neuron and its axon together represent the dominant partner in the relationship, the Schwann cell primarily functioning as the recipient and responding partner.

EVIDENCE FOR NEURONAL REGULATION OF MYELINOGENESIS

Independent studies in two laboratories recently established that the myelinating behavior of the Schwann cell is regulated by the axon with which it is associated (2,44,45). Both groups of investigators employed the technique of nerve cross-anastomosis by which Schwann

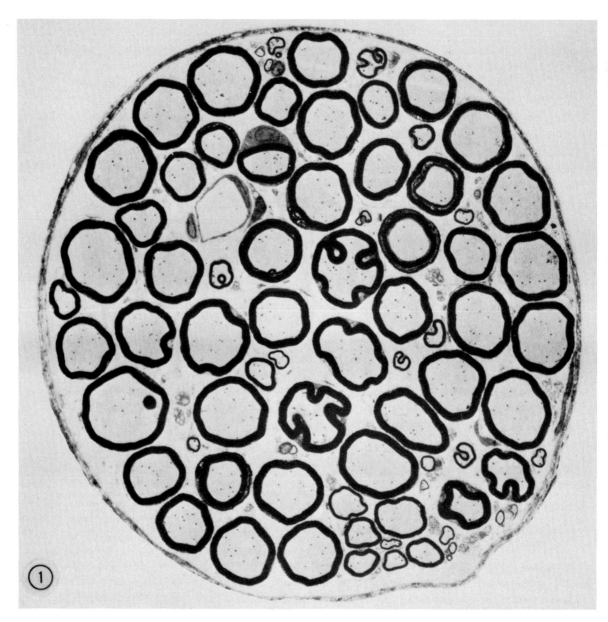

FIG. 1. Normal myelinated nerve (sternohyoid) used as the proximal stump in the cross-anastomosis experiment. Figures 1–3 are electron micrographs of beam-thinned 0.25 μm unstained epoxy cross sections. ×2,000. (From ref. 44.)

cells derived from unmyelinated nerves could be confronted by axons regenerating from myelinated nerves. In our investigations the proximal stump of a transected rat sternohyoid nerve (myelinated) was anastomosed in a Silastic tube to the distal stump of an adjacent severed cervical sympathetic trunk (unmyelinated) (Figs. 1 and 2). Fibers in the myelinated nerve stump underwent regeneration and penetrated into the unmyelinated distal stump where Schwann cells were dividing to form a dedifferentiated population as a consequence of Wallerian degeneration. These cells associated normally with the foreign regenerating

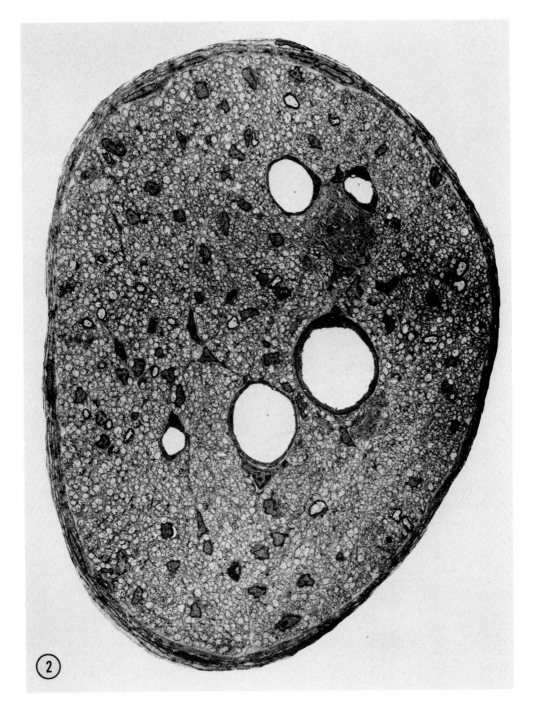

FIG. 2. Normal unmyelinated nerve (cervical sympathetic trunk) used as the distal stump in the cross-anastomosis experiment. ×1,600. (From ref. 44.)

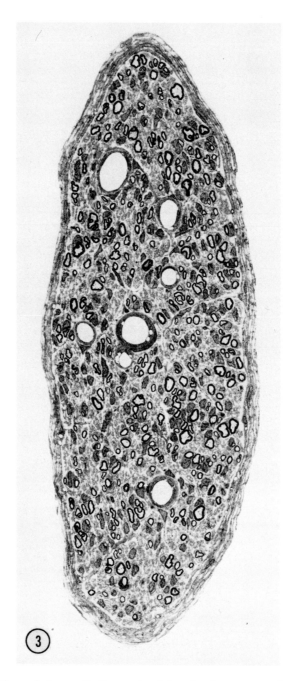

FIG. 3. Distal stump of the cervical sympathetic nerve trunk 6 weeks after anastomosis with a sternohyoid nerve. The formerly unmyelinated nerve (Fig. 2) now contains a large number of regenerating myelinated fibers. ×900. (From ref. 44.)

axons and were able to elaborate myelin sheaths (Fig. 3). This was evident from quantitative electron microscope examination of the anastomosed distal stump several weeks after anastomosis when there was a significant increase in the number of myelinated fibers compared with that of the normal cervical sympathetic trunk. The origin of the myelinating cells in the formerly unmyelinated nerve was studied by following the behavior of Schwann cells that had been labeled selectively in either nerve stump. By examining the distribution of the labeled cells after anastomosis, it was demonstrated that the newly myelinating cells were derived from the original cell population of the unmyelinated nerve. These data allowed us to conclude that peripheral nerves contain a uniform population of Schwann cells, the formation of myelin being dictated by the type of axon with which the ensheathing cell is associated.

PUTATIVE MECHANISMS OF NEURONAL REGULATION

Several theories have been proposed relating neuronal influences to the onset and degree of myelination. One hypothesis developed from the concept that a trophic factor, secreted by the neuron and distributed along the axon, functioned in the maintenance of the myelin sheath. From the observations that myelin development is dependent on neuronal maturation *in vitro* and that Schwann cells become associated with the growing tips of myelinated axons in preference to those of unmyelinated axons *in vivo,* it was suggested that the critical stimulus switching on Schwann cells to form myelin might be a chemical messenger derived from the neuronal perikaryon and transported via the axon to instruct the Schwann cell (30, 37–39).

Another hypothesis suggested that the alterations in axonal size which accompany growth mediate the neuronal regulation of myelinogenesis. One such proposal was that shrinkage of the axon would remove contact inhibition from the Schwann cell, thereby allowing rotational growth to commence (34). Others suggested that myelin thickness was influenced by the amount the Schwann cell was stretched during longitudinal growth of the axon. A detailed theory relating incremental changes in

axonal caliber to the rate and amount of myelin formation was proposed by Friede (18). This involved a three-step process: stretching and elongation of the Schwann cell plasmalemma at the mesaxon to accommodate axonal expansion, the transformation of each unit of plasmalemma into three units of myelin to produce new lamellae, and slippage between existing lamellae to adjust the sheath to further axonal enlargement. Much of the impetus for this theory was the concept of a critical axonal diameter at which myelination would proceed, and the existence of a linear relationship between axon circumference and myelin thickness in the adult animal (12,18). More recent studies, however, pointed out that myelinogenesis commences about axons of varying diameter, and that it is inappropriate to extrapolate data obtained from the adult to the developing animal (16,17).

Although Friede's theory has met with opposition (7,43), it has served to focus attention on the likely importance of surface membrane interaction in the neuronal regulation of myelin production. Any new theory of myelination should relate this mechanism of communication to the cellular control of myelinogenesis. The latter is generally assumed to occur at the level of nuclear DNA, the cell which forms myelin having differentiated considerably from the nonmyelin-forming cell (28). One interesting view is that the biogenesis of myelin is a coordinated phenomenon in which a series of enzymes is transcribed at a particular stage of nervous system development. The regulation of this transcription is envisaged either as an induction of myelin enzyme operon or by sequential transcription, where the synthesis of one enzyme or its products regulates the transcription of enzymes involved in later stages of biosynthesis (25).

INTERCELLULAR COMMUNICATION AND REGULATION OF INTRACELLULAR METABOLISM

Before discussing an alternative theory for the neuronal regulation of Schwann cell behavior, it is pertinent briefly to consider some contemporary concepts of intercellular communication—how information is received on cell surfaces and how it is transmitted to the level of nuclear DNA. The mechanism by which communication occurs between spatially related cells is poorly understood. Some dissociated cells seem able to use soluble factors to promote cell aggregation (4,5). Theoreticians have suggested that specific cell recognition occurs by complementary molecular interaction at cell surfaces. This idea has been extended in the "cell ligand" hypothesis in which glycoprotein complexes serve as cell receptor sites, specificity of cellular interaction being determined by varied topographic arrangements of the ligands. According to this idea, apposed cells with high ligand complementarity become linked whereas those with low complementarity adhere poorly if at all (27). Roseman (35) modified the ligand theory by suggesting that the protein–carbohydrate interaction at the cell surface might involve a specific enzymatic reaction. This model suggests that one (A) of two interacting cells (A and B) has a certain incomplete chain of monosaccharides on a surface membrane glycoprotein. The second cell has the appropriate enzyme (glycosyl transferase) to transfer an appropriate sugar nucleotide (UDP–glycose) from its cytoplasm to the glycoprotein on A. An absence of sugar nucleotide would allow enzyme and substrate to remain combined, thereby promoting cellular adhesion; conversely, the presence of the nucleotide would result in separation effected by transfer of the sugar nucleotide.

The detection of a glycoprotein in myelin has led to speculation that it might function in the cell recognition and contact phenomena assumed to be involved in myelinogenesis (32). Brady and Quarles suggested a role for both glycoproteins and gangliosides in myelination (9). According to this idea, the CNS neuron (whose axon is to be myelinated) exports an activator or inducer of hydrolytic enzymes, which changes the composition of the plasma membrane of the myelinating cell and/or the axon. This leads to a complementary ganglioside pattern which promotes adhesion of apposing cell surfaces. Brady and Quarles further suggested that glycoproteins and glycosyl transferases on the surface membranes might also interact as proposed in the Roseman model.

How do signals arriving on the cell surface regulate cellular metabolism? In considering this problem, Roseman suggested that plasma-

lemmae contain a variety of specific receptors which, after binding with informational molecules, release specific intracellular messenger substances such as a protein or a messenger RNA. One important and widespread mediator of intracellular metabolism is the cyclic nucleotide adenosine 3'5'-monophosphate (cyclic AMP). The concentration of cyclic AMP within the cell is regulated by two apposing enzymes: adenylate cyclase, which catalyzes the formation of cyclic AMP from adenosine triphosphate, and cAMP phosphodiesterase, which breaks down cyclic AMP. The significant feature of this system for the purposes of the present discussion is that adenylate cyclase may be activated by exogenous signals arriving on cell surface receptors, thereby promoting the formation of cyclic AMP. This molecule modulates cell metabolism by stimulating the phosphorylation of proteins by protein kinases, one important method of regulating intracellular function. For example, cyclic AMP-dependent phosphorylation and dephosphorylation of histones and acidic proteins of chromatin might provide a method for regulating nuclear fractions and genome expression (3). Cyclic AMP-dependent protein kinase stimulation of protein phosphorylation has been recognized in CNS and, in our laboratory, in PNS myelin (22,26). This is relevant to the control of myelination because developmental differences in the phosphorylation of certain peripheral myelin proteins have been noted during the period of myelinogenesis. It now seems reasonable to explore the possibility that a cyclic AMP-dependent kinase system exists in the plasmalemma of the Schwann cell, thereby possibly providing the cell with a mechanism by which to respond to exogenous axonal stimuli. Preliminary studies in our laboratory have pointed to the existence of such a system in crude plasma membrane fractions obtained from dedifferentiated Schwann cells (51) (*vide infra*).

A UNITARY THEORY OF NEURONAL REGULATION OF SCHWANN CELL FUNCTION

A satisfactory theory of neuronal regulation of Schwann cell function should not only consider the control of myelination but also ac-

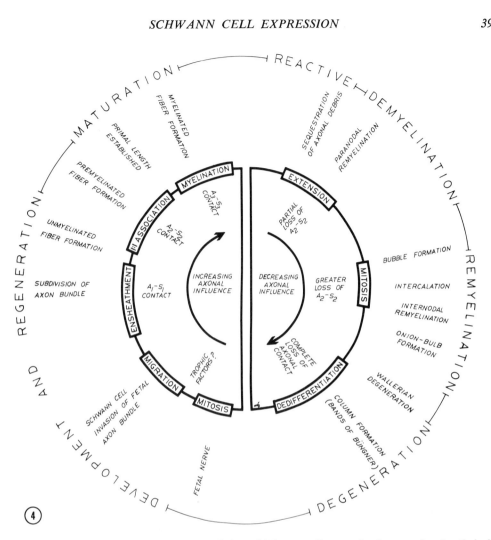

FIG. 4. A working hypothesis of the axonal regulation of Schwann cell expression in normal and pathological states. See text for explanation.

count for the entire gamut of axon–Schwann cell interactions in normal and pathological states. The unitary theory tentatively presented here attempts to correlate contemporary theories of cell sorting, interaction, and metabolic regulation with available data on the behavior of axons and Schwann cells during development and in a wide range of pathological states (Fig. 4). The model is based on three principal assumptions. First, it is assumed that Schwann cells form a single, undifferentiated population in the fetal nerve, a reasonable extrapolation from results of the cross-anastomosis experiments discussed above. The second assumption proposes that complementary molecular sites exist on the axolemma (i.e., instructors A_{1-3}), and the plasmalemma of the Schwann cell (i.e., receptors S_{1-3}), their interaction variably bestowing on the Schwann cell the property of adhesiveness to the axon, contact inhibition, and myelin production. The final assumption considers that during fetal development the axolemma of axons to be myelinated progresses from an undifferentiated to a differentiated (premyelinated) state. This is envisioned to result from neuronal production of membrane instructors, which are transported via the axon for insertion into the axolemma. Axons destined to remain unmyelinated fail to differentiate in this manner.

PERIPHERAL NERVE FIBER DEVELOPMENT

The Myelinated Fiber

Several phases of the process of myelination must be considered: the partitioning of axon bundles by migrating and mitosing Schwann cells, the establishment of a 1:1 axon/Schwann cell relationship, the production of myelin-specific components, the phenomena of membrane spiralization and compaction, and the cessation of production of new myelin lamellae. The fetal nerve is composed of a bundle of contiguous naked axons surrounded by undifferentiated Schwann cells. It is proposed that the initial phase of interaction between these two populations involves either a surface-surface interaction between axons and Schwann cells, or release from the axon of a soluble molecule serving to attract the surrounding Schwann cells. This might be a metabolic product (e.g., carbon dioxide) or a specific trophic substance. Schwann cells would respond by mitosing and migrating along a gradient of concentration of the attracting molecule. The daughter cells would invade the fetal nerve and partition groups of axons. The pattern of Schwann cell movement around the axons would be dictated by interaction between instructors and receptors located on the axolemma (A_1) and Schwann cell plasmalemma (S_1), respectively. At this stage, partitioning would be arbitrary because Schwann cells would display equal affinity to all axons within the bundle.

The second phase of cellular interaction—establishment of a unitary relationship between axon and Schwann cell—would occur at a stage of neuronal maturation when a new membrane component (A_2) would be produced and incorporated into the axolemma. This represents the committed step in the formation of a premyelinated axon. The new instructor molecule would interact with pre-existing Schwann cell receptors (S_2), the A_2–S_2 bond increasing cellular adhesiveness and causing retraction and separation from other Schwann cells and undifferentiated axons. Once the 1:1 relationship between axon and Schwann cell is established, the Schwann cell would extend longitudinally until a specific number of receptor/instructor interactions results in contact inhibition and the prevention of further extension. The Schwann cell would then be extended to its "primitive length," at which point it would occupy the minimal territory required for myelination to commence.

The next phase preparatory to myelin formation requires the production of myelin components by the Schwann cell. This might involve another axolemmal instructor (A_3), which would interact with a third, pre-existing Schwann cell receptor (S_3). Such interaction (A_3–S_3) would activate intracellular regulatory systems capable of inducing the sequential synthesis of myelin components. The production of one component might precipitate the formation of enzymes required to synthesize the next component in the sequence. Following synthesis and assembly, membrane components would be transported to the plasmalemma, perhaps via the Golgi apparatus (19). Insertion of membrane components would enlarge the plasmalemma and cause growth of the free edges of the Schwann cell adjacent to the mesaxon. Spiralization would be effected by surface recognition between the growing edge of the Schwann cell and either the adjacent axolemma or Schwann cell plasmalemma. [The ability of oligodendrocytes in a denervated optic nerve to elaborate myelin around astrocytic processes indicates that the myelinating cells in the CNS do not require an axolemma to effect spiralization (Weinberg and Spencer, *unpublished*).] Compaction would then follow the insertion of appropriate myelin components into apposed Schwann cell plasmalemmae. Spiralization would commence at the inner mesaxon and continue at that site until compaction of myelin lamellae impedes transfer of membrane components from the Golgi apparatus (located in the adaxonal cytoplasm) to this site. Membrane components would be diverted to the outer mesaxon, which would then continue and complete the spiralization process. Myelin membrane redistribution or slippage would be required to accommodate the growing axon. The amount of myelin components manufactured by the Schwann cell, and therefore the ultimate thickness of the myelin sheath, would depend on the amount of intracellular messenger released, which in turn would depend on the number of A_3–S_3 interactions. The number of axolemmal instructors, which would determine the potential A_3–S_3 interactions, would be proportional to the *surface area* of the axon contact. As the axon increased in diameter and internodal length, its surface area would enlarge, allowing additional surface molecular interaction and the production of new myelin components. In this way, a linear relationship would develop between axon caliber and myelin thickness or total fiber diameter. Since the ratio (g) between the former and latter quantities varies in different parts of the PNS (48), the density or arrangement of instructor molecules on the axolemma should be neuron-specific.

After the elaboration of new turns of myelin has ceased, the Schwann cell must provide a continuous supply of myelin precursors in order to maintain the integrity of the myelin sheath. The control mechanisms for this process might involve a self-regulating system in which an excess production of precursors would lead to their accumulation in the cytoplasm and consequential inhibition of the responsible synthetic mechanisms.

The Unmyelinated Fiber

Unlike the myelinated fiber, the mature unmyelinated fiber is characterized by multiple small axons lying separately in surface furrows of regularly spaced but longitudinally overlapping Schwann cells. Development of the unmyelinated fiber would differ from that of the myelinated fiber because the enveloped axons would fail to elaborate the specific axolemmal signals (instructors A_2, A_3) required for myelination. Schwann cells interacting with preunmyelinated axons would continue to divide until contact inhibition was achieved by interaction between overlapping Schwann cells and by Schwann cell/axon apposition. Cessation of longitudinal growth might promote the formation of laterally directed processes, which would partition and envelop each axon. The final arrangement of axons at any one level would reflect the shape assumed by the

Schwann cell when its growth and cytoplasmic redistribution ceased.

Initial and Terminal Regions of Myelinated Fibers

Two regions of the PNS require special consideration. One is the somatic sensory neuron and the initial (prebifurcation) portion of its axon (Fig. 5). Satellite cells surround the neuronal cyton and nonmyelinated axon hillock. As the axon egresses distally, the ensheathing cells adopt the features of myelinating Schwann cells. The pattern of myelination in this area is distinguished by short internodes, which increase in myelin thickness stepwise at each node of Ranvier (39). The g value is unusually large in the initial portion of the axon because myelin is thin relative to axon diameter, but at the position of axonal bifurcation the fiber parameters adopt the stereotyped pattern seen in peripheral nerves. The terminal portions of peripheral nerve fibers also display an unusual relationship between axon and Schwann cell. The precise configuration varies with the type of nerve terminal, but in general there is a shortening of internodal length, a stepwise decrease in myelin thickness, and a naked terminal axon.

The unitary theory presented here suggests that the stepwise alterations in myelin thickness in these regions simply reflect the number (or density) of instructor molecules the Schwann cells see on the axolemma. The sensory neuronal cyton and axon hillock, as well as the axon terminal, would lack myelinating instructor molecules, permitting the ensheathing cells to adopt the characteristics dictated by their local environment. However, the spatial changes in the pattern of myelination in the initial and preterminal regions may be related to differential growth of the nerve fiber during development. If growth occurred uniformly throughout the nerve fiber but decreased progressively at the proximal and distal ends, the territories of Schwann cells in these areas would approximate their premyelin lengths. The short internodal lengths would allow an unusually low number of instructor-receptor interactions because this would depend on the total area of axon–Schwann cell

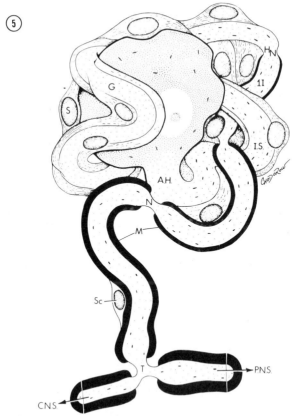

FIG. 5. The initial complex of a dorsal root ganglion cell comprises the neuron cell body, which gives rise to the axon hillock (A.H.). Distally, the "initial segment" (I.S.) begins to wind around the neuronal soma. Satellite cells (S) ensheath the neuron, axon hillock, and initial segment. A nonmyelinated extension of the initial segment entwines the perikaryon to form a glomerulus (G). The first short internode (1I) begins at a heminode (H.N.) and is ensheathed by a Schwann cell with a few myelin lamellae. This heminode forms the boundary between the satellite-type and Schwann-type ensheathing cell. Subsequent internodes may be longer with a progressive increase in myelin thickness (N), each increase demarcated by a node of Ranvier. The final internode of the initial complex terminates at a bifurcating node of Ranvier (T), where the fiber branches centrally and peripherally. The two fiber branches have relatively attenuated axons but thicker myelin sheaths characteristic of fibers on peripheral nerves. The axon directed along the dorsal root to the spinal cord (→C.N.S.) is thinner when compared with the fiber branch passing distally to the peripheral nerve (→P.N.S.). (From ref. 39.)

apposition. In the initial and terminal portions of the fiber, the Schwann cells would therefore interact, respectively, with progressively increasing and decreasing numbers of axolemmal myelinating instructor molecules. The paucity of interaction would eventually result in the production of atypically thin myelin relative to axonal diameter but proportional to cellular surface contact area.

CNS/PNS Transitional Region

As a myelinated nerve fiber passes from the CNS and enters the PNS, it penetrates a frilled astroglial dome studded with blood vessels (6) (Fig. 6). The basal lamina of the astrocytic dome is continuous with that of the Schwann cells myelinating the peripheral portion of the fiber. This region characteristically also has unusually short internodes (probably a growth-related phenomenon) and sometimes differences in myelin thickness and axonal size relative to its CNS counterpart (Berthold, *this volume*). The abrupt change in myelin thickness at the transitional region might merely reflect differences in degree of membrane elaboration by the oligodendrocyte and the Schwann cell. The variation in axonal caliber

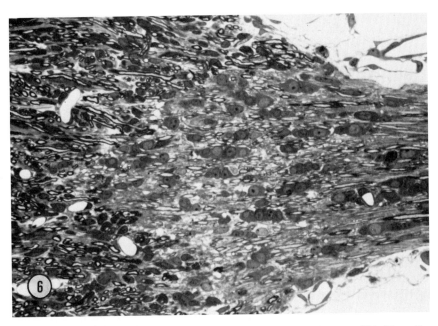

FIG. 6. Transition region between CNS (*right*) and PNS (*left*) of a rabbit spinal root. ×300. (From Gown, Raine, and Spencer, *unpublished data*.)

might also be controlled by the type of cellular ensheathment. The possibility that myelinating Schwann cells somehow promote axonal expansion seems reasonable from the results of nerve grafting experiments between normal and trembler mice (*vide supra*) and from the observation of focal changes in axonal size which accompany demyelination and remyelination (Raine, *this volume*).

The CNS/PNS transition region also raises a question of major importance—whether the axonal factors regulating myelination are common throughout the entire nervous system. The recent suggestion that fibers can transform from unmyelinated to myelinated axons on entry to the CNS is difficult to reconcile with this notion and requires confirmation (11). On the other hand, two lines of evidence do suggest the existence of a common neuronal regulation of both Schwann cell and oligodendrocyte myelination. Firstly, it is known from studies of human and experimental spinal cord demyelination that Schwann cells invade demyelinated plaques and perform normal *peripheral* myelination around denuded CNS axons (Raine, *this volume*). A similar result is encountered if desheathed peripheral nerves

are deliberately implanted in the spinal cord following induced demyelination and prevention of central remyelination (8). Secondly, it has been demonstrated in the spinal roots of dystrophic mice (which contain large numbers of naked axons) that ectopic oligodendrocytes elaborate normal *central* myelin around these PNS axons (47). Direct evidence of a common nervous system signal for the axonal regulation of myelination is currently being sought in our laboratory by grafting an optic nerve explant between a transected peripheral nerve. A few of the regenerating peripheral axons penetrate the optic nerve and become myelinated by oligodendrocytes (43a).

NONAXONAL MYELINATION

Although attempts to produce myelin around artificial conduits *in vitro* have been unsuccessful, despite an earlier claim to the contrary (14,15), there are several instances in which myelin has been observed around structures other than axons. Examples are provided by the myelinated neuronal somata of ciliary and spiral ganglia, and of the granular layer of the cerebellum (33). In these instances it seems likely that the neuronal plasmalemma has undergone a similar type of differentiation postulated for the axon during its transition from a fetal to a premyelinated state. The subsequent myelinating behavior of the ensheathing cell would then be dictated by the number and spatial arrangement of instructor molecules in the neuronal plasmalemma. Those instances in the CNS in which myelin is formed around nonneuronal structures (e.g., oligodendrocytes, astrocytes) are readily understandable if the myelinating cells have formed some contact with an instructing axon.

PUTATIVE AXON–SCHWANN CELL INTERACTIONS IN PATHOLOGICAL STATES

The proposed theory of axonal regulation of Schwann cell behavior may also be employed to explain the biological basis of several special axon/Schwann cell relationships seen in a variety of reactive and pathological states.

Demyelination and Remyelination

There are many unrelated conditions in which the first manifestation of demyelination occurs at the paranodal region. For example, in states of primary demyelination, phagocytic cells frequently penetrate the paranodal myelin sheath as a first step in stripping the internode (Raine, *this volume*). Another example is provided by the demyelination which accompanies axonal disease; here the paranodal axon may enlarge focally, causing mechanical retraction of the paranodal myelin sheath (Spencer and Schaumburg, *this volume*). A third example of paranodal demyelination is seen in compression and entrapment injuries of peripheral nerves (29). Irrespective of the etiology of paranodal demyelination, repair is effected either by paranodal extension of the myelin sheath (if the length for repair is short) or by creation of a new, intercalated internode formed by a newly arrived Schwann cell. Although the origin of such Schwann cells has not been rigorously examined, there is some evidence to suggest their derivation as daughter cells from the Schwann cell which is maintaining the adjacent, partially affected internode of myelin (20). Such daughter cells presumably

migrate under the basal lamina of the nerve fiber to the denuded axon and there elaborate myelin. When the damage involves two adjacent paranodes, the Schwann cells engaged in the repair process may sometimes compete for axonal contact. This results in a bizarre pattern of double myelination in which one myelin sheath traverses the nodal gap and overrides the sheath of the adjacent internode (21).

All of these phenomena may be explained by proposing that the process of paranodal demyelination results in a partial loss of contact inhibition between axon and Schwann cell, thereby stimulating cellular movement (lateral extension) and, with major loss of contact, Schwann cell mitosis. Mitosis would yield a dedifferentiated daughter cell, which would employ the same directional signaling to reach the axon as that used during fetal nerve development (*vide supra*). After reaching the denuded axon, the Schwann cell would extend longitudinally, become contact-inhibited at its primitive length, and interact with existing axolemmal instructors to commence myelinogenesis. The thickness of the myelin sheath (commonly abnormally thin) would be controlled by the number of *existing* axolemmal instructors, which would be smaller than adjacent, unaffected internodes because of the abnormally short length of surface contact between the axon and the remyelinating Schwann cell. Such a local mechanism for the control of remyelination would obviate the need for intercourse between the neuronal perikaryon and the affected part of the axon.

Chronic Demyelination—Myelin Bubble Formation

An unusual type of incomplete demyelination may be observed in the proximal stump of a permanently severed nerve trunk that develops a terminal neuroma. The myelin perturbations, which take the form of single or multiple intramyelinic or adaxonal vacuous swellings of giant proportions, develop proximal to the position of axonal sprouting. These myelin bubbles develop slowly and seem to be stable for prolonged periods. The axon within the myelin bubble is commonly shrunken and naked (40). This latter feature distinguishes these bubbles from the intramyelinic swellings seen in triethyltin and hexachlorophene intoxications. A remarkable feature of myelin bubbling is the development of large numbers of undifferentiated Schwann cells along the perimeter of the swollen fiber (24). Most of these supernumerary Schwann cells form a separate collar of overlapping processes around the fiber although a few may be retained beneath the original basal lamina.

It seems likely that the supernumerary Schwann cells represent daughter cells derived from division of the Schwann cell maintaining the myelin bubble. This may be the consequence of a prolonged partial loss of contact inhibition associated with separation of axon and adaxonal Schwann cell within the bubble region. The Schwann cells might accumulate along the perimeter of the fiber because of inaccessibility to the denuded internodal axon surface. When bubbling causes retraction of the paranodal myelin sheath and consequential axonal denudation, there is repair by remyelination.

Repetitive Demyelination

The collar of Schwann cell cytoplasm which commonly develops around positions of demyelination and remyelination is reminiscent of the onion skin formation seen in a variety of hypertrophic interstitial neuropathies (13). The nerve pathology of such diseases is characterized by multiple concentric collars of Schwann cell cytoplasm surrounding single damaged nerve fibers. Such changes are believed to develop by repeated demyelination and remyelination, phenomena which may also occur secondary to a disease process within the axon (e.g., distal axonopathy). Repetitive loss and restoration of contact inhibition between axon and Schwann cell would accompany repeated demyelination. This would repeatedly stimulate the production of daughter Schwann cells, which would gradually pile up around affected regions of the fiber.

Schwann Cell Sequestration

The phenomenon of adaxonal sequestration of axonal debris (Spencer and Schaumburg, *this volume*) represents another type of interaction between the axon and its ensheathing cell. The presence of abnormal or effete organelles within the axoplasm is spatially and temporally associated with the development of a coated, focal depression of the axon surface. At this position there is loss of the normal, close apposition between axolemma and Schwann cell plasmalemma. This event might reduce contact inhibition, promote local movement and redistribution of ensheathing cell cytoplasm, and allow a sheet of cytoplasm to invaginate the axonal surface and perform its sequestering function. Schwann cell deymelination and mitosis are not associated with this process.

Axonal Degeneration

During wallerian degeneration of the distal stump of a severed nerve, all fibers undergo dissolution of axoplasm, loss of axolemma, collapse and breakdown of the myelin sheath (if present), and Schwann cell division (42). Contact inhibition between axon and Schwann cell would be totally lost concomitant with axolemmal degeneration, an event that might trigger mitosis of the Schwann cell within the basal lamina of the fiber. In the absence of axons, the dedifferentiated daughter Schwann cells assemble within the original basal lamina into overlapping longitudinal columns of cytoplasmic processes (Fig. 7). These Schwann cells represent a stable and nonmigratory population capable of surviving for months in a dedifferentiated state in the absence of axonal influence.

Distal axonopathy, another type of axonal degeneration, is associated with slow retrograde nerve fiber breakdown (Spencer and Schaumburg, *this volume*). Because axons degenerate at different times, it is frequently possible to encounter an unmyelinated fiber with a partial loss of its axonal population. In such cases the associated Schwann cells seem to separate from their basal lamina. This has been interpreted to indicate local movements of the Schwann cell, perhaps a consequence of a partial loss of contact inhibition.

Axonal and Fiber Regeneration

The reinnervation of a degenerated nerve stump has been studied in detail for myelinated

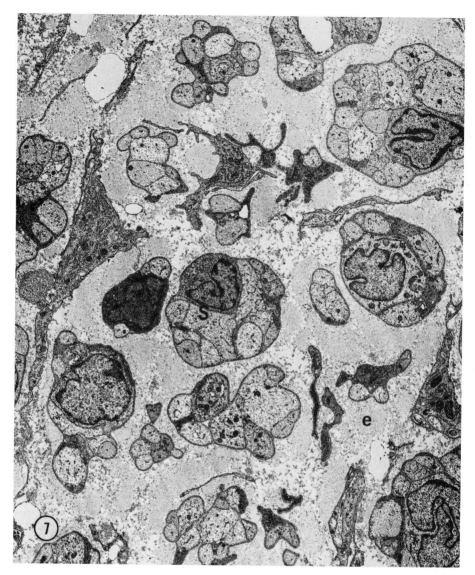

FIG. 7. Denervated distal stump of a rabbit tibial nerve 8–9 weeks after transection. The nerve contains nu merous Schwann cell columns (S) embedded in an endoneurial collagen matrix (e). ×6,000. (From ref. 46.

fibers. The process is characterized by pene- tration of naked, regenerating axon sprouts between the overlapping Schwann cell proc- esses within a Schwann cell column. After en- veloping the axon sprouts, the Schwann cells retract from each other in a lateral plane and form a cluster of regenerating myelinated fi- bers. During this process, much of the interac- tion between axons and Schwann cell appears to recapitulate that which occurs during de-

velopment. Myelination commences only when a 1:1 relationship between axon and Schwann cell is achieved. However, during the process of myelination of regenerating axons, inter- nodal distances remain foreshortened (36), each approximating the primitive length of the Schwann cell. The contrast between this situ- ation and that following development may be explained by postulating that it is the elonga- tion of the nerve trunk during body growth (and not elongation of the axon) which is responsible for lengthening the internode.

PROBING SCHWANN CELL BEHAVIOR

An important frontier in the study of axon–Schwann cell interaction and myelination is the isolation and characterization of purified preparations of Schwann cells and their plasma membranes. Two methods were employed in other laboratories to study the isolated Schwann cell. One approach is to separate cells from schwannomas (31), but these may differ radically from normal Schwann cells. Another approach which yields normal Schwann cells utilizes an elegant tissue culture technique (49). Unfortunately, this method is limited because of its technical difficulty and the low yield of Schwann cells for biochemical studies.

To surmount these problems we have used the phenomenon of wallerian degeneration to prepare a high yield of normal, dedifferentiated Schwann cells that are completely free of axonal contamination and largely devoid of myelination (46). Preparation of Schwann cells by this method commences with surgical transection of the (rabbit) sciatic nerve close to the sciatic notch. The cut ends are tightly ligated to discourage regenerating axons from entering the distal stump. After surgery the nerve is allowed to undergo wallerian degeneration for periods of 7–12 weeks. During this time, there is breakdown and removal of axons and myelin and alignment of Schwann cells into longitudinal columns. (Fig. 7). The nerve is then removed from the animal and the endoneurial contents (containing the Schwann cells) plucked from the perineurial and epineurial connective tissue ensheathment (10).

Schwann cells prepared by this method are currently being employed for a number of studies. One approach involves transplantation of Schwann cells to the anterior compartment of the eye, to either the anterior chamber or the posterior stroma of the cornea. This might provide an opportunity to establish a colony of Schwann cells *in vivo* with which to test their response to neuronal factors. In another series of biochemical experiments, Schwann cell plasma membranes are being prepared by differential and density centrifugation from these naturally enriched Schwann cell pools (51). It is hoped to employ such preparations to search for molecular receptor mechanisms which might interact with putative axonal instructor molecules.

SUMMARY

This chapter has discussed the role of the axon in regulating the biological expression of the Schwann cell and presented a speculative theory of the control mechanism based on specific molecular interaction between apposed surface membranes. This theory differs from that presented by previous authors in that it attempts to integrate a wide variety of axon-Schwann cell interactions in normal and pathological states. Furthermore, the discussion of the control of myelinogenesis and the regulation of myelin thickness considers not only the role of axon diameter (the subject of previous theories) but rather the surface area of contact between axon and Schwann cell. Our purpose is not to present a dogma but merely to suggest new approaches for exploration of the biology of the nerve fiber and myelination. It remains our conviction that peripheral nerves provide the ideal site to study these problems because of their relatively simple organization and accessibility, and that the elucidation of cellular relationships in this locus may prove relevant to those present in the brain.

ACKNOWLEDGMENTS

This work was supported by NIH training grant 5T5 GM1674 and 5T32 GM7288; in part by grants OH 00535, NS 13106, NS 08952, and NS 03356 from the USPHS; and a Joseph P. Kennedy, Jr. Fellowship in the Neurosciences to P.S.S.

REFERENCES

1. Aguayo, A. J., Attiwell, M., Trecarten, J., Perkins, S., and Bray, G. M. (1977): Abnormal myelination in transplanted trembler mouse Schwann cells. *Nature* (Lond), 265: 73–74.
2. Aguayo, A., Charron, L., and Bray, G. M. (1976): Potential of Schwann cells from unmyelinated nerves to produce myelin: A quantitative ultrastructural and radioautographic study. *J. Neurocytol.*, 5:565–573.

3. Allfrey, V. G., Johnson, E. M., Kain, J., and Vidali, G. (1973): In: *Protein Phosphorylation Control Mechanisms, Miami Winter Symposium,* Vol. 5, p. 217.
4. Barondes, S. H. (1975): Toward a molecular basis of neuronal recognition. In: *The Nervous System, Vol. 1: The Basic Neurosciences,* edited by D. B. Tower. Raven Press, New York.
5. Barondes, S. H. (1976): *Neuronal Recognition.* Plenum Press, New York.
6. Berthold, C-H., and Carlstedt, T. (1977): Observations on the morphology at the transition between the peripheral and central nervous system in the cat. II. General organization of the transitional region in S₁ dorsal rootlets. *Acta Physiol. Scand. [Suppl.],* 446:28–42.
7. Bischoff, A., and Thomas, P. K. (1976): Microscopic anatomy of myelinated nerve fibres. In: *Peripheral Neuropathy,* edited by P. J. Dyck, P. K. Thomas, and E. H. Lambert. Saunders, Philadelphia.
8. Blakemore, W. F. (1977): Remyelination of CNS axons by Schwann cells transplanted from the sciatic nerve. *Nature (Lond),* 266:68–69.
9. Brady, R. O., and Quarles, R. H. (1973): The enzymology of myelination. *Mol. Cell Biochem.,* 2:23–29.
10. Brown, M. J., Pleasure, D. E., and Asbury, A. K. (1976): Microdissection of peripheral nerve. *J. Neurol. Sci.,* 29:361–369.
11. Carlstedt, T. (1977): Observations on the morphology at the transition between the peripheral and central nervous system in the cat: Unmyelinated fibres in S₁ dorsal rootlets. *Acta Physiol. Scand. [Suppl.],* 446:61–71.
12. Duncan, D. (1934): A relation between axone diameter and myelination determined by measurements of myelinated spinal root fibers. *J. Comp. Neurol.,* 60:437–471.
13. Dyck, P. J., Thomas, P. K., and Lambert, E. H. (1975): *Peripheral Neuropathy.* Saunders, Philadelphia.
14. Ernyei, S., and Young, M. R. (1966): Pulsatile and myelin-forming activities of Schwann cells in vitro. *J. Physiol. (Lond),* 183:469–480.
15. Field, E. J., Raine, C. S., and Hughes, D. (1969): Failure to induce myelin sheath formation around artificial fibres; with a note on toxicity of polyester fibres for nervous tissue in vitro. *J. Neurol. Sci.,* 8:129–142.
16. Fraher, J. P. (1972): A quantitative study of anterior root fibres during early myelination. *J. Anat.,* 112:99–129.
17. Fraher, J. P. (1973): A quantitative study of anterior root fibres during early myelination. II. Longitudinal variation in sheath thickness and axon circumference. *J. Anat.,* 115:421–444.
18. Friede, R. L. (1972): Control of myelin formation by axon caliber (with a model of the control mechanism). *J. Comp. Neurol.,* 144:233–252.
19. Gould, R. (1977): Incorporation of newly-formed glycoprotein into peripheral nerve myelin. *J. Cell Biol. (in press).*
20. Jacobs, J. (1977): Personal communication.
21. King, R. H. M., Pollard, J. D., and Thomas, P. K. (1975): Aberrant remyelination in chronic relapsing experimental allergic neuritis. *Neuropath. Appl. Neurobiol.,* 1:367–378.
22. Krygier-Brévart, V., Zabrenetzky, V. S., and Spencer, P. S. (1977): Cyclic AMP stimulation of a peripheral myelin protein kinase. *Trans. Am. Soc. Neurochem.,* 8 (abstract).
23. Landon, D. N. (1976): *The Peripheral Nerve.* Chapman and Hall, London.
24. Lubińska, L. (1961): Demyelination and remyelination in the proximal parts of regenerating nerve fibers. *J. Comp. Neurol.,* 117:275–289.
25. Mandel, P., Nussbaum, J. L., Neskovic, N. M., Sarlieve, L. L., and Kurihara, T. (1972): Regulation of myelinogenesis. *Adv. Enzyme Regul.,* 10:101–117.
26. Miyamoto, E., and Kakiuchi, S. (1974): In vitro and in vivo phosphorylation of myelin basic protein by exogenous and endogenous adenosine 3′:5′-monophosphate-dependent-protein kinases in brain. *J. Biol. Chem.,* 249:2769–2777.
27. Moscona, A. A. (1973): Surface specification of embryonic cells: lectin receptors, cell recognition, and specific cell ligands. In: *The Cell Surface in Development.* Wiley, New York.
28. Norton, W. T. (1975): The myelin sheath. In: *The Cellular and Molecular Basis of Neurologic Disease,* edited by G. M. Shy, E. S. Goldensohn, and S. H. Appel. Lea & Febiger, Philadelphia.
29. Ochoa, J., Fowler, T. J., and Gilliatt, R. W. (1972): Anatomical changes in peripheral nerves compressed by a pneumatic tourniquet. *J. Anat.,* 113:433–455.
30. Peterson, E. R., and Murray, M. R. (1955): Myelin sheath formation in cultures of avian spinal ganglia. *Am. J. Anat.,* 96:319–355.
31. Pfeiffer, S. E., and Wechsler, W. (1972): Biochemically differentiated neoplastic clone of Schwann cells. *Proc. Natl. Acad. Sci. USA,* 69:2885–2889.
32. Quarles, R. H. (1976): Glycoproteins in the nervous system. In: *The Nervous System, Vol. I: The Basic Neurosciences,* edited by D. B. Tower. Raven Press, New York.
33. Raine, C. S. (1977): Morphological aspects of myelin and myelination. In: *Myelin,* edited by P. Morell. Plenum Press, New York.
34. Robertson, J. D. (1962): The unit membrane of cells and mechanisms of myelin formation. In: *Proc. Assoc. Res. Nerv. Ment. Dis., Vol. 40: Ultrastructure and Metabolism of the*

Nervous System. Williams & Wilkins, Baltimore.

35. Roseman, S. (1973): Complex carbohydrates and intercellular adhesion. In: *The Cell Surface in Development,* edited by A. A. Moscona. Wiley, New York.

36. Schröder, J. M. (1972): Altered ratio between axon diameter and myelin thickness in regenerated nerve fibers. *Brain Res., 45*:49–65.

37. Singer, M. (1968): Penetration of labelled amino acids into the peripheral nerve fibre from surrounding body fluids. In: *CIBA Foundation Symposium on Growth of the Nervous System,* edited by G. E. W. Wolstenholme and M. O'Connor. Churchill, London.

38. Speidel, C. C. (1964): In vivo studies of myelinated nerve fibers. *Int. Rev. Cytol., 16*:173–231.

39. Spencer, P. S., Raine, C. S., and Wiśniewski, H. (1973): Axon diameter and myelin thickness—unusual relationships in dorsal root ganglia. *Anat. Rec., 176*:225–244.

40. Spencer, P. S., and Thomas, P. K. (1976): The examination of isolated nerve fibres by light electron microscopy, with observations on demyelination proximal to neuromas. *Acta Neuropathol. (Berl), 16*:177–186.

41. Sunderland, S. (1968): *Nerves and Nerve Injuries.* Churchill, London.

42. Thomas, P. K. (1974): Nerve injury. In: *Essays on the Nervous System,* edited by R. Bellairs and E. G. Gray. Clarendon Press, Oxford.

43. Webster, H. deF. (1975): Development of peripheral myelinated and unmyelinated nerve fibers. In: *Peripheral Neuropathy,* edited by P. J. Dyck, P. K. Thomas, and E. H. Lambert. Saunders, Philadelphia.

43a. Weinberg, E. L., and Spencer, P. S. Signalling of central myelination by regenerating peripheral axons. (*In preparation.*)

44. Weinberg, H., and Spencer, P. S. (1975): Studies on the control of myelinogenesis. I. Myelination of regenerating axons after entry into a foreign unmyelinated nerve. *J. Neurocytol., 4*:395–418.

45. Weinberg, H., and Spencer, P. S. (1976): Studies on the control of myelinogenesis. II. Evidence for neuronal regulation of myelination. *Brain Res., 113*:363–378.

46. Weinberg, H., and Spencer, P. S. (1977): Studies on the control of myelinogenesis. III. The preparation of large numbers of dedifferentiated Schwann cells. *In preparation.*

47. Weinberg, H. J., Spencer, P. S., and Raine, C. S. (1975): Aberrant PNS development in dystrophic mice. *Brain Res., 88*:532–537.

48. Williams, P. L., and Wendell-Smith, C. P. (1971): Some additional parametric variations between peripheral nerve fibre populations. *J. Anat., 109*:505–526.

49. Wood, P. M. (1976): Separation of functional Schwann cells and neurons from normal peripheral nervous tissue. *Brain Res., 115*:361–375.

50. Wood, P. M., and Bunge, R. P. (1975): Evidence that sensory axons are mitogenic for Schwann cells. *Nature (Lond), 256*:662–664.

51. Zabrenetsky, V. S., Krygier-Brévart, V., and Spencer, P. S. (1977): Cyclic AMP stimulated protein phosphorylation in peripheral myelin and Schwann cell plasma membranes. In: *Proceedings: 6th International Meeting of the International Society for Neurochemistry, Copenhagen.*

Physiology and Pathobiology of Axons, edited by
S. G. Waxman. Raven Press, New York © 1978.

Spinal Cord Regeneration and Axonal Sprouting in Mammals

Jerald J. Bernstein, Mary E. Bernstein, and Michael R. Wells

Department of Neuroscience and Ophthalmology, University of Florida, College of Medicine, Gainesville, Florida 32610

As with many fields that have sustained long-term medical and scientific scrutiny, the field of spinal cord regeneration is replete with terms and definitions interpreted in the light of the state of the art at that time. This is particularly true in the field of central nervous system (CNS) regeneration. Regeneration is defined as "the renewal or repair of lost tissue or parts" (38). This immediately presents a problem. If regeneration is a reduplication of the organ involved, it would imply that the entire system must be reconstituted as originally generated and that exact anatomical reconstitution occurs. However, this does not seem to be the case even in lower vertebrates such as goldfish (10) or salamanders (87) where there is the return of function but aberrant anatomy. Perhaps regeneration which results in a return of function with indeterminate degrees of electrophysiological regeneration but with aberrant anatomical regeneration could be defined as functional regeneration. Thus anatomy may not return as generated, but the function of the animal after the regenerative process can be restored without testable deficits. There must also be neurochemical correlates of the regenerative process which may or may not result in an anatomical or electrophysiological effect that can be resolved with current methodologies.

The morphological appearance of CNS regeneration has commonly been interpreted to be regenerated nerve fibers derived from transected central nerve fibers. Although usually not specified, the implication is that growth is from the proximal tip of the transected axon.

However, axonal sprouts from the transected axon should be included in this category.

The problem is further complicated by the fact that new synaptic complex formation has been described on α-motoneurons in spinal cord and can be considered as part of the regenerative phenomenon. The source of the axons forming individual complexes cannot be described precisely (11) since the new synapses can be derived from regenerated transected axons, axonal sprouts from transected axons, or axonal sprouts from intact or uninjured axons.

The most recently recognized component of the regenerative process is axonal sprouting (7, 91,105). This phenomenon is the response of intact remaining neuronal afferents sprouting into areas of partial neuronal deafferentation (due presumably to trophic influences). These axonal sprouts act as new members of synaptic complexes in the septal area of the brain (91,94), the hippocampus (70,105), nucleus gracilis (99), and spinal cord (7,11,15). In general, this phenomenon has been termed "plasticity." Since axonal sprouting is part of the regenerative process in the CNS, the plasticity of the nervous system in current usage represents part of the regenerative repertoire of the spinal cord.

If the important factor in regeneration is the restoration of function, the anatomical, electrophysiological, and neurochemical components of the regenerative process are only indices of the possible return of function. The number of nerve fibers necessary to restore different degrees of function may be small but remain unknown. After lesions of sensory systems the large majority of nerve fibers can be deleted from a system before massive deficits are reported. Although there is the danger of comparing different systems, there is the implication that return of function in the regenerated spinal cord would require relatively small numbers of nerve fibers derived from various sources (transected axons and sprouts or interneurons) which would make new, viable, electrophysiologically meaningful synapses in spinal cord distal to the lesion. This combination of events would result in varying degrees of functional restitution distal to the site of transection of the spinal cord.

In order to understand the regenerative process, all of the components described should be taken into account. It is in these contexts that the regeneration process of the spinal cord is briefly reviewed. Anatomical, neurochemical, and functional components are discussed. At this point in time, the electrophysiological component of regeneration is difficult to discuss since the reinnervated neuron has not been a topic of extensive electrophysiological research. This seems to be related to the fact that the phenomenon of axonal sprouting as a source of reafferentation has been described only recently, and the precise time course and sources of reinnervation for the neurons are obscure.

SOURCES OF AXONS FOR REGENERATION OF THE SPINAL CORD

If an analysis of the long tracts in the spinal cord is carried out on the basis of motor and sensory control of movement at the spinal level, surprisingly few tracts would be involved in brain-mediated movement via cortical, subcortical, cerebellar, and brainstem control of the spinal cord. Not only are the number of tracts limited, but the connectivity of the tracts is discrete by spinal cord zone for α-motoneuron. On the rat and cat α-motoneuron, afferents are derived from segmental interneurons (28,58,84,112) usually lying approximately 0.5 to 1.5 segments rostral to the α-motoneuron innervated. In primates approximately 10% of the descending corticospinal system can directly innervate the peripheral dendrites of α-motoneurons (106). These data are still

consistent with the fact that to date the overwhelming majority of afferents to α-motoneurons in mammals are known to be derived from secondary sources, the spinal interneurons. The problem is compounded by the fact that in the rat, which appears to be a totally interneuron to α-motoneuron model (28,106), the regeneration occurring in the first segment rostral to a hemisection appears to have only a minor reafferentation component from long descending tracts (6,7). The total input that is long-tract-derived in this segment is less than 10% of the total segmental input into the area of the α-motoneuron in the segment. There is, however, ample evidence that the long tracts of the spinal cord do have extensive axonal sprouts above the site of lesion. This phenomenon was discussed by Ramón y Cajal in 1910 and in more recent experiments on axonal sprouting of descending rubrospinal nerve fibers in the rat (88,89). However, it is not known if these sprouts are available in the first segment rostral to the hemisection.

What are the remaining sources of nerve fibers for the synaptic renewal described earlier? The dorsal root fibers that remain intact after hemisection could be a source of nerve fibers into the ventral horn. This may be the case in segments farther rostral to the hemisection, but the distribution of sprouted dorsal roots appears to be restricted in axonal sprouting patterns and has a minor contribution to the α-motoneuron (49,68,82). However, the contribution of dorsal roots to α-motoneurons can be defined by the neurotransmitter (GABA) through immunohistochemistry of the enzyme glutamate decarboxylase (GAD) (76). This analysis shows that there are dorsal root axons in the ventral horn that could be available as sprouts for reafferented α-motoneurons. The synaptic apparatus for the myotactic reflex (M bulb with associated P complex) (26,34–36,73–75) that is found in the lumbar enlargement of the spinal cord could be a source of nerve fibers following spinal cord lesion. Following peripheral nerve hemisection, there is a switching from somatic to peripheral input electrophysiologically over time (79). Since loss of presynaptic terminals from the soma of axotomized neurons occurs (3,107), these results may represent an unmasking of peripheral Ia afferents. Since spinal cord hemisection results in a chronically de-afferented α-motoneuron (7), this state of the neuron might result in the loss of terminals responsible for the myotactic reflex. Because of numbers these large afferent fibers could only be a minor input to the deafferented α-motoneuron (unless axonal sprouting is greater on a per-axon basis than suspected).

The pattern of distribution of the dorsal roots in the spinal cord after selective rhizotomy shows a pattern of reinnervation into restricted zones in the spinal cord (49,68,82). There are also specified territories for the afferents to the nucleus gracilis following partial deafferentation of the nucleus (99). The distribution of areas occupied by axonal sprouts in the CNS is not a generalized process but is orderly and occurs with specific patterns of reinnervation which are supplied by specific groups of axons. This also appears to be the case in the ventral horn of thoracic spinal cord following hemi- or transection. From the discussion thus far and recent work on the subject, the large majority of axonal sprouts in the spinal cord in the first segment rostral to a hemi- or transection appear to be derived from lamina VII interneurons (16). The regeneration in this segment appears to be from the original source of axons which normally innervated the α-motoneuron (16,28,112).

INTERPRETIVE PROBLEMS IN IDENTIFICATION OF CNS AXONS

One of the basic problems in spinal cord regeneration is identification of the source of axons. Following lesions of the CNS, nerve fibers can be derived from central, peripheral, or autonomic sources (9). The morphological distinction of nerve fibers derived from these sources is baffling. Making the assumption that there are nerve fibers in the site of lesion following hemi- or transection of the spinal cord, what criteria would be utilized to establish the source of axons, with the knowledge that single fibers cannot be traced with any certainty?

The myelinating satellite cell may well be an indicator of nerve fiber origin after injury. If the myelin sheath has an external cytoplasmic process that completely surrounds the nerve fiber, with or without a nucleus, is surrounded by basement membrane and has

Schmidt–Lanterman incisures, it may be assumed that the satellite cell of the myelinated nerve fiber is a Schwann cell. Schwann or Schwann-like satellite cells have been observed as myelinating cells in the CNS following pathological spontaneous lesions or experimentally induced lesions of the spinal cord (9,21–24,33,47,48,56). It is interesting that the lesion can be totally noninvasive, e.g., vitamin B deficiency (33); relatively noninvasive, e.g., x-ray injuries (48); invasive via toxic drugs (21); or pathologically invasive (9). From this evidence, one might conclude such a nerve fiber is peripheral (9). However, this does not mean the axis cylinder in the sheath is peripheral in origin. Vitamin B deficiency in rats results in demyelination of the nerve fiber in the CNS and remyelination by Schwann-like cells (33). What are the sources of Schwann cells in the spinal cord? Schwann cells are continuous through the dorsal root into the dorsal columns and white matter that is associated with the dorsal afferent systems. During regeneration of these peripheral systems in the CNS (dorsal columns), the myelinating satellite cells are Schwann cells (61). In addition, Schwann cells are found normally throughout many parts of the CNS (90). Thus, Schwann cells are available for both peripheral and central axis cylinders.

The relative differences in the frequency of the dense and interperiod lines in a given linear area has been used as a criterion for differentiating central versus peripheral origin of the satellite cell. This determination for central versus peripheral satellite has been interpreted with caution (86), since there appear to be only specific areas of the CNS where these criteria are valid. In spinal cord myelin, periodicity differences cannot be statistically verified. This is due to myelin dense and interperiod line frequency variability in normal spinal cord. Myelin periodicity therefore must be discarded as a morphological criterion following injury.

Without entering into the argument of the name or classification of the axis cylinder satellite cell, since the various cells may represent a continuum (86), astrocytes can ensheath (with pentalaminate junctions but without myelin formation) axons and dendrites after spinal cord injury, demonstrating that the satellite may not always be the traditional oligodendrocyte (2,13). These data show that following injury the satellite cell cannot be utilized as a criterion for the central or peripheral origin of a nerve fiber.

Can the axis cylinder be used as a central, peripheral, or autonomic indicator of origin? The microtubule/neurofilament ratio can be utilized as an index of relative age of an axis cylinder (generate versus mature) but not as to its location (peripheral or central).

There does not appear to be a morphological criterion which definitely establishes if a nerve fiber in the cicatrix of a regenerated CNS is centrally or peripherally derived. Perhaps the most reliable method is an experimental surgical approach that is carefully designed to demonstrate degenerating distal axons (16).

SYNAPTIC RENEWAL DURING SPINAL CORD REGENERATION

Perhaps one of the most important processes in the regeneration of the spinal cord after an available source of nerve fibers has been discovered is synaptic renewal. Synaptic renewal has been found in the septal nuclei in the brain after section of the fimbria or medial forebrain bundle (91,94). The denervated sites in this case are reoccupied by axonal or bouton sprouts. Thus the septal neurons are completely reafferented. Reafferentation also takes place in the hippocampus following a variety of deafferenting lesions (69,71). The reafferentation of hippocampal neurons occurs in specified and now-predictable patterns. The hippocampal and septal models have a common factor—the stability of the synaptic profile of the reafferented neurons. The reafferentation process proceeds in these brain areas from approximately 6 to 30 days and stabilizes after this period of time.

Another model for central reafferentation has been the use of peripheral nerve axotomy followed by loss of presynaptic afferents to the axotomized neuron. This loss of boutons occurs not only on the soma (25) but also on the injured neuronal dendrite. These models of the severed facial and hypoglossal nerve have yielded exciting results. The injured neurons appear to loose a specific profile of boutons (107). Boutons classified as S (spherical presynaptic vesicles) type (8,16,107,111) are selec-

tively lost over time. However, these boutons on hypoglossal neurons are restored by 84 days postoperation if the target muscle is reinnervated. The lost complement of S (spherical, clear synaptic vesicles with symmetrical or asymmetrical synaptic membrane specialization) is not restored by 98 days postaxotomy if the hypoglossal nerve is not allowed to reinnervate the tongue (107). This model shows the capacity for CNS neurons to remodel and yields the important fact (if it can be extended to entirely central intrinsic neurons) that reinnervation by the axon is in part critical to synaptic remodeling on the neuron soma and dendrite (postsynaptic innervation influences of the afferent synaptic profile of the same neuron).

These data indicate that there may well be synaptic remodeling of the long-tract neurons following spinal cord lesion. This is the case since red nucleus neurons permanently loose afferents after axotomy (3). This correlation is complicated by the fact that the long tracts play only a minor role in the regenerative capacity of the nervous system (6,7). This is a critical difference between central and peripheral axotomy. If the specificity of reafferentation is in part determined by reinnervation by the original neuron (which is not known at present), the exciting possibility exists for exact remodeling of the CNS if long-tract nerve fibers can be induced to grow into and reinnervate neurons in the distal spinal cord stump.

It has been firmly established that synaptic renewal can take place in the brain and brainstem of mammals following partial deafferentation of peripheral or central axons. This can also be accomplished via axotomy of the peripheral nerve or axotomy of various afferent sources. In the spinal cord there is electrophysiological (79) and anatomical evidence that there is synaptic modification of afferents following partial peripheral axotomy (monosynaptic) and cyclic renewal of synapses on interneurons (lamina VII of Rexed) and α-motoneurons following spinal cord hemisection (11).

Hemisection of the spinal cord at the T1–T2 interface results in a consistent deafferentation–reafferentation pattern on sensory, ventral horn interneurons and α-motoneurons (11).

These data indicate that there may be a 30-day cycle of synaptic turnover with maximal numbers at 30 and 90 days, and minimal numbers at the time of greatest deafferentation 10–20 days and 60 days posthemisection (11). As discussed in a previous section, the majority of the afferents to α-motoneurons appear to be interneuronal. This is consistent with the hypothesis of local sprouting of axons and boutons within the zone of deafferentation. In addition, these data show that there is an axonal pool that can reinnervate spinal cord neurons with presynaptic boutons which appear to be functional (based on morphological criteria). These findings also show that there is an available source of axons that could be utilized in the regeneration of axons across the site of spinal cord lesion which have the capacity to form presumably functional synapses.

NEUROCHEMICAL AND DRUG-INDUCED CORRELATES OF MAMMALIAN SPINAL CORD REGENERATION

Although extensive neurochemical study of acute spinal cord trauma has been made in recent years (83,85,100), the chemical events that might be associated with the abortive regeneration or synaptic remodeling of injured spinal cord has received little attention. This is probably due to the difficulty in approaching the injury of a tissue as complex as nervous system chemically, and the fact that any regenerative response of spinal cord or other CNS areas in mammals can be demonstrated only with difficulty (30,52,53,120).

Reaction of the Central Neuron to Axotomy

Although the reaction of the central neuron to axotomy is of importance in understanding the processes associated with the failure of long tracts in the spinal cord to regenerate, very little is known about the process. Major studies of the response of the neuron to axotomy have utilized peripherally projecting axons which do show regeneration (37,50,65).

The perikaryal response of the peripheral neuron after axotomy is generally described as regenerative. As with the morphological aspects of the axonal reaction, chemical alterations (65) are dependent on the type and age of animal studied, the area of nervous system, the position of the lesion in reference to the cell body, and the type of lesion (e.g., scissor transection, crush). The general chemical aspects, however, may be described as follows: The axotomized neuron exhibits an early decrease in RNA and protein synthesis followed by an increase in RNA and protein synthesis 2–20 days postlesion (27,114–116). The timing of this response is dependent on the distance of the lesion from the cell soma (114). It has also been suggested that the turnover of proteins synthesized in the soma may be altered (60) and that the types of proteins made may come to resemble that of the immature neuron (51). Other chemical responses of the soma include (65) a biphasic reaction leading to a decrease in transmitter-associated enzymes and transmitter substances (e.g., acetylcholinesterase, dopamine-β-hydroxylase, monoamine oxidase, or tyrosine hydroxylase) (50) and increases in glycolytic and other metabolic enzymes, lipofuscin granules, cytoplasmic acid phosphatase, lysosomes, and autophagic granules. These chemical alterations approach near-normal levels as axonal regrowth and reconnection is complete.

Many of these changes may be interpreted as either regenerative or degenerative. It has been argued that histological chromatolysis is actually an injury reaction of the cell rather than a regenerative response (32,40,41). Severe chromatolysis is often associated with cell death (65,103). However, it seems likely (50) that the chemical processes underlying the morphology are a combination of anabolic and catabolic processes, perhaps under separate control. The predominating reaction might depend, then, on the genome of the neuron in relation to its ability to respond, as well as the extent of the injury.

Another factor which may enter into the axon reaction and subsequent regeneration of the cell process has been suggested (118,119) in studies of [³H]lysine uptake into spinal cord and brain protein after sciatic nerve lesions in the rat. It has been observed (54,78) that peripheral nerves may regenerate at a greater rate if they are subjected to a priming lesion 2 weeks prior to the final lesion. Using similar designs (118), rats subjected to either a simultaneous double lesion (cut and crush) or an interval double lesion with 2 weeks separating the lesion (cut, 2-week interval, crush) have greater growth rates after interval lesions. It was observed that, in addition to a faster rate of regeneration of the sciatic nerve, interval-lesioned animals exhibited marked differences in the overall rate of incorporation of [^{3}H]lysine into brain and spinal cord trichloroacetic acid (TCA)-precipitable protein and soluble fractions (118). These data indicate that general changes in CNS metabolism may also contribute to regenerative processes.

In contrast to the peripherally projecting neuron, the general response of the intrinsic neuron to axotomy may be described as atrophy and/or cell death (50,65), although there is no consistent response over different areas of the nervous system. Some intrinsic central neurons react with an apparently typical chromatolysis in areas as varied as Clark's nucleus (67), pyramidal cells of the cortex (59,63), red nucleus, and lateral geniculate (3–5). Central neurons undergoing histological chromatolysis may or may not show evidence of recovery (4). Other central neurons—such as those in the thalamic sensory relay nuclei (29, 113) and retinal ganglion cells (39,57)—may show rapid degeneration. Some chromalytic neurons may atrophy and persist in an atrophied form with reduced amounts of Nissl substance (113). Still other central neurons exhibit minimal histological changes such as those of the locus ceruleus (96,98). The interpretation of many of these reactions is confused by the presence of transneuronal degeneration and deafferentation or the existence of sustaining collaterals. In general, the chromalytic response appears to be, in part, regenerative in nature.

Biochemical correlates of the above histological responses are very limited (65). Studies on the axotomized locus ceruleus neurons (96, 98) indicate the fluctuations of transmitter-associated materials in these neurons similar to reactions of neurons in the periphery. However, these neurons may not be a typical model for other reacting central neurons since they represent neurons with enormous axonal arborizations, diffuse innervation, and a specific

transmitter. This propensity for regeneration may be the case for central noradrenergic neurons in general (18,19,52,81,104) and selected other tracts such as those of the hypothalamic hypophyseal tract (92,93). In the dorsal column nuclei (32,80) there are reductions of reduced nicotinamide adenine dinucleotide phosphate (NADPH) associated with lesions of the medial lemniscus. Such reductions of NADPH were not noted after control lesions of the hypoglossal and facial nerves. In the red nucleus of the cat (4), there are decreases in lysosome-related acid phosphatase and a consistently lower incorporation of tritiated amino acid into the nucleus and cytoplasm of reacting neurons of the axotomized side compared to the control side. Cytochemical evaluation of RNA in the red nucleus under similar conditions of axotomy (101) indicate a transient elevation of RNA content in axotomized rubral neurons followed by a prolonged decrease in RNA. These observations were made in addition to histological data and suggest that the response of the red nucleus to axotomy is sequentially regressive but may have regenerative aspects.

The above data suggest that the central neuronal reaction to axotomy is generally regressive, and that central intrinsic neurons may be unable to make appropriate metabolic responses to regenerate axons (50,65). However, there is great variability in response of central neurons to axotomy, and the variability of regeneration or abortive attempts at regeneration by central fibers under various conditions does not allow a clear resolution of the regressive or regenerative nature of the response. In addition, regressive reactions following axotomy are found on peripherally projecting neurons where regeneration is prevented or blocked (1, 65,107). The nature of the experimental designs show the neuronal response as linearly regressive. However, if this were not the case and the neuronal response actually peaked and troughed after axotomy, parts of the response could be considered regenerative.

It has been a common tenet of CNS regeneration research during past years that the formation of the thick glial–pial scar at the site of a spinal cord or other CNS lesion prevents the regrowth of central fibers (30,52,72,120).

By this argument, central neurons might exhibit a different reaction to axotomy and perhaps regeneration if the proper conditions for regrowth existed at the site of injury. The resolution of this problem awaits further research on the cell biology of the injured CNS and lesion cicatrix.

General Metabolic Studies

Spinal cord and brain metabolism were studied after spinal cord injury during the time periods in which synaptic reorganization had recently occurred. Alterations of the protein amino acid incorporation in lesioned spinal cord were investigated in the rat (69,117) and monkey (119). In the rat a spinal hemisection at T1–T2 results in significant increases in the incorporation of [^{14}C]leucine into the TCA-precipitable protein of lesioned and adjacent spinal cord segments 7 and 30 days postoperation. Increases in the amino acid incorporation of left and right somatomotor cortex were observed 30 days postoperation, whereas incorporation in the left somatomotor cortex decreased to less than that in controls by 70 days postoperation.

In the Cebus monkey increases were noted in the uptake of [^{3}H]lysine into spinal cord TCA-precipitable protein as early as 3 days after spinal hemisection at T2 (117). Increases in overall uptake of amino acid into spinal cord protein were noted in addition to local increases at the site of the lesion. The overall increases seemed to be related to surgical stress during the early time periods, as the average levels of incorporation into protein decreased 3–6 days postoperation. However, a subsequent increase in the overall levels of amino acid incorporation 6–13 days postoperation did not seem consistent with a stress model. Local increases of [^{3}H]lysine into protein in the area of the lesion increase progressively over time and become more restricted to the area and side of the lesion. In the brain of the hemisected monkey (12), there are significant left (lesioned side)–right differences (L > R) in the radioactivity of protein in the leg area of motor cortex, occipital cortex, and superior colliculus. Fluctuations of amino acid uptake into TCA-precipitable protein of brain (averaged overall

samples) seemed generally to parallel those of the spinal cord. In these studies, an increase in radioactivity in brain and spinal cord protein were attributed to stress and unknown, perhaps blood-borne factors. Local increases in the area of spinal lesions were attributed to gliosis, neuronal reaction, regenerative responses, and infiltrating cells from the periphery. Focal laterality differences in brain were attributed to synaptic depletion, alterations in blood flow, sprouting of axons, or increased metabolic demand on the intact side.

Drug therapy studies in injured CNS tissues designed to induce regeneration give some insight into biochemical processes involved in regeneration or its failure. Some of the primary drugs utilized include Piromen, nerve growth factor, adrenocorticotropic hormone (ACTH), triiodothyronine, hydrolytic enzymes, cyclophosphamide, and puromycin (13,14,30,52, 120).

Piromen and associated bacterial polysaccharides have been utilized in numerous studies in rats (45,120) and cats (45,66). Some return of function after spinal transection and Piromen treatment has been noted in both species, but with low success rates. The limited success of the bacterial pyrogens has been attributed to an ability to stimulate the growth of severed fibers and to "loosen" or otherwise alter the formation of the neuroglial scar, which may act as a barrier to the regrowth of nerve fibers.

Nerve growth factor (62) has been noted to stimulate the growth of cell processes from sensory neurons and ganglia *in vitro* and *in vivo* (102). It is believed to produce its effects by stimulating RNA production in nerve cells. Nerve growth factor has been utilized to promote regeneration of the spinal cord in kittens after dorsal column lesions (102). Regrowth of nerve fibers across the site of lesion is noted with the continued administration of the drug. More recently it was demonstrated that nerve growth factor could significantly increase the degree and rate of regeneration of rat brain catecholaminergic pathways (20). It does not, however, seem to stimulate other types of fiber growth.

ACTH was used to induce regeneration of nerve fibers within the spinal cord of the rat (77). If ACTH is administered after cord transection, there is regeneration with the return of sensation in a small number of animals. Anatomically, the growth of nerve fibers could be demonstrated, but the number of fibers regenerated is small, and the sources of the nerve fibers are not known. The regrowth of axons in brain-lesioned rats was also noted after ACTH treatment (44). ACTH and/or its induced release of corticosteroids is believed to reduce inflammation and connective tissue scarring.

Intraperitoneal injections of ACTH into rats, after somatomotor cortex lesions, enhances growth into lesioned areas (52). In the same set of experiments, triiodothyronine (intraperitoneal injection) did seem to enhance the regeneration of unmyelinated axons even into the area of lesion. This supported earlier observations (55) that L-thyroxine might enhance axon regrowth and functional recovery after spinal cord compression in rats. This further supported the observation suggesting that triiodothyronine might enhance regeneration in rat brain after lesions with only slight effects on scarring (44). Enhancement of peripheral nerve regeneration in the rat by exogenous triiodothyronine has also been noted (31). Triiodothyronine and thyroxine may stimulate protein synthesis in injured nerve cells directly to enhance growth (97) but may also have effects on satellite cells and scarring.

Hydrolytic enzymes have been used to enhance regeneration in studies of spinal cord lesions in dogs (46). In these experiments a modified trypsin treatment reduces scarring in spinal lesions and enhances regeneration. Further studies (72) utilize treatments of hyaluronidase, trypsin, elastase, pyrogeneal prosenine, lidase, and combinations of these drugs. These authors obtain a high degree of functional, electrophysiological, and anatomical regeneration after hemisection and transection of the rat spinal cord. The use of these enzymes is reported to reduce the formation of the scar matrix and aid in the removal of debris to allow the regrowth of fibers. Further study is necessary to evaluate the usefulness of this treatment and applicability to other species.

An immunological model for the failure of CNS fibers to regenerate has been postulated (17). In the model, autoantibodies to brain or spinal cord antigens are formed after injury. These complexes or other lymphocyte products

are transported from the axon lesion to the cell body where they may alter protein synthesis. This hypothesis has been tested to some extent with the use of cyclophosphamide in spinal-transected rats as an immunosuppressive agent (43). Histological and electrophysiological evidence indicates an enhanced regrowth of fibers across the site of lesion in treated rats in the apparent absence of any effects on the neuroglial scar. However, the incidence of regrowth was slight, and functional regeneration was not obtained.

Puromycin and other protein synthesis inhibitors have been utilized to enhance the regeneration of spinal cord in the hemisected spinal cord of the rat (14). The application of puromycin in a Gelfoam sponge into the site of hemisection results in the transient growth of CNS nerve fibers into the site of the lesion. Puromycin treatment also delays the formation of dendritic varicosities and the reduction of dendritic field typical of neurons after spinal lesion (13). These observations indicate that puromycin could delay the morphological changes of injured neurons (presumably through its protein synthesis-inhibiting capacity) and enhance the regrowth of fibers. This evidence suggests that some of the chemical processes leading to observed morphological injury of neurons are active: protein synthesis, linked and regenerative. These data are supported by the fact that histological changes induced by axotomy in the motoneurons of the mouse can be delayed if actinomycin D is applied within 9–12 hr after axotomy (108–110). The mechanism of the protective effect is not known but appears to be related to the protein synthetic responses of neurons (42,64).

The regeneration of nerve fibers in the spinal cord appear to be enhanced by both locally acting drugs and systemically administered drugs with unspecified sites of action. Nonetheless, these factors are involved in scar formation and in the intrinsic ability of the neuron soma of the long tracts and local interneurons to regenerate axons. Such factors are known to contribute in the prognosis of peripheral nerve injuries and eventual return of function. Thus, it is not unreasonable that central neurons may be affected by similar factors, perhaps on a different scale. The extent to which the processes determining the capacity of central fibers to grow can be controlled externally remains to be determined by future research.

DISCUSSION

Regeneration of the spinal cord of mammals includes many processes, including axonal regenerative processes that have been placed by different authors into varying disciplines. The varying terminologies make it difficult to determine if the mammalian spinal cord does regenerate following lesion. Perhaps better stated, are there regenerative processes following spinal cord injury?

This brief review attempts to correlate the regenerative properties of neurons in the CNS utilizing neurochemical, electrophysiological, and anatomical studies which analyze central alterations following peripheral or central lesions. If one defines these changes in the context of the processes discussed, it can be stated that the spinal cord of mammals regenerates in a limited manner. This is based on several lines of evidence. New synaptic complexes are cyclically renewed in numbers and morphologically patterned (perhaps by availability) after spinal cord hemisection (11). These data are confined to the first segment rostral to T1–T2 interface spinal hemisection in rats and also appear to be valid for monkeys (15). It is also possible that these processes are occurring distal to the lesion.

There is synaptic loss on red nucleus neurons following central axotomy of the rubrospinal tract (3). Although the lost boutons from the soma degenerate, it is an indication that there is a higher center neuronal synaptic reorganization following spinal injury which may play a role in the regenerative processes. In addition, axotomy of rubospinal neurons results in sprouting of the tract rostral to the lesion which can also play an important role as sources of axons and boutons in spinal cord regeneration (88,89,95).

There are also neurochemical indices in the spinal cord and brain which again demonstrate that a limited amount of regeneration and metabolic restitution may occur following injury. The regrowth of nerve fibers in these instances is usually correlated with alterations of the properties of the neuroglial-pial cicatrix at the site of lesion by drugs or

enzymes, although direct influence on cell bodies within the nervous system cannot be ruled out.

The use of Piromen, ACTH, triiodothyronine, puromycin, and hydrolytic enzymes can produce alterations in the formation of the glial cicatrix. These alterations are generally described as a "loosening" of the scar, increased vascularity, or a general reduction of scar density. Other drugs, nerve factor, cyclophosphamide, and to some extent ACTH and triiodothyronine may have systemic effects or scar alteration too subtle to be detected morphologically. It is interesting in this respect that in some studies where temporary regrowth of fibers and/or functional recovery is induced the loss of nerve fibers and function may be correlated with the normalization or maturation of the scar cicatrix (14,45,120). These studies strongly suggest that the formation of the scar and the subsequent microenvironment in which severed axons must regenerate is of great importance in determining whether fibers grow through the area of a spinal lesion.

General metabolic studies of spinal cord injury over time periods in which regenerative changes occur (12,117) may correlate with the anatomical studies. These studies demonstrate that, in addition to increased amino acid uptake into protein in the area of spinal injury, overall changes in CNS metabolism occur in spinal cord and brain associated with the injury and operative trauma. The manner in which general changes in CNS metabolism interact with local cell responses is not known.

These studies are in contrast to neurochemical and histochemical studies of the axotomized central neuron, which suggest that most of these neurons are incapable of regrowing severed axon stumps. However, the origin of regrowing fibers in the spinal cord has not been defined, nor has the reaction of the central neuron under conditions favorable for regeneration been studied. It may be possible, therefore, that the functional recovery noted in experimental treatment results from regrowth of dorsal roots, interneurons, or selected tracts into interneuronal pools below the site of lesion, rather than a general long-tract regeneration (16). On the other hand, central neurons subtending long tracts may show altered metabolic responses and exhibit regeneration when the conditions are proper for axon growth within the lesion.

It appears that the mammalian spinal cord does regenerate by operational definition. The process lacks at least one critical factor to meet the classic definition of the term, the regeneration of transected nerve fibers across the site of lesion. This problem has not been solved. However, the spinal interneuron is a possible source of nerve fibers for regeneration because of copious sprouting after spinal cord lesion (16). Perhaps this source of nerve fibers can be utilized to alleviate the enigma of spinal cord regeneration and paraplegia.

ACKNOWLEDGMENTS

Supported in part by a grant from the National Institutes of Health, NINCDS (NS-06164). M.W. is a National Science Foundation predoctoral fellow. The authors thank Ms. G. Hunter and Mr. M. Zanakis for their aid.

REFERENCES

1. Barr, M. L., and Hamilton, J. D. (1948): A quantitative study of certain morphological changes in spinal motor neurons during axon reaction. *J. Comp. Neurol.,* 89:93–121.
2. Barron, K. D., Chiang, T. Y., Daniels, A. C., and Dollin, P F. (1971): Subcellular accompaniment of axon reaction in cervical motoneurons of the cat. In: *Progress in Neuropathology,* Vol. 1, edited by H. M. Zimmerman, pp. 255–280. Grune & Stratton, New York.
3. Barron, K. D., Dentinger, M. P., Nelson, L. R., and Mincy, J. E. (1975): Ultrastructure of axonal reaction in red nucleus of cat. *J. Neuropathol. Exp. Neurol.,* 34:222–248.
4. Barron, K. D., Dentinger, M. P., Nelson, L. R., and Scheibly, M. E. (1976): Incorporation of tritiated leucine by axotomized rubral neurons. *Brain Res.,* 116:251–266.
5. Barron, K. D., Doolin, P. F., and Oldershaw, J. B. (1967): Ultrastructural observations on retrograde atrophy of lateral geniculate body. I. Neuronal alterations. *J. Neuropathol. Exp. Neurol.,* 26:300–326.
6. Bernstein, J. J., and Bernstein, M. E. (1971): Axonal regeneration and formation of synapses proximal to the site of lesion following hemisection of the rat spinal cord. *Exp. Neurol.,* 30:336–351.
7. Bernstein, J. J., and Bernstein, M. E. (1973): Neuronal alteration and reinnervation following axonal regeneration and sprouting in the mammalian spinal cord. *Brain Behav. Evol.,* 8:135–161.
8. Bernstein, J. J., and Bernstein, M. E. (1976): Ventral horn synaptology in the rat. *J. Neurocytol.,* 5:109–123.
9. Bernstein, J. J., Bernstein, M. E., and Collins, G. (1973): Ultrastructure of a human spinal neuroma. *J. Neurol. Sci.,* 18:489–492.
10. Bernstein, J. J., and Gelderd, J. B. (1973): Synaptic reorganization following regeneration of goldfish spinal cord. *Exp. Neurol.,* 41:402–410.
11. Bernstein, J. J., Gelderd, J. B., and Bernstein, M. E. (1974): Alteration of neuronal synaptic complement during regeneration and axonal sprouting of rat spinal cord. *Exp. Neurol.,* 44:470–482.
12. Bernstein, J. J., and Wells, M. R. (1977): Amino acid incorporation in medulla, pons, midbrain and cortex following spinal cord hemisection in the cebus monkey (Cebus appella). *Brain Res.,* 122:475–483.
13. Bernstein, J. J., Wells, M. R., and Bernstein, M. E. (1975): Dendrites and neuroglia following hemisection of rat spinal cord: Effects of puromycin. *Adv. Neurol.,* 12:439–451.
14. Bernstein, J. J., Wells, M. R., and Bernstein, M. E. (1978): Effect of puromycin treatment on the regeneration of hemisected and transected spinal cord. *J. Neuropathol. (in press).*
15. Bernstein, M. E., and Bernstein, J. J. (1973): Regeneration of axons and synaptic complex formation rostral to the site of hemisection in the spinal cord of the monkey. *Int. J. Neurosci.,* 5:15–26.
16. Bernstein, M. E., and Bernstein, J. J. (1977): Synaptic frequency alteration on rat ventral horn neurons in the first segment proximal to spinal cord hemisection: An ultrastructural statistical study of regenerative capacity. *J. Neurocytol.,* 6:85–102.
17. Berry, M., and Riches, A. C. (1974): An immunological approach to regeneration in the central nervous system. *Br. Med. Bull.,* 30:135–140.
18. Bjorklund, A., Johansson, B., Stenevi, U., and Avendgaard, N. E. (1975): Re-establishment of functional connections by regenerating central adrenergic and cholinergic axons. *Nature (Lond),* 253:446–448.
19. Bjorklund, A., Katzman, R., Stenevi, U., and West, K. A. (1971): Development and growth of axonal sprouts from noradrenaline and 5-hydroxytryptamine neurons in the rat spinal cord. *Brain Res.,* 31:21–33.
20. Bjorklund, A., and Stenevi, U. (1972): Nerve growth factor: Stimulation of regenerative growth of central noradrenergic neurons. *Science,* 175:1251–1253.
21. Blakemore, W. F. (1973): Remyelination of the cerebellar peduncle in the mouse fol-

lowing demyelination induced by feeding cuprizone. *J. Neurol. Sci.*, 20:73–83.

22. Blakemore, W. F. (1974): Pattern of remyelination in the CNS. *Nature (Lond)*, 249: 557–578.

23. Blakemore, W. F. (1976): Invasion of Schwann cells into the spinal cord of the rat following local injections of lysolecithin. *Neuropathol. Appl. Neurobiol.*, 2:21–39.

24. Blakemore, W. F., and Patterson, R. C. (1975): Observations on the interactions of Schwann cells and astrocytes following x-irradiation of neonatal rat spinal cord. *J. Neurocytol.*, 4:573–585.

25. Blinzinger, K., and Kreutzberg, G. (1968): Displacement of synaptic terminals from regenerating motoneurons by microglial cells. *Z. Zellforsch. Mikrosk. Anat.*, 85:145–157.

26. Bodian, D. (1975): Origin of specific synaptic types in the motoneuron neuropil of the monkey. *J. Comp. Neurol.*, 159:225–243.

27. Brattgard, S. O., Edstrom, J. E., and Hydén, H. (1957): The chemical changes in regenerating neurons. *J. Neurochem.*, 1:316–325.

28. Brown, L. T. (1971): Projections and termination of the corticospinal tract in rodents. *Exp. Brain Res.*, 13:432–450.

29. Chow, K. L., and Dewson, J. H., III (1966): Numerical estimates of neurons and glia in lateral geniculate body during retrograde degeneration. *J. Comp. Neurol.*, 128:63–74.

30. Clemente, C. D. (1964): Regeneration in the vertebrate central nervous system. *Int. Rev. Neurobiol.*, 6:257–293.

31. Cockett, S. A., and Kiernan, J. A. (1973): Acceleration of peripheral nervous regeneration in the rat by exogenous triiodothyronine. *Exp. Neurol.*, 39:389–394.

32. Cole, M. (1968): Retrograde degeneration of axon and soma in the nervous system. In: *The Structure and Function of Nervous Tissue*, Vol. 1, edited by G. Bourne, pp. 269–300. Academic Press, New York.

33. Collins, G. H. (1966): An electron microscopic study of remyelination in the brainstem of thiamine deficient rats. *Am. J. Anat.*, 48:259–275.

34. Conradi, S. (1969): Ultrastructure and distribution of neuronal and glial elements on the motoneuron surface in the lumbosacral spinal cord of the adult rat. *Acta Physiol. Scand. [Suppl.]*, 332:5–48.

35. Conradi, S. (1969): Ultrastructure and distribution of neuronal and glial elements on the surface of the proximal part of a motoneuron dendrite, as analyzed by serial sections. *Acta Physiol. Scand. [Suppl.]*, 332: 49–64.

36. Conradi, S. (1969): Ultrastructure of dorsal root boutons on lumbosacral motoneurons of the adult cat, as revealed by dorsal root section. *Acta Physiol. Scand. [Suppl.]*, 332:85–115.

37. Cragg, B. G. (1970): What is the signal for chromatolysis? *Brain Res.*, 23:1–21.

38. Dorland (1959): *Medical Dictionary*, p. 1172. Saunders, Philadelphia.

39. Eayrs, J. T. (1952): Relationship between the ganglion cell layer of the retina and optic nerve in the rat. *Br. J. Ophthalmol.*, 36:453.

40. Engh, C. A., and Schofield, B. H. (1972): A review of central response to peripheral nerve injury and its significance in nerve regeneration. *J. Neurosurg.*, 37:195–203.

41. Engh, C. A., Schofield, B. H., Doty, S. B., and Robinson, R. A. (1971): Perikaryal synthetic function following reversible and irreversible peripheral injuries as shown by radioautograph. *J. Comp. Neurol.*, 142: 465–480.

42. Farber, E., Verbin, R. S., and Lieberman, M. (1971): Cell suicide and cell death. In: *Mechanisms of Toxicity*, edited by W. N. Aldridge, pp. 163–173. Macmillan, London.

43. Feringa, E. R., Johnson, R. D., and Wendt, J. S. (1975): Spinal cord regeneration in rats after immunosuppressive treatment. *Arch. Neurol.*, 32:676–683.

44. Fertig, A., Kiernan, J. A., and Seyan, S. S. A. S. (1971): Enhancement of axonal regeneration in the brain of the rat by corticotrophin and triiodothyronine. *Exp. Neurol.*, 33:372–385.

45. Freeman, L. W. (1955): Functional recovery in spinal rats. In: *Regeneration in the Central Nervous System*, edited by W. F. Windle, pp. 195–207. Charles C Thomas, Springfield, Ill.

46. Freeman, L. W., MacDougall, J., Turbes, C. A., and Bowman, D. E. (1960): The treatment of experimental lesions of the spinal cord of dogs with trypsin. *J. Neurosurg.*, 17:259–265.

47. Gilmore, S. A. (1973): Long-term effects of ionizing radiation on rat spinal cord: Intramedullary connective tissue formation. *Am. J. Anat.*, 137:1–18.

48. Gilmore, S. A., and Duncan, D. (1968): On the presence of peripheral-like nervous and connective tissue within irradiated spinal cord. *Anat. Rec.*, 160:675–690.

49. Goldberger, M. E., and Murray, M. (1974): Restitution of function and collateral sprouting in the rat spinal cord: The deafferented animal. *J. Comp. Neurol.*, 158:37–54.

50. Grafstein, B. (1975): The nerve cell body response to axotomy. *Exp. Neurol.*, 48: 32–51.

51. Griffith, A., and LaVelle, A. (1971): Developmental protein changes in normal and chromatolytic facial nuclear regions. *Exp. Neurol.*, 33:360–371.

52. Guth, L. (1974): Axonal regeneration and functional plasticity in the central nervous system. *Exp. Neurol.*, 45:606–654.

53. Guth, L., and Clemente, C. D. (1975):

Growth and regeneration in the central nervous system. *Exp. Neurol.*, 48:1–251.

54. Gutmann, E. (1942): Factors affecting recovery of motor function after nerve lesions. *J. Neurol. Psychiatry*, 5:81–95.

55. Harvey, J. E., and Srebnik, H. H. (1967): Locomotor activity and axon regeneration following spinal cord compression in rats treated with L-thyroxine. *J. Neuropathol. Exp. Neurol.*, 26:661–668.

56. Hirano, A., Zimmerman, H. M., and Levine, S. (1969): Electron microscope observations of peripheral myelin in the central nervous system lesion. *Acta Neuropathol. (Berl)*, 12:348–365.

57. James, G. R. (1933): Degeneration of ganglion cell following axonal injury. *Arch. Ophthalmol.*, 9:338.

58. Kaizawa, J., and Takhashi, I. (1970): Motor cell columns in rat lumbar spinal cord. *Tohoku J. Exp. Med.*, 101:25–34.

59. Kalil, K., and Schneider, G. E. (1975): Retrograde cortical and axonal changes following lesions of the pyramidal tract. *Brain Res.*, 89:15–27.

60. Kung, S. H. (1971): Incorporation of tritiated precursors in the cytoplasm of normal and chromatolytic sensory neurons as shown by autoradiography. *Brain Res.*, 25:656–660.

61. Lampert, P., and Cressman, M. (1964): Axonal regeneration in the dorsal column of the spinal cords of adult rats. *Lab. Invest.*, 13:825–839.

62. Levi-Montalcini, R., and Angeletti, P. U. (1968): Nerve growth factor. *Physiol. Rev.*, 48:534–569.

63. Levin, P. M., and Bradford, F. K. (1938): The exact origin of the corticospinal tract of the monkey. *J. Comp. Neurol.*, 68:411–422.

64. Lieberman, M. W., Verbin, R. S., Landay, M., Liang, H., Farber, E., Lee, T., and Starr, R. (1970): A probable role for protein synthesis in intestinal epithelial cell damage induced in vivo by cytosine arabinoside, nitrogen mustard or x-irradiation. *Cancer Res.*, 30:942–951.

65. Lieberman, A. R. (1971): The axon reaction: A review of the principal features of perikaryal responses to axon injury. *Int. Rev. Neurobiol.*, 14:49–124.

66. Litrell, J. L. (1955): Apparent functional restitution in Piromen treated spinal cats. In: *Regeneration in the Central Nervous System*, edited by W. F. Windle. Charles C Thomas, Springfield, Ill.

67. Liu, C. N. (1955): Time pattern in retrograde degeneration after trauma of central nervous system of mammals. In: *Regeneration in the Central Nervous System*, edited by W. F. Windle, pp. 84–93, Charles C Thomas, Springfield, Ill.

68. Liu, C. N., and Chambers, W. W. (1958): Intraspinal sprouting of dorsal root axons. *Arch. Neurol. Psychiatry*, 79:46–61.

69. Luttge, W., Mannis, M., and Bernstein, J. J. (1975): Alterations of central nervous system protein systhesis in response to spinal cord hemisection. *J. Neurosci. Res.*, 1:77–82.

70. Lynch, G., and Cotman, C. W. (1975): The hippocampus as a model for studying anatomical plasticity in the adult brain. In: *The Hippocampus, Vol. 1: Structure and Development*, edited by R. L. Isaacson and K. H. Pribram, pp. 123–154. Plenum, New York.

71. Lynch, G., Stanfield, B., and Cotman, C. (1973): Developmental differences in post-lesion axonal growth in the hippocampus. *Brain Res.*, 59:155–168.

72. Martinian, L. A., and Ardreasian A. S. (1976): Enzyme therapy in organic lesions of the spinal cord. Translated by E. Tanasescu. Brain Inf. Ser., UCLA, Los Angeles.

73. McLaughlin, B. (1972): The fine structure of neurons and synapses in the motor nuclei of the cat spinal cord. *J. Comp. Neurol.*, 144:429–460.

74. McLaughlin, B. (1972): Dorsal root projections to the motor nuclei in the cat spinal cord. *J. Comp. Neurol.*, 144:461–474.

75. McLaughlin, B. (1972): Propriospinal and supraspinal projections to the motor nuclei of the cat spinal cord. *J. Comp. Neurol.*, 144:475–500.

76. McLaughlin, B. J., Barber, R., Saito, K., Roberts, E., and Wu, J. Y. (1975): Immunocytochemical localization of glutamate decarboxylase in rat spinal cord. *J. Comp. Neurol.*, 164:305–322.

77. McMasters, R. E. (1962): Regeneration of the spinal cord in the rat: Effects of Piromen and ACTH upon the regenerative capacity. *J. Comp. Neurol.*, 119:113–116.

78. McQuarrie, I. G., and Grafstein, B. (1973): Axon outgrowth enhanced by a previous nerve injury. *Arch. Neurol.*, 29:53–55.

79. Mendell, L. M., Munson, J. B., and Scott, J. G. (1976): Alterations of synapses on axotomized motoneurones. *J. Physiol. (Lond)*, 255:67–79.

80. Meyer, D. D., and Cole, M. (1970): Comparison of certain retrograde oxidative reactions after section of axons in central and peripheral nervous systems. *Neurology (Minneap)*, 20:918.

81. Moore, R. Y., Bjorklund, A., and Stenevi, U. (1971): Plastic changes in the adrenergic innervation of the rat septal area in response to denervation. *Brain Res.*, 33:13–35.

82. Murray, M., and Goldberger, M. E. (1974): Restitution of function and collateral sprouting in the cat spinal cord: The partially hemisected animal. *J. Comp. Neurol.*, 158:19–36.

83. Naftchi, E., Demeny, M., De Crescito, V., Tomasula, J., Flamm, E., and Campbell, J. (1974): Biogenic amine concentrations in

traumatized spinal cords of cats. *J. Neurosurg.*, 40:52–57.

84. Nyberg-Hansen, R., and Brodal, A. (1963): Sites of termination of corticospinal fibers in the cat: An experimental study with silver impregnation methods. *J. Comp. Neurol.*, 129:369–391.

85. Osterholm, J. L. (1974): The pathophysiological response to spinal cord injury: The current status of related research. *J. Neurosurg.*, 40:5–33.

86. Peters, A., Palay, S., and Webster, H. de F. (1976): *The Fine Structure of the Nervous System: The Neurons and Supporting Cells*, p. 406. Saunders, Philadelphia.

87. Piatt, J. (1955): Regeneration of the spinal cord of the salamander. *J. Exp. Zool.*, 129: 177–207.

88. Prendergast, J., and Stelzner, D. J. (1976): Changes in the magnocellular portion of the red nucleus following thoracic hemisection in the neonatal and adult rat. *J. Comp. Neurol.*, 166:163–172.

89. Prendergast, J., and Stelzner, D. J. (1976): Increases in collateral axon growth rostral to a thoracic hemisection in neonatal and weanling rat. *J. Comp. Neurol.*, 166:145–162.

90. Raine, C. S. (1976): On the occurrence of Schwann cells within the normal central nervous system. *J. Neurocytol.*, 5:371–380.

91. Raisman, G. (1969): Neuronal plasticity in the septal nuceli of the adult rat. *Brain Res.*, 14:25–48.

92. Raisman, G. (1973): An ultrastructural study of the effects of hypophysectomy on the supraoptic nucleus of the rat. *J. Comp. Neurol.*, 147:181–208.

93. Raisman, G. (1973): Electron microscopic studies of the development of new neurohaemal contacts in the median eminence of the rat after hypophysectomy. *Brain Res.*, 55:256–261.

94. Raisman, G., and Field, P. (1973): A quantitative investigation of the development of collateral reinnervation after partial deafferentation of the septal nuclei. *Brain Res.*, 50:241–264.

95. Ramón y Cajal, S. (1959): In: *Degeneration and Regeneration of the Nervous System*, edited by R. M. May, p. 769. Hafner, New York.

96. Reis, D. J., and Ross, R. A. (1973): Dynamic changes in brain dopamine-β-hydroxylase activity during anterograde and retrograde reactions to injury of central noradrenergic neurons. *Brain Res.*, 57:307–326.

97. Rhodes, A., Ford, D., and Rhines, R. (1964): Comparative uptake of DL-lysine-³H by normal and regenerative hypoglossal nerve cells in euthyroid, hypothyroid and hyperthyroid male rats. *Exp. Neurol.*, 10; 251–263.

98. Ross, R. A., Joh, T. H., and Rees, D. J. (1975): Reversible changes in the accumulation and activities of tyrosine hydroxylase and dopamine-β-hydroxylase in neurons of nucleus locus coeruleus during the retrograde reaction. *Brain Res.*, 92:57–72.

99. Rustioni, A., and Sotelo, C. (1974): Some effects of chronic deafferentation on the ultrastructure of the nucleus gracilis of the cat. *Brain Res.*, 73:527–533.

100. Schoultz, T. W., DeLuca, D. C., and Reding, D. (1976): Norepinephrine levels in traumatized spinal cord of catecholamine depleted cats. *Brain Res.*, 109:367–374.

101. Schreiber, S., and Barron, K. D. (1975): Quantitative cytochemistry of RNA in rubral neurons during axon reaction. *Neurosci. Abstr.*, 1:104.

102. Scott, D., and Liu, C. N. (1964): Factors promoting regeneration of spinal neurons: Positive influence of nerve growth factor. *Prog. Brain Res.*, 13:127–150.

103. Shapovalov, A. I., and Grantyn, A. A. (1968): Suprasegmental synaptic influences on chromatolysed motor neurones. *Biophys. J.*, 13:308–319.

104. Stenevi, U., Bjorklund, A., and Moore, R. Y. (1972): Growth of intact central adrenergic axons in the denervated lateral geniculate body. *Exp. Neurol.*, 35:290–299.

105. Stewart, O., Cotman, C., and Lynch, G. (1973): Re-establishment of electrophysiologically functional entorhinal cortical input to the dentate gyrus deafferented by ipsilateral entorhinal lesions: Innervation by the contralateral entorhinal cortex. *Exp. Brain Res.*, 18:396–414.

106. Stoney, S. D. (1971): Motor mechanisms: The role of the pyramidal system in motor control. *Annu. Rev. Physiol.*, 33:337–392.

107. Sumner, B. E. H. (1976): Quantitative ultrastructural observations on the inhibited recovery of the hypoglossal nucleus from the axotomy response when regeneration of the hypoglossal nerve is prevented. *Exp. Brain Res.*, 26:141–150.

108. Torvik, A., and Heding, A. (1967): Histological studies on the effect of actinomycin D on retrograde nerve cell reaction in the facial nucleus of mice. *Acta Neuropathol. (Berl)*, 9:146–157.

109. Torvik, A., and Heding, A. (1969): Effect of actinomycin D on the retrograde nerve cell reaction: Further observations. *Acta Neuropathol. (Berl)*, 14:62–71.

110. Torvik, A., and Skjorten, F. (1974): The effect of actinomycin D upon normal neurons and retrograde nerve cell reaction. *J. Neurocytol.*, 3:87–97.

111. Uchizono, K. (1966): Excitatory and inhibitory synapses in the cat spinal cord. *Jpn. J. Physiol.*, 16:570–575.

112. Valverde, F. (1966): The pyramidal tract

of rodents, a study of its relations with posterior column nuclei, dorsal lateral reticular formation of the medulla oblongata, and cervical spinal cord (Golgi and electron microscopic observations). *Z. Zellforsch. Mikrosk. Anat.*, 71:297–363.

113. Walker, A. E. (1938): *The Primate Thalamus.* University of Chicago Press, Chicago.

114. Watson, W. E. (1965): An autoradiographic study of the incorporation of nucleic acid precursors by neurones and glia during nerve regeneration. *J. Physiol. (Lond)*, 180:741–753.

115. Watson, W. E. (1968): Observations on the nucleolar and total cell body nucleic acid content of injured nerve cells. *J. Physiol. (Lond)*, 196:655–676.

116. Watson, W. E. (1974): Cellular responses to axotomy and to related procedures. *Br. Med. Bull.*, 30:112–115.

117. Wells, M. R., and Bernstein, J. J. (1976): Early changes in protein synthesis following spinal cord hemisection in the cebus monkey (Cebus apella). *Brain Res.*, 111:31–40.

118. Wells, M. R., and Bernstein, J. J. (1977): Amino acid incorporation in the rat spinal cord and brain after simultaneous and interval sciatic nerve lesions. *Brain Res. (in press).*

119. Wells, M. R., and Bernstein, J. J. (1977): Amino acid uptake in the spinal cord and brain of the short term spinal hemisected rat. *Exp. Neurol. (in press).*

120. Windle, W. F. (1955): *Regeneration in the Central Nervous System.* Charles C Thomas, Springfield, Ill.

Physiology and Pathobiology of Axons, edited by
S. G. Waxman. Raven Press, New York © 1978.

Evoked Potentials in Demyelinating Disease

Norman S. Namerow

*Department of Neurology, School of Medicine, UCLA Center for the Health Sciences,
Los Angeles, California 90024*

Following the initial report by Dawson (7)
on the recording of brain responses to peripheral nerve stimulation, numerous investigators sought clinical use for this neurophysiological technique. The recording of brain
evoked potentials has subsequently found application in patients with trauma, vascular
disease, mass lesions, psychiatric disorders, and
demyelinating disease. It is in this latter category that the method has been of unique value,
for it provided for the first time insight into
pathophysiological mechanisms in this disease.
Early studies concentrated on the somatosensory evoked response, although subsequently a
large body of data has been compiled using
visual and auditory responses as well as brainstem reflexes as a means of evaluating patients.
The results from somatosensory stimulation,
however, have proved of greatest value in the
study of axonal conduction characteristics
following demyelination.

The problem of measuring nerve conduction
in the central nervous system (CNS) of man is
formidable. One must deal with tracts or fiber
bundles rather than single nerve fibers. For
routine evaluation, one must stimulate and detect responses at a distance because of the
intervening skin, subcutaneous tissue, bone,
and meninges. Concerning demyelinating disease or multiple sclerosis (MS) in particular,
this approach is all that is available as the
disease is uniquely human and affects only the
brain and spinal cord. Despite the indirect
measures to be discussed, the method of evoking a brain response to peripheral stimulation
has given some clarity to our understanding
of this disease and in some instances has offered an aid in diagnosis.

SOMATOSENSORY EVOKED RESPONSES

The first report concerning the somatosensory evoked response (SER) in patients with
demyelinating disease was that of Halliday and
Wakefield (9). They demonstrated an abnormal SER in two patients with dissociated sensory loss: These patients had impaired vibration
and joint position sense but normal pain and
light touch perception. Giblin (8) and Larson
et al. (15) also reported abnormal responses
in patients with this type of sensory loss. The
fact that the SER was mediated primarily over
proprioceptive pathways was confirmed in a
report by Namerow (21) that showed the responses of three patients following cervical
cordotomy for intractable pain. In each instance there was an excellent surgical result
with hypalgesia and hypesthesia below the level
of cordotomy, yet the SER on median nerve
stimulation was normal in both latency and
configuration.

The intent of the initial papers dealing with
MS patients was to point out that the SER was
transmitted over proprioceptive pathways or
those that subserved vibration and position
sense. It was left to others to study systematically the findings in patients with demyelinating disease.

The first series of MS patients was that of
Baker et al. (2) who reported delayed-onset
latencies and a monophasic response in those
patients with proprioceptive impairment. These
findings were confirmed by Namerow (19)
(Fig. 1) who studied a group of 32 MS patients. In this report patients were divided into
three groups depending on their clinical sensory examination. One group had vibration

NORMAL

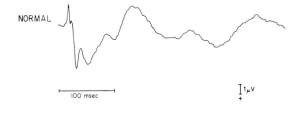

|—————————|
100 msec

$\mathop{\mathrm{I}}\limits_{+}$ 1 µV

PATIENT

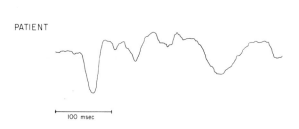

|—————————|
100 msec

FIG. 1. Upper tracing is the SER from a normal subject. The lower tracing is from an MS patient with severe vibration and position sense impairment in the hand being stimulated. Note the loss of the early sharp negative deflection and the marked delay in onset and peak of the major positive wave. (From ref. 23.)

and/or position sense impairment at the time of the study. The second group had such impairment at some time in the past but not at the time of testing. The third group never had such sensory loss despite frequent examinations in an MS clinic. This study demonstrated a correlation between the degree of sensory loss and the prolongation of response latencies, as measured to the onset of the response, and the peak of the major positive wave. The study was of particular interest in that abnormal responses were noted in patients with normal clinical sensory examinations. Even some patients who had never experienced sensory symptoms gave responses that were delayed in onset and of abnormal configuration. Silent demyelinated lesions could therefore be demonstrated and the method of evoking a brain potential gained recognition as a neurophysiological technique sensitive enough to study axonal conduction and to offer a diagnostic capability.

These early results suggested that the abnormal response was produced by slowed conduction across areas of demyelination. Occasional profound delays in response onset further suggested that the larger and fastest conducting fibers might be more selectively damaged by demyelination, leaving transmission to persist over smaller and slower fibers. Such slow conduction, variable from fiber to fiber depending on the degree or extent of demyelination, would then produce temporal

dispersion of arriving cortical impulses. Thus an area of demyelination could account for the delayed as well as the broadened appearance of the evoked potentials. This was a demonstration in man's CNS of the animal observations of Mayer (16) and McDonald (17). They had previously shown reduced axonal conduction velocity in experimental demyelination of central axons.

In a subsequent report (20) a good correlation between the degree of sensory loss and response latencies was confirmed. In this study, evoked responses were obtained as patients experienced an attack of sensory symptoms. These results demonstrated that conduction changes could be documented as the patient passed through such an attack. The study also revealed that recovery of response latencies to more normal values lagged behind clinical improvement. This finding is similar to recoverable peripheral neuropathies where, despite return to a normal clinical examination, nerve conduction velocities may still be quite abnormal. In the case of MS, the evoked response latencies continued to shorten for months following resolution of an attack and long after the patient had returned to a normal clinical sensory examination. These results suggested that recovery from an attack of MS may be a two-phased event. On the one hand, adaptive mechanisms allow for normal function despite impaired nerve conduction. In essence, the brain may properly interpret a "noisy" signal, allowing the patient to give normal sensory responses. The long-term progressive reduction of latencies implies that longer-term repair and perhaps remyelination is also a factor.

The above studies abundantly demonstrated that one could get a reasonably accurate assessment of central axonal conduction in humans, and offered for the first time a means of objectively measuring that which is universally accepted as the cause of symptoms in MS, the demyelination of axons. Using a classic approach to the study of nerve fibers, the evoked response recovery function was next studied in normal subjects and MS patients (22). In normal subjects test response latencies were not significantly different from the conditioning response latencies until one reached interstimulus times of 10 msec or less. At the shorter stimulation separations, the test response latencies were slightly longer, a picture similar to that seen with direct stimulation of individual nerve fibers. In contrast, however, test stimulus latencies from MS patients became shorter as the interstimulus times were reduced. This paradoxical response could be explained by considering that after a conditioning stimulus conduction in the most demyelinated fibers would be blocked. The more severely demyelinated fibers ordinarily would contribute last to the evoked response owing to the slower conduction along these fibers. As one gradually reduces the interstimulus times, there would be successive blocking of less-affected fibers and the resultant evoked potential would have a progressively shorter latency. This study suggested that diseased or demyelinated axons could not effectively respond to a test stimulus that followed a conditioning stimulus by short intervals (less than 60 msec). The results also suggested that the more heavily myelinated and faster-conducting fibers were more affected by the demyelinating process.

Based on the recovery function results and the animal studies of Cragg and Thomas (4), McDonald and Sears (17), and Davis (5), it became apparent that a repetitive train of stimuli might have much to offer in the study of central axon conduction following demyelination.

Cragg and Thomas showed a posttetanic depression in peripheral demyelinated nerves following a 2-min tetanus at 368 Hz. McDonald and Sears, on the other hand, demonstrated central fiber inability to follow each

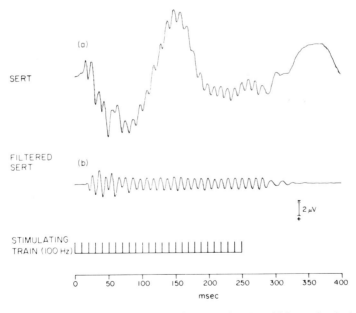

FIG. 2. Upper tracing is the SERT to a train of stimuli at 100 Hz. The middle tracing is the SERT response passed through a band pass filter peaked at 100 Hz prior to summating. The lower trace represents the stimuli presented during a 250-msec interval. The total duration of the plotted response is 400 msec. (From ref. 24.)

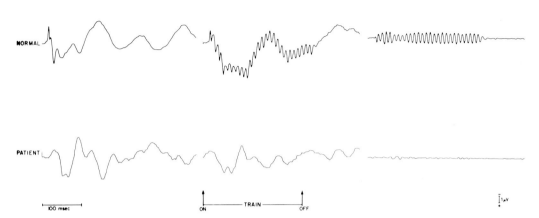

FIG. 3. Upper middle tracing is the SERT at 100 Hz, showing a rhythmical response detectable on the scalp. The effect of demyelination in the patient was to prevent transmission of these 100-Hz stimuli, leaving the response unchanged from that obtained at 1 Hz. The last column demonstrates the effect of band pass filtering There is virtually no 100-Hz activity detected on the scalp. (From ref. 23.)

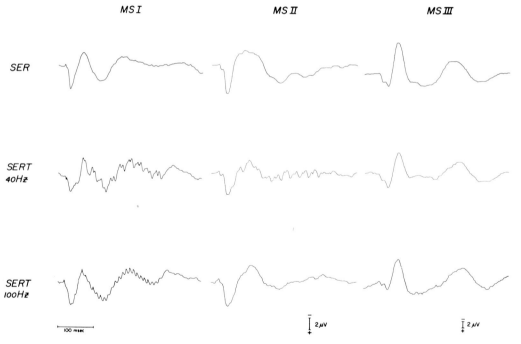

FIG. 4. SER and SERTs at 40 and 100 Hz are shown from three subjects. The patient in the group MS I had no vibration or position sense impairment at the time of study. The MS II patient had mild to moderate loss of such sensation, and the patient in group MS III had severe vibration and position sense loss. This illustrates the ability of patients to transmit stimulating trains as a function of the degree of demyelination. The normal or minimally affected patient can transmit all stimulating frequencies up to and greater than 100 Hz. The MS II patient is unable to allow passage of a 100-Hz train but does allow passage of the 40-Hz train. The more severely affected patient (of group MS III) is unable to transmit any repetitive activity, even below 40 Hz. The demyelinated area acts as a high-frequency filter, with the more extensive lesions preventing all except the slowest repetitions to produce an evoked brain potential. (From ref. 30.)

stimulus of a train at frequencies as low as 290 Hz. The next step was to investigate the human SER following repetitive high-frequency stimulation of the median nerve. This somatosensory evoked response to trains of stimuli (SERT) proved to be an easily observed and consistent brain response (Fig. 2). As with the SER, the peak amplitude of this response was over the contralateral parietal scalp. Analysis of the data suggested that the rhythmical potentials seen at higher frequencies may be due to subcortical activity with the cortical or postsynaptic contributions refractory at the higher stimulation frequencies. The data also supported the conclusion that the SERT was mediated over the same proprioceptive pathways that subserved the SER. It is of particular interest that the method of train stimulation and the data analysis method of filtering and single-cycle averaging significantly improved the signal/noise ratio of the cortical responses. Latencies could still be measured but now averaged single-cycle amplitudes could also be used as a means of measuring pathway competency. This is in part shown in Fig. 3 where, after filtering, there was virtually no 100-Hz activity in the patient's brain response.

Following demonstration of the feasibility of the SERT in evaluating human central conduction, a group of 33 MS patients were studied. The results were strikingly different from normal subjects. There was a close qualitative correlation between the degree of SERT change and the degree of clinical involvement as a function of the train stimulating frequency. Patients who had severe sensory loss revealed an impaired response at all stimulating frequencies. Individuals with mild to moderate sensory deficits showed a deterioration of their SERT response at midrange stimulating frequencies (Fig. 4). Those patients with no sensory loss had, at all frequencies, a response which appeared normal. In brief, the SERT appeared to be a sensitive measure of axonal function. The results indicated a markedly impaired ability to transmit trains of stimuli in patients suffering with demyelination in the appropriate afferent pathways. This impaired ability was quantitatively described by the filtered single-cycle peak-to-peak amplitude over a range of stimulating frequencies, and there was a direct correlation between the amplitudes of these responses and the severity of clinical sensory impairment (Fig. 5). This inability to conduct repetitive stimuli may be clinically reflected in the fre-

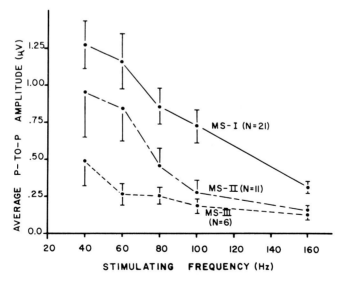

FIG. 5. Plot of the average peak-to-peak voltages of the repetitive response as a function of stimulating frequency for three MS subgroups (MS I none, MS II mild–moderate, MS III severe vibration and position sense loss). The flat response of the MS III group indicates virtually no transmitted repetitive activity at stimulation frequencies above 40 Hz. At each stimulating frequency, the response of normal individuals was well above the mean for all MS patients, to a highly significant degree. (From ref. 30.)

quently observed decline in function as a repetitive motor act is performed by patients with clinical pyramidal tract signs.

It should be stressed at this point that the abnormal evoked responses have always been assumed to be related to the process of central demyelination. There are many conducting structures intervening between the point of stimulation at the wrist and the point of detection on the scalp. However, there are no known significant peripheral nerve lesions in MS, and the occasional encroachment of MS plaques into the cortical gray matter appears to be too spotty in extent, marginal in location, and mild in degree to affect the cortical response. This leaves the central nerve tracts with their well-documented pathology of demyelination as the most likely contributor to the abnormal responses. The role of the central synapse is not so easily ignored. The possibility of a synaptic factor has been periodically raised and answered, yet the issue is still in question (3,6, 29). A synaptic influence has not been considered in the results discussed, and indeed the weight of evidence points toward this being a safe position to take. The technique described, however, would clearly be of great value in investigating such a phenomenon, and may be the only way to measure directly this influence in man.

Finally, there is no evidence to suggest that the SERs and SERTs are due to a generalized defect in conduction, ubiquitous in the MS patient. Rather, the results have always been approached and explained in the light of a specific area of demyelination producing specific conduction impairment.

VISUAL EVOKED RESPONSES

The SER has provided the greatest insight into neurophysiological mechanisms in MS. However, to date, the visual evoked response (VER) has offered the most clinically useful application of the averaged evoked response technique.

VER responses in MS patients were first reported by Rouher et al. (28). Richey et al. (27) and Namerow and Enns (25) also demonstrated VER changes secondary to optic nerve lesions in MS. These latter results demonstrated a correlation between latencies of the VER wave peaks and the degree of visual impairment. In this regard, the results were quite

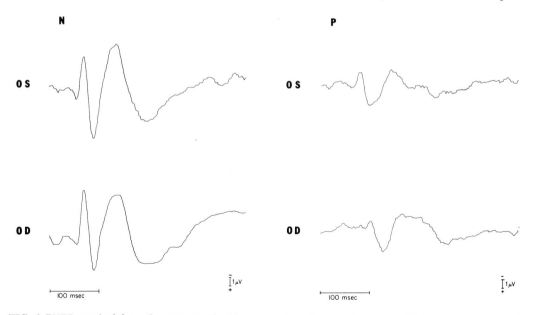

FIG. 6. PVERs to the left are from a normal subject. The alternating checkerboard of light was presented at 1 meter. Individual squares subtended 25′ of the arc. Responses were obtained from an electrode placed on the midline at a point 5 cm above the inion, referenced to the vertex. To the right are responses from a patient with progressive spinal cord signs but no history of visual symptoms. The response from the right eye is significantly prolonged, indicating an optic pathway lesion. In our laboratory, utilizing 36 normal subjects, a normal response is 106 msec or less (mean 95.8 msec + 2 SD).

similar to those reported for the SER. However, the latencies of the visual response appeared to be much more variable than the results using direct median nerve stimulation. It was felt this reflected an increased difficulty in controlling pertinent parameters (e.g., ocular fixation in patients with central field defects) as well as involuntary eye movements (e.g., nystagmus) typically seen in these patients. These initial visual studies employed a single flash for VER production. As indicated, although correlations could be made, the method appeared too gross or variable for routine clinical use in detecting subtle visual pathway lesions.

Halliday et al. (11) next reported on the use of an alternating checkerboard pattern of light as a sensitive means of generating a VER from the central visual field. This was followed by reports by Milner et al. (18) and Asselman et al. (1), each of whom confirmed the high degree of sensitivity and the ability of this method to detect subclinical or silent optic pathway lesions. Halliday et al. reported that 86% of MS patients without symptoms of optic involvement demonstrated an abnormal response. Other laboratories have not reported as high a percentage of abnormalities. However, the technique is of sufficient sensitivity that many medical centers currently employ the procedure as a means of evaluating patients with possible optic pathway demyelination. This use of the pattern VER (PVER) in the diagnosis and management of MS patients has been well documented. As an example, a recent patient in our clinic had progressive spinal cord signs but gave no history of optic symptoms. This patient was studied by the PVER technique, and responses from the right eye had latencies well beyond the normal range (Fig. 6). This identified a second, previously unrecognized neurological lesion, thereby confirming the probable diagnosis of MS.

Recently Halliday et al. (10) demonstrated that the delay of the evoked response was not specific to MS and optic neuritis. They reported an abnormal response in 18 of 19 patients with surgically proved lesions compressing the optic nerve, chiasm, or optic tract. The responses, however, were abnormal in a fashion somewhat different from that seen in patients with demyelinating disease. The incidence of delayed responses was much lower and the

amplitude of the response smaller. In particular, an absent response was characteristic of patients with an intracranial meningioma.

It has been demonstrated that the PVER is mainly subserved by central vision pathways, and the high sensitivity for MS lesion detection, using this method, probably reflects the fact that optic neuritis characteristically affects central vision.

BRAINSTEM EVOKED RESPONSES

Jewett et al. (12,13) first described the technique of far-field averaging of auditory brainstem evoked potentials. Subsequently Starr and Achor (31) reported on auditory abnormalities in patients with neurological disease, including four patients with MS. These patients had brainstem symptoms and signs, and all four gave abnormal responses. In three cases there was a reduction in amplitude of all wave peaks except for wave I, and the fourth patient had an absent wave V. Starr and Hamilton (32) subsequently demonstrated specific wave peak changes correlated to localized brainstem lesions. Although MS patients have not been systematically studied, the technique clearly holds promise as yet another objective means of assessing axonal function in demyelinating disease. In this same category would also have to be placed the more recent studies demonstrating the far-field somatosensory brainstem evoked potentials. These methods clearly extend the usefulness of the evoked potential approach and offer a new dimension to MS patient evaluation.

Other neurophysiological techniques have been used to evaluate MS patients. These approaches include the orbicularis oculi reflex (14,26) and the electro-oculogram (33). However, a discussion concerning these techniques would go beyond the intended scope of this chapter. It should suffice to say that each of these methods has reconfirmed the observation of delayed responses, observations consistent with slowed or blocked axonal conduction following demyelination.

SUMMARY

The various methods of brain and brainstem evoked response analysis have clearly been of value in understanding the pathophysiology of demyelinating disease. Future utilization rests with refinement of the techniques to aid in diagnosis in addition to obtaining objective indices of conduction. This latter point becomes critical as we approach a possible era of treatment evaluation in MS. The frequent, vague clinical presentation of MS and the extreme variability of lesion localization and severity indicate it would be of great value to have these objective measures.

In summary, the evoked response technique as applied to patients with demyelinating disease has provided a means of assessing central axonal function. The developed techniques have frequently proved to be more sensitive than clinical sensory examination. Indeed the evoked response approach has shown that silent MS lesions exist, and that they are a common feature of this disease. These methods directly measure the primary defect in MS, axonal demyelination, and therefore assume importance.

The reported results have demonstrated slowed and blocked conduction in the presence of demyelination. Further, the recovery function of the demyelinated axon has been shown to be prolonged and the demyelinated axon has been demonstrated to have a marked inability to respond to trains of stimuli. The studies have indicated an ability for conduction improvement following a bout of MS, but the improvement appears to lag behind the clinical course. The results have also shown that long-term repair or remyelination probably occurs.

Finally, the PVER has proved sufficiently sensitive and reliable to offer an aid in demyelinating disease diagnosis. The far-field methods of analysis, although only of preliminary interest, offer a new dimension for subcortical or brainstem conduction evaluation that should prove valuable in the future assessment of MS patients.

ACKNOWLEDGMENTS

Material presented was in part supported by National Multiple Sclerosis Society grant 516-C-3, United States Public Health Service grant NSO8711, and the Joe Gheen Barbeque Research Fund. Computing assistance was obtained from the Health Sciences Computing Facility, UCLA, sponsored by NIH Special Resources Grant FR3. The author wishes to acknowledge the significant contributions of Dr. Robert Sclabassi and Mr. Nelson Enns.

REFERENCES

1. Asselman, P., Chadwick, D. W., and Marsden, C. D. (1975): Visual evoked responses in the diagnosis and management of patients suspected of multiple sclerosis. *Brain*, 98:261–282.
2. Baker, J. B., Sances, A., and Larson, S. J. (1966): Neurophysiological evaluation of patients with multiple sclerosis. *Marquette Med. Rev.*, 32:37.
3. Bornstein, M. D., and Crain, S. M. (1965): Functional studies of cultured brain tissues as related to demyelinating disorders. *Science*, 148:1242–1244.
4. Cragg, B. G., and Thomas, P. K. (1964): Changes in nerve conduction in experimental allergic neuritis. *J. Neurol. Neurosurg. Psychiatry*, 4:537–544.
5. Davis, F. A. (1972): Impairment of repetitive impulse conduction in experimentally demyelinated and pressure injured nerves. *J. Neurol. Neurosurg. Psychiatry*, 35:537–544.
6. Davis, F. A., and Schauf, C. L. (1976): Neural blocking activity of multiple sclerosis and EAE sera. *Neurology (Minneap)*, 26:43–44.
7. Dawson, G. D. (1974): Cerebral responses to electrical stimulation of peripheral nerve in man. *J. Neurol. Neurosurg. Psychiatry*, 10:134–140.
8. Giblin, D. R. (1964): Somatosensory evoked potentials in healthy subjects and in patients with lesions of the nervous system. *Ann. NY Acad. Sci.*, 112:93–142.
9. Halliday, A. M., and Wakefield, G. S. (1963): Cerebral evoked potentials in patients with dissociated sensory loss. *J. Neurol. Neurosurg. Psychiatry*, 26:311–363.
10. Halliday, A. M., Halliday, E., Kriss, A., McDonald, W. I., and Mushin, J. (1976): The pattern evoked potentials in compression of the anterior visual pathways. *Brain*, 99:357–374.
11. Halliday, A. M., McDonald, W. I., and Mushin, J. (1973): Visual evoked response of multiple sclerosis. *Br. Med. J.*, 4:661–664.
12. Jewett, D. L. (1970): Volume conducted potentials in response to auditory stimuli as detected by averaging in the cat. *Electroencephalogr. Clin. Neurophysiol.*, 28:609–618.
13. Jewett, D. L., Romano, M. N., and Williston, J. S. (1970): Human auditory evoked potentials: Possible brain stem components detected on the scalp. *Science*, 167:1517–1518.
14. Kimura, J. (1973): The blink reflex as a test for brain stem and higher nervous system function. In: *New Developments in Electro-*

myography and Clinical Neurophysiology, Vol. 3, edited by J. E. Desmedt, pp. 682–691. Karger, Basel.

15. Larson, S. J., Sances, A., and Christenson, P. C. (1966): Evoked somatosensory potentials in man. *Arch. Neurol.,* 15:88–93.

16. Mayer, R. F. (1966): Conduction velocity in spinal cord during experimental demyelination in the cat. *Trans. Am. Neurol. Assoc.,* 91: 294–296.

17. McDonald, W. I., and Sears, T. A. (1970): The effects of experimental demyelination on conduction in the central nervous system. *Brain,* 93:583–598.

18. Milner, B. A., Regan, D., and Heron, J. R. (1974): Differential diagnosis of multiple sclerosis by visual evoked potential recording. *Brain,* 97:755–772.

19. Namerow, N. S. (1968): Somatosensory evoked responses in multiple sclerosis. *Bull. Los Angeles Neurol. Soc.,* 33:74–81.

20. Namerow, N. S. (1968b): Somatosensory evoked responses in multiple sclerosis patients with varying sensory loss. *Neurology, (Minneap),* 18:1197–1204.

21. Namerow, N. S. (1969): Somatosensory evoked responses following cervical cordotomy. *Bull. Los Angeles Neurol. Soc.,* 34:184–187.

22. Namerow, N. S. (1970): Somatosensory recovery functions in multiple sclerosis patients. *Neurology (Minneap),* 20:813–817.

23. Namerow, N. S. (1972): In: *Multiple Sclerosis, Immunology, Virology, and Ultrastructure,* edited by F. Wolfram, G. Ellison, J. G. Stevens, and J. Andrews. Academic Press, New York.

24. Namerow, N. S., Sclabossi, R. J., and Enns,

N. F. (1974): Somatosensory responses to stimulus trains: normative data. *EEG Journal* 37:11–41.

25. Namerow, N. S., and Enns, N. (1972): Visual evoked responses in patients with multiple sclerosis. *J. Neurol. Neurosurg. Psychiatry,* 35:829–833.

26. Namerow, N. S., and Entemadi, A. (1970): The orbicularis oculi reflex in multiple sclerosis. *Neurology (Minneap),* 20:1200–1203.

27. Richey, E. T., Kooi, K. A., and Tourtellotte, W. W. (1971): Visually evoked responses in multiple sclerosis. *J. Neurol. Neurosurg. Psychiatry,* 34:275–280.

28. Rouher, F., Plane, C., and Sole, P. (1968): Interet des potentiels evoques visuals daus les, affections du nerf optique. *Arch Ophthalmol. Rev. Gen. Ophthalmol.,* 2a:555–564.

29. Seil, F. J., Leiman, A. L., and Kelly, J. M. (1975): Neuroelectric blocking factors in multiple sclerosis and normal human sera. *Arch. Neurol.,* 33:418–422.

30. Sclabossi, R. J., Namerow, N. S., and Enns, N. F. (1974): Somatosensory responses to stimulus trains in patients with multiple sclerosis. *EEG Journal,* 27:23–33.

31. Starr, A., and Achor, L. J. (1975): Auditory brain stem responses in neurological disease. *Arch. Neurol.,* 32:761–768.

32. Starr, A., and Hamilton, A. E. (1976): Correlation between confirmed sites of neurological lesions and abnormalities of far field auditory brain stem responses. *Electroencephalogr. Clin. Neurophysiol.,* 41:595–608.

33. Solinger, L. D., Baloh, R. W., Myers, L., and Ellison, G. (1977): Subclinical eye movement disorders in patients with multiple sclerosis. *Neurology (Minneap)* *(in press).*

Physiology and Pathobiology of Axons, edited by
S. G. Waxman. Raven Press, New York © 1978.

Patterns of Clinical Deficits in Peripheral Nerve Disease

Thomas D. Sabin, Norman Geschwind, and Stephen G. Waxman

Departments of Neurology, Boston City Hospital, Boston, Massachusetts 02118; and Beth Israel Hospital, Boston, Massachusetts 02215

Localization of disease processes has often provided a fruitful starting point for the clinician and neuroscientist to learn more about how the nervous system functions. Certain problems such as aphasia are primarily limited to study within the clinical setting. The topography of such higher cortical functions has attracted great interest and study; the localization of peripheral nerve disease is by contrast usually assumed to be a simple by-product of the beginning course in gross anatomy. The ancients must have been astonished that a battle wound of the supraclavicular fossa could result in numbness of the hand. Such wonderment probably led to the development of acupuncture when early practitioners attempted to reproduce the analgesic effects of battle wounds with needle punctures. The more rigorous systematization of the nerve-by-nerve approach to localization is epitomized in the work of Sunderland (16). Indeed, this elegant millimeter by millimeter exposition of funicular arrangement within the major nerves might cause us to doubt a need for further inquiry.

However, when the clinician scrutinizes with care the nontraumatic diseases of peripheral nerves, he finds the classic root–plexus–nerve approach to analysis to be inadequate. The study of these neuropathies can provide not only new information on pathogenesis of these various diseases but even some further insights into the way the nervous system functions.

LEPROSY NEUROPATHY

Leprosy neuropathy is an excellent example of a disorder of sensation, the pattern of which is clearly explainable in terms of pathogenesis.

In the lepromatous type of leprosy there is minimal host resistance to the proliferation and dissemination of *Mycobacterium leprae*. Bacteremia with subsequent bacterial invasion of nerve results in a fairly symmetrical and extensive form of sensory loss with especial involvement of the extremities. This pattern is usually categorized as "stocking–glove" sensory loss. The paralysis has been interpreted as a mononeuropathy multiplex due to the increased liability to trauma of the enlarged nerves. However, when detailed mapping of the sensory changes in patients with lepromatous leprosy is carried out, one finds definite differences from the stocking–glove sensory loss of other neuropathies. Figure 1 illustrates the unique pattern of sensory loss in lepromatous leprosy. The regional variations in the extremities, early loss of sensation over the ears (helices), nose, and malar areas differentiate the picture from other neuropathies. Analyses of tissue temperatures and sensory thresholds shows that sensory loss begins in the coolest tissues and progresses to less cool areas as the disease advances (14). In addition, the major mixed motor and sensory nerves are affected in the segments that course closest to the surface and are therefore cooler than deeper lying portions. Only these portions of the nerves develop marked enlargement, and bacilli are most numerous in these segments. *M. leprae* have a highly thermosensitive growth rate (15). They proliferate optimally at 27°–30°C and not at all at core body temperature. Leprosy is then a disease of skin, superficial nerves, testes, upper respiratory tract, and the most anterior structures of the eye, in which the pattern of sensory loss is determined by thermal gradients.

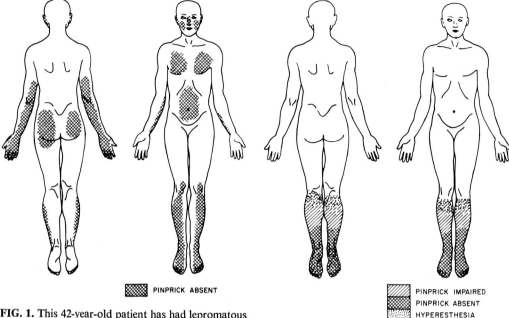

PINPRICK ABSENT

PINPRICK IMPAIRED
PINPRICK ABSENT
HYPERESTHESIA

FIG. 1. This 42-year-old patient has had lepromatous leprosy for at least 4 years. The sensory loss has affected "cool" areas on the extremities and face as well as the "cooler" skin which overlies relatively greater adipose tissue of the buttocks, breasts, and abdomen. The sensory loss usually is halted but not reversed by effective antibacterial treatment.

FIG. 2. This 51-year-old male had a long history of alcoholism and entered the hospital complaining of painful burning sensations in his soles. The dysesthesias may make accurate sensory examination difficult. The ankle reflexes are absent.

NEUROPATHIES WITH DISTAL PATTERNS OF SENSORY LOSS

Despite the frequency with which it is clinically observed, even the ubiquitous stocking–glove pattern of sensory loss which characterizes a variety of toxic, metabolic, nutritional, and hereditary neuropathies has not been fully explored. The term stocking–glove can be misleading since sensory loss in the hands and feet with a sharp boundary line at the ankles and wrists appears only as a manifestation of psychiatric disturbances. In most true polyneuropathies, sensory loss is apparent in the foot and leg before any sensory loss appears in the hand (Fig. 2). Progression of the disease is marked by a characteristic spatial pattern. Sensory abnormality extends above the knee before the hand is affected. In addition, the change from lost to normal sensation occurs not over a distinct line; it gradually shades off to normal across a fairly broad zone, as depicted in Fig. 2. Another band in which repeated stimuli lead to hyperpathia can often be

delineated within this transitional zone. Therefore the examiner who uses too rapid a series of stimuli may evoke severe dysesthesias and thus has difficulty in establishing the extent of the sensory loss. The soles and later in the course of a neuropathy the palms may have marked hyperpathia even though the dorsa of the feet and hands are insensitive. Hyperpathia seems to occur in areas of partial denervation, a finding which may reflect qualitative or quantitative differences between nerve supply to the palms and soles and that to the dorsum of the hand or foot.[1] Theoretical models for the stocking–glove sensory loss should account for these regions of hyperpathia which develop in some of the polyneuropathies.

With progression of the neuropathy, the upper extremities are affected, by which time the

[1] There is also relative sparing of the palms and soles in the temperature-linked sensory loss of lepromatous leprosy. The insulating effect of the corium at these sites makes for a bacillary milieu that is warmer than the dorsa of the hands and feet.

lower-extremity neuropathy has extended well above the knees (Fig. 3). Sensory fibers lose function according to their length, regardless of which of the named peripheral nerves they traverse in their course into the limbs. The clinician has often been told that the longest fibers are affected first, but the consistency and precision with which this occurs has not been widely appreciated. If one makes a practice of measuring the length of preserved fibers by placing one end of a tape measure at the proximal border of the sensory loss and the other end at the estimated spinal cord level of fiber origin for that region, the measurements for all four limbs are often within centimeters of each other. These measurements provide a useful quantitative measure for following the progress of a polyneuropathy.

This distal pattern of sensory loss is not limited to the limbs. When the sensory loss has progressed to involve proximal portions of the limbs, the next "longest" population of fibers

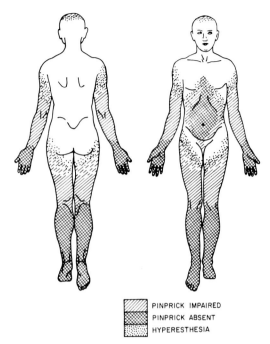

PINPRICK IMPAIRED
PINPRICK ABSENT
HYPERESTHESIA

FIG. 4. This 35-year-old juvenile diabetic had long-standing neuropathy, severe retinopathy, postural hypotension, and nocturnal diarrhea with fecal incontinence. She also had irregular pupils with a poor response to light. There is a area of sensory loss in the most distal portions of the trigeminal distributions.

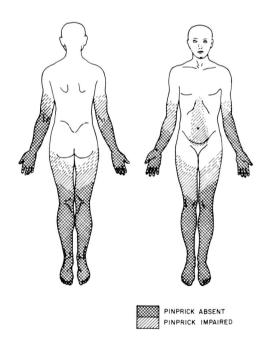

PINPRICK ABSENT
PINPRICK IMPAIRED

FIG. 3. This 43-year-old male is a member of a family with dominantly inherited amyloid neuropathy. This illness began at age 30 with "tingling" in his feet, and there was subsequent development of chronic plantar ulcers. Ankle and knee jerks are absent. The sensory loss over the abdomen reflects dysfunction in the nerves traversing the body wall. The lengths of preserved sensory nerves were 34–40 cm.

to be affected are those which traverse the body wall. These nerves increase in length along with the ribs downward along the thoracic cage, but the longest of these fibers take an oblique course to the lower abdomen. This dysfunction in these fibers causes a "teardrop" pattern of sensory loss over the lower abdomen (Fig. 3). This abdominal sensory loss is consistently found in diabetic pseudotabes and may be matched by a concomitant disturbance in abdominal autonomic fibers. These patients have bladder symptoms, nocturnal diarrhea, gastric "crises," and impotence (Fig. 4). This sensory loss widens with progression of the neuropathy and can ultimately encroach on the midline of the back. When the spared fiber length becomes less than 24 cm, the distance from the gasserian ganglion to the terminals of the first division is surpassed, and the "beanie cap" of sensory loss appears on the scalp (Fig. 5). The theme throughout this progression is the relative invariance all over the body surface of the distances, from the

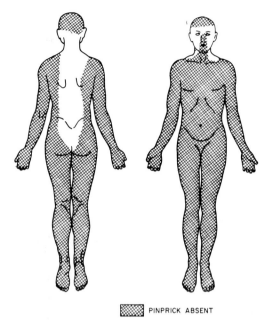

PINPRICK ABSENT

FIG. 5. This 14-year-old boy and his sister developed sensory neuropathy at age 2–3 with severe absorption of distal extremities. The length of spared fibers is 10–12 cm.

appropriate level of the spinal cord to the points where abnormal sensation is found.

This distal-to-proximal sequence of sensory loss is precisely paralleled by certain motor neuropathies. In Charcot–Marie–Tooth disease, for example, paralysis begins in the intrinsic muscles of the foot. The anterior tibial group is then affected, and the patient has significant disability due to bilateral footdrop. The center of muscle mass for the anterior tibial group is approximately 8 cm more distal than that for the gastrocnemius–soleus group. When progression does eventually affect these ankle extensors, the patient develops the classical "inverted champagne bottle" legs. After some time lag, atrophy and weakness of the intrinsic muscles of the hand can be identified.

There are several possible mechanisms to explain these deficits, which begin distally and progress proximally. A process which impairs metabolic function in the nucleus or neuronal cell body could be first reflected in the longest fibers. A derangement in axoplasmic transport systems would also first disrupt the function of the longest nerves. These mechanisms may be the basis for the "dying-back" neuropathies,

which have been carefully described from morphological and physiological points of view (Spencer and Schaumburg, *this volume;* Sumner, *this volume*).

The stocking–glove pattern might also be explained by random scattering of a myriad of microscopic lesions within the peripheral nervous system. If lesions are placed randomly, a longer fiber is more likely to have a lesion on it. Erlanger and Schoepfle (3) discussed this possibility as early as 1946. In the case of alcoholic and uremic polyneuropathies, a clinical electrophysiological studies on the H-reflex demonstrate a significant correlation between proximal and distal impairment of conduction velocity, and are consistent with the hypothesis that there are demyelinating lesions diffused along the whole length (proximal and distal) of the affected nerves (5). We previously discussed the possible significance of randomly distributed lesions located throughout the entire length of a nerve (17).

Segmental demyelination (Rasminsky, *this volume*) could affect peripheral nerve function by a number of mechanisms. Slowing of conduction has been demonstrated in demyelinated fibers in both the peripheral (8,9) and central (10) nervous systems. Gilliatt and Willison (4) observed loss of nerve action potentials in some diabetic patients with motor conduction velocities close to the lower limit of the normal range, and suggested that unequal slowing of conduction in the component axons within a nerve could lead to temporal dispersion of conduction times with a consequent abnormality of temporal summation of impulses. Conduction block (12) has also been demonstrated at sites of demyelination. Finally, it was suggested (17) that weak interactions between fibers may occur at sites of low safety factor and may perturb information transfer along the nerve. There is, in fact, experimental evidence for transmission of nerve impulses from fiber to fiber in the abnormally myelinated nerve roots of dystrophic mice (6); (see also Rasminsky, *this volume*).

The frequency with which any of the above abnormalities would be encountered would be expected to be related to the probability of pathology within a given nerve fiber or ensemble of fibers. Figure 6 shows the probability that a lesion will occur along a fiber, as a func-

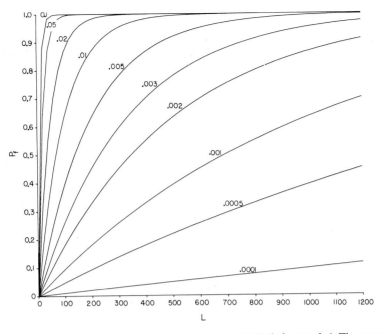

FIG. 6. Probability (P_f) of axonal pathology as related to fiber length (L) (in internodes). The curves were plotted for the indicated values of the probability that pathology will occur at any given internode. The curves here and in Figs. 7 and 8 were plotted from digital data calculated for values of L between 0 and 1,200 at increments of 20.

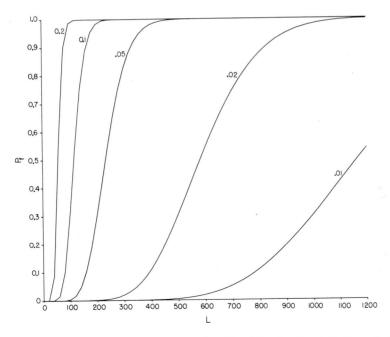

FIG. 7. Probability of 12 or more affected internodes as a function of fiber length, plotted from the binomial expansion for various values (indicated adjacent to curves) of pathological involvement of a single internode. Temporal divergence and the degree of weak interaction between fibers should increase with the number of demyelinated internodes. Note the inflection points in the curves here and in Fig. 8.

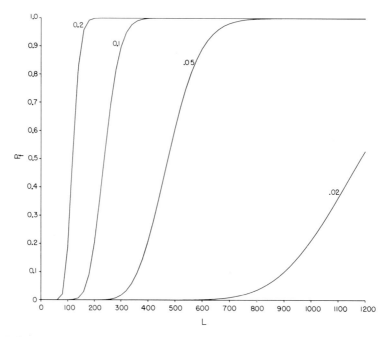

FIG. 8. Probability of 24 or more affected internodes as a function of fiber length.

tion of fiber length. The different curves were computed for the indicated values of the probability (next to each curve) that pathology would occur at any given internode. The probability of dysfunction increases with increasing fiber length. Figures 7 and 8 show, respectively, the probability that there will be 12 or more or 24 or more affected internodes along an axon, as functions of axonal length. These curves exhibit distinct inflection points and thus predict a more clearly defined boundary between areas of normal and abnormal sensory function (17).

As noted in preceding chapters of this volume, it is clear that in some polyneuropathies dying-back processes may account in large part for the clinical deficit. There is also evidence that in some neuropathies regions of segmental demyelination are clustered, with differences between affection of proximal and distal portions of the nerve (2). However, as shown in Figs. 6–8, randomly distributed lesions can also account for the proximodistal gradient of clinical deficit, and there is, in fact, electrophysiological evidence to support this hypothesis (5).

As illustrated in Figs. 2–5, clinical dysfunc-

tion in the polyneuropathies may, at least in some patients, exhibit a remarkably stereotyped progression in which there is a relative invariance in the length of nerves which subserve normal function. As commented on above, the spatial pattern of sensory loss may provide a useful measure on which to grade quantitatively the progression of peripheral nerve disease.

OTHER PATTERNS OF NEUROPATHIC DEFICIT

Although the clinical deficits in leprosy and the distal polyneuropathies are at least partially understood, there are many other clinical entities which have defied analysis. The pattern of *proximal sensory loss,* which has been observed in porphyria (13) and Tangier disease (7), exemplify this problem. This sensory loss affects the torso and proximal limbs, much as an old-fashioned bathing costume covered the body. This "bathing trunk" neuropathy implies a selective dysfunction in short fibers and makes any analysis based on randomized lesions in nerves or nerve roots untenable. Nothing is known about short nerves which might render them more vulnerable than longer nerves.

The syndrome of diabetic amyotrophy is another selective, clinically stereotyped condition which eludes analysis. The elderly mildly diabetic patient experiences the onset of intense, debilitating aching, boring, or burning pain in one thigh. Profound weakness with extensive atrophy appears in the muscles of the hip and thigh on the affected side. Detailed motor examination shows the greatest weakness in the muscles innervated by the femoral nerve, but less severe weakness in the distribution of the gluteal nerves, obturator nerve, and sciatic nerve can be documented. Knee jerk is absent, but ankle jerk is preserved. Although pain is usually the most distressing part of the disorder, a meticulous sensory examination shows only the poorly defined areas of slightly diminished pain and temperature sensation over anterior and lateral aspects of the affected thigh. The most confusing feature is the extensive involvement of muscles supplied by several nerves in the thigh with sparing of all the muscles below the knee. How do sensory fibers and the peroneal–anterior tibial innervated muscles escape? Peripheral nerve, spinal cord, and muscular lesions have been postulated. A vascular lesion would perhaps be the most convenient explanation. Raff et al. (11) found scattered foci of ischemic necrosis within the femoral and obturator nerves 15–25 cm into the thigh. No vascular occlusions could be found to explain the infarcts. The two cases of very painful muscle infarction in the same level of the thigh described by Banker and Chester (1) lend support to the suggestion that this area of the thigh has some special vascular vulnerability similar to the border zone areas of the cerebrum (11).

Neuralgic amyotrophy is an equally puzzling disorder that affects the upper extremity, usually predominantly or exclusively on one side. The patients are generally healthy adults, but approximately half provide a history of some antecedent nonspecific infectious disease or immunization. Severe, acute pain in the shoulder, neck, or arm often wakes the patient from sleep. As the pain diminishes over the next 2–14 days, paralysis and atrophy appear. The paralysis is always in a nerve distribution. The long thoracic, axillary, and suprascapular nerves are most commonly affected. This is another painful neuropathy in which sensory

loss can only rarely be documented. The lesions are usually limited to specific peripheral nerves, and detailed examination reveals that the roots of origin for the affected nerve(s) are spared. Since this is the type of neuropathy that accompanies serum sickness, one might expect it to appear diffusely and symmetrically rather than unilaterally in the upper extremity. No explanation for the remarkable selectivity or severe pain has been found.

This brief discussion of clinical problems is intended to motivate the asking of a number of questions which, although outside the realm of axonology in its restricted sense, are of obvious importance to our understanding of the nervous system. In what ways do peripheral axons code information—by simple frequency coding or by fine temporal patterning of impulse trains? To what degree do the constituent fibers of a nerve trunk function as independent channels, rather than as components of an ensemble in which information is signaled by the average rate of firing? What are the relative roles of slowed conduction, conduction block, and weak interactions between fibers? These questions, although dealing with pathophysiological mechanism, are of direct relevance to clinical questions, and may be answered in part by careful clinical studies. One approach, which has not been explored, would be the development of radionuclide technology appropriate for "nerve scanning." Such an approach might allow direct visualization of the sites of axonal pathology. Finally, we believe that much information can be obtained, and pathophysiological questions at least in part answered, by careful observation at the bedside.

REFERENCES

1. Banker, B. Q., and Chester, S. (1973): Infarction of thigh muscle in the diabetic patient. *Neurology (Minneap)*, 23:667–677.
2. Dyck, P. J., Lais, A. C., and Offord, K. P. (1974): The nature of myelinated nerve fiber degeneration in dominantly inherited hypertrophic neuropathy. *Proc. Mayo Clin.*, 49:34–39.
3. Erlanger, I., and Schoepfle, G. M. (1946): A study of nerve degeneration and regeneration. *Am. J. Physiol.*, 147:550–581.
4. Gilliatt, R. W., and Willison, R. G. (1962): Peripheral nerve conduction in diabetic neu-

ropathy. *J. Neurol. Neurosurg. Psychiatry,* 25: 11–18.

5. Guiheneuc, P., and Bathien, N. (1976): Two patterns of results in polyneuropathies investigated with the H reflex. *J. Neurol. Sci.,* 30:83–94.

6. Huizar, P., Kuno, M., and Miyata, Y. (1975): Electrophysiological properties of spinal motoneurons of normal and dystrophic mice. *J. Physiol. (Lond),* 248:231–246.

7. Kocen, R. S., Lloyd, J. K., Lascelles, P. T., Fosbrooke, A. S., and Williams, D. (1967): Familial alpha-lipoprotein deficiency (Tangier disease) with neurological abnormalities. *Lancet,* 1:1341.

8. Mayer, R. F., and Denny-Brown, D. (1964): Conduction velocity in peripheral nerve during experimental demyelination in the cat. *Neurology (Minneap),* 14:714–726.

9. McDonald, W. I. (1963): Effects of experimental demyelination on conduction in peripheral nerve: a histological and electrophysiological study. II. Electrophysiological observations. *Brain,* 86:501–524.

10. McDonald, W. I., and Sears, T. A. (1970): The effects of experimental demyelination on conduction in the central nervous system. *Brain,* 93:583–598.

11. Raff, M. C., Sangalang, V., and Asbury, A. K. (1968): Ischemic mononeuropathy multiplex associated with diabetes mellitus. *Arch. Neurol.,* 18:487–499.

12. Rasminsky, M., and Sears, T. A. (1972): Internodal conduction in undissected demyelinated nerve fibers. *J. Physiol. (Lond),* 227:323–350.

13. Ridley, A. (1969): The neuropathy of acute intermittent porphyria. *Q. J. Med.,* 38:307–333.

14. Sabin, T. D. (1969): Temperature-linked sensory loss: A unique pattern in leprosy. *Arch. Neurol.,* 20:257–262.

15. Shepard, C. C. (1965): Temperature optimum of Mycobacterium leprae in mice. *J. Bacteriol.,* 90:1271–1275.

16. Sunderland, S. (1968): *Nerves and Nerve Injuries.* Livingstone, Edinburgh.

17. Waxman, S., Brill, M. H., Geschwind, N., Sabin, T. D., and Lettvin, J. Y. (1976): Probability of conduction deficit as related to fiber length in random-distribution models of peripheral neuropathies. *J. Neurol. Sci.,* 29:39–53.

Subject Index

Accommodation, in motor and sensory fibers, 135
Acetylcholinesterase, 30
Aconitine, as modifier of sodium channel gating, 163
Acrylamide neuropathy, 350-356
    axoplasmic transport in, 258, 265, 269
    and regeneration of nerves, 357
    single-fiber studies in, 351-356
ACTH
    in multiple sclerosis, 328
    and spinal cord regeneration, 413-414
Actin filaments, of peripheral axons, 8
Adrenoleukodystrophy, 301, 341
Aequorin, as calcium-sensitive probe, 248
Alcoholic neuropathy, 259, 357, 434
Alexander's disease, abnormal myelination in, 301
Amino acid uptake, in spinal cord regeneration, 413
6-Aminonicotinamide, demyelination from, 301
cAMP, and intercellular communication, 394
Amyotrophy
    diabetic, 437
    neuralgic, 437
Anesthetics, local, as conductance blocking agents, 162-163
Anoxia, myelin loss in, 301
Antibody factors, in demyelination, 288, 318-319
Antidromic activation, 200
Astrocytes
    and myelination, 66
    phagocytic activity in demyelination, 288, 322, 324
Axoglial junction, paranodal, 99-105
    axonal membrane properties, 102-103
    glial membrane properties, 102
    role in conduction, 101, 105
Axogliosis, 304
Axolemma
    of central myelinated axons, 68
        undercoating of, 70
    of initial segment, undercoating of, 126
    internodal, 105-106, 111
    of myelin sheath attachment segment, 21-22
    at node of Ranvier, 106, 112-115, 155
        in central axons, 23
        compared to internodal membrane, 174-176
        corrugations of, 22
        dense bodies in, 369
        in peripheral axons, 22, 42, 47
        undercoating of, 174
    optical probes of, 237-249

    at paranodal axoglial junction, 103
    of peripheral axons, 5, 15
    structural differences in myelinated axons, 174-176
Axonopathies, distal, 349-358
    and acrylamide neuropathy, 350-356
    axonal degeneration in, 269, 401
    axonal swelling in, 272
    axoplasmic transport in, 258, 275, 280, 357, 434
    central-peripheral, 258, 266
    enzyme inactivation in, 280
    and evolution of fiber degeneration, 270-272
    experimental, 268-280
    fiber vulnerability in, 269-270
        and diameter of axon, 270
        and length of axon, 269
    and hypothesis of dying-back process, 280-281
    metabolic lesion in, 278-280
    nerve conduction in, 350
    from neurotoxins, 265-267
    Ranvier nodes in, 272-275
    regeneration in, 356-357
    Schwann cell sequestration in, 275-278, 401
Axoplasm
    of central myelinated axons, 68
    of nodal segments of peripheral axons, 23-24
        bulk flow in, 26
    of peripheral axons, 5-6, 15, 33; see also Peripheral axons
    sequestered areas in distal axonopathy, 275-278
Axoplasmic transport, 251-259
    in acrylamide neuropathy, 258, 265, 269
    batrachotoxin affecting, 257-258
    blocking of, 257
    bulk flow through nodal segments, 26
    calcium role in, 256-257
    characteristics of, 251-254
    in distal axonopathy, 258, 275, 280, 357, 434
    energetics of, 255
    fast, 255
    materials transported in, 254
    mechanisms in, 255-256
    microtubules in, 257
    pathology related to, 258-259
    in peripheral axons, 6, 8
    rate of, 251-252
    retrograde, 254-255, 258
    slow, 255
    temperature affecting, 257